Psychiatric Disorders Late in Life

Rajesh R. Tampi • Deena J. Tampi
Lisa L. Boyle
Editors

Psychiatric Disorders Late in Life

A Comprehensive Review

Springer

Editors
Rajesh R. Tampi, MD, MS, DFAPA
Professor of Psychiatry
Case Western Reserve University School of Medicine, Vice Chairman for Education and Faculty Development
Residency Program Director and Chief of Geriatric Psychiatry, MetroHealth
Cleveland, OH
USA

Associate Clinical Professor of Psychiatry
Yale School of Medicine
New Haven, CT
USA

Deena J. Tampi, MSN, MBA-HCA, RN
Executive Vice President
Clinical Services, Diamond Healthcare
Richmond, VA
USA

Lisa L. Boyle, MD, MPH
Associate Clinical Professor of Psychiatry, University of Wisconsin School of Medicine and Public Health
Program Director
Geriatric Psychiatry Fellowship
Madison, WI
USA

ISBN 978-3-030-10311-8 ISBN 978-3-319-73078-3 (eBook)
https://doi.org/10.1007/978-3-319-73078-3

Printed on acid-free paper

This Springer imprint is published by the registered company Springer International Publishing AG part of Springer Nature
The registered company address is: Gewerbestrasse 11, 6330 Cham, Switzerland

Contents

Contributors

Vimal M. Aga, M.D., F.A.P.A. Department of Neurology, Oregon Health and Science University, Portland, OR, USA

Poorvanshi Alag, M.D. Case Western Reserve University School of Medicine and Metrohealth, Cleveland, OH, USA

Ali Ahsan Ali, M.D. Ican School of Medicine at Mount Sinai (Elmhurst), Queens, NY, USA

Ali Abbas Asghar-Ali, M.D. Department of Psychiatry and Behavioral Sciences, Baylor College of Medicine, Michael E. DeBakey VA Medical Center, Houston, TX, USA

Sarah J. De Asis, M.D. Department of Psychiatry, Yale University, New Haven, CT, USA

Jimmy Avari, M.D. Department of Psychiatry, Weill Cornell Medical College, White Plains, NY, USA

Gayle Ayers, D.O. Department of Psychiatry, Dell Medical School — The University of Texas at Austin, Seton Healthcare Family, Austin, TX, USA

Silpa Balachandran, M.D. Case Western Reserve University School of Medicine and Metrohealth, Cleveland, OH, USA

Meera Balasubramaniam, M.D., M.P.H. Department of Psychiatry, New York University School of Medicine, New York, NY, USA

Ashmita Banerjee, M.D. Case Western Reserve University School of Medicine and Metrohealth, Cleveland, OH, USA

Azziza Oluwakemi Bankole, M.D. Department of Psychiatry and Behavioral Medicine, Virginia Tech Carilion School of Medicine, Roanoke, VA, USA

Laurel J. Bessey, M.D. Department of Psychiatry, University of Wisconsin School of Medicine and Public Health, Madison, WI, USA

Lisa L. Boyle, M.D., M.P.H. Department of Psychiatry, University of Wisconsin School of Medicine and Public Health, Madison, WI, USA

William S. Middleton Memorial Veterans Hospital, Madison, WI, USA

Cheryl Bradas, PhDc, APRN, CHPN, CNRN Department of Nursing, The MetroHealth System, Cleveland, OH, USA

Wynnelena C. Canio, M.D. Semel Institute for Neuroscience and Human Behavior, UCLA School of Medicine, Los Angeles, CA, USA

Evan N. Caporaso, M.D. Directorate for Mental Health, Naval Medical Center San Diego, San Diego, CA, USA

Suneela Cherlopalle, M.D. Case Western Reserve University School of Medicine and Metrohealth, Cleveland, OH, USA

Ravi Chivukula, M.D., M.P.H. West Virginia University School of Medicine, Morgantown, WV, USA

Carl Cohen, M.D. SUNY Downstate Medical Center, Brooklyn, NY, USA

Dhweeja Dasarathy Harvard University, Cambridge, MA, USA

Joel P. Dey, M.D. Metrohealth, Cleveland, OH, USA

Nery A. Diaz, D.O. Washington Heights Community Services of the New York State Psychiatric Institute, Columbia University Medical Center, New York, NY, USA

Erica C. Garcia-Pittman, M.D. Department of Psychiatry, Dell Medical School — The University of Texas at Austin, Seton Healthcare Family, Austin, TX, USA

Garima Garg, M.D. Case Western Reserve University School of Medicine, Cleveland, OH, USA

Metrohealth, Cleveland, OH, USA

Dina Ghoneim, M.D. SUNY Downstate Medical Center, Brooklyn, NY, USA

Katherine Rice Goettsche, M.D. Department of Psychiatry, Weill Cornell Medical College, New York, NY, USA

Aarti Gupta, M.D. Department of Psychiatry, Connecticut Valley Hospital, Middletown, CT, USA

Department of Psychiatry, Yale Univeristy School of Medicine, New Haven, CT, USA

Michael C. Hann, M.D., M.B.A., M.S. Directorate for Mental Health, Naval Medical Center San Diego, San Diego, CA, USA

Bronwyn Huggins, M.D. SUNY Downstate Medical Center, Brooklyn, NY, USA

Jennifer Jacobson, M.D. Department of Psychiatry, Dell Medical School — The University of Texas at Austin, Seton Healthcare Family, Austin, TX, USA

Pallavi Joshi, D.O., M.A. Hofstra-Northwell School of Medicine-Staten Island University Hospital, Staten Island, NY, USA

Karin Kerfoot, M.D., F.R.C.P.C. Department of Psychiatry, Western University, London, ON, Canada

Thomas Wolfgang Klotz, M.D. Directorate for Mental Health, Naval Medical Center San Diego, San Diego, CA, USA

Jessica Koenig, M.D. Department of Psychiatry, Dell Medical School — The University of Texas at Austin, Seton Healthcare Family, Austin, TX, USA

Ashley Trust, M.D. Department of Psychiatry, Dell Medical School — The University of Texas at Austin, Seton Healthcare Family, Austin, TX, USA

Mallika Lavakumar, M.D. Case Western Reserve University School of Medicine and Metrohealth, Cleveland, OH, USA

Joanna C. Lim, M.D. Veterans Affairs Medical Center, Washington, DC, USA

Anup Mani, D.O. SUNY Downstate Medical Center, Brooklyn, NY, USA

Geetha Manikkara, M.D. Metrohealth, Cleveland, OH, USA

Rachel D. Maree, M.D., M.P.H. Department of Psychiatry, University of Pittsburgh School of Medicine, Western Psychiatric Institute and Clinic, Pittsburgh, PA, USA

Raman Marwaha, M.D. Case Western Reserve University School of Medicine, MetroHealth Medical Center, Cleveland, OH, USA

Nisha Mehta-Naik, M.D. Department of Psychiatry, New York Presbyterian-Weill Cornell Medical College, New York, NY, USA

Aaron Meyer, M.D. Department of Psychiatry, University of California, San Diego, San Diego, CA, USA

Tessa Murante, D.O. SUNY Downstate Medical Center, Brooklyn, NY, USA

Aurora Osteen, M.D. Department of Psychiatry, Dell Medical School — The University of Texas at Austin, Seton Healthcare Family, Austin, TX, USA

Rosanne M. Radziewicz, MSN, APRN-CNS Department of Nursing, The MetroHealth System, Cleveland, OH, USA

Michael Reinhardt, M.D. SUNY Downstate Medical Center, Brooklyn, NY, USA

Craig A. Riccelli, M.D. Department of Psychiatry, University of Pittsburgh School of Medicine, Western Psychiatric Institute and Clinic, Pittsburgh, PA, USA

Mamta Sapra, M.D. Department of Psychiatry and Behavioral Medicine, Virginia Tech Carilion School of Medicine, Roanoke, VA, USA

Salem Veteran Affairs Medical Center, Salem, VA, USA

Caitlin Snow, M.D., M.B.A. Department of Psychiatry, Weill Cornell Medical College, New York, NY, USA

Deena J. Tampi, M.S.N., M.B.A.-H.C.A., R.N. Diamond Healthcare, Richmond, VA, USA

Rajesh R. Tampi, M.D., M.S., D.F.A.P.A. Case Western Reserve University School of Medicine and Metrohealth, Cleveland, OH, USA

Amit Thour, M.B.B.S. Primary Health Center, Rampur, Himachal Pradesh, India

Kalya Vardi, M.D. Department of Psychiatry, University of California, San Diego (UCSD), San Diego, CA, USA

M. Ingre Walters, M.D. Lewis Katz School of Medicine at Temple University, Philadelphia, PA, USA

Sophia Wang, M.D. Department of Psychiatry, Indiana University School of Medicine, Indianapolis, IN, USA

Brandon C. Yarns, M.D. Division of General Internal Medicine, Department of Medicine, University of California, Los Angeles, CA, USA

Department of Psychiatry/Mental Health, VA Greater Los Angeles Healthcare System, Los Angeles, CA, USA

Part I

Developmental, Psychological and Social Aspects of Aging

1 Life Course: Developmental and Transitional Events

Nisha Mehta-Naik

Introduction

A life transition is defined by a significant shift in social circumstances, which is often accompanied by a period of emotional and social instability as one moves from one life stage to another [1]. Although life transitions can often be perceived as planned events that carry a positive connotation, such as marriage and joining the workforce, many life transitions are marked by unpredictability and upheaval. Nonetheless, all life transitions can result in a disruption of social networks, coping skills, finances, and health [1]. As a result, success in life transitions requires individuals to demonstrate resilience by cultivating new coping skills, utilizing different social supports and accepting a change in identity [1]. Some research suggests that such transitions could be risk factors for depression in older adults [2]. Although each older adult has a unique experience of aging, as a group, the geriatric population shares several life transitions such as retirement, bereavement, relocation, changes in the caregiver role, and changes in medical health. Some of these topics—including caregiver stress and psychological factors affecting medical conditions—will be featured in subsequent chapters. This section will highlight two key geriatric life transitions: retirement and bereavement.

Retirement

Retirement has been defined in multiple ways. Feldman defines retirement as the "exit from labor force taken by individuals after middle age and taken with the intention of reduced psychological commitment to work thereafter [3]." This definition indicates that retirement is an individual and a deliberate decision. Sociologist Angela M. O'Rand states that retirement is an "age-related and permanent transition from an income status based on employment to one based on transfers and assets at the end of the work career" which highlights a shift from depending on individual income to larger economic institutions [4]. Such definitions of retirement suggest that this life transition is abrupt, marked by the single decision to retire from the workforce. Organizational psychologists Wang and Shultz suggest that retirement can also be a dynamic process often involving multiple, stepwise decisions resulting in a gradual transition out of the workforce through part-time work and alternate work opportunities [5]. Strict definitions of retirement often do not capture the conditions surrounding retirement—namely, if retirement was voluntary, involuntary, or regulatory/statutory—retirement that is mandated at a set age [6]. The lack of standard definitions of retirement highlights that there are key differences in how individuals

R. R. Tampi et al. (eds.), *Psychiatric Disorders Late in Life*, https://doi.org/10.1007/978-3-319-73078-3_1

experience retirement, the retirement decision-making process, and how retirement is studied by different professional groups.

Despite the significance of this life transition, there is little conclusive data regarding impact of retirement on one's emotional and physical well-being [6]. Limitations of research include lack of universal definitions regarding retirement, as well as a difference in conditions surrounding retirement. A population's outlook on retirement may be impacted by national policies on retirement, insurance, and pension, thus making it difficult to generalize results to an international population [7]. As women historically comprised of a lower portion of the labor force, there is limited data regarding women's experience of retirement, as well as that of dual-income households [8].

In this section, trends in American retirement, data regarding impact of retirement on health, as well as psychosocial interventions to improve retirement experiences will be reviewed.

Trends in American Retirement

Older adult participation in the American labor force (including full-time and part-time employment) notably decreases between ages 60 and 70. Per 2010 US Census data, 60% of men in the 60–64 age group are engaged in the workforce, though only 36.5% of older men in the 65–69 age group are employed [9]. Similarly, female participation decreases from 50.7% in the 60–64 age group to 27% in the 65–69 age group. Following age 69 years, the workforce participation decreases by approximately 10–12% every 5 years [9].

Patterns of retirement behavior have changed significantly over the course of the twentieth and twenty-first centuries. While approximately 10% of women over age 65 maintained employment from 1950 to 1990, older male rates of employment steadily decreased over the majority of the twentieth century [9]. Approximately 45.8% of American men over age 65 maintained employment in 1950, but only 15% of older men remained active in the workforce by 1993 [9]. The development of Social Security, as well as the strengthening of pension programs, has contributed to increased older adult retirement in the twentieth century.

The twenty-first century was marked by a rebound in older adult engagement in the workforce—with 22.1% of men and 13.8% of women over the age of 65 maintaining employment in 2010 [9]. Multiple hypotheses have been offered to explain why older adults are remaining in the workforce at increasing rates, namely, decreased financial security in light of the 2007–2009 economic recession [10], as well as the decreased quality and availability of pension programs [11], rising age of Social Security eligibility [11], and increased life expectancy [11].

Retirement and Health

Different studies have investigated the relationship between retirement and health, and the available data is varied. We will review some of the key international studies that shed light on this topic in the next few paragraphs.

Much of the literature suggests that retirement is associated with an improvement in both physical and mental health. Depressive symptoms, as measured by the quantity of antidepressant prescriptions distributed to a Finnish cohort, were noted to decrease following retirement [12]. Data from the Whitehall II study, a large longitudinal prospective study conducted in England, corroborated these findings. Self-report of general mental health improved for all employees following statutory retirement, though most noticeably for those of higher socioeconomic status [13]. Similar findings regarding a decrease in depressive symptoms following retirement were noted in a Canadian population study [14] as well as a Swiss population study [15]. The GAZEL project, a French longitudinal prospective cohort, demonstrated evidence of decreased sleep disturbances in the years following statutory retirement [16]. It seems that affective and anxiety symptoms surrounding retirement may peak when individuals are in the process of preparing for retirement and upon initiation of retirement itself. A series of interviews demonstrated that many individuals experienced pre-retirement anxiety in the setting of uncertainty and change, followed by post-retirement satisfaction and happiness as they adjusted to a new phase of life [17]. In spite of a significant shift in identity during the process of retirement, a study of American individuals found that self-esteem remained steady before and after retirement [18].

Many studies also suggest that retirement is correlated with improvements in physical health. Further data from the GAZEL cohort demonstrated that the chronic disease prevalence was not impacted by retirement itself, but rather by normal aging [19]. Moreover, self-report of physical and mental fatigue decreased following retirement. GAZEL cohort data also found a decreased prevalence of headaches [20], increased physical activity [21], and decreased report of "suboptimum health" following retirement [22]. Several studies have noted that the level of somatic complaints [23] and self-report of health [24] do not change significantly for individuals following retirement when compared to age-matched adults who remained in the workforce.

Despite overwhelming data supporting improvements in mental and physical health following retirement, some data suggests that retirement is correlated with worse health outcomes. One study found that early retirement was correlated with higher prevalence of depression and anxiety [25]. Although a study of the Swiss Household Panel found that the majority of individuals experience improvements or stability in self-reported general health and mood following retirement, the study also notes that approximately 25% of individuals experience worsening of mood and anxiety following retirement [15]. Additional data from the GAZEL cohort suggested that the prevalence of heavy alcohol consumption increased around the retirement period [26]. Although many studies suggested that retirement was correlated with an increase in physical activity, one study found that the loss of physical activity related to work commutes was not compensated for by recreational physical activity in retirement [27].

Several studies emphasize that individual characteristics, and external factors which exist prior to retirement may impact one's experience of retirement. Data from the GAZEL cohort found that the presence of Type A and aggressive personality traits prior to retirement is correlated with worsened mood following retirement [28]. Results from the Whitehall II study propose that hardship faced in the workplace in the years prior to retirement including workplace satisfaction and perceived workload is correlated with symptoms of depression post-retirement [29]. Such data highlights the complexity of this life transition and the multitude of factors that influence individual retirement experiences.

Psychosocial Interventions

Although many older adults seem to thrive both physically and mentally after retirement, available data suggests that many older adults experience worsening mood and physical health correlated with retirement. Several interventions have been proposed to help older adults transition to retirement, focusing on reshaping older adults' social identities following retirement by providing new responsibilities, fostering environments that promote socialization, and helping structure time. Several initiatives encouraged older adults to serve as mentors to young adults [30] or adopted grandparents [31] (Foster Grandparent Program) to young adults and children and were noted to have positive effects.

Future Directions

Despite European studies regarding retirement demonstrating overall improvements in mental and physical health following this life transition, there is limited data regarding the American experience of retirement. As the average age of retirement rises in the United States and pension plans and benefits diminish, it is possible that Americans will experience increased stress in the setting of retirement. Further research on health outcomes following retirement in the United States would help elucidate this effect. Although retirement has commonly been perceived as a positive life transition, there remains a subset of individuals who struggle with this change. Incorporating aspects of positive psychiatry and interpersonal psychotherapy may alleviate distress related to retirement.

Bereavement

The death of a loved one and the subsequent mourning of loss is a process that impacts the geriatric population immensely. Loss is an inevitable part of life for older adults—the average life expectancy in 2009 was found to be 75 years for men and 80.9 years for women [32]. Approximately 28.1% of individuals over age 65 are widowed, and 59.6% of individuals over age 85 are widowed [32]. The prevalence of spousal loss is higher in women—39.9% of women over 65 and 72.9% of women over 85 are widows [32]. This data does not encapsulate other major losses that older adults face including but not limited to the death of parents, friends, siblings, and in rarer circumstances children.

Despite the universality of bereavement, individuals seem to have varied responses to loss ranging from exhibiting minimal psychiatric symptoms to experiencing significant dysfunction. Psychiatrists and psychologists have long discussed the range of responses to loss, often wondering where to draw the fine line between expected bereavement and a pathological response to loss. In the classic paper *Mourning and Melancholia* [33], Freud defines mourning as "the reaction to the loss of a loved person, or to the loss of some abstraction which has taken the place of one, such as one's country, liberty, an ideal and so on [33]." In this statement, Freud highlights that mourning is a process of coming to terms with object loss. He draws the distinction between mourning and melancholia, noting that "although mourning involves grave departures from the normal attitude to life, it never occurs to us to regard it as a pathological condition and to refer it to medical treatment. We rely on mourning being overcome after a certain lapse of time, and we look upon any interference with that process as useless or even harmful [33]." Psychoanalyst Otto Kernberg questioned whether the mourning process is a time-limited one as Freud proposed or a lifelong process that "may bring about a permanent alteration of psychological structures that affect various aspects of the mourning persons' lives [34]."

The dialogue regarding the course of expected bereavement and defining its pathological variants has continued in the twenty-first century with the DSM-5 and the decision to remove the bereavement exclusion from diagnostic criteria of major depressive disorder [35]. The next section will explore the complexities of categorizing pathological vs. non-pathological bereavement, biological responses to grief, and management of bereavement.

The Biology of Loss

Bereavement is not only a psychological and social process but also a physiological one. Widowhood has been correlated with increased morbidity and mortality from a broad range of health conditions—including increased risk of mortality from accidents, strokes, heart disease, and cancer [36]. Although the etiology of increased morbidity and mortality is unclear, there are known endocrine and immunologic changes associated with bereavement [37]. The acute period following spousal loss has been associated with decreased T lymphocyte activity [38], decreased NK cell reactions [39], and increased neutrophil count [40]. Widows and widowers were found to have elevations in cortisol levels 2 weeks and 6 months after loss of a spouse [41]. Research has also demonstrated that there is increased heart rate and elevated blood pressures in the period following significant loss [42]. Such neuroendocrine and immunologic changes represent a physiologic response to the stress of acute grief, which may have downstream effects [37].

Current Categorization of Bereavement

The clinical range of responses to loss has most recently been separated into three distinct categories by Zisook and Shear: uncomplicated grief, complicated grief, and grief-related major depression [43].

Uncomplicated grief is a fluctuating and dynamic process, which for some does not come to a complete resolution. Individuals will have varying responses to loss, ranging from minimal psychological distress to time-limited significant dysfunction. Zisook and Shear describe that uncomplicated grief usually begins with a phase of "acute grief," during which an individual experiences heightened sadness and psychological pain and increased longing for the lost individual [43]. Symptoms of depression are often present during this acute period including low mood, anhedonia, and diminished motivation and focus although individuals do not meet full criteria for a major depressive episode. As acute grief fades, individuals face a period of "integrated grief." This phase is characterized by holding onto memories of lost loved ones and continuing to miss them without any concomitant changes in functioning [43].

Although many individuals experience depressive symptoms in the context of bereavement, most do not meet criteria for a major depressive episode. However, a subset of individuals experience "grief-related major depression"— a major depressive episode in the setting of loss and bereavement [43]. While the precise prevalence rates of bereavement-related depressive episodes are unclear, one study found that 7.7% of all depressive episodes in a population were related to bereavement [44]. Depressive episodes in the setting of bereavement when compared to general depressive episodes have been correlated with lower rates of suicidal ideations and feelings of worthlessness [44]. Individuals with bereavement-related depression often report decreased need for sleep, rather than increased need for sleep [44]. Additionally, those who experienced a grief-related depressive episode do not carry an increased risk of subsequent depressive episodes [44].

Complicated grief is defined as a syndrome of prolonged and intense grief that is associated with substantial impairment in work, health, and social functioning [43]. When compared to its normal variant, complicated grief is marked by ongoing distress, persistent guilt for finding enjoyment in the absence of deceased loved one, and inability to come to terms with the loss [43]. The prevalence of complicated grief has been estimated to be approximately 2.5 [45] to 5.0% [46] in the general population and is estimated to occur in approximately 10% [43] to 25% [46] of those grieving a loss. Complicated grief has been associated with increased comorbidity with major depressive disorder and anxiety disorders [46]. However, complicated grief can occur in the absence of comorbid major depressive episode. Ages between 75 and 84 years, the loss of a child or spouse, and female gender have been correlated with increased prevalence of complicated grief [46]. Unexpected loss, death of a loved one who passed away in an inpatient facility, and increased time spent with loved ones in the week prior to their death were also found to carry increased risk of complicated bereavement [45].

Management of Bereavement

Appropriate categorization of a patient's response to grief is critical, as specific interventions—and in some cases no intervention—have been found to be effective for uncomplicated grief, grief-related major depression, and complicated bereavement.

No intervention has been found to be helpful in managing uncomplicated grief. Although individuals may continue to miss the deceased, they are able to find enjoyment in activities and report less psychological distress within 6–18 months of a significant loss without any intervention [47].

Grief-related major depression improves with psychotherapy and antidepressants. Several small studies have demonstrated improvements in depressive and grief symptoms with the use of antidepressants [48, 49]. One study found that interpersonal psychotherapy when combined with nortriptyline was more effective than nortriptyline alone in the treatment of grief-related major depression [49].

Many interventions have been proposed for the treatment of complicated bereavement. There is little data to support the use of antidepressants or other psychiatric medications in the treatment of complicated grief [50]. Cognitive behavioral therapy [51], interpersonal psychotherapy [52], and behavioral activation [53] have all demonstrated some efficacy in treating complicated grief. However, complicated grief therapy, a therapy which incorporates strategies from exposure therapy, motivational interviewing, and interpersonal therapy, has been found to be the most effective in reducing symptoms of complicated grief [52]. Complicated grief therapy has specifically been found to alleviate symptoms of complicated grief among older adults [54].

Bereavement and Suicidality

Bereavement is correlated with an increased prevalence of suicidal ideations and suicide attempts. Widowed individuals had higher rates of suicidal ideations than non-widowed individuals [55]. Rates of suicidal ideations were higher in those who had high scores on the Beck Depression Inventory [55]. In another study, complicated grief was associated with passive suicidal ideations in 65% of individuals and 38% of individuals admitted to self-injurious behavior [56]. In the same study, 9% of individuals suffering from complicated bereavement had attempted suicide [56]. Given the concern for suicidality in the setting of bereavement—particularly grief-related depressive episode and complicated bereavement—psychiatrists should take more initiative in evaluating and treating the pathological variants of depression.

Summary

Bereavement is a psychological, social, and physiological process associated with changes in acute immune, cardiovascular, and endocrine function. Bereavement can be differentiated into three categories: uncomplicated grief, complicated grief, and grief-related major depression. Uncomplicated grief does not benefit from treatment. However, research suggests that complicated grief improves with psychotherapy, particularly complicated grief therapy. Furthermore, grief-related major depression can improve with antidepressant use and with psychotherapy. Appropriately diagnosing and treating pathological variants of bereavement are critical, as complicated grief and grief-related major depression are associated with increased risk for suicide.

Disclosures. I have no financial interests/arrangements to disclose that could be perceived as a real or apparent conflict of interest.

References

1. Schumacher KL, Jones PS, Meleis AI. Helping elderly persons in transition: a framework for research and practice. In: Swanson A, Tripp-Reimer T, editors. Life transitions in the older adult: issues for nurses and other health professionals. New York: Springer; 1999. p. 1–26.
2. Arean PA, Reynolds CF. The impact of psychosocial factors on late-life depression. Biol Psychiatry. 2005;58:277–82.
3. Feldman DC. The decision to retire early: a review and conceptualization. Academy of 6. Manag Rev. 1994;19:285–311.
4. Ritzer, George (ed). Blackwell encyclopedia of sociology. New Jersey: Blackwell Publishing. 2007. http://www.blackwellreference.com/public/book.html?id=g9781405124331_9781405124331. Accessed 20 Mar 2016.
5. Wang M, Shultz KS. Employee retirement: a review and recommendations for future investigation. J Manag. 2010;36(1):172–206.
6. Van der Heide I, van Rijn RM, Robroek SJW, Burdorf A, Proper KI. Is retirement good for your health? A systematic review of longitudinal studies. BMC Public Health. 2013;13:1180.
7. Taylor AW, Pilkington R, Feist H, Dal Grande E, Graeme H. A survey of retirement intentions of baby boomers: an overview on health, social and economic determinants. BMC Public Health. 2014;14:355.
8. Kim JE, Moen P. Retirement transitions, gender, and psychological well-being: a life-course, ecological model. J Gerontol. 2002;57B(3):212–22.
9. West LA, Cole S, Goodkind D, He W. 65+ in the United States: 2010. In: U.S. Census Bureau, editor. Special studies: current population reports. U.S. government printing office. Washington, D.C.: U.S. Government Printing Office; 2014. p. 23–212.
10. Szinovacz ME, Martin L, Davey A. Recession and expected retirement age: another look at the evidence. The Gerontologist. 2014;54(2):245–57.
11. Ekerdt DJ. Frontiers of research on work and retirement. J Gerontol. 2010;65B(1):69–80.
12. Oksanen T, Vahtera J, Westerlund H, et al. Is retirement beneficial for mental health? Antidepressant use before and after retirement. Epidemiology. 2011;22:553–9.

13. Mein G, Martikainen P, Hemingway H, Stansfeld S, Marmot M. Is retirement good or bad for mental and physical health functioning? Whitehall II longitudinal study of civil servants. J Epidemiol Community Health. 2003;57:46–9.
14. Latif E. The impact of retirement on psychological well-being in Canada. J Socio-Econ. 2011;40:373–80.
15. Mojon-Azzi S, Sousa-Poza A, Widmer R. The effect of retirement on health: a panel analysis using data from the Swiss Household Panel. Swiss Med Wkly. 2007;137:581–5.
16. Vahtera J, Westerlund H, Hall M, Sjosten N, Kivimaki M, Salo P. Effect of retirement on sleep disturbances: the GAZEL prospective cohort study. Sleep. 2009;32(11):1459–66.
17. Nuttman-Shwartz O. Like a high wave: adjustment to retirement. The Gerontologist. 2004;44(2):229–36.
18. Reitzes DC, Mutran EJ, Fernandez ME. Does retirement hurt well-being? Factors influencing self-esteem and depression among retirees and workers. The Gerontologist. 1996;35(5):649–56.
19. Westerlund H, Vahtera J, Ferrie JE, Singh-Manoux A, Pentti J, Melchior M, et al. Effect of retirement on major chronic conditions and fatigue: French GAZEL occupational cohort study. BMJ. 2010;341:c6149.
20. Sjosten N, Nabi H, Westerlund H, Singh-Manoux A, Dartigues JF, Goldberg M, et al. Influence of Retirement and work stress on headache prevalence: a longitudinal Modelling study from the GAZEL cohort. Cephalagia. 2011;31(6):696–705.
21. Sjosten N, Kivimaki M, Singh-Manoux A, Ferrie JE, Goldberg M, Zins M, et al. Change in physical activity and weight in relation to retirement: the French GAZEL cohort study. BMJ Open. 2012;2:e000522.
22. Westerlund H, Kivikami M, Singh-Manoux A, Melchior M, Ferrie JE, Pentti J, et al. Self-rated health before and after retirement in France (GAZEL): a cohort study. Lancet. 2009;374(5):1889–96.
23. Ekerdt DJ, Bosse R, Goldie C. The effect of retirement on somatic complaints. J Psychosom Res. 1983;27(1):61–7.
24. Ekerdt DJ, Baden L, Bosse R, Dibbs E. The effect of retirement on physical health. Am J Public Health. 1983;73(7):779–83.
25. Buxton JW, Singleton N, Melzer D. The mental health of early retirees—national interview survey in Britain. Soc Psychiatry Psychiatr Epidemiol. 2005;40(2):99–105.
26. Zins M, Gueguen A, Kivimaki M, Singh-Manoux A, Leclerc A, Vahtera J, et al. Effect of retirement on alcohol consumption: longitudinal evidence from the French Gazel cohort study. PLoS One. 2011;6(10):e26531.
27. Slingerland AS, van Lenthe FJ, Jukema JW, Kamphuis CB, Looman C, Giskes K, et al. Aging, retirement, and changes in physical activity: prospective cohort findings from the GLOBE study. Am J Epidemiol. 2007;165(12):1356–63.
28. Airagnes G, Lemogne C, Consoli SM, Schuster JP, Zins M, Limosin F. Personality moderates the improvement of depressive symptoms after retirement: evidence from the GAZEL cohort. Am J Geriatr Psychiatr. 2015;23(9):941–9.
29. Virtanen M, Ferrie JE, Batty GD, Elovainio M, Jokela M, Vahtera J. Socioeconomic and psychosocial adversity in midlife and depressive symptoms post retirement: a 21-year follow-up of the Whitehall II study. Am J Geriatr Psychiatr. 2015;23(1):99–109.
30. Stevens-Roseman ES. Older mentors for newer workers: impact of a worker-driven intervention on later life satisfaction. J Workplace Behav Health. 2009;24(4):419–26.
31. Saltz R. Research evaluation of a Foster-grandparent program. J Child Contemp Soc. 1989;20:205–16.
32. Federal Interagency Forum on Aging-Related Statistics. Older Americans 2012: key indicators of well-being. Federal Interagency Forum on aging-related statistics. Washington, DC: U.S. Government Printing Office; 2012.
33. Freud S. Mourning and melancholia. In: The standard edition of the complete psychological works of Sigmund Freud, volume XIV (1914–1916): on the history of the psycho-analytic movement, papers on metapsychology and other works. London: The Hogarth Press and the Institute of Psycho-Analysis; 1917. p. 237–58.
34. Kernberg O. Some observations on the process of mourning. Int J Psychoanal. 2010;91:601–19.
35. American Psychiatric Association. Diagnostic and statistical manual of mental disorders: DSM-5. Washington, D.C: American Psychiatric Publishing; 2015.
36. Hart CL, Hole DJ, Lawlor DA, Smith GD, Lever TF. Effect of conjugal bereavement on mortality of the bereaved spouse in participants of the Renfrew/paisley study. J Epidemiol Community Health. 2007;61(5):455–60.
37. Buckley T, Sunari D, Marshall A, Bartrop R, McKinley S, Tofler G. Physiological corre-

lates of bereavement and the impact of bereavement interventions. Dialogues Clin Neurosci. 2012;14(2):129–39.
38. Bartrop RW, Luckhurst E, Lazarus L, Kiloh LG, Penny R. Depressed lymphocyte function after bereavement. Lancet. 1977;1:834–6.
39. Gerra G, Monti D, Panerai AE, Sacerdote P, Anderlini R, Avanzini P, et al. Long-term immune-endocrine effects of bereavement: relationships with anxiety levels and mood. Psychiatry Res. 2003;121:145–58.
40. Buckley T, Morel-Kopp MC, Ward C, Bartrop R, McKinley S, Mihailidou AS, et al. Inflammatory and thrombotic changes in early bereavement: a prospective evaluation. Eur J Prev Cardiol. 2012;19(5):1145–52.
41. Buckley T, Bartrop R, McKinley S, Ward C, Bramwell M, Roche D, et al. Prospective study of early bereavement on psychological and behavioural cardiac risk factors. Intern Med J. 2009;39(6):370–8.
42. Buckley T, Mihaildou A, Bartrop R, McKinley S, Ward C, Morel-Kopp MC, et al. Haemodynamic changes during early bereavement: potential contribution to increased cardiovascular risk. Heart Lung Circ. 2011;20(2):91–8.
43. Zisook S, Shear K. Grief and bereavement: what psychiatrists need to know. World Psychiatry. 2009;6:67–74.
44. Mojitbai R. Bereavement-related depressive episodes: characteristics, 3-year course, and implications for the DSM-5. Arch Gen Psychiatry. 2011;68(9):920–8.
45. Fujisawa D, Miyashita M, Nakajima S, Ito M, Kato M, Kim Y. Prevalence and determinants of complicated grief in general population. J Affect Disord. 2010;127:352–8.
46. Newson RS, Boelen PA, Hek K, Hofman A, Tiemeier H. The prevalence and characteristics of complicated grief in older adults. J Affect Disord. 2011;132:231–8.
47. Bonanno GA, Wortman CB, Nesse RM. Prospective patterns of resilience and maladjustment during widowhood. Psychol Aging. 2004;19(2):260–71.
48. Hensley PL, Slonimski CK, Uhlenhuth EH, Clayton PJ. Escitalopram: an open-label study of bereavement-related depression and grief. J Affect Disord. 2009;113:142–9.
49. Reynolds CF 3rd, Miller MD, Pasternak RE, Frank E, Perel JM, Cornes C, et al. Treatment of bereavement-related major depressive episodes in later life: a controlled study of acute and continuation treatment with nortriptyline and interpersonal therapy. Am J Psychiatr. 1999;156:202–8.
50. Simon NM. Treating complicated grief. JAMA. 2013;310:416–23.
51. Boelen PA, de Keijser J, van den Hout MA, van den Bout J. Treatment of complicated grief: a comparison between cognitive-behavioral therapy and supportive counseling. J Consult Clin Psychol. 2007;75:277–84.
52. Shear K, Frank E, Houck PR, Reynolds CF. Treatment of complicated grief: a randomized controlled trial. JAMA. 2005;293:2601–8.
53. Papa A, Sewell MT, Garrison-Diehn C, Rummel C. A randomized open trial assessing the feasibility of behavioral activation for pathological grief responding. Behav Ther. 2013;44:639–50.
54. Shear K, Wang Y, Skritskaya N, Duan N, Mauro C, Ghesquiere A. Treatment of complicated grief in elderly persons: a randomized clinical trial. JAMA Psychiat. 2014;71:1287–95.
55. Stroebe M, Stroebe W, Abakoumkin G. The broken heart: suicidal ideation in bereavement. Am J Psychiatr. 2005;162:2178–80.
56. Szanto K, Shear MK, Houck PR, Reynolds CF III, Frank E, Caroff K, et al. Indirect self-destructive behavior and overt Suicidality in patients with complicated grief. J Clin Psychiatry. 2006;67(2):233–9.

2 Demography and Epidemiology

Sarah J. De Asis

Introduction

Demography is defined as the analysis of the population size and its structure especially in relation to its determinants, fertility, mortality, and migration [1]. Demography also identifies many major social and policy issues including the growth of the population, the challenges of an aging population, and the implications of migration on the population.

The World Health Organization (WHO) defines epidemiology as the study of the distribution and determinants of health-related states or events (including disease) and the application of this study to the control of diseases and other health problems [2]. According to Morris, epidemiology may be further defined as the study of health and disease of populations in relation to their environment and ways of living [3]. It provides the facts about community health; it describes the nature and relative size of the problems to be dealt with, and "maps" are produced of such scales as are required or possible. The main function of epidemiology is to discover groups in the population with high or low rates of diseases, so that causes of disease and reasons for freedom from disease can be postulated.

The Aging Population

In late life, the epidemiology of psychiatric disorders is the study of the distribution of psychiatric symptoms and disorders and the variables that affect their distribution [4]. In 2010, approximately 40 million persons aged 65 years and older lived in the United States, accounting for 13% of the population. With the aging of the baby boomer cohort (those born between 1946 and 1964), the size of the elderly population is projected to reach 72.1 million by the year 2030 and 88.5 million by 2050 accounting for an estimated 20.2% of the total population [4, 5]. The current older population of the United States is predominantly female and white. In 2010, women accounted for 57% of the population aged 65 years and older and 67% of those aged 85 years and older [4].

Life expectancy in the United States was 80.9 years for women and 76.0 for men [4]. According to Blazer, life expectancy at age 65 is 15.5 years for men and 19.1 years for women, so reaching age 80 is becoming the usual rather than the exceptional event [6]. The life expectancy for people 80 years old and older is greater in the United States than in Sweden, France, England, and Japan and is increasing. It is estimated that the number of people older than 65 years with psychiatric disorders in the United States will increase from about 4 million in 1970 to 15 million in 2030 [7].

Psychiatric Disorders Among Older Adults

The National Institute of Mental Health (NIMH) Epidemiologic Catchment Area (ECA) study used the Diagnostic Interview Schedule (DIS) based on DSM-III as the case-identification

R. R. Tampi et al. (eds.), *Psychiatric Disorders Late in Life*, https://doi.org/10.1007/978-3-319-73078-3_2

instrument to report on the 1-month prevalence rates of mental disorders from five sites across the United States [8]. The investigators found that for individuals aged ≥65 years, the prevalence of psychiatric according to the DIS was 12.3%. Jeste and colleagues consider this as underestimation of the prevalence of psychiatric disorders among older adults secondary to factors such as misattribution of psychiatric symptoms to cognitive impairment, physical disorders, or normal aging, lack of age-appropriate diagnostic criteria, and the underreporting due to forgetfulness and social stigma [7]. They opined that the "real" prevalence of psychiatric disorders other than dementia in elderly persons to be at least 25% higher than what is reported in the ECA study.

The ECA study found that the prevalence of alcohol abuse/dependence was 0.9% among older adults with it being more common among men (1.8%) than among women (0.3%) [8]. The prevalence of schizophrenia was found to be 0.1% for both sexes, and the prevalence of schizophreniform disorder was 0.0%. The prevalence of affective disorders was 2.5%; 3.3% in women and 1.4% in men. Dysthymia was found to be more common (1.8%) than major depressive episode (0.7%) and manic episode at (0.0%). Anxiety disorders were the most prevalent disorders at 5.5%; 6.8% and 3.6% in women and men, respectively. The prevalence of phobia was 4.8%, obsessive-compulsive disorder was 0.8%, and panic disorder was 0.1% in both sexes. The prevalence of somatization disorder was 0.1% and antisocial personality 0.0%. Cognitive impairment increased with age; it was seen in 2.9% of individuals 65–74 years in age, 6.8% of individuals 75–84 years in age, and 15.8% of individuals ≥85 years in age. Higher rates of almost all psychiatric disorders were found in younger age group individuals with the exception of severe cognitive impairment. Excess mortality (from suicide or physical comorbidity) in early life among individuals with schizophrenia, depression, substance dependence, and other psychiatric disorders was thought to be an important reason for the lower prevalence of serious mental illness among older adults when compared to younger adults [7].

Shapiro et al. reported that the most common diagnoses for women were phobias and affective disorders, whereas for men the predominant disorder was substance abuse and/or dependence [9]. The total rates of psychiatric disorders drop after the age of 45 years and particularly so after age 65 years with the exception of cognitive impairment.

The Australian National Mental Health and Well-Being Survey by Trollor et al. described the 1–12-month prevalence of mental disorders, their demographic correlates, and their impact on service utilization and disability among individuals ≥65 years [10]. The Composite International Diagnostic Interview (CIDI) was used to determine the presence of mental disorders using the International Classification of Diseases (ICD-10) and the *Diagnostic and Statistical Manual of Mental Disorders, Fourth Edition* (DSM-IV) diagnostic criteria. About 12.9% of the individuals met the criteria for a psychiatric disorder in the past 1 month, and 15.8% of the respondents met the criteria for a psychiatric disorder in the past 12 months. The most prevalent diagnostic category was cognitive impairment, followed by anxiety disorders and personality disorders. Major depression and generalized anxiety disorder (GAD) were the two most common individual ICD-10 defined 12-month diagnoses. Older women were more than twice as likely as older men to have experienced ICD-10 major depression and GAD in the preceding 12 months. The 12-month prevalence for major depression was (ICD-10, 2.4%; DSM-IV, 2.2%). The reported prevalence rate of cognitive impairment (7.4%) was based on the mini-mental state examination (MMSE) score and was greater than the 1-month prevalence data from the ECA study (4.9%). An association was noted between cognitive impairment and a higher prevalence of affective disorders. After cognitive impairment, anxiety disorders were the most prevalent diagnostic group in this survey. There were no significant differences in the overall rates of mental health disorders between males and females. However, there were specific sex differences in the rates for certain diagnostic groups like affective disorders where major depression was twice as prevalent among elderly females when compared to elderly males. There was also a marked female predominance for GAD. Male predominance was noted for substance use disorders, particularly alcohol abuse and dependence. Marital status was associated with affective disorders with those individuals who had never married being twice as likely to experience an affective disorder. In addition, those individuals with a physical health disorder were more than twice as likely to experience a mental health disorder. Lastly, among those individuals experiencing a mental health disorder within the past 12 months, only one-quarter had consulted a mental health professional. Even among those with multiple disorders, only about one-third had consulted a mental health professional.

Nationally representative data for community-dwelling older Americans had been limited until the ECA study from the 1980s comprehensively investigated rates of psychiatric disorders among a representative sample of older Americans from multiple communities [8]. The National Comorbidity Study Replication (NCS-R) is the most current nationally representative study of the epidemiology of psychiatric disorders in the United States [11]. Among the NCS-R respondents, there were 1461 individuals who were ≥65 years in age. The mean age of the participants was 74 years. Approximately 58% of the participants were women, 70.5% had 12 or more years of education, 54.3% were married, and 82.8% were non-Latino White. A total of 22.8% of all respondents received a diagnosis of at least one DSM-IV disorder. Among older adults, 8.5% of the individuals met the criteria for a psychiatric disorder. The 12-month prevalence was 7.0% for anxiety disorder, 2.6% for mood disorders, and 0% for any substance abuse disorder. Specific phobia was the most common diagnosis for the whole sample (8.7%), and for those individuals ≥ 65 years in age, the rate was 4.7%. Regardless of age, women had a higher rate of any psychiatric diagnoses. Among older adults, women were four times more likely to have a psychiatric diagnosis than men (12.6% vs. 2.9%). The lifetime prevalence for any DSM-IV disorder among older adults was 20.9%. The most prevalent diagnosis across all age groups was MDD (16.6%), with 9.3% for older adults meeting the criteria for MDD. Respondents aged 75 years and older were less likely than those aged 65–69 years to be diagnosed with a lifetime anxiety disorder, with no significant difference in those aged between 70–74 and 65–69 years. Individuals aged 65 years and older had lower rates of 12-month and lifetime mood, anxiety, and substance use disorder diagnoses when compared with that of younger and middle-aged adults. Those aged 75 years and older had the lowest prevalence particularly for lifetime psychiatric disorders. Within the last 12 months, 8.5% of older adults were diagnosed with at least one psychiatric disorder. Specific phobia was the most prevalent 12-month diagnosis (4.7%), followed by social phobia (2.3%) and MDD (2.3%).

The study by Rovner found that among nursing home residents, the prevalence of psychiatric disorders was approximately 75% [12]. Primary degenerative dementia accounted for 56% of the cases followed by vascular dementia (18%) and Parkinson's dementia (4%).

In the next section of the chapter, we describe the epidemiology of some common psychiatric disorders among older adults in greater detail.

Cognitive Disorders

The H70 study or the Longitudinal Gerontological and Geriatric Population Study in Göthenburg, Sweden, was a comprehensive population study that was started in 1971 [13]. This study found the prevalence of dementia at age 70 to be 6.6% in men and 3.1% in women. The prevalence of severe dementia increased from 1% at age 70 years to 2% at age 75 years and 7% at age 79 years. The prevalence of mild to moderate dementia increased from 2% to 4% and 9%, respectively. Almost one-third of the 85-year-olds had dementia (30%), and the prevalence rates were similar between men and women. The prevalence of dementia increased in women but not in men from age 85 to 88 years. The increase was attributed to higher rates of new cases in women. Individuals with Alzheimer's disease (AD) and vascular dementia (VD) had a higher prevalence of white matter lesions than did non-demented subjects. The 7-year survival rate in 85-year-olds was higher in women (35%) than in men (20%).

One community-based study showed that the estimated annual incidence of AD in the population was 0.6% for persons aged 65–69 years, 1.0% for persons aged 70–74 years, 2.0% for persons aged 75–79 years, 3.3% for persons aged 80–84 years, and 8.4% for persons aged 85 years and older [14]. This incidence is approximately 14 times higher among persons older than 85 years of age when compared with those between 65 and 69 years of age.

It is estimated that 5.4 million people or 22.2% of the population of the United States in 2002 aged 71 years or older have cognitive impairment without dementia [15]. Prominent subtypes included prodromal AD (8.2%) and cerebrovascular disease (5.7%). Among participants who completed follow-up assessments, 11.7% of individuals with cognitive impairment but without dementia progressed to dementia annually, whereas those with subtypes of prodromal AD and stroke progressed at annual rates of 17 to 20%. The prevalence of dementia in the United States among individuals aged 71 and older was 13.9%. Dementia prevalence increased with age from 5.0% among those aged 71 to 79 years to 37.4% of those aged 90 and older.

Evans et al. sampled 467 residents 65 years of age and older of a defined community. Of those with probable AD, 26% had severe cognitive impairment, 51% moderate cognitive impairment, and 23% mild cognitive impairment [16]. Among those 65–74 years old, the prevalence rate of probable AD was 3.0%. For those 75–84 years of age, the prevalence rate of probable AD was 18.7% and among those 85 years or older, it was 47.2%. Conditions other than AD that caused moderate to severe cognitive impairment including multiple cerebral infarcts, alcohol-induced dementia, Parkinsonian dementia, depression, psychosis, mental retardation, and subacute combined degeneration, were uncommon in this community sample. Of the 113 persons with moderate to severe cognitive impairment and a probable diagnosis, 84.1% had AD alone. Approximately 8.8% had only a cause of dementia other than AD, and 7.1% had both AD and another cause of dementia. The overall estimate of AD prevalence of 10.3% among those over the age of 65 years in this study was somewhat higher than reported in previous reports.

Prevalence and incidence rates of mild cognitive impairment (MCI) vary as a result of different diagnostic criteria as well as different sampling and assessment procedures [17]. The results of the Leipzig Longitudinal Study of the Aged (LEILA 75+) showed that the prevalence rates of MCI ranged from 3 to 20%. Rates of conversion to dementia over 2.6 years ranged from 23% to 47%. The study stated that people with MCI develop dementia at a rate of 10–15% per year, while the rate of healthy controls is 1–2% per year. The pre-dementia syndrome identifies conditions with age-related deficits in cognitive functioning. There are age-associated memory impairment (AAMI), aging-associated cognitive decline (AACD), age-related cognitive decline (ARCD), and mild cognitive impairment (MCI). The prevalence of AAMI among people aged 65 and older ranges from 7% to 38.4% [18]. People who meet AACD criteria show more extensive cognitive impairment. In another study, the prevalence of AACD was 26.6% in people aged 60 and older [19]. The incidence rate of pre-dementia syndromes appear to be increasing with age and is higher in subjects with less education. MCI is a prodromal phase of dementia, particularly AD type. Annual conversion rates of dementia for subjects classified according to the AAMI criteria vary from 3% to 24%. The individuals who meet the AACD criteria are more homogenous than those characterized by the MCI criteria and progressed to dementia at a rate of 28.6% over a 3-year follow-up period, contrary to the idea that AACD is a stable, non-pathologic entity. Approximately 28% of subjects with ARCD developed dementia after 2 years. Furthermore, 15% of subjects aged 65 years and older in age and 15 to 25% of subjects 75 years and older in age who are classified as having minimal dementia developed clinical dementia after 1 year. Annual conversion rates for pre-dementia syndromes to dementia vary between 4% and 40%. The annual conversion rates for MCI to AD vary between 10% and 15% per year.

An epidemiologic study by Ganguli et al. showed that among individuals with a diagnosis of MCI, 27% developed dementia over the next 10 years [20]. Over each 2-year interval, MCI persons showed increased risk for dementia:

11.1–16.7% progressed to Alzheimer disease, and 0–5.0% progressed to other dementias. Over the same time intervals, 11.1–21.2% of those with MCI remained at the MCI stage, and 33.3–55.6% no longer had MCI.

Anxiety Disorders

Anxiety disorders are one of the most common psychiatric disorders in the elderly, yet there are very few studies about epidemiology of these disorders. Smalbrugge et al. found that the prevalence of anxiety disorders among nursing home residents varied between 0% and 20% [21]. A Dutch community-based study found the overall prevalence of anxiety disorders among elderly to be 10.2%. Female sex, living without a partner, low level of education, somatic comorbidity, functional impairments, psychiatric comorbidity, and loneliness were found to be associated with anxiety disorders among the community-dwelling older adults. Phobias were the most prevalent anxiety disorder at 3.6%, followed by panic disorder at 1.5%, and generalized anxiety disorder at 1.2%. Approximately 29.7% of the individuals had one or more anxiety symptoms. A mini-mental state examination score of greater than 23, depression, stroke, more than 6-year education, impaired vision, pain, negative life events in the past year, serious functional impairments, loneliness, and perceived inadequacy of care were significantly associated with anxiety symptoms [21].

Two studies by Grant et al. showed that the prevalence of social anxiety disorder (SAD) in national and international epidemiologic surveys conducted since the early 1980s have varied widely [22, 23]. Overall, the 12-month and lifetime prevalence of SAD among all age groups were noted to be 2.8 and 5.0%, respectively. For ages ≥ 65 years, the 12-month and lifetime prevalence of SAD were 1.6 and 3.0%, respectively. The onset of SAD was typically during childhood and adolescence, and the onset after the age of 24 years was relatively uncommon. Among those individuals with SAD, in the prior 12 months, 13.1% had an alcohol use disorder, 5.5% had a drug use disorder, and 27.1% had nicotine dependence. Among those with lifetime history of SAD, 48.2% had an alcohol use disorder, 22.3% had a drug use disorder, 33.0% had nicotine dependence, 54.1% had any other anxiety disorders, 56.3% had a mood disorder, and 55.4% had a personality disorder. Bipolar I disorder was more strongly associated with SAD than either major depressive disorder, bipolar II, or persistent depressive disorder. The association of 12-month SAD with GAD was somewhat greater than with panic disorder and specific phobia. Avoidant personality disorder was more strongly related with SAD than any other personality disorder. Over 80% of individuals with SAD received no treatment [22, 23].

Depressive Disorders

Depression is a common and disabling psychiatric disorder in later life [24]. Results from the National Epidemiologic Survey on alcoholism and related conditions showed that being female, Native American, middle-aged, widowed, separated, divorced, and of low-income group increased the risk of becoming depressed [25]. Being of Asian, Hispanic, or Black race decreased the risk for being depressed. The Australian Longitudinal Study of Ageing by Anstey et al. showed that the prevalence of depression in residential care facilities was 32% when compared to 14.4% in the community [26]. Functional impairment and cognitive decline were associated with increasing risk of depression in late life. Blazer et al. reported that the prevalence of major depression in the community-dwelling elderly to be less than 5% [27]. The prevalence of primary depressive disorder was reported at 1.8% and of secondary depressive disorder at 1.9%.

Approximately 13.5% of older adults followed by a traditional visiting nurse agency were diagnosed with major depression [28]. Of these, 71% of the individuals were experiencing their first episode of depression, and the episode had lasted for more than 2 months in 78% of the individuals. Approximately 22% of the depressed individuals were receiving antidepressant treatment, but none were receiving psychotherapy. Approximately 31% of individuals receiving antidepressants were prescribed subtherapeutic doses, and 18% who were prescribed appropriate doses reported not complying with their antidepressant treatment. Teresi et al. found that 14.4% of nursing home residents met the criteria for probable and or definite major depressive disorder [29]. The estimate for significant depressive symptomatology among these individuals was 44.2%.

The AGED (Amsterdam Groningen Elderly Depression) study showed prevalence of major depression among elderly nursing home residents to be 8.1% and the prevalence of minor depression to be at 14.1% [24]. Approximately 24% of the individuals suffered from subclinical depression. Risk indicators for major depression were found to be pain, functional limitations, visual impairment, stroke, being lonely, the lack of social support, negative life events, and perceived inadequacy of care [24]. Another study found that 40% of institutionalized older adults met the criteria for depression [30]. Approximately 12% of these individuals met the DSM-III-R criteria for major depression, and almost half of them suffered significant cognitive deficits [30].

Data from the West Friesland Study showed that the prevalence of major depression among older adults consulting their general practitioner in the Netherlands was 13.7%, and the prevalence for minor depression was 10.2% [31]. Patients with major depression were younger and more often female than those with minor depression. Only 22.9% of the individuals with major depression were treated with antidepressants. In the Aging, Demographics, and Memory Study (ADAMS) where the participants were aged ≥71 years, the overall prevalence for depression was 11.19% [32]. The prevalence of depression was similar for men and women. Whites and Hispanics had nearly three times the prevalence of depression when compared to African-Americans. Dementia diagnosis and pain severity were associated with increased depression prevalence, while black race was associated with lower rates of depression. The H70 study found that the prevalence of depression among 70- to 74-year-old women was 12% when individuals with dementia were included in the denominator and 13% when they were excluded [13]. Among the 85-year-old women, the prevalence of depression was 13% when individuals with dementia were included in the denominator and 19% when demented were excluded.

Depression in old age may also be a symptom of incipient dementia [13]. The elderly have a disproportionally high rate of suicide worldwide, with a peak above the age of 80 [13]. There is also a greater degree of lethal intent. Among mentally healthy 85-year-olds, only 4% had thought during the last month that life is not worth living, 4% had death wishes, and 1% had thought about taking their lives. None had seriously considered suicide. Among those individuals with mental disorders 29% had thought that life is not worth living, 28% had death wishes, 9% had thought about taking their lives, and 2% had seriously considered suicide [13].

Substance Use Disorders

Large-scale US and international surveys conducted in the early 1980s using the DSM-III criteria showed that among individuals 65 years older, the 12-month prevalence of alcohol abuse was 1.2%, and alcohol dependence was 0.2% [33]. The 12-month prevalence for any alcohol use disorder in this age group was 1.5%. The lifetime prevalence of alcohol abuse and dependence among individuals 65 years older was 12.7% and 3.4%, respectively; for any alcohol use disorder, it was 16.1%. The 12-month alcohol abuse remained strongly and significantly associated with substance use disorders (OR ≥ 1.8). The 12-month alcohol dependence remained strongly associated with substance use disorders, specific phobias, and bipolar disorders but with lower ORs and was significantly associated with histrionic and antisocial personality disorders. Mean ages for onset of alcohol abuse and dependence were 22.5 and 21.9 years, respectively. Hazard rates for onset of both disorders peaked at 19 years and decreased thereafter. The duration of alcohol use disorder was often chronic with a mean of nearly 4 years for alcohol dependence. Men were at greater risk of alcohol use disorder than women. African-Americans and Asians were at lower risk than Caucasians for alcohol abuse and dependence.

Blazer and Wu in their two studies evaluated the epidemiology of substance use disorders among middle-aged and older adults [34, 35]. In the first study, they reported that the number of older adults needing treatment for SUD is estimated to increase from 1.7 million in 2000–2001 to 4.4 million in 2020 [34]. In the two large surveys, Epidemiologic Catchment Area (ECA study) and the National Comorbidity Study Replication (NCS-R), the prevalence of drug use was very low among middle-aged and older adults. In the ECA study, 7% of individuals 45–64 years and 1.6% of individuals ≥65 years in age had a lifetime prevalence of illegal drug use. Active use of illegal drugs occurred in 0.8% of subjects 45–64 years and 0.1% of individuals ≥ 65 years in age. In another study of older adults who were referred to a hospital substance abuse consultation service, older adults when compared to younger adults were more likely to use alcohol and less likely to be injection drug users and users of heroin, cocaine, or multiple substances. Nearly 60% of subjects used alcohol during the past year, 2.6% used marijuana, and 0.41% used cocaine. Both alcohol and drug use were far more frequent in subjects 50 to 64 years in age and among men. Drug use in contrast to alcohol use was not associated with the level of education but was more common among those who were not married and among those with major depression. The prevalence of drug abuse or dependence in the ≥50 age group was very low at only 0.33% for any abuse or dependence, 0.12% for marijuana abuse or dependence, and 0.18% for cocaine abuse or dependence, respectively. Nevertheless, the use of marijuana approached 4% in the 50–64 age groups in comparison to 0.7% in the ≥65 age group.

Psychotic Disorders

Psychotic symptoms are reported to be uncommon among older adults, although they are substantially more common among individuals with dementia [13]. The prevalence of schizophrenic and paranoid syndromes are 0.5, 1.7, and 2.5% at 70, 75, and 79 years, respectively. It was noted that 10% of non-demented 85-year-olds had psychotic symptoms, and 7% had paranoid ideation during the preceding year. Hallucinations were found in 7% and delusions in 6%. Hallucinations, delusions, and paranoid ideation at age 85 were each related to an increased incidence of dementia from 85 to 88 years, but only a minority of those individuals with these symptoms developed dementia.

There are only a limited number of studies about epidemiology of psychosis among the elderly. In a study done by Christenson et al. in a community sample of elderly individuals in San Francisco, the investigators found that 17% of those rated as psychiatrically impaired had symptoms of suspiciousness and 13% had delusions [36]. When the entire sample was considered, 2.5% showed suspiciousness, and 2% had paranoid delusions. In the community-based elderly population, the prevalence of generalized persecutory ideation was 4%. There were no significant differences in age, sex, race, or education between individuals who exhibited persecutory ideations versus those who did not exhibit these symptoms. Sensory and cognitive impairments appeared to be significant risk factors for developing persecutory ideations in this study.

According to Meesters et al., the estimated proportion of individuals developing schizophrenia after the age of 40 years is thought to be 23.5% [37]. On a lifetime basis, the risk of developing schizophrenia for men relative to women is estimated to be 1.32. In this study, the estimated 1-year prevalence of all disorders (schizophrenia, schizoaffective disorder, or delusional disorder) was 0.71%. The prevalence was 0.55% for schizophrenia, 0.14% for schizoaffective disorder, and 0.03% for delusional disorder. Estimated prevalence of schizophrenia in women aged 60–79 years was higher than in women aged 80 years and older. Estimated prevalence of schizophrenia was higher in women than in men for age groups 60–69 years and 70–79 years. Delusional disorder was found only in women aged 70 years and older. With regards to age of onset, the estimated 1-year prevalence of late-onset schizophrenia (LOS) was 0.14% and that of very late-onset schizophrenia (VLS) was 0.05%. Among individuals aged 40 years or older who developed schizophrenia, 76.5% were women. This figure rose to 92.9% for those individuals who developed symptoms of schizophrenia after 60 years of age. Delusional disorder was found only in women aged 40 years or older at onset. Individuals with LOS have better premorbid social functioning and display less executive impairment and higher levels of everyday functioning. Also, affective flattening and social withdrawal were reported to be less prominent in LOS individuals.

A study by Östling and Skoog reported that the prevalence of psychotic symptoms in the elderly might be underrated because of reluctance to report psychotic symptoms [38]. In a study of non-demented individuals aged 85 years living in a community or in institutions in Göthenburg, Sweden, psychotic symptoms were identified in 10.1% of the individuals. Hallucinations were seen in 6.9% of the participants, delusions in 5.5%, and paranoid ideations in 6.9%. Individuals with hallucinations had an increased frequency of depressed mood, anxiety, irritability, suicidal ideation, and paranoid personality traits. These symptoms were often associated with major depressive syndrome, disability in daily life, and visual deficits. Individuals with delusions had an increased frequency of depressed mood, blunted affect, and paranoid personality traits and were associated with disability in life. Individuals with paranoid ideation had an increased frequency of depressed mood, irritability, and paranoid personality traits and were associated with visual deficits and myocardial infarction. Among individuals with hallucinations or delusions, 20.0% were prescribed neuroleptics, 17.1% antidepressants, 22.9% anxiolytics or sedatives, and 37.1% any psychotropic drug. No individuals with paranoid ideation without concomitant hallucinations or delusions were prescribed neuroleptics. The 3-year mortality rate was increased in women with hallucinations (40.0%) and paranoid ideations (36.8%) when compared to women without these symptoms. Hallucinations, delusions, and paranoid ideation were not associated with mortality in men. In addition, hallucinations, delusions, and paranoid ideation were each related to an increased 3-year incidence of dementia from 85 to 88 years. Sensory impairments were associated with late life psychosis and paranoid symptoms.

The study by Östling et al. on cognitively intact individuals aged 70 and above found that the cumulative incidence of psychotic symptoms during the 3.6-year follow-up period was 4.8% [39]. The incidence rate for schizophrenia was 0.03/1000 person-years and for delusional disorder was 0.16/1000 person-years. The investigators found a double mortality risk in individuals aged above 70 years with psychotic symptoms at baseline during the 3.6-year follow-up period. In this study 8% of non-demented 70-year-olds developed first-onset psychotic symptoms during a 20-year follow-up period. There were no significant sex differences in the incidence of first-onset psychotic symptoms in the study. The cumulative incidence for hallucinations and delusions among individuals with probable Alzheimer's disease was 51% in 4 years. Hallucinations were in most cases visual. Delusions were related to an increased risk for developing dementia at a later time period. Approximately 60% of individuals with hallucinations, 30% with delusions, and 45% of those with any psychotic symptom developed dementia.

Conclusions

Epidemiology of psychiatric disorders in late life indicates that with the exception of cognitive disorders, these disorders are more common among younger adults. Cognitive impairment is the most prevalent diagnostic category followed by anxiety disorders among older adults. The prevalence of dementia is noted to increase with age. Alzheimer's disease is the most common form of dementia. The rate of conversion of mild cognitive impairment to dementia is approximately 10–15% per year. Phobias and affective disorders are more common among elderly women, and substance use disorders are more common among elderly men. Phobia is the most common anxiety disorder among older adults. Depression is a common psychiatric disorder in late life, and it is more prevalent among females and Caucasian and Hispanic races. Psychotic symptoms are uncommon among the elderly but are often seen in individuals with dementia especially women. The most common psychotic symptoms are visual hallucinations and persecutory delusions. Alcohol use disorders are more common in elderly men, and its rate of onset decreases with age. Illicit drug use appears to be rare among the elderly. The elderly also have higher rates of suicides especially among older Caucasian men. Knowledge of epidemiologic data regarding psychiatric illness among the elderly can aid in the appropriate planning and treatment of these disorders.

References

1. Demography and health. http://www.lse.ac.uk/LSEHealthAndSocialCare/research/LSEHealth/DemographyandHealth.aspx. Accessed 30 Jan 2017.
2. Epidemiology. http://www.who.int/topics/epidemiology/en/. Accessed 30 Jan 2017.
3. Morris JN. Uses of epidemiology. Int J Epidemiol. 2007;36:1165–72.
4. Hybels CF, Blazer DG. Demography and epidemiology of psychiatric disorders in late life. In: Steffens D, Blazer D, Thakur M, editors. The American Psychiatric Publishing textbook of geriatric psychiatry. Arlington: American Psychiatric Publishing; 2015.
5. Plassman BL, Langa KM, Fisher GG, Heeringa SG, Weir DR, Ofstedal MB, Burke JR, Hurd MD, Potter GG, Rodgers WL, Steffens DC, Willis RJ, Wallace RB. Prevalence of dementia in the United States: the aging, demographics, and memory study. Neuroepidemiology. 2007;29:125–32.
6. Blazer DG. Psychiatry and the oldest old. Am J Psychiatry. 2000;157:1915–24.
7. Jeste DV, Alexopoulos GS, Bartels SJ, Cummings JL, Gallo JJ, Gottlieb GL, Halpain MC, Palmer BW, Patterson TL, Reynolds CF, Lebowitz BD. Consensus statement on the upcoming crisis in geriatric mental health. Arch Gen Psychiatry. 1999;56:848–53.
8. Regier DA, Boyd JH, Burke JD, Rae DS, Myers JK, Kramer M, Robins LN, George LK, Karno M, Locke BZ. One-month prevalence of mental disorders in the United States. Arch Gen Psychiatry. 1988;45:977–86.
9. Shapiro S, Skinner EA, Kessler LG, Von Korff M, German PS, Tischler GL, Leaf PJ, Benham L, Cottler L, Regier DA. Utilization of health and mental health services. Arch Gen Psychiatry. 1984;41:971–8.
10. Trollor JN, Anderson TM, Sachdev PS, Brodaty H, Andrews G. Prevalence of mental disorders in the elderly: the Australian National Mental Health and well-being survey. Am J Geriatr Psychiatry. 2007;15:455–66.
11. Gum AM, King-Kallimanis B, Kohn R. Prevalence of mood, anxiety, and substance use disorders for older Americans in the National Comorbidity Survey-Replication. Am J Geriatr Psychiatry. 2009;17:769–81.
12. Rovner BW, Kafonek S, Filipp L, Lucas MJ, Folstein MF. Prevalence of mental illness in a community nursing home. Am J Psychiatry. 1986;143:1446–9.
13. Skoog I. Psychiatric epidemiology of old age: the H70 study–the NAPE lecture 2003. Acta Psychiatr Scand. 2004;109:4–18.
14. Hebert LE, Scherr PA, Beckett LA, Albert MS, Pilgrim DM, Chown MJ, Funkenstein HH, Evans DA. Age-specific incidence of Alzheimer's disease in a community population. JAMA. 1995;273:1354–9.
15. Plassman BL, Langa KM, Fisher GG, Heeringa SG, Weir DR, Ofstedal MB, Burke JR, Hurd MD, Potter GG, Rodgers WL, Steffens DC, McArdle JJ, Willis RJ, Wallace RB. Prevalence of cognitive impairment without dementia in the United States. Ann Intern Med. 2008;148:427–34.
16. Evans DA, Funkenstein HH, Albert MS, Scherr PA, Cook NR, Chown MJ, Hebert LE, Hennekens CH, Taylor JO. Prevalence of Alzheimer's disease in a community population of older persons. JAMA. 1989;262:2551–6.
17. Busse A, Bischkopf J, Riedel-Heller SG, Angermeyer MC. Mild cognitive impairment: prevalence and incidence according to different diagnostic criteria. Br J Psychiatry. 2003;182:449–54.
18. Hänninen T, Hallikainen M, Tuomainen S, Vanhanen M, Soininen H. Prevalence of mild cognitive impairment: a population based study in elderly subjects. Acta Neurol Scand. 2002;106:148–54.
19. Panza F, D'Introno A, Colacicco AM, Capurso C, Del Parigi A, Caselli RJ, Pilotto A, Argentieri G, Scapicchio PL, Scafato E, Capurso A, Solfrizzi V. Current epidemiology of mild cognitive impairment and other Predementia syndromes. Am J Geriatr Psychiatry. 2005;13:633–44.
20. Ganguli M, Dodge HH, Shen C, DeKosky ST. Mild cognitive impairment, amnestic type. Neurology. 2004;63:115–21.
21. Smalbrugge M, Pot AM, Jongenelis K, Beekman ATF, Eefsting JA. Prevalance and correlates of anxiety among nursing home patients. J Affect Disord. 2005;88:145–53.
22. Grant BF, Hasin DS, Blanco C, Stinson FS, Chou SP, Goldstein RB, Dawson DA, Smith S, Saha TD, Huang B. The epidemiology of social anxiety disorder in the United States: results from the National Epidemiologic Survey on alcohol and related conditions. J Clin Psychiatry. 2005;66:1351–61.
23. Grant BF, Hasin DS, Stinson FS, Dawson DA, Goldstein RB, Smith S, Huang B, Saha TD. The epidemiology of DSM-IV panic disorder and agoraphobia in the United States: results from the National Epidemiologic Survey on alco-

hol and related conditions. J Clin Psychiatry. 2006;67:363–74.
24. Jongenelis K, Pot AM, Eisses AMH, Beekman ATF, Kluiter H, Ribbe MW. Prevalence and risk indicators of depression in elderly nursing home patients: the AGED study. J Affect Disord. 2004;83:135–42.
25. Hasin DS, Goodwin RD, Stinson FS, Grant BF. Epidemiology of major depressive disorder. Arch Gen Psychiatry. 2005;62:1097–106.
26. Anstey KJ, von Sanden C, Sargent-Cox K, Luszcz MA. Prevalence and risk factors for depression in a longitudinal, population-based study including individuals in the community and residential care. Am J Geriatr Psychiatry. 2007;15:497–505.
27. Blazer D, Hughes DC, George LK. The epidemiology of depression in an elderly community population. The Gerontological Society of America. 1987;27:281–7.
28. Bruce ML, McAvay GJ, Raue PJ, Brown EL, Meyers BS, Keohane DJ, Jagoda DR, Weber C. Major depression in elderly home health care patients. Am J Psychiatry. 2002;159:1367–74.
29. Teresi J, Abrams R, Holmes D, Ramirez M, Eimicke J. Prevalance of depression and depression recognition in nursing homes. Soc Psychiatry Pyschiatr Epidemiol. 2001;36:613–20.
30. Parmelee PA, Katz IR, Lawton MP. Depression among institutionalized aged: assessment and prevalence estimation. J Gerontol. 1989;44:M22–9.
31. Licht-Strunk E, van der Kooij KG, van Schaik DJF, van Marwijk HWJ, van Hout HPJ, de Haan M, Beekman ATF. Prevalence of depression in older patients consulting their general practitioner in the Netherlands. Int J Geriatr Psychiatry. 2005;20:1013–9.
32. Steffens DC, Fisher GG, Langa KM, Potter GG, Plassman BL. Prevalence of depression among older Americans: the aging, demographics and memory study. Int Psychogeriatr. 2009;21:879–88.
33. Hasin DS, Stinson FS, Ogburn E, Grant BF. Prevalence, correlates, disability, and comorbidity of DSM-IV alcohol abuse and dependence in the United States. Arch Gen Psychiatry. 2007;64:830–42.
34. Blazer DG, Wu LT. The epidemiology of alcohol use disorders and subthreshold dependence in a middle-aged and elderly community sample. Am J Geriatr Psychiatry. 2011;19:685–94.
35. Blazer DG, Wu LT. The epidemiology of substance use and disorders among middle aged and elderly community adults: National Survey on drug use and health (NSDUH). Am J Geriatr Psychiatry. 2009;17:237–45.
36. Christenson R, Blazer D. Epidemiology of persecutory ideation in an elderly population in the community. Am J Psychiatry. 1984;141:1088–91.
37. Meesters PD, de Haan L, Comijs HC, Stek ML, Smeets-Janssen MMJ, Weeda MR, Eikelenboom P, Smit JH, Beekman ATF. Schizophrenia Spectrum disorders in later life: Prevalance and distribution of age at onset and sex in a Dutch catchment area. Am J Geriatr Psychiatry. 2012;20:18–28.
38. Östling S, Skoog I. Psychotic symptoms and paranoid ideation in a nondemented population-based sample of the very old. Arch Gen Psychiatry. 2002;59:53–9.
39. Östling S, Pálsson SP, Skoog I. The incidence of first-onset psychotic symptoms and paranoid ideation in a representative population sample followed from age 70-90 years. Relation to mortality and later development of dementia. Int J Geriatr Psychiatry. 2007;22:520–8.

3 Culture and Gender

Brandon C. Yarns

Introduction

Culture is defined as "the integrated patterns of human behavior that include the language, thoughts, communications, actions, customs, beliefs, values and institutions of racial, ethnic, religious or social groups" [1]. Thus, culture can be thought of as a complicated term which incorporates many facets of human experience and applies broadly to a variety of different social groups. For example, veterans may be considered as a cultural group which struggles with health disparities resulting from posttraumatic stress disorder, depression, and substance abuse [2]. The smallest unit of culture in any society is the culture of individual families, wherein a family's culture may, for example, promote or limit options for its female members [3]. The American Psychological Association, in a 2009 report on multicultural competency for older adults, called for age itself to be considered as having cultural ramifications, given that cohorts of different ages had exceptionally different experiences and life events, attitudes, and values [1].

The DSM-5 states that, "mental disorders are defined in relation to cultural, social, and familial norms and values. Culture provides interpretive frameworks that shape the experience and expression of the symptoms, signs, and behaviors that are criteria for diagnosis. Culture is transmitted, revised and recreated within the family and other social systems and institutions" [4]. The field of cultural psychiatry is aimed at "the comparative study of mental health and mental illness among different societies, nations and cultures and the interrelationships of mental disorders with cultural environments" [5]. Thus, culture has been a central focus in the diagnosis and treatment of mental disorders for some time.

As a result of the importance of considering culture in providing health and mental health services, the US Department of Health and Human Services Office of Minority Health calls for cultural and linguistic competence or "a set of congruent behaviors, attitudes and policies that come together in a system, agency or among professionals that enables effective work in cross-cultural situations" [1]. Given the broad definition of what may account for cultural situations, a geriatric mental health provider who strives for "cultural competence" may, therefore, consider the many ways in which a patient's culture differs from their own.

Acknowledging the broad definitions of culture, cultural psychiatry, and cultural competence, the remainder of this chapter describes some of the important disparities in geriatric mental health and mental health care evident when considering three specific categories of cultures—race/ethnicity, gender, and sexual minority status—and provides recommendations for geriatric mental health providers to become more culturally competent in working with these unique groups of older adults.

R. R. Tampi et al. (eds.), *Psychiatric Disorders Late in Life*, https://doi.org/10.1007/978-3-319-73078-3_3

Racial/Ethnic Geriatric Mental Health Disparities

For more than two decades, racial/ethnic minority elders have represented the fastest growing segments of the aging population of the United States [6]. Prevalence rates of psychiatric disorders tend to be similar or lower in ethnic minority elders when compared to their White counterparts, although access to and utilization of mental health services is significantly less in minority elders than among Whites [7].

Several studies have been conducted which evaluate the prevalence of psychiatric diagnoses across ethnically diverse older adults based on data from the National Institute of Mental Health's Collaborative Psychiatric Epidemiology Surveys (CPES) [7–11]. CPES combined data from three multistage area probability samples with a common set of objectives and instrumentation: data for older non-Latino Whites in the National Comorbidity Survey Replication, older African Americans and Afro-Caribbean older adults from the National Survey of American Life, and Latino and Asian American older adults from the National Latino and Asian American Study [11]. Twelve-month and lifetime psychiatric diagnoses were determined using the World Mental Health Composite International Diagnostic Interview [11].

In these studies, older Asian American, African American, and Afro-Caribbean respondents exhibited lower lifetime rates of depression and anxiety diagnoses than among older non-Latino Whites, although no differences were found in 12-month diagnoses. However, older Latinos had the same lifetime rates of depression and anxiety diagnoses as older non-Latino Whites and had higher 12-month rates of depressive disorders than non-Latino Whites. The authors of one study concluded that previously described "protective effects of ethnicity" may not extend in all ethnicities, particularly among Latinos, into old age [7].

Similarly, the Aging, Demographics, and Memory Study (ADAMS) , which included a population-representative sample drawn from the larger Health and Retirement Study, found that among ADAMS participants aged 71 years and older, non-Latino Whites and Latinos had nearly three times the prevalence of depression as African Americans measured with the Composite International Diagnostic Interview—Short Form and the informant depression section of the Neuropsychiatric Inventory [12].

Another interesting finding is the effects of "nativity" or the distinction between US-born and immigrant populations. Although there were no significant differences in the aggregate categories of psychiatric illness according to nativity, immigrant Latinos and Asian Americans had higher rates of some individual disorders, such as generalized anxiety disorder, than their US-born counterparts [7].

In a small study of depression rates in home health-care nurse depression assessment, rates of positive depression screening using the Patient Health Questionnaire 2-item were also lower among older African Americans and Latinos than older non-Latino Whites; however, when two key clinical indicators from the patients' charts were included in analyses, preexisting depression diagnosis, and presence of antidepressant medication on patient medication lists, African Americans had significantly more positive screens when compared with older non-Latino Whites and Latinos [13]. The authors concluded that special attention should be applied to diagnosing depression in African Americans with depression risk factors [13].

In spite of these findings of lower rates of depression and anxiety among some ethnically diverse elders, a 2009 study using data from the California Health Interview Survey revealed that African American, Asian American, and Latino elders in California were significantly more likely to have mental distress than non-Latino Whites (21.2–24.2% vs. 14.4%) and had significantly higher prevalence of serious mental illness (4.1–7.7% vs. 2.5%) [14].

Ethnic minority elders also have poorer access to mental health services than non-Latino Whites. In a study of depression treatment among older ethnically diverse home health-care patients, the odds of receiving an antidepressant among those who screened positive for depression were lower for African Americans and Latinos when compared to non-Latino Whites [15]. In the aforementioned study using data from the California Health Interview Survey, African American, Asian American, and Latino older adults had worse access to mental health services even after adjusting for health insurance status [14].

Because of these lower rates of access and utilization of geriatric mental health-care services, it is important to understand the cultural beliefs and mental health treatment preferences of ethnic minority elders in order to best provide culturally competent geriatric mental health care. In a study of cultural beliefs and mental health treatment preferences among ethnically diverse older adults who participated in the Primary Care Research in Substance Abuse and Mental Health for the Elderly (PRISM-E) randomized trial of integrated care versus referral, older African Americans tended to view mental illness as caused by the loss of family or friends, stress over money, and stress or worry in general than non-Latino Whites [16]. Older African Americans and Asian Americans were also less willing to speak to psychiatrist or psychologists than older non-Latino Whites, although Latinos were more willing to speak to a psychologist and less likely to speak to a medical doctor than non-Latino Whites [16]. Finally, older African Americans preferred more for their health-care providers to understand their culture when compared to non-Latino Whites, and older Asian Americans preferred more for their health-care providers to be of the same racial/ethnic group [16].

In a follow-up study, older PRISM-E patients completed the Substance Abuse and Mental Health Services Administration Mental Health and Alcohol Abuse Stigma Assessment. This assessment found that no significant differences in shame or embarrassment at having a mental illness were observed between older African Americans and non-Latino Whites, but older Asian Americans and Latinos felt significantly more shame or embarrassment with regard to having a mental illness than did non-Latino Whites [17]. Older Asian Americans also stated they had greater difficulty engaging in mental health treatment if others knew, were less comfortable in speaking with their primary care providers about mental health issues, and had greater difficulty seeking mental health treatment in specialty mental health clinics. However, older African Americans and Latinos expressed greater comfort in speaking with primary care providers and mental health professionals than older non-Latino Whites [17].

Studies also have been conducted to determine ethnic differences in the experience of dementia diagnosis across immigrants in the United States and the United Kingdom [18, 19]. While many similarities exist, African American caregivers noted special concerns about racism, while Latino caregivers worried about their loved ones' institutionalization, and Chinese caregivers reported concerns that the stigmatization associated with mental illness in their culture may extend to dementia as well [19].

Gender Geriatric Mental Health Disparities

Most evidence on gender disparities among older adults have been derived from studies of depression. Although some epidemiological studies have found depression to be more common in women across age groups, older women may have rates closer to those of older men [12, 20]. Using data from the National Comorbidity Study Replication, a nationally representative study of the epidemiology of psychiatric disorders in the United States, among those 65 years and older, women had higher lifetime and 12-month prevalence rates than men for all psychiatric disorders, 24% vs. 16.7% and 12.6% vs. 2.9%, respectively [21]. However, in the Aging, Demographics, and Memory Study, prevalence of depression was similar for older men (10.19%) and older women (11.44%) [12].

Men have significantly lower rates of correct depression identification and lower rates of treatment when compared to women. In two studies of depression diagnosis in primary care settings, depression in older men was less likely to be recognized than depression in older women [22, 23]. In a survey of 9585 adults from 60 US communities, clinically depressed older men had significantly lower rates of treatment when compared to older women [24]. Older men also have significantly higher rates of completed suicide than older women (31.8 per 100,000 in men age 65 years and older when compared to 4.1 per

100,000 in older women), emphasizing the critical importance for correct identification and treatment of depression in older men [25].

Studies have investigated potential causes for depression due to gender disparities. In particular, men have been identified as having more negative attitudes toward help-seeking for mental health services, lower disclosure rates of depressive symptoms, lower rates of health service utilization, and more "atypical" presentations of depression [26–29]. In a mixed-method investigation of gender disparities in IMPACT, older men were significantly less likely to be referred to IMPACT, to endorse core depressive symptoms, and to have had prior depression treatment when compared to older women, and qualitative themes identified as important contributors to these disparities included differences in how men experienced and expressed depression, traditional masculine values, and the stigma of mental illness [20]. In a survey of elderly Korean Americans, living alone was significantly correlated with depressive symptoms and suicidal ideation in men but not in women, whereas living in a multigenerational family without a spouse and having a lower household income were significantly associated with poorer mental health in both men and women [30].

Apart from depression disparities, there is evidence that men's brains may lose gray matter faster as they age when compared to women, which may increase the likelihood in men versus women of functional consequences such as cognitive impairment and dementia [31, 32]. Nonetheless, incidences of dementia in men and women have been shown to be similar in several large epidemiologic studies [33–36]. Since women tend to live longer on average than men, a larger portion of women than men have Alzheimer's disease and dementia overall [37].

Finally, predictors for mild cognitive impairment (MCI) differ between older men and older women. In a study of Malaysian older adults, hypercholesterolemia, age, ethnicity, and total years of education predicted MCI in men, but in women, MCI was best predicted by married status, less exercise, and higher weight [38]. The authors concluded that special care should be taken by geriatric mental health-care providers to evaluate gender-specific risk factors in older men and women [38].

Lesbian, Gay, Bisexual, and Transgender Geriatric Mental Health Disparities

The Centers for Disease Control and Prevention in their landmark report *The State of Aging and Health in America 2013* announced a call for action to address lesbian, gay, bisexual, and transgender (LGBT) aging and health issues as LGBT elders continue to have higher levels of illness, disability, and premature deaths [39]. Additionally, aging services and the health needs of LGBT elders are often not adequately addressed in policies, research, and services.

A recent review article estimates that the current population of older LGBT adults in the USA numbers close to 1 million [40]. This was based in part on a Gallup Poll in which 2% of individuals 65 years and older were identified as LGBT. The authors note that the 2% in the Gallup Poll may be an underestimate of the true population of older LGBT adults, given that poll and survey respondents need to ensure that they feel safe in order to report their gender identities and sexual orientations [40].

Cohort differences may be especially important when considering the mental health of older LGBT adults because of the rapid changes in social attitudes toward LGBT individuals that have occurred in the late 20th and early 21st centuries. The findings from *Caring and Aging with Pride*, a population-based survey which investigated the disparities and resilience among over 2000 LGBT older adults, indicated that the rates of victimization and internalized stigma were higher for LGBT respondents aged 80 years and older when compared to those aged 50–79 years [41].

Until recently, very little empirical evidence existed on the prevalence of psychiatric disorders in the older LGBT population. The Institute of Medicine Report, *The Health of Lesbian, Gay, Bisexual, and Transgender People: Building a Foundation for Better Understanding*, summarizes data on the topic prior to 2011 [42]. Since then, a population-based survey of LGBT elders in the USA, *Caring and Aging with Pride*, and a YouGov survey in the United Kingdom comparing older LGBT and heterosexual individuals have both shown that the rates of depression, anxiety, suicidal ideation, and alcohol and substance misuse were as much as two to three times higher among older LGBT respondents when compared to older heterosexual respondents or age-matched population norms [41, 43]. In the US survey, rates of anxiety, depression, and mental distress were highest among the transgender respondents, and 71% of transgender elders reported a lifetime history of suicidal ideation [41]. Among the respondents with a history of suicidal ideation, 39% reported that they had become suicidal in relation to their sexual orientation or gender identity [41].

Although no surveys have been completed specifically to investigate disparities in health-care access and utilization in older LGBT individuals, disparities in access and utilization were noted among men and women in the same-sex relationships across age groups in a study using data from the 2000 to 2007 iterations of the Behavioral Risk Factor Surveillance System [44]. The study found that men and women in same-sex relationships were less likely to have health insurance and more likely to report unmet medical needs than men and women in opposite-sex relationships; women in same-sex relationships were also less likely to have had a checkup within the last year and less likely to have had a recent mammogram or Pap test, although men in same-sex relationships were more likely to have had a checkup in the past year [44].

"Coming out," a developmental process for all LGBT individuals in which one's sexual orientation or gender identity is realized internally and then disclosed to others, has been emphasized as a significant stressor for older LGBT individuals who must often repeatedly come out to health-care providers and caregivers as they age [40]. Concerns among gay and lesbian caregivers of individuals living with dementia identify the lack of cultural competence of health-care service providers as a major concern, and caregivers of gay and lesbian seniors in Canada also point to concerns about anticipated discrimination and the complex process of coming out in health-care situations [45, 46].

In spite of these concerning findings, there is also some evidence that older LGBT individuals have many strengths and resilience factors and that many are aging successfully. Physical and mental health quality of life using the Short Form 8-item were investigated among older LGBT respondents in the US population-representative *Caring and Aging with Pride* study, and many older LGBT adults had high physical and mental health quality of life [47]. In a subsequent editorial, the lead investigator of *Caring and Aging with Pride* noted that despite disparities, most LGBT elders are aging well [48].

Understanding basic terminology may be a good start for geriatric mental health providers who want to reduce disparities and promote successful aging by becoming more culturally competent in caring for older LGBT patients. *Sex* is assigned at birth and refers to one's biological status as male or female and is associated primarily with physical attributes such as chromosomes, hormones, and anatomy. *Gender* refers to socially constructed roles, behaviors, and attributes that a given society sees as appropriate for men versus women [49]. *Gender identity* refers to one's personal sense of being male, female, or something else; *cisgender* is used to describe an individual whose sex and gender identity are the same, whereas *transgender* describes an individual whose gender identity conflicts with biological sex [49].

In contrast, *sexual orientation* refers to the nature of emotional and sexual attraction for others; one is said to be *homosexual* if one is primarily attracted to members of the same sex, whereas one is said to be *heterosexual* if one is primarily attracted to members of the opposite sex; individuals who have attractions to members of both sexes are *bisexual* [50]. Both cisgender and transgender individuals may be homosexual, heterosexual, or bisexual [40].

Conclusions

"Culture" refers broadly to an array of characteristics which define various social groups. In order to provide high-quality mental health care, a geriatric mental health-care provider should be sensitive to the many ways in which an older patient's culture may differ from their own. Research points to certain geriatric mental health and health-care disparities which exist among certain racial/ethnic groups, between older men and older women and in sexual minority populations. Older African Americans and Asian Americans may have lower rates of depression and anxiety than older Latinos and non-Latino Whites, but racial/ethnic minority groups tend to have poorer access to and utilization of geriatric mental health-care services compared to non-Latino Whites. Rates of depression may be higher in older women than in older men, although epidemiologic evidence is mixed, but older men tend to receive less correct identification of depression and less appropriate treatment for depression when compared to older women. LGBT elders have higher rates of depression, anxiety, alcohol and substance misuse, and suicidal ideation than their heterosexual counterparts, with older transgender individuals having the highest rates of all. Cultural competence in geriatric mental health-care providers has been cited repeatedly in studies as something that older adult minorities want and expect from those taking care of them.

Acknowledgments. Dr. Yarns was supported by the VA Office of Academic Affiliations through the VA National Clinician Scholars Program.

Disclaimer These contents do not represent the views of the US Department of Veterans Affairs or the United States Government.

References

1. Crowther MR, David S, DiGilio D, Elmore D, Molinari V, Qualls SH, Tazeau YN. Multicultural competency in Geropsychology. Washington, DC: American Psychological Association; 2009.
2. Keynan Hobbs M. Reflections on the culture of veterans. Workplace Health & Safety. 2008;56(8):337.
3. Hollander BS, Bukowitz WR. Women, family culture, and family business. Fam Bus Rev. 1990;3(2):139–51. https://doi.org/10.1111/j.1741-6248.1990.00139.x.
4. APA. Introduction *Diagnostic and Statistical Manual of Mental Disorders*. 5th ed. Arlington, VA: American Psychiatric Association; 2013. p. 5–17.
5. Sakauye K. Cultural psychiatry considerations in older adults. Am J Geriatr Psychiatry. 2012;20(11):911–4. https://doi.org/10.1097/JGP.0b013e3182702c18.
6. Angel JL, Hogan DP. The demography of minority aging populations. J Fam Hist. 1992;17(1):95–115.
7. Jimenez DE, Alegria M, Chen CN, Chan D, Laderman M. Prevalence of psychiatric illnesses in older ethnic minority adults. J Am Geriatr Soc. 2010;58(2):256–64. https://doi.org/10.1111/j.1532-5415.2009.02685.x.
8. Ford BC, Bullard KM, Taylor RJ, Toler AK, Neighbors HW, Jackson JS. Lifetime and 12-month prevalence of diagnostic and statistical manual of mental disorders, disorders among older African Americans: findings from the National Survey of American life. Am J Geriatr Psychiatry. 2007;15(8):652–9.
9. González HM, Tarraf W, Whitfield KE, Vega WA. The epidemiology of major depression and ethnicity in the United States. J Psychiatr Res. 2010;44(15):1043–51.
10. Williams DR, Gonzalez HM, Neighbors H, Nesse R, Abelson JM, Sweetman J, Jackson JS. Prevalence and distribution of major depressive disorder in African Americans, Caribbean blacks, and non-Hispanic whites: results from the National Survey of American life. Arch Gen Psychiatry. 2007;64(3):305–15. https://doi.org/10.1001/archpsyc.64.3.305.
11. Woodward AT, Taylor RJ, Bullard KM, Aranda MP, Lincoln KD, Chatters LM. Prevalence of lifetime DSM-IV affective disorders among older African Americans, black Caribbeans, Latinos, Asians and non-Hispanic white people. Int J Geriatr Psychiatry. 2012;27(8):816–27. https://doi.org/10.1002/gps.2790.
12. Steffens DC, Fisher GG, Langa KM, Potter GG, Plassman BL. Prevalence of depression among older Americans: the aging, demographics and memory study. Int Psychogeriatr. 2009;21(5):879–88. https://doi.org/10.1017/s1041610209990044.
13. Pickett YR, Bazelais KN, Greenberg RL, Bruce ML. Racial and ethnic variation in home healthcare nurse depression assessment of older minority patients. Int J Geriatr Psychiatry. 2014a;29(11):1140–4. https://doi.org/10.1002/gps.4001.
14. Sorkin DH, Pham E, Ngo-Metzger Q. Racial and ethnic differences in the mental health needs and access to care of older adults in california. J Am Geriatr Soc. 2009;57(12):2311–7. https://doi.org/10.1111/j.1532-5415.2009.02573.x.
15. Pickett YR, Greenberg RL, Bazelais KN, Bruce ML. Depression treatment disparities among older minority home healthcare patients. Am J Geriatr Psychiatry. 2014b;22(5):519–22. https://doi.org/10.1016/j.jagp.2013.01.078.

16. Jimenez DE, Bartels SJ, Cardenas V, Daliwal SS, Alegría M. Cultural beliefs and mental health treatment preferences of ethnically diverse older adult consumers in primary care. Am J Geriatr Psychiatry. 2012;20(6):533–42. https://doi.org/10.1097/JGP.0b013e318227f876.
17. Jimenez DE, Bartels SJ, Cardenas V, Alegria M. Stigmatizing attitudes toward mental illness among racial/ethnic older adults in primary care. Int J Geriatr Psychiatry. 2013;28(10):1061–8. https://doi.org/10.1002/gps.3928.
18. Lawrence V, Samsi K, Banerjee S, Morgan C, Murray J. Threat to valued elements of life: the experience of dementia across three ethnic groups. The Gerontologist. 2011;51(1):39–50. https://doi.org/10.1093/geront/gnq073.
19. Mahoney DF, Cloutterbuck J, Neary S, Zhan L. African American, Chinese, and Latino family caregivers' impressions of the onset and diagnosis of dementia: cross-cultural similarities and differences. The Gerontologist. 2005;45(6):783–92.
20. Hinton L, Zweifach M, Tang L, Unützer J, Oishi S. Gender disparities in the treatment of late-life depression: qualitative and quantitative findings from the IMPACT trial. Am J Geriatr Psychiatry. 2006;14(10):884–92.
21. Gum AM, King-Kallimanis B, Kohn R. Prevalence of mood, anxiety, and substance-abuse disorders for older Americans in the national comorbidity survey-replication. Am J Geriatr Psychiatry. 2009;17(9):769–81.
22. Callahan CM, Kesterson JG, Tierney WM. Association of symptoms of depression with diagnostic test charges among older adults. Ann Intern Med. 1997;126(6):426–32.
23. Crawford M, Prince M, Menezes P, Mann A. The recognition and treatment of depression in older people in primary care. Int J Geriatr Psychiatry. 1998;13(3):172–6.
24. Klap R, Unroe KT, Unützer J. Caring for mental illness in the United States: a focus on older adults. Am J Geriatr Psychiatry. 2003;11(5):517–24.
25. Kochanek KD, Murphy SL, Anderson RN, Scott C. Deaths: final data for 2002. Natl Vital Stat Rep. 2004;53(5):1–115.
26. Addis ME, Mahalik JR. Men, masculinity, and the contexts of help seeking. Am Psychol. 2003;58(1):5.
27. Cleary PD, Burns BJ, Nycz GR. The identification of psychiatric illness by primary care physicians. J Gen Intern Med. 1990;5(4):355–60.
28. Kockler M, Heun R. Gender differences of depressive symptoms in depressed and nondepressed elderly persons. Int J Geriatr Psychiatry. 2002;17(1):65–72.
29. Möller-Leimkühler AM. Barriers to help-seeking by men: a review of sociocultural and clinical literature with particular reference to depression. J Affect Disord. 2002;71:1), 1–9.
30. Jeon G-S, Jang S-N, Rhee S-J, Kawachi I, Cho S-I. Gender differences in correlates of mental health among elderly Koreans. J Gerontol Ser B Psychol Sci Soc Sci. 2007;62(5):S323–9.
31. Kiraly A, Szabo N, Toth E, Csete G, Farago P, Kocsis K, et al. Male brain ages faster: the age and gender dependence of subcortical volumes. Brain Imaging Behav. 2016;10(3):901–10. https://doi.org/10.1007/s11682-015-9468-3.
32. Nemeth VL, Must A, Horvath S, Kiraly A, Kincses ZT, Vecsei L. Gender-specific degeneration of dementia-related subcortical structures throughout the lifespan. J Alzheimers Dis. 2017;55(3):865–80. https://doi.org/10.3233/jad-160812.
33. Bachman D, Wolf PA, Linn R, Knoefel J, Cobb J, Belanger A, et al. Incidence of dementia and probable Alzheimer's disease in a general population the Framingham study. Neurology. 1993;43(3 Part 1):515–9.
34. Barnes L, Wilson R, Schneider J, Bienias J, Evans D, Bennett D. Gender, cognitive decline, and risk of AD in older persons. Neurology. 2003;60(11):1777–81.
35. Kukull WA, Higdon R, Bowen JD, McCormick WC, Teri L, Schellenberg GD, et al. Dementia and Alzheimer disease incidence: a prospective cohort study. Arch Neurol. 2002;59(11):1737–46.
36. Rocca WA, Cha RH, Waring SC, Kokmen E. Incidence of dementia and Alzheimer's disease a reanalysis of data from Rochester, Minnesota, 1975–1984. Am J Epidemiol. 1998;148(1):51–62.
37. Seshadri S, Wolf P, Beiser A, Au R, McNulty K, White R, D'agostino R. Lifetime risk of dementia and Alzheimer's disease the impact of mortality on risk estimates in the Framingham study. Neurology. 1997;49(6):1498–504.
38. Lee LK, Shahar S, Chin A-V, Mohd Yusoff NA, Rajab N, Aziz SA. Prevalence of gender disparities and predictors affecting the occurrence of mild cognitive impairment (MCI). Arch Gerontol Geriatr. 2012;54(1):185–91. https://doi.org/10.1016/j.archger.2011.03.015
39. CDC. The state of aging and health in America 2013. Atlanta, GA: Centers for Disease Control and Prevention, U.S. Dept of Health and Human Services; 2013.
40. Yarns BC, Abrams JM, Meeks TW, Sewell DD. The mental health of older LGBT adults. Curr Psychiatry Rep. 2016;18(6):60. https://doi.org/10.1007/s11920-016-0697-y.

41. Fredriksen-Goldsen KI, Kim H-J, Emlet CA, Muraco A, Erosheva EA, Hoy-Ellis CP, et al. The aging and health report. Seattle, WA: Institute for Multigenerational Health; 2011.
42. Graham R, Berkowitz B, Blum R, Bockting W, Bradford J, de Vries B, et al. The health of lesbian, gay, bisexual, and transgender people: building a foundation for better understanding. Washington, DC: Institute of Medicine; 2011.
43. Guasp A. Lesbian, gay & bisexual people in later life. London: Stonewall; 2011.
44. Buchmueller T, Carpenter CS. Disparities in health insurance coverage, access, and outcomes for individuals in same-sex versus different-sex relationships, 2000-2007. Am J Public Health. 2010;100(3):489–95.
45. Brotman S, Ryan B, Collins S, Chamberland L, Cormier R, Julien D, et al. Coming out to care: caregivers of gay and lesbian seniors in Canada. Gerontologist. 2007;47(4):490–503.
46. Price E. Coming out to care: gay and lesbian carers' experiences of dementia services. Health Soc Care Community. 2010;18(2):160–8.
47. Fredriksen-Goldsen KI, Kim HJ, Shiu C, Goldsen J, Emlet CA. Successful aging among LGBT older adults: physical and mental health-related quality of life by age group. Gerontologist. 2015;55(1):154–68. https://doi.org/10.1093/geront/gnu081.
48. Fredriksen-Goldsen KI. Despite disparities, most LGBT elders are aging well. Aging Today. 2014;35(3)
49. Munoz V, Nadal K, Hendricks ML, Davidson J, Perry JR, Singh A. Answers to your questions about transgender people, gender identity, and gender expression (Vol. 2016). Washington, DC: The American Psychological Association; 2011.
50. APA. Answers to your questions: for a better understanding of sexual orientation and homosexuality. Washington, DC: The American Psychological Association; 2008.

4 Family and Community

Jessica Koenig, Aurora Osteen, and Erica C. Garcia-Pittman

Introduction

Advances in medicine and societal trends contributing to an increasing lifespan and declining fertility rate are two significant factors that contribute to the growing population of aging individuals [1]. The aging population is predicted to continue to grow and potentially accelerate, with people ages 65 and older predicted to soon outnumber children under 5 years old for the first time in known history [2]. Other trends in aging include females having an average longer lifespan than males but being in poorer health [1]. While it is now known that individuals can sustain health and independence into old age, it is also known that the prevalence of dementia, particularly Alzheimer's dementia, increases with age [1]. The risk of developing Alzheimer's dementia doubles every 5 years after age 65 [1]. There are differing thoughts on whether the prevalence of disability will increase or decrease with the expanding aging population. One idea refers to a "compression of morbidity" or that the occurrence of physical or mental disability will decrease as the average lifespan increases [1]. This is contrasted with the idea that, as lifespan increases and medical advancements manage chronic diseases, the prevalence of disability will increase as the degree of disability decreases [1]. Alzheimer's dementia is particularly associated with a range of disabilities [1]. Greater disability is likely to be associated with a greater need for caregiving, which traditionally has included family members and, more recently, social entitlement programs such as Social Security and Medicare [3].

Family and Community Supports

Caregiving for the aging population may include community support, assisted living, residential living, medical care through nursing, and prolonged hospital stays [1]. Caregiving also provides support for physical or cognitive impairment that ranges from moderate difficulties to more significant loss of functioning and independence [1]. It is estimated that 52 million adults in the United States, or one in three adults, voluntarily provide care to disabled family or friends without receiving compensation [4]. Recent changes and trends in social structure play a role in anticipated changes in both the aging and caregiving populations. People are now moving to cities and presumably benefitting from more available resources than what metropolitan areas can provide [1]. Rapidly developing technology and the globalization of the economy are impacting people of all ages and generations [1]. There is evidence that suggests that remaining individuals who are active in the workplace maintain their cognitive functioning [1]. However, as a result of an increased life expectancy, a greater proportion of one's life is likely

R. R. Tampi et al. (eds.), *Psychiatric Disorders Late in Life*, https://doi.org/10.1007/978-3-319-73078-3_4

to be spent in retirement, resulting in a greater burden on some social entitlement programs [2]. Females who are not married are less likely than unmarried males to have assets or pensions, while males have less propensity to maintain social networks [2].

In addition to changes in the demographics of the population, changes in the family structure, a significant provider of care for the aging population, are occurring as well [1]. With people living longer and having fewer children, there are more likely to be a greater number of generations made up of fewer members [1] and therefore fewer family members able to care for the aging population. Negative aspects of this trend impact both caregiving families and older individuals, who mutually benefit from sharing resources and supports [1]. Despite these changes, family and friends not only provide approximately 75% of care given to Americans with Alzheimer's dementia, who remain at home, but they also are the main purchasers of the remainder of services needed [3]. The most common caregiver for adults with dementia is usually a single individual who is most likely to be a spouse [3]. The next most common caregivers are typically adult children, with daughters and daughters-in-law more likely to spend time caregiving [3].

The trends discussed in the earlier paragraph have been found to be happening at a faster pace than in the past [1]. In the concept of successful aging, the goal is to keep the aging individual in the community as long as possible. Rowe and Kahn [5] describe successful aging as maintaining a low probability of disease and associated disability with a high cognitive and physical functional capacity and an active engagement with life. Maintaining a low probability of disease requires maintaining few disease risk factors and diseases [5]. Active engagement in life describes the maintenance of relationships with others through a mutual transferring of information, emotional support, and assistance [5]. It also includes maintaining activities that have value to society [5]. Active engagement is important as isolation is found to be a risk factor for negative health consequences, and the emotional and instrumental support of others can have positive effects on health [5].

One Canadian study found successful aging is associated with marriage, a university-level education, income, regular alcohol use, never smoking, exercising regularly, taking calcium supplements, perceiving themselves as having better health, and satisfaction with life [6]. This study further found that achieving successful aging decreases with age [6]. Predictors specific for maintaining cognitive ability included education, strenuous activity around the home, peak pulmonary flow rate, and one's own perceived self-efficacy [7]. Individuals living with either a significant other or children are associated with having the highest levels of functioning, while single adults living with non-relatives have the lowest [8]. Not surprisingly, remaining active in the community and in relationships as well as maintaining activities of daily living (ADLs) and instrumental activities of daily living (iADLs) can contribute to longer periods of functioning and decrease the likelihood of entering a nursing home to receive care [8]. Common comorbidities in dementia that impact successful aging include depression, which affects between 20% and 24% of the individuals [9, 10] with dementia. The Health and Retirement Study also found an association between an individual's connections with family and their economic status, depression status, and health advantages [8]. Families and other resources help keep the aging population in the community.

By providing physical and emotional support, caregivers support successful aging and independence. Caregivers are often a strong source of collateral information and provide insights regarding behavioral and functional changes that they have observed at home. Additionally, they typically bear the responsibility to implement treatment interventions that family members with disabilities are requiring. This involvement is crucial for the appropriate diagnosis and treatment of patients with disabilities, including dementia. Anecdotal reports point to dementia care as the most stressful type of family caregiving, and the demands of the caregiver can lead to negative impacts on the entire family [11]. National organizations (American Association for Retired Persons (AARP) and the National Association for Caregiving) support this report with findings that indicate dementia caregivers provide more assistance and have more associated stress including work-related difficulties and having to give up more vacation, hobbies, and family time [12]. However, it is known that caregiving can be akin to a severe, long-term chronic stressor with effects dependent on degree of physical and cognitive impairment, frequency of problem behaviors, and length and intensity of caregiving provided [13].

Caregiver Stress

Effects of caregiving on individuals can be measured and examined by the amount of psychological distress, psychiatric and physical morbidity, and impact of reduced work hours or leaving the workforce on the economy [14, 15]. These effects are also moderated by the caregiver's gender, personality, coping skills, relationship to the care recipient, economic status, and the availability of supportive resources [13, 16, 17]. Caregivers of patients with dementia are at risk for developing depression, anxiety, and dementia, especially the female caregivers [13, 17–20]. Caregivers are also more likely to have an increased risk of illness [21, 22] and mortality [23] and to take fewer preventative health measures [19]. They may have a less robust immune response [18, 21, 24], greater cardiovascular reactivity [25], and slower wound healing [26]. Furthermore, the relationship between the caregiver and the recipient declines in the context of a caregiving relationship [3].

Addressing caregiver's modifiable factors can lower the risk of negative outcomes that are directly related to caregiving. Examples of these modifiable factors include providing an age-friendly environment, support networks within the community, and coping skills for caregivers. Ideal age-friendly environments would take into consideration health, communication, transportation, labor, housing, safety, and long-term care [27]. Providing sufficient coping strategies for caregivers will not only help reduce stress for the caregiver but could also improve the quality of life of the patient. Caregivers have to adjust to changes that they may not have anticipated including a care recipient's cognitive impairments, behavioral problems, increased need for physical assistance, and navigating a complicated healthcare system. Individual and community interventions that utilize a broad range of interventions have been shown to be more effective than targeting only caregiver knowledge about caregiving and social support resources. These interventions include addressing "individual or family counseling, care management, skills training, environmental modification and behavioral management strategies" [3]. Providing diverse services and addressing multiple stressors have been shown to improve support for caregivers and occasionally patient symptom severity in individuals with dementia. These strategies could be applicable to the challenges all caregivers face when dealing with aging family members. When these services are not available, case studies have found that single interventions have greater impact if they are implemented with higher frequency and for longer duration [3].

One dementia caregiver intervention trial termed the Resources for Advancing Alzheimer's Caregiver Health tested several different social and behavioral interventions. The results across different sites and different interventions consistently showed that interventions that targeted behavior skills training "had the greatest impact in reducing caregiver depression" [28].

Caregivers have daily contact with clients and are often the best sources of information regarding effectiveness of interventions. They are also the ones most likely to be implementing treatments and behavioral interventions, so supporting them is vital to the success of the patient's care. The best outcomes are likely to arise from the involvement of caregivers and patients rather than treating either one alone. Since clinicians have direct contact with family and patient, they are essential in helping coordinate non-pharmacological treatment plans. For instance, they can assist in recruiting other family members to help with caregiving to help alleviate the burden on a single family member. Clinicians can assess the needs of the family and patient to be able to provide the most appropriate individualized care. Referrals for case management or instructions on how to access local resources would be very impactful for families that are not aware of resources in the community.

Guidelines published by the American Medical Association (AMA) and American Psychiatric Association (APA) attempt to address these concerns and advocates for stronger caregiver support and partnerships. The AMA has produced a Caregiver Self-Assessment Tool to help providers identify the most vulnerable caregivers and begin to implement support networks [29].

Age-Friendly Environments

Ideal age-friendly environments would take into consideration health, communication, transportation, labor, housing, safety, and long-term care [27]. Having such support promotes greater adaptation to negative incidents [30]. The AARP and WHO have gathered multiple community initiatives that contribute to environments that foster healthy aging and provide adequate accommodations. These ideals focus on prohibiting barriers to accessible community resources to support independence and successful aging. These may include wheelchair-accessible pavements and toilets, lower curb height, and safe and accessible public seating and transportation, all well-marked and well-lit with visual and audio cues [27].

Benefits of maintaining environments where elderly people are mobile and have access are numerous. Financially, institutional care is significantly more expensive than care in the community. By allowing older adults to be geographically mobile, it increases their ability to remain engaged with their own community. As people age, they begin to have physical and sensory limitations that may prohibit them from driving. Implementing resources that make it easier to move around will reduce isolation and increase community involvement. Without certain community accommodations, older adults would struggle to be adequately mobile and independent. Ultimately this may result in older adults having to leave their communities to gain these important support systems elsewhere, such as through assisted care facilities.

Placement into nursing homes has been associated with reduced quality of life and increased risk of mortality for older individuals. It can also increase distress felt by family members that provide care for these older adults [31]. Allowing elderly to stay within the communities allows them to interact as neighbors and volunteers, thus enabling them to make positive contributions to the community around them. Appropriate housing that is safe and affordable is also vital to building age-friendly cities. By allowing people to age safely and be comfortable in their community, it enables them to stay independent at their home for longer time period.

Disaster Management

Older adults can be at higher risk for poor outcomes during disasters because of vulnerabilities that come with aging. Circumstances that can occur during a disaster can worsen chronic conditions and increase long-term morbidity. With age comes a higher likelihood of physical impairments and mobility restrictions. More than half of adults have a functional limitation that contributes to this increased vulnerability [32]. Loss of medications during a disaster period can increase the likelihood of conditions relapsing and resulting in bad outcomes. Lack of clean food and water and exposure to extreme temperatures and to infection affect all age groups, but their effects to the vulnerable elderly can be devastating. Chronic medical conditions and mental functioning can result in reduced information processing capabilities and sensory awareness. Social support systems are often restricted in this age group by limited family networks and geographic isolation from direct family contact. Elderly individuals are often retired or unemployed and have a fixed financial income that limits their ability to afford last minute travel, housing expenses, or medical treatment that would assist them in disaster situations.

In addition to recommendations that can help assist all age groups in disasters, there are some specific things that can be done for the elderly population that can minimize adverse events. These recommendations include [32]:

- Having stock supplies of ready to eat food, water, and batteries for emergency
- Having an evacuation plan for people and for pets
- Having a personalized emergency plan

- Having a personalized list of medications, doctors, and pharmacies
- Having a photocopy of prescriptions to make it easier to get refills in another location
- Having a preidentified meeting place for families
- Having the identity of shelters and special needs shelters to use if needed

The above recommendations are ways to help prepare this population during a disaster to lessen the negative impact these unexpected situations can cause.

Conclusion

Aging and caregiving can be very isolating, and without proper support, it can negatively impact the quality of life of both the older individual and their caregivers. Incorporating community and family involvement has been shown to have positive impacts on the health and quality of life of both the elderly as well as their caregivers. Taking care of the elderly should include exposing patients and their families to local and national organizations that can help provide the best care for the elderly population.

References

1. World Health Organization. Global health and aging. 2011. https://d2cauhfh6h4x0p.cloudfront.net/s3fs-public/global_health_and_aging.pdf. NIH publication no. 11-7737. Accessed 24 May 2016.
2. U.S. Department of Health and Human Services. Why population aging matters: A global perspective. 2007. https://www.nia.nih.gov/research/publication/why-population-aging-matters-global-perspective. NIH publication no. 07-6134. Accessed 27 May 2016.
3. Schulz R, Matire LM. Family caregiving of persons with dementia. Am J Geriatr Psychiatry. 2004;12:240–9.
4. Department of Health and Human Services. Informal caregiving: compassion in action. 1998. https://aspe.hhs.gov/sites/default/files/pdf/73286/carebro2.pdf. Accessed 27 May 2016.
5. Rowe JW, Kahn RL. Successful aging. The Gerontologist. 1997;37(4):433–40.
6. Meng X, D'Arcy C. Successful aging in Canada: prevalence and predictors from a population-based sample of older adults. Gerontology. 2014;60:65–72.
7. Albert MS, Savage CR, Jones K, et al. Predictors of cognitive change in older persons: MacArthur studies of successful aging. Psychol Aging. 1995;70:578–89.
8. The Health and Retirement Study Online. Aging in the 21st century: challenges and opportunities for Americans. 2007. http://hrsonline.isr.umich.edu/sitedocs/databook/?_ga=2.43096101.1453392178.1497231370-720073253.1497231370. Accessed 11 Jun 2017.
9. Lyketsos CG, Steinberg M, Tschanz TT, et al. Mental and behavioral disturbances in dementia: findings from the Cache County study on memory in aging. Am J Psychiatry. 2000;157:708–14.
10. Meyers BS. Depression and dementia: comorbidities, identification and treatment. J Geriatr Psychiatry Neurol. 1998;11:201–5.
11. Tierney MC, Herrmann N, Geslani DM, et al. Contribution of informant and patient ratings to the accuracy of the mini-mental state exam in predicting probable Alzheimer's disease. J Am Geriatr Soc. 2003;51:813–8.
12. Ory MG, Hoffman RR, Yee JL, et al. Prevalence and impact of caregiving: a detailed comparison between dementia and non-dementia caregivers. Gerontologist. 1999;39:177–85.
13. Schulz R, O'Brien AT, Bookwala J, et al. Psychiatric and physical morbidity effects of Alzheimer's disease caregiving: prevalence, correlates, and causes. Gerontologist. 1995;35:771–91.
14. Biegel D, Sales E, Schulz R. Family caregiving in chronic illness: Alzheimer's disease, cancer, heart disease, mental illness, and stroke. Newbury Park, CA: Sage Publications; 1991.
15. Schulz R, editor. Handbook on dementia caregiving: evidence-based interventions for family caregivers. New York, NY: Springer; 2000.
16. Haley WE, Roth DL, Coleton MI, et al. Appraisal, coping, and social support as mediators of well-being in black and white family caregivers of patients with Alzheimer's disease. J Consult Clin Psychol. 1996;64:121–9.
17. Yee J, Schulz R. Gender differences in psychiatric morbidity among family caregivers: a review and analysis. Gerontologist. 2000;40:147–64.
18. Kiecolt-Glaser JK, Dura JR, Speicher CE, et al. Spousal caregivers of dementia victims: longitudinal changes in immunity and health. Psychosom Med. 1991;53:345–62.
19. Schulz R, Newsom J, Mittelmark M, et al. Health effects of caregiving: the caregiver health effects

study: an ancillary study of the cardiovascular health study. Ann Behav Med. 1997;19:110–6.
20. Miller B, Cafasso L. Gender differences in caregiving: fact or artifact? Gerontologist. 1992;32:498–507.
21. Kiecolt-Glaser J, Glaser R, Gravenstein S, et al. Chronic stress alters the immune response to influenza virus vaccine in older adults. Proc Natl Acad Sci. 1996;93:3043–7.
22. Shaw WS, Patterson TL, Semples SJ, et al. Longitudinal analysis of multiple indicators of health declines among spousal caregivers. Ann Behav Med. 1997;19:101–9.
23. Schulz R, Beach S. Caregiving as a risk factor for mortality: the caregiver health effects study. J Am Med Assoc. 1999;282:2215–9.
24. Glaser R, Kiecolt-Glaser JK. Chronic stress modulates the virus- specific immune response to latent herpes simplex virus type 1. Ann Behav Med. 1997;19:78–82.
25. King AC, Oka RK, Young DR. Ambulatory blood pressure and heart rate responses to the stress of work and caregiving in older women. J Gerontol A Biol Sci Med Sci. 1994;49:239–45.
26. Kiecolt-Glaser JK, Marucha PT, Malarkey WB, et al. Slowing of wound healing by psychological stress. Lancet. 1995;346:194–6.
27. World Health Organization. Checklist of essential features of age-friendly cities. World Health Organization Web site. 2007. http://www.who.int/ageing/publications/Age_friendly_cities_checklist.pdf. Accessed 24 May 2016.
28. Schulz R, Burgio L, Burns R, et al. Resources for enhancing Alzheimer's caregiver health (REACH): overview, site-specific outcomes, and future directions. Gerontologist. 2003;43(4):514–20.
29. American medical association Web site. Caregiver self-assessment questionnaire. 2015. http://www.healthinaging.org/files/documents/caregiver.self_assessment.pdf. Accessed 11 Jun 2017.
30. National Research Council. Preparing for an aging world: the case for cross-National Research. Washington, DC: National Academies Press; 2001.
31. Lehning, A, Harmon, A. Livable community indicators for sustainable aging in place. Stanford Center on Longevity and MetLife Mature Market Web site. 2013. http://longevity3.stanford.edu/wp-content/uploads/2013/03/mmi-livable-communities-study. Accessed 11 Jun 2017.
32. Aldrich, N., Benson, W. F. Disaster planning tips for older adults and their families. Centers for Disease Control and Prevention (CDC) Healthy Aging Program. 2013. www.cdc.gov/aging/pdf/disaster_planning_tips.pdf. Accessed 11 Jun 2017.

5
Economics and Health Policy

Rajesh R. Tampi, Deena J. Tampi, Ashmita Banerjee, and Ravi Chivukula

Introduction

Available data indicates that the population of individuals 65 years and older in the United States will grow from 46.2 million or 14.5% of the total population to roughly 21.7% of the US population by 2040 [1]. As the population ages, the total healthcare costs escalate, and this results in a greater burden on an already strained healthcare system [2]. To minimize the healthcare costs, the use of available resources should be closely monitored. In this chapter we review important aspects of Medicare and Medicaid and also recent policies and legislation that clinicians caring for older adults with psychiatric disorders should be aware of so as to improve the care of their patients.

Medicare and Medicaid

Medicare and Medicaid are the two major payers for healthcare among older adults [3]. These two major healthcare programs were signed into law on July 30, 1965. The Medicare Modernization Act (MMA) that was signed into law by President George W. Bush on December 8, 2003 added an outpatient prescription drug benefit to Medicare.

In 2010, President Obama signed the Affordable Care Act which created a national Medicaid minimum eligibility level of 133% of the federal poverty level (FPL) for nearly all Americans who were ≤65 years in age [4]. In 2016 President Obama signed into law the Twenty-First Century Cures Act that expedites the discovery, development, and delivery of new treatments and cures so as to maintain America's global status as the leader in biomedical innovations [5].

Medicare

Medicare provides health insurance programs for the following individuals [6]:

1. Individuals ≥65 years
2. Individuals ≤65 years with certain types of disabilities
3. Individuals of all ages with disabilities
4. Individuals of all ages with end-stage renal disease

Medicare programs are divided into three parts:

Medicare Part A: It is the hospital insurance program that covers inpatient care in hospitals. It includes care in critical access hospitals and skilled nursing facilities. Part A also covers hospice care and some home healthcare, but it does not cover custodial or long-term care. It is paid for by individuals from their payroll taxes while working, and hence no premiums have to be paid.

Medicare Part B: This plan covers physician services, outpatient care, physical and occupational therapy services, and some home health-

R. R. Tampi et al. (eds.), *Psychiatric Disorders Late in Life*, https://doi.org/10.1007/978-3-319-73078-3_5

care when deemed medically necessary. It also pays for medical supplies when necessary. The funds for Part B are levied as monthly premiums from individuals.

Medicare Part C (Advantage Plan): This is an insurance plan where individuals pay a monthly premium to buy drug plans from private companies. Beneficiaries may have to pay a penalty if they decide not to enroll in a drug plan when they are first eligible but choose to join later.

Medicare Part D Coverage Gap Discount Program: Manufacturer discounts on covered Part D drugs are made available to eligible beneficiaries while in the coverage gap with this program.

The Centers for Medicare & Medicaid Services which is a branch of the Department of Health and Human Services runs the Medicare Program. Medicare is funded by two trust funds, the Hospital Insurance (HI) Trust Fund and Supplementary Medical Insurance (SMI) Trust Fund. Medicare spending as of 2014 was $618.7 billion [7].

Medicaid

Health coverage to nearly 69 million Americans is provided by Medicaid [8]. It is the single largest source of health coverage in the United States. Medicaid provides healthcare coverage for children, pregnant women, parents, and seniors and to individuals with disabilities. It is funded jointly by the federal and the state governments. Medicaid programs are established and administered by each state. The states using broad federal guidelines determine the type, amount, duration, and scope of the Medicaid services. The federal government however requires the state governments to cover certain mandatory benefits. Mandatory benefits include services like inpatient and outpatient hospital services, physician services, laboratory and x-ray services, and home health services. The states can then choose to provide additional/optional benefits. These additional/optional benefits include services like prescription drugs, case management, physical therapy, occupational therapy, and the payment for prescription drugs. The federal government provides the states with matching funds to provide these benefits to individuals. It is required under federal law that states need to cover certain population groups called the "mandatory eligibility groups" in order to participate in Medicaid. Low-income families, qualified pregnant women and children, and individuals receiving the Supplemental Security Income (SSI) are examples of mandatory eligibility groups. The law also gives the states the flexibility to cover other population groups also called "optional eligibility groups." Examples of optional eligibility groups include individuals receiving home- and community-based services and children in foster care who are not otherwise eligible. The states are allowed to set individual eligibility criteria within federal minimum standards.

The Affordable Care Act helped states expand Medicaid to cover nearly all low-income Americans under age 65 [8]. The Act extended the eligibility for children to at least 133% of the federal poverty level (FPL) in every state. In addition, the states were given the option to extend eligibility to adults with income at or below 133% of the FPL. The states are paid a specified percentage of program expenditures called the Federal Medical Assistance Percentage (FMAP) by the federal government. The states calculate the income for many eligibility groups using a percentage of FPL, e.g., 100% of FPL in 2017 for a family of four in the 48 contiguous states is $22,350 [9]. Income standards are based on income or other nonfinancial criteria standards such as the Supplemental Security Income (SSI) program for the other groups [10]. The federal law gives the states the option to charge premiums and to establish out-of-pocket spending (cost sharing) requirements for Medicaid enrollees [8]. The out-of-pocket costs may include copayments, coinsurance, deductibles, etc. Although the maximum out-of-pocket costs are limited, the states can choose to impose higher charges for certain higher income groups. Certain vulnerable groups such as children and pregnant women are exempt from most out-of-pocket costs.

In order to be eligible for Medicaid, individuals need to satisfy federal and state requirements regarding residency, immigration status, and documentation of US citizenship [8]. The Medicaid beneficiaries must generally be residing in the state in which they are receiving Medicaid. They must be citizens of the United States or be certainly qualified noncitizens, such as lawful permanent residents. Medicaid coverage is effective either on the date of application or the first day of the month of application. There may be retroactive coverage for up to 3 months prior to the month of application, if the individual would have been eligible during that period had they applied for coverage. Coverage is terminated at the end of the month at which an individual no longer meets the eligibility requirements.

The law allows states to have the option to establish a "medically needy program" for individuals who have significant health needs but whose income is too high to otherwise qualify for Medicaid [8]. These individuals can become eligible by "spending down" the amount of income that is above a particular state's medically needy income standard. They spend down by incurring expenses for medical and remedial care for which they do not have health insurance. Once these individual's incurred expenses have exceed the difference between the individual's income and the state's medically needy income level, i.e., the "spend down" amount, then they can become eligible for Medicaid programs. The Medicaid program then pays the cost of services that are in excess of what the individual had to incur in the way of expenses in order to become eligible.

Medicaid is the single largest payer for mental health services in the United States [8]. Its role is being expanded to play an increasingly larger role in the reimbursement of substance use disorder services.

The Mental Health Parity and Addiction Equity Act (MHPAEA) enables Americans with mental health and substance use disorders to get the care that they need [8]. This Act prohibits certain discriminatory practices that limit insurance coverage for behavioral health treatment and services. The MHPAEA requires coverage for mental health and substance use disorders to be no more restrictive than the coverage that available for medical and surgical conditions. This requirement applies to copays, coinsurance, and out-of-pocket maximums; limitations on services utilization such as limits on the number of inpatient days or outpatient visits that are covered; and the use of care management tools and criteria for medical necessity determinations. The federal statutes require Medicaid programs to comply with mental health and substance use disorder parity requirements.

More than 4.6 million low-income seniors most of whom are also enrolled in Medicare get healthcare coverage through Medicaid [8]. In addition, Medicaid provides coverage to 3.7 million people with disabilities who are also enrolled in Medicare. A total of 8.3 million individuals are "dually eligible" and enrolled in both Medicaid and Medicare. These individuals comprise more than 17% of all the Medicaid enrollees. Under federal statute those individuals who are enrolled in both Medicaid and Medicare can be covered under both optional and mandatory categories. Those Medicare enrollees who have limited income and access to resources can use Medicaid to pay for their premiums and out-of-pocket medical expenses. In addition, Medicaid also covers additional services that are not usually covered under Medicare. These services include skilled nursing facility care beyond the 100-day limit or custodial care in skilled nursing facilities, prescription drugs, eyeglasses, and hearing aids. Those services that are dually covered are usually first paid by Medicare with Medicaid filling in the difference up to the state's payment limit.

Affordable Care Act

The Affordable Care Act (ACA), comprising the Patient Protection and Affordable Care Act (P.L. 111–148) and the Health Care and Education Reconciliation Act of 2010 (P.L. 111–152), expanded Medicaid coverage for the poorest Americans by creating an opportunity for states to provide Medicaid eligibility, effective January 1, 2014, for individuals under 65 years of age with incomes effectively up to 138% of the federal poverty level (FPL, $27,310 for family of three in 2014; federal statute up to 133% with mandatory income disregard up to 5% FPL) [11, 12]. However, in 2012 the Supreme Court ruled that expansion could not be enforced by withholding funds for a state's entire Medicaid program, and this made the program optional for the various states. According to the Kaiser Family Foundation, as of January 2017, 32 states including the District of Columbia implemented the ACA Medicaid expansion to the adults. In 2015, about 14 million Medicaid enrollees were adults in the expansion group representing 18% of total Medicaid enrollees [13].

The ACA instituted several key changes to Medicare, which broadly included significantly decreased cost sharing in the Part D coverage gap, increased coverage of preventative care and screenings (including an annual Medicare Wellness Visit), and provider payment and health delivery reform. The Medicare provisions of the ACA were estimated to result in a net reduction of $428 billion in Medicare spending between 2010 and 2019 [14]. The life of the Medicare Trust fund was extended to at least 2029—a 12-year extension due to reductions in waste, fraud and abuse, and Medicare costs [15].

The Affordable Care Act also made several provisions for increased coordination of care of those eligible for both Medicare and Medicaid [16]. These individuals are, by definition, among the sickest and poorest covered by either the Medicaid or Medicare programs. Medicare primarily pays for acute and hospital care and prescription drugs, while Medicaid generally helps to pay for Medicare premiums, cost sharing, and long-term care, as well as other nonmedical services. The law increased federal support for state efforts to expand home- and community-based services and support for long-term care.

Twenty-First Century Cures Act

The Twenty-First Century Cures Act constituted a landmark attempt at the overhaul of the mental healthcare system in the United States. Signed by President Obama into law in December 2016, this Act drew upon mental health, substance use, and criminal justice provisions from the Helping Families in Mental Health Crisis Act (H.R. 2646), the Mental Health Reform Act of 2016 (S. 2680), the Mental Health and Safe Communities Act (S. 2002), as well as the Comprehensive Justice and Mental Health Act (S. 993) [17]. It sought to organize a fragmented mental healthcare delivery system by creating visible leadership positions, namely, the Assistant Secretary for Mental Health and Substance Use (ASMH), who would work in collaboration with a newly appointed Chief Medical Officer (CMO) at the Substance Abuse and Mental Health Services Administration (SAMHSA). The ASMH, CMO, and Assistant Secretary for Planning and Evaluation (ASPE) would be tasked with incorporating evidence-based medicine into SAMHSA-administered programs; recruiting and retaining a mental health workforce, including psychiatrists; and collaborating with other federal agencies such as the Departments of Veterans Affairs, Labor, Housing and Urban Development, and Defense to improve care for veterans and address chronic homelessness. The Act provided funding and grants for multifaceted approaches to enhance education, training, and innovation in mental health and substance abuse disorders. Most notably, it provided $1 billion over 2 years for opioid prevention and treatment programs. The Act renewed focus on strengthening the enforcement of the Mental Health Parity and Addiction Equity Act of 2008.

The Act also put a spotlight on research and innovation elucidating the biological basis of major mental health and substance abuse disorders by providing $4.8 billion over 10 years to the National Institutes of Health [18]. This includes $1.5 billion for the Brain Research Through Advancing Innovative Neurotechnologies (BRAIN) Initiative that revolutionizes collaborative approaches to find cures for disorders of the brain, including schizophrenia, epilepsy, autism, and Alzheimer's, through the development and application of innovative technologies.

CHIP Reauthorization Act of 2015

The Medicare Access and CHIP Reauthorization Act of 2015 (MACRA) was signed into law on April 26, 2015 [19]. This Act addressed delivery system and Medicare payment reform. It prioritized value over volume of care for Medicare/CHIP enrollees by addressing provider payment reform in Medicare/CHIP reimbursements. Multiple quality and value programs for Medicare physicians and practitioners were combined into a Merit-Based Incentive Payment System (MIPS) and alternative payment models (APMs) to incentivize quality and value were strongly promoted.

Conclusion

In the United States, Medicare and Medicaid provide majority of the funding for the healthcare for older adults. These two systems cover a range of services including inpatient and outpatient care, medication prescriptions, home care, and also skilled nursing facility care. Recent legislations have been enacted by the federal government to improve the care of individuals with psychiatric disorders and the care of older adults.

References

1. Aging statistics. https://aoa.acl.gov/Aging_Statistics/index.aspx. Accessed 14 Jun 2017.
2. Walaszek A. Clinical ethics issues in geriatric psychiatry. Psychiatr Clin North Am. 2009;32(2):343–59.
3. http://www.cms.gov/About-CMS/Agency-Information/History/index.html?redirect=/history/. Accessed 14 Jun 2017.
4. http://www.medicaid.gov/Medicaid-CHIP-Program-Information/By-Topics/Eligibility/Eligibility.html. Accessed 14 Jun 2017.
5. https://energycommerce.house.gov/sites/republicans.energycommerce.house.gov/files/documents/114/analysis/20161128%20Cures%20Fact%20Sheet.pdf. Accessed 14 Jun 2017.
6. https://www.cms.gov/Medicare/Medicare.html. Accessed 18 Jun 2017.
7. https://www.cms.gov/research-statistics-data-and-systems/statistics-trends-and-reports/nationalhealthexpenddata/nhe-fact-sheet.htm. Accessed 18 Jun 2017
8. https://www.medicaid.gov/. Accessed 18 Jun2017.
9. https://aspe.hhs.gov/2011-hhs-poverty-guidelines. Accessed 23 Jun 2017.
10. https://www.ssa.gov/disabilityssi/ssi.html. Accessed 23 Jun 2017.
11. Medicaid and CHIP in the context of the APA. https://www.macpac.gov/subtopic/overview-of-the-affordable-care-act-and-medicaid. Accessed 25 Jun 2017.
12. https://www.medicaid.gov/affordable-care-act/index.html. Accessed 25 Jun 2017.
13. http://www.kff.org/interactive/interactive-maps-estimates-of-enrollment-in-aca-marketplaces-and-medicaid-expansion/. Accessed 25 Jun 2017.
14. http://www.kff.org/health-reform/issue-brief/summary-of-key-changes-to-medicare-in/. Accessed 26 Jun 2017.
15. https://www.medicare.gov/about-us/affordable-care-act/affordable-care-act.html. Accessed 26 Jun 2017.
16. Affordable care act provisions relating to the care of dually eligible medicare and medicaid beneficiaries. http://www.kff.org/health-reform/issue-brief/affordable-care-act-provisions-relating-to-the/. Accessed June 25, 2017.
17. Mental health reform provisions in H.R. 34, the 21st Century Cures Act. American Psychiatric Association. https://www.psychiatry.org/psychiatrists/advocacy/federal-affairs/comprehensive-mental-health-reform. Accessed 26 Jun 2017.
18. Hudson KA, Collins FS. The 21st century cures act—a view from the NIH. N Engl J Med. 2017;376(2):111–3.
19. MACRA. https://www.cms.gov/Medicare/Quality-Initiatives-Patient-Assessment-Instruments/Value-Based-Programs/MACRA-MIPS-and-APMs/MACRA-MIPS-and-APMs.html. Accessed 26 Jun 2017.

Part II
Biological Aspects of Aging

6 Neuroanatomy and Neuropathology

Katherine Rice Goettsche, Caitlin Snow, and Jimmy Avari

Aging is associated with stereotypical neuroanatomical and physiologic changes and constitutes a significant risk factor for neurodegenerative disorders, particularly Alzheimer's disease [1]. As with most biological processes, there is variability in the degree to which aging adult brains undergo characteristic age-related changes. Furthermore the burden of medical and neurologic comorbidity in the elderly, including neurocognitive disorders, ischemia, and inflammation, can lead to pathological findings that overlap with neuropathological changes of normal aging. Differentiating age-related changes from the early stages of neurocognitive disorders can be confounding [2, 3]. While neuroanatomical and neuropathological changes associated with age have long been studied and are well documented, the relationship between the cognitive and structural changes associated with increasing age and the underlying mechanisms of normal and pathologic aging remain incompletely understood [4].

Neuroanatomy

Some cognitive functions are relatively unaffected by age. Procedural, primary, and semantic memory are preserved in healthy aging [5]. Cognitive abilities that decline with normal aging include processing speed, executive function, episodic memory, spatial memory, and both short-term and delayed recall [6, 7]. Processing speed is generally impacted the most, and one way this manifests is that the ability to learn and remember is preserved but slow [3, 4, 7].

Functional neuroimaging studies reveal trajectories of age-related changes in neural activity that may underlie executive function impairment. With increasing age, abnormal patterns of activation are seen in the prefrontal cortex and hippocampus [4]. Specifically, activation in these areas is less coordinated and more delocalized, in contrast to activation patterns in young adults which are more integrated and discrete [1, 4]. The changes in activation patterns in nonpathologic aging are likely a downstream effect of alterations in mechanisms that affect systems level functioning [1]. The driving forces underlying functional cognitive decline of nonpathologic aging include altered signaling through disruption of myelin fibers, changes in synaptic physiology, and alterations in gene expression [1].

Structural changes associated with age are observable at the gross level. Although the size of the brain typically decreases with age, as many as 30–50% of aging brains will not demonstrate typical age-related anatomical or pathological changes, including atrophy [3]. The average weight of a male adult brain is 1400 g [3], which is approximately 10% higher than female brain weight [8]. Brain weight and volume are thought to peak by the third decade, and evidence of age-related gyral atrophy can be visible on CT scan as early as age 40 [2]. By

R. R. Tampi et al. (eds.), *Psychiatric Disorders Late in Life*, https://doi.org/10.1007/978-3-319-73078-3_6

the mid-1980s, brain weight declines by 11% of the weight in young adulthood [8]. There is a consensus that brain weight declines at a fairly constant rate through young and middle adulthood and that atrophy begins to accelerate at a nonlinear rate around age 70 [9]. Loss of brain weight is reflected on neuroimaging as both ventricular enlargement, which can be multifactorial in etiology though likely also reflects an independent process of healthy aging, and also as gyral atrophy [2]. Accelerated volume change in normal aging is seen in ventricular CSF; frontal gray matter; superior, middle, and medial frontal; and superior parietal regions; in contrast, areas demonstrating accelerated volume change in the setting of mild cognitive impairment include whole brain volume, ventricular cerebrospinal fluid, temporal gray matter, and orbitofrontal and temporal association cortices including hippocampus [10]. Differential patterns of accelerated volume loss may distinguish mild cognitive impairment from normal aging [10].

Structural brain changes have variable effect on changes in cognitive function; 25–100% of the differences in select cognitive function between young and old age may be accounted for by structural brain changes, and consistent with this is the observation that patterns of age-related changes in size are heterogeneous [6]. Alzheimer's disease is associated with significant atrophy in the medial temporal lobes and especially in the entorhinal cortex; however, in normally aging brains, these areas typically do not demonstrate as significant volume loss [4].

The adult human brain has approximately 20 billion neurons [3]. Age-related reduction in brain size is driven in only part by neuronal cell death [11] with an estimated loss of 10% of neurons from age 20 to age 90 [12]. More sophisticated techniques for quantifying neurons have shown that the number of neurons in the cortex and hippocampus actually does not significantly decline with age, and in fact neuronal loss in those areas may even be minimal [1, 4]. Historically, neuron cell loss was thought to occur widely throughout the cortex and hippocampus, with more focal areas of loss in subcortical structures, the brainstem and the cerebellum [2, 4]. Similarly, contrary to older findings [2, 13], dendritic branching in the hippocampus may remain constant or increase with age [4, 14]. While apoptosis accounts for some of the volume loss, the majority of age-related volume loss is likely through shrinkage of neurons, reductions in synaptic spines, and fewer numbers of synapses [6]. Synaptic density is reduced in the frontal lobes of aged brains [15], and this finding correlates with less activation in the prefrontal cortex in performing executive processing tasks [4].

Structural changes are downstream of age-related genetic and molecular changes. Calcium channel signaling, a process central to synaptic plasticity [4], is affected by age-related reduction in expression of proteins involved in calcium channel signaling [16].

Additional molecular mechanisms that may contribute to aging include mitochondrial dysfunction, oxidative stress, epigenetic changes, autophagy and protein turnover, and insulin and IGF-1 signaling [1].

There are additional quantifiable changes in brain size that occur in the course of normal aging. Cortical width can reduce by 0.5–1% per year [6]; however, this measurement is not consistently observed to be affected by aging [2]. There have been findings of age-related loss of myelin staining in association cortices in the forebrain and in corticocortical tracts in the centrum semiovale [2]. Total length of myelinated fibers studied through neurostereology has been found to be reduced with age [12], and reductions in length may be by as much as 50% [6]. Normal aging is associated with a greater loss of white matter than of gray matter [4, 13]. Loss of white matter density with age is observable on neuroimaging in the prefrontal cortex and anterior corpus callosum [14, 17] and correlates with declines in measures of executive function including processing speed and short-term recall [18] possibly by impairing signaling through the prefrontal cortex, hippocampus, and striatum [4]. The number of glial cells is not thought to change significantly with age [2, 12].

Table 6-1 summarizes common age-related neuroanatomical changes and corresponding functional changes that can be expected [19].

TABLE 6-1. Neuroanatomical locations: age-related changes and their effects [19]

Location	*Changes seen with age*	*Effects of age-related changes*
Thalamus	Reduction in size	Slower processing speed
Hypothalamus	Decreased hormone production (e.g., reduced estrogen from decreased gonadotropin-releasing factor) Disruption of circadian rhythm	Physical changes associated with changes in hormone level Disruption in sleep wake cycle
Cerebrum	Reduction in brain weight (gray and white matter) Increase CSF volume	Far reaching effects on learning, memory, language, communication, sensory processing, movement, planning, organizing, intelligence, personality
Cerebral cortex	Atrophy particularly in prefrontal cortex, motor and sensory association areas affected more and earlier than primary sensory; neuron number relatively preserved	Effects on executive function, vision and color recognition, visuospatial recognition, emotional responses, memory and speech
Cerebellum	Volume of vermis declines more than volume of medial hemisphere Lateral hemisphere volume unaffected by age	Coordination and timing of movements
Basal ganglia	Dopaminergic neuron drop out in nigrostriatal pathway (less marked in normal aging than seen in Parkinson's disease); high levels of deleted mitochondrial DNA and somatic mitochondrial DNA deletions associated with selective neuron loss in healthy aging and Parkinson's disease	Effects on voluntary movement and mood regulation
Olfactory bulb and olfactory cortex	Age-dependent cell death in olfactory cortex, reduced volume in sensory neuroepithelium (due to cumulative effects of viral infections), replacement of olfactory neuroepithelium with nonsensory columnar epithelium in olfactory clefts in nose, diminution of central neurotransmitters	Decline in sense of smell
Amygdala	(1) Decreased reactivity to negative information and maintained or increased reactivity to positive information. (2) Greater functional connectivity between right amygdala and ventral anterior cingulate cortex. (3) Decreased functional connectivity with posterior brain regions	(1) Experience less negative emotion, pay less attention to negative than positive emotional stimuli, less likely to remember negative than positive emotional content. (2) Possible correlate with increased emotional regulation. (3) Decreased perceptual processing
Cingulate gyrus	Age-related loss in gray matter	Sensory input regarding emotions and regulation of aggressive behavior
Fornix	Linear rate of degeneration starting in 20s–30s	Decline in recall
Hippocampus	Anterior hippocampal size relatively preserved in normal aging compared with Alzheimer's disease	Learning and memory
Pineal gland	Age-related decrease in central and peripheral levels of melatonin	Effects on immune response, biologic rhythms
Pituitary gland	Smaller and more fibrous more so in men than women	Reduction in hormone secretion with end organ effects

Neuropathology

Neuropathological changes that result from normal aging processes are seen in most but not all elderly individuals [3]. The relatively more common age-related pathological findings in cognitively intact elderly individuals include senile neuritic plaques and neurofibrillary tangles [3]. Neuritic plaques and neurofibrillary tangles are also evident in various stages and subtypes of neurocognitive disorders and are pathological hallmarks of Alzheimer's disease in particular

[20]. There are images implicating neurons as the initial nidus of plaque formation [21]. Senile plaques initially develop in the neutropil as small focal structures consisting of an immunoreactive beta-amyloid core in a non-fibrillar form. These so-called diffuse plaques are possible findings in normal aging and can also appear early in the course of Alzheimer's disease [3, 20]. Diffuse or pre-amyloid plaques mature into neuritic plaques consisting of accumulations of neurites containing fibrillar amyloid among other proteinaceous structures surrounding the beta-amyloid core [3, 20]. These mature neuritic plaques can distort the neutropil [2] and may even be a common to frequent incidental finding in healthy aging [3]. With increasing maturity, plaques become small and more compact; an effect of these "burned out" plaques is that axons are displaced by beta-amyloid. The presence of neuritic plaques does not necessarily predict decline in cognitive function [3]. There are some interesting correlations between plaque formation and age. The prevalence of senile plaques in the temporal neocortex has been found to correlate with age, although the density of senile plaques was not found to increase with age, meaning that senile plaques stabilize instead of steadily progressing with time. Increasing age was also associated with a higher proportion of neuritic to senile plaque ratio, suggesting that evolution of individual plaques may be a more meaningful metric than total number of senile plaques in normal aging [20].

Neuritic senile plaques that are distributed throughout the cortex and in Alzheimer's disease are similarly present in the cortex and also more focally in the hippocampus, amygdala, and other subcortical structures. Plaques are associated with dystrophic neuritis and reactive astrocytic and microglial responses [2]. In Alzheimer's disease, as in normal aging, plaque burden does not increase significantly with time [22]. Effecting toxicity in the neutropil [22] and structural axonal injury associated with abnormal sprouting [23] are proposed mechanisms of plaques in the pathophysiology of cognitive decline.

Neurofibrillary tangles (NFTs) are intracellular accumulations of hyperphosphorylated tau, a microtubule-associated protein. As NFTs grow in size, the neuron cell bodies become distorted, and the nucleus is displaced. NFTs remain visible after the neuronal cell death has occurred. NFTs are associated with expression of fetal antigens and abnormal proliferation of dendrites, synaptic spines, and axons [2]. NFTs can be seen in cognitively intact elderly individuals as with neuritic plaques; however, unlike neuritic plaque burden, NFT frequency and distribution do correlate with cognitive status [3]. Aged adults without cognitive impairment will have fewer NFTs than those who have Alzheimer's disease. There is a characteristic pattern of development and distribution of neurofibrillary tangles in Alzheimer's disease. NFTs initially develop in the hippocampus, entorhinal cortex, and adjacent limbic structures. As they increase in number, NFTs begin to appear in the adjacent temporal neocortex. NFTs continue to develop and cluster and become more widely distributed with time, emerging finally in the frontal and parietal lobes with more advanced disease [24]. Neurofibrillary tangles in the ventromedial temporal lobe are evident in the brains of older adults with amnestic mild cognitive impairment, suggesting that amnestic mild cognitive impairment may in fact represent early Alzheimer's disease [25]. The presence of neurofibrillary tangles in the medial temporal lobe, before Alzheimer's disease is diagnosed clinically, is consistent with the hypothesis that NFTs are a substrate for memory loss in normal aging, mild cognitive impairment, and Alzheimer's disease [24].

Additional pathophysiologic findings in the aging brain have variable significance with regard to normal aging. Granulovacuolar degeneration is a pathological finding marked by large double membrane-bound vacuoles containing a central granule that tend to develop in neurons in the CA [1] region of the hippocampus. Granulovacuolar degeneration is seen in less than 10% of hippocampal neurons in a normal aged brain and at higher frequency in brains with Alzheimer's disease [2, 26]. Granulovacuolar degeneration may be associated with other neurocognitive disorders; they may be associated with NFTs and neuritic plaques, but they may also be independent of these pathologic findings [2]. Accumulation of granulovacuolar bodies may be connected to incomplete autolysosome formation [26].

Hirano bodies are eosinophilic, spindle shaped, and cytoplasmic inclusion bodies that are rich in actin arranged in highly refractile paracrystalline arrays [2, 27]. Unlike other intraneuronal inclusion bodies including Negri bodies, Lewy bodies, and Pick bodies which are pathognomonic for specific disease states, the Hirano body is more newly identified, less specific finding that is more generally associated with aging than other named inclusion bodies [28]. Hirano bodies are associated with various neurocognitive disorders including Alzheimer's disease, Pick's disease, amyotrophic lateral sclerosis, and parkinsonism-dementia complex, as well as chronic alcoholism and normal aging [27]. Hirano bodies likely originate from age-related changes in the microfilamentous system [28].

Pigments in the brain demonstrate classic changes with age. Lipofuscin, the "wear and tear" pigment, accumulates in the lysosomes of postmitotic cells and consists of undegradable oxidized, cross-linked protein residues [2]. Lipofuscin accumulates linearly with age, and correlates inversely with longevity [29]. In addition to being an indicator of age, lipofuscin accumulation may contribute directly to cellular degeneration by acting as a magnet of sorts for newly produced lysosomal enzymes thus impeding regular recycling of cellular components [29]. Melanin is a pigment in the locus ceruleus and substantia nigra that increases until age 60 and then decreases as neurons in those regions are lost [29].

Conclusions

In summary, neuroanatomical age-related changes in the brain include reduced brain weight, gyral atrophy, greater loss of white matter than gray matter, ventricular dilation, and loss of myelin staining. Apoptosis accounts for only a small percentage of neuronal volume loss. Activation of signaling pathways become delocalized and disintegrated in normal aging. There are various hypotheses about genetic and molecular mechanisms that underlie and contribute to these changes.

Investigating the processes of normal and pathological aging invites the central query: what encourages healthy aging? Physical exercise and caloric restriction have beneficial effects on life span and minimizing age-related pathology [4], with caloric restriction without causing malnutrition found to be associated with increasing lifespan [1]. Studies have investigated techniques to prevent oxidative damage through dietary vitamin E, selegiline, and coenzyme Q; cyclooxygenase-2 inhibitors and omega-3 fatty acids have been studied to target inflammation [4]. Despite wide inquiry, the evidence base for interventions to promote healthy aging is mixed [1].

References

1. Bishop NA, Lu T, Yankner BA. Neural mechanisms of ageing and cognitive decline. Nature. 2010;464:529–35.
2. Kemper TL. Neuroanatomical and Neuropathological changes during aging and dementia. In: Albert ML, Knoefel JE, editors. Clinical neurology of aging. 2nd ed. New York, NY: Oxford University Press; 1994. p. 3–67.
3. Taylor WD, Moore SD, Chin SS. Neuroanatomy, neurophysiology, and neuropathology of aging. In: Blazer DG, Steffens DC, editors. The American Psychiatric Publishing textbook of geriatric psychiatry. 4th ed. Arlington, VA: American Psychiatric Publishing; 2009. p. 63–95.
4. Yankner BA, Lu T, Loerch P. The aging brain. Annu Rev Pathol Mech Dis. 2008;3:41–66.
5. Wilson RS, Beckett LA, Barnes LL, Schneider JA, Bach J, Evans DA, Bennett DA. Individual differences in rates of change in cognitive abilities of older persons. Psychol Aging. 2002;17(2):179–93.
6. Fjell AM, Walhoyd KB. Structural brain changes in aging: courses, causes and cognitive consequences. Rev Neurosci. 2010;21(3):187–221.
7. Petersen RC, Smith G, Kokmen E, Ivnik RJ, Tangalos EG. Memory function in normal aging. Neurology. 1992;42:396–401.
8. Dekabon AS. Changes in brain weights during the span of human life: relation of brain weights to body heights and body weights. Ann Neurol. 1978;4:345–35.
9. Scahill RI, Frost C, Jenkins R, Whitwell JL, Rossor MN, Fox NC. A longitudinal study of brain volume changes in normal aging using serial registered magnetic resonance imaging. Arch Neurol. 2003;60(7):989–94.
10. Driscol I, Davatizikos C, An Y, Wu X, Shen D, Kraut M, Resnick SM. Longitudinal pattern of regional brain volume change differentiates normal aging from MCI. Neurology. 2009;72(22):1906–13.

11. Sastry PS, Rao KSJ. Apoptosis and the nervous system. J Neurochem. 2000;74(1):1–20.
12. Pakkenberg B, Pelvid D, Marner L, Bungaard MJ, Gundersen HJ, Nyengaard JR, Regeur L. Aging and the human neocortex. Exp Gerontol. 2003;38(1–2):95–9.
13. Salat DH, Kaye JA, Janowsky JS. Prefrontal gray and white matter volumes in healthy aging and Alzheimer disease. Arch Neurol. 1999;56(3):338–44.
14. Burke SN, Barnes CA. Neural plasticity in the ageing brain. Nat Rev Neurosci. 2006;7:30–40.
15. Liu X, Erikson C, Brun A. Cortical synaptic changes and gliosis in normal aging, Alzheimer's disease and frontal lobe degeneration. Dementia. 1996;7(3):128–34.
16. Lu T, Pan Y, Kao SY, Li C, Kohane I, et al. Gene regulation and DNA damage in the ageing human brain. Nature. 2004;429:883–91.
17. Bartzokis G, Cummings JL, Sultzer D, Henderson VW, Nuechterlein KH, Mintz J. White matter structural integrity in healthy aging adults and patients with Alzheimer disease: a magnetic resonance imaging study. Arch Neurol. 2003;60(3):393–8.
18. Gunning-Dizon FM, Raz N. The cognitive correlates of white matter abnormalities in normal aging: a quantitative review. Neuropsychology. 2000;14:224–32.
19. Brisibe T, De Asis SJ. Neurobiological changes in aging. In: Tampi RR, Williamson D, editors. Fundamentals of geriatric psychiatry. New York, NY: Nova Science Publisher; 2013. p. 55–65.
20. Mackenzie IR. Senile plaques do not progressively accumulate with normal aging. Acta Neuropathol. 1994;87:520–5.
21. Pappolla MA, Omar RA, Sambamurti K, Anderson JP, Robakis NK. The genesis of the senile plaque. Further evidence in support of its neuronal origin. Am J Pathol. 1992;141(5):1151–9.
22. Serrano-Pozo A, Betensky RA, Frosch M, Hyman BT. Plaque-associated local toxicity increases over the clinical course of Alzheimer disease. Am J Pathol. 2016;186(2):375–84.
23. Woodhouse A, West AK, Chuckowree JA, Vickers JC, Dickson TC. Does beta-amyloid plaque formation cause structural injury to neuronal processes? Neurotox Res. 2005;7(1–2):5–15.
24. Guillozet AL, Weintraub S, Mash DC, Mesulam MM. Neurofibrillary tangles, amyloid, and memory in aging and mild cognitive impairment. Arch Neurol. 2003;60(5):729–36.
25. Markesbery WR, Schmitt FA, Kryscio RJ, Davis DG, Smith CD, Wekstein DR. Neuropathologic substrate of mild cognitive impairment. JAMA Neurol. 2006;63(1):38–46.
26. Funk KE, Mrak RE, Kuret J. Granulovacuolar degeneration (GVD) bodies of Alzheimer's disease (AD) resemble late-stage autophagic organelles. Neuropathol Appl Neurobiol. 2011;37(3): 295–306.
27. Griffin P, Furukawa R, Piggott C, Maselli A, Fechheimer M. Requirements for Hirano body formation. Eukaryot Cell. 2014;13(5):625–34.
28. Hirano A. Hirano bodies and related neuronal inclusions. Neuropathol Appl Neurobiol. 1994; 20:3–11.
29. Brunk UT, Terman A. Lipofuscin: mechanisms of age-related accumulation and influence on cell function. Free Radic Biol Med. 2002;33(5):611–9.

7 Biochemistry and Neuropharmacology

Jimmy Avari, Katherine Rice Goettsche, and Caitlin Snow

The aging brain undergoes a variety of biochemical changes consistent with normal aging that may be primarily rooted in heredity. Many of these changes are time related and may be etiologically relatively independent of stress, trauma, or disease. Senescence from Latin *senescere*, meaning "to grow old," from *senex* is a term that describes permanent proliferative arrest of cells that has implications in the process of aging. More than 50 years ago, cellular senescence was described as "the limited in vitro lifetime of human diploid cell strains." It was observed that human cells cultured in vitro ceased to proliferate after a limited number of proliferations; these cells remained metabolically active [1]. It is commonly believed that cellular senescence underlies the larger organismal senescence.

The theories of wear and tear, oxidative damage, DNA damage, and telomere shortening will be introduced. While multiple theories of aging have been proposed, there is no consensus on this issue. Instead, many of the proposed theories likely interact in a tangled way.

Wear-and-Tear Theory

The wear-and-tear theory suggests that cells and tissues have vital parts that wear out resulting in aging. Dr. August Weismann introduced this theory in 1882. He postulates that the daily grind of life, in particular abuse or overuse, literally wears the body out and can result in disease states. This is generally thought to happen with organs. Toxins in our diet and in the environment wear down the liver, stomach, kidneys, skin, and so on. However, wear and tear can take place on a cellular level or on an organ system level [2].

Oxidative Damage

The role of reactive oxygen species (ROS) has been implicated in the process of aging and senescence. More specifically, if there is an imbalance between ROS and antioxidants, the result is oxidative stress. Severe oxidative stress can cause cell death; moderate oxidation can trigger apoptosis, and even more intense stresses may cause necrosis [3].

A free radical is a molecule or atom with unpaired electron in the outer shell. They are unstable, highly reactive, and energized molecules. There are many types of free radicals, but most related to biological systems are derived from oxygen and thus termed ROS. They can be classified into oxygen-centered radicals and oxygen-centered nonradicals. Oxygen-centered radicals are superoxide ion, hydroxyl radical, alkoxyl radical, and peroxyl radical. Oxygen-centered nonradicals are hydrogen peroxide and singlet oxygen. The free radicals commonly described in aging are superoxide ion, hydroxyl radical, and hydrogen peroxide. The formation of these radicals can lead to harmful cellular effects, including damage of DNA, oxidations of polyunsaturated

R. R. Tampi et al. (eds.), *Psychiatric Disorders Late in Life*, https://doi.org/10.1007/978-3-319-73078-3_7

fatty acids in lipids, oxidations of amino acids in proteins, and oxidative deactivation of specific enzymes by oxidation of cofactors [4].

Early evidence for this theory includes the observation that the overexpression of catalase, the enzyme that degrades peroxide and superoxide dismutase, was protective in Drosophila. Those that overexpressed the antioxidant live 30–40% longer than controls [5]. More recent studies in animal models have confirmed that ROS production increases with age [6]. Other studies, looking at aging rats, demonstrated a significant increase in superoxide radical formation in the mitochondria of the brain and heart tissue. Furthermore, elevation in the level of lipid peroxidation was found in tissue of the brain and the liver [7]. Similarly in humans, overproduction of the superoxide radical is associated with impaired endothelial function in hypertension and aging [8].

The free radical theory has developed to include aging and age-related diseases. Oxidative stress and free radical damage have been associated with many neurodegenerative disorders, such as Parkinson's disease, Alzheimer's disease, Huntington's disease, and amyotrophic lateral sclerosis. There are increases in markers of lipid oxidation and an increase in oxidative damage of proteins [9].

DNA Damage Theory

Deoxyribonucleic acid (DNA) is a molecule that carries most of the genetic instructions used in the growth, development, functioning, and reproduction of all known living organisms. DNA stores biological information. Remarkably, DNA is the only biologic molecule that relies solely on repair of existing molecules, without any remanufacture. It accumulates damage over a lifetime and is represented by only one copy in most cells [10].

DNA damages occur continuously in cells of living organisms. The DNA damage theory proposes that aging is a consequence of unrepaired accumulation of naturally occurring DNA damages. Damages can occur because of many agents, including oxidizing agents, alkylating agents, and ultraviolet light. The damage is specific to the offending agent. UV light can damage DNA by producing thymine dimers, which are cross-links between pyrimidine bases [11]. Free radicals may cause multiple types of damage, including base modifications and double-strand breaks [12].

DNA damages due to normal cellular processes occur frequently. DNA repair processes have evolved to compensate for this damage; however, damage may remain even after the repair process. It is this accumulation of residual damage that may result in aging. Elevated levels of DNA damage can also accelerate physiological decline and the development of age-related diseases. The damage may reduce the expression of selectively vulnerable genes involved in areas of learning, memory, and neuronal survival, which promotes brain aging early in adult life. Furthermore, higher DNA damage may trigger cellular signaling pathways that result in a faster depletion of stem cells [13, 14].

The accumulation of unrepaired DNA damage is more prevalent in slowly replicating cells like the brain, skeletal, and cardiac muscle. With DNA damage, transcription of a gene can be prevented, and translation into a protein will be blocked.

The Telomere Shortening Theory

A telomere is a region of repetitive nucleotide sequences at each end of a chromosome. It protects the end of the chromosome from deterioration or from fusion with neighboring chromosomes. The nucleotide sequence of a telomere is "TTAGGG."

When chromosomes replicate, the duplication does not include the entire length of the chromosome. This leads to shortening of the ends of chromosomes. The telomeres are the buffers at the ends of chromosomes, which are reduced during cell division, thus protecting the DNA. Every time the cell divides, the telomeres get shorter. When they get too short, the cell can no longer divide, and it becomes inactive.

Counteracting telomere shortening is the enzyme telomerase. Telomerase lengthens telomeres in DNA strands and leads to longer cell life. Telomerase, which is active in normal stem cells, is normally absent from, or at very low levels in, most somatic cells [15]. If a cell were missing telomerase and dividing repeatedly, the progeny would at some point reach their "Hayflick limit." The "Hayflick limit" is the number of times a normal human cell population will divide until cell division stops. The telomerase absent cell's Hayflick limit is believed to be between 50 and 70 cell divisions. Once the limit is reached, cell division stops [1]. Telomerase does not completely prevent telomere shortening after extensive stem cell division either, providing a proposed mechanism for the limit of stem cell replicative history [16].

In 2003, Richard Cawthon discovered that those with longer telomeres lead longer lives than those with short telomeres [17]. Short telomeres have also been linked to age-related diseases and premature aging syndromes, including Werner syndrome, ataxia-telangiectasia, ataxia-telangiectasia-like disorder, Bloom syndrome, Fanconi anemia, and Nijmegen breakage syndrome [18].

Telomerase mutations have also been studied. When mice are engineered to lack telomerase, their telomeres progressively shorten over several generations. These animals age much faster than normal mice. The telomerase-deficient mice are barely fertile; suffer from age-related conditions such as osteoporosis, diabetes, and neurodegeneration; and die young [19].

In humans, we see the role of telomerase in cancer cells. These cells are often "immortal," and in about 85% of tumors, their immortality is the result of up-activation of their telomerase genes [20].

Neuropharmacology

The therapeutic targets of pharmacology are most often neurotransmitters, or chemical messengers, that transmit signals across a chemical synapse, such as a neuromuscular junction, from one neuron to another "target" neuron. We discuss the effect of aging on the neurotransmitters dopamine, serotonin, glutamate, *gamma*-aminobutyric acid, norepinephrine, and acetylcholine, common targets of pharmacologic intervention. We must keep in mind that age-related changes in the neurotransmitter systems of the brain are not a global phenomenon of normal aging, they are brain region specific and cell type specific.

Dopamine

Dopamine is a catecholamine neurotransmitter that has many roles in the brain and body. In the brain, there are many dopamine pathways related to reward, pleasure, and motor control. Dopamine is one of the most well-understood neurotransmitters with regard to aging. Dopamine levels decline by nearly 10% per decade from early adulthood and have been associated with declines in cognitive and motor performance [21]. Many studies have shown age-dependent dopamine decline in production and in receptor density [22].

More specifically, D1-like receptors decrease by 7–9% per decade in caudate, putamen, and occipital cortex [23], and D2-like receptors decrease by 6–12% per decade in thalamus, temporal cortex, and frontal cortex [24]. Compounding this is the age-related reduction in dopamine transporters [25]. The loss of dopamine with age is likely responsible for many neurological symptoms that are more commonly seen in the elderly, including decreased arm swing and increased rigidity.

Serotonin

Serotonin is a monoamine neurotransmitter found primarily in the gastrointestinal tract (approximately 90%), platelets, and the central nervous system. Serotonin in the brain is thought to regulate mood, appetite, and sleep. It is also thought to have a role in cognition, including memory and learning. Medications targeting serotonin at synapses are thought to have antidepressant effect.

Broadly, serotonin levels, receptors, and transporters are sensitive to aging. With increased age come decreasing levels of serotonin receptors and serotonin transporters. There is a decrease in serotonin receptors, with 5-hydroxytryptamine (5HT) 2A receptor decrease in the caudate nucleus, putamen, and frontal cerebral cortex [26]. The 5HT 1A receptors decrease at a rate of approximately 10% per decade [27]. The serotonin transporter, 5HT, has also been shown to have a decreased binding capacity in the thalamus and the midbrain in the aging brain [28].

Glutamate

Glutamate is the main excitatory neurotransmitter in the nervous system. Glutamates activity is at postsynaptic N-methyl-D-aspartate (NMDA) receptors and α-amino-3-hydroxy-5-methyl-4-isoxazolepropionic acid (AMPA) receptors. It is thought to have a role in synaptic plasticity and cognitive functions [29]. Disruptions of the glutamate system, like excess release of glutamate, can lead to hyperexcitability in postsynaptic neurons, to the point of excitotoxicity and cell death [30].

The glutamate system, too, is also affected by age. There is an age-related decline in glutamate concentrations in the parietal gray matter and basal ganglia of men [31]. The parietal and basal ganglia regions are often the areas affected in degenerative brain diseases. This suggests that glutamate may have a role as a marker in brain diseases that are affected by aging [32].

This is supported by the use of memantine, a noncompetitive NMDA antagonist, that has shown benefit in cognition, function, and global outcome in patients with moderate to severe AD [33].

Gamma-Aminobutyric Acid

Gamma-aminobutyric acid (GABA) is the chief inhibitory neurotransmitter in the brain. GABA is synthesized from glutamate by the enzyme L-glutamic acid decarboxylase (GAD). To date, three subtypes of GABA-specific receptors have been identified: GABAA, GABAB, and GABAC. Both GABAA and GABAB receptors are localized in the central nervous system [34].

The GABAA receptor is pre- and postsynaptic, with modulatory sites for benzodiazepines, barbiturates, steroids, and ethanol. GABAB is also found both presynaptically and postsynaptically, which decreases neuronal excitability and may be linked to cognition.

In the aging brain, GAD decreases by roughly 20–30% in the cortex and thalamus of postmortem human brains. There is also a decrease in GABA receptor binding sites and GAD mRNA levels in the aged rodent brain [35].

Examining the brains of people with Alzheimer's disease has led to theories of GABAergic regional disruptions. In Alzheimer's disease, GABA concentrations are reduced in frontal, temporal, and parietal areas. When combined with GABA and benzodiazepine binding studies, the temporal region is most affected. Neuroimaging studies have identified the parietal cortex as having reduced GABAergic binding [36].

Norepinephrine

Norepinephrine (NE) is the main neurotransmitter used by the sympathetic nervous system. Its release is lowest during sleep and rises during wakefulness, reaching higher levels during stress or danger (the fight-or-flight response). NE promotes arousal, vigilance, formation and retrieval of memory, and attention. Two broad families of norepinephrine receptors have been identified, known as alpha- and beta-adrenergic receptors. Alpha receptors are divided into subtypes α_1 and α_2 and beta receptors into subtypes β_1, β_2, and β_3.

The locus coeruleus is the primary site for brain synthesis of norepinephrine. The locus coeruleus is a small nucleus in the pons on the lateral edge of the fourth ventricle. The locus coeruleus appears to be the first brain region where Alzheimer's disease pathology emerges. Lesions in this NE-producing area exaggerate AD-related pathology, and augmentation of the brain's norepinephrine transmission reduces neuroinflammation and cognitive decline [37]. Furthermore, evidence suggests that maintaining the neural density of the NE nuclei can prevent cognitive decline in aging [38]. AD has also been linked to a 30–60% reduction in α-2 adrenergic receptors in the frontal cortex, hypothalamus, and cerebellum [39].

Acetylcholine

Acetylcholine (Ach) is synthesized from its two immediate precursors, choline and acetyl coenzyme A. It has functions both in the peripheral nervous system and central nervous system. There are two main classes of acetylcholine receptor, nicotinic and muscarinic. Nicotinic receptors are ligand-gated ion channels that have the receptor site on the channel itself. Muscarinic receptors work via a second messenger system and increase intracellular levels of IP_3 and calcium by activating phospholipase C. A group of cholinergic neurons in the nucleus basalis of Meynert projects to the cerebral cortex and limbic system. In the reticular system, neurons project to the cerebral cortex, limbic system, hypothalamus, and thalamus.

ACh plays an important role in sustaining attention, learning, and memory. Human studies have demonstrated that blocking muscarinic receptors impairs the encoding of new memories but not the retrieval of previously stored memories [40, 41] and impairs working memory for some stimuli [42]. Conversely, drugs which activate nicotinic receptors enhance the programming of new information [43]. Cholinergic abnormalities have been observed in AD brains [44]. It has been reported that the level of acetylcholine receptors is reduced in AD and that dysfunction of cholinergic signal transmission could be responsible for the symptoms of AD [45]. This has led to the development of cholinergic therapy; treatments based on the assumption that low levels of acetylcholine are responsible for the cognitive decline associated with AD. Cholinesterase inhibitors effectiveness is in part through direct activation of the nicotinic receptors and through a direct activation of the allosteric site on the receptor [46]. Further support for this nicotinic receptor stimulation in AD is based upon the fact that nicotine improves memory in animals, healthy subjects, and AD patients [47].

Conclusions

In this section, the biological theories of aging were explored. Each provides a scientific explanation for age-related changes, but none is recognized as irrefutable. Also, the most common neurotransmitters that are targets for pharmacologic interventions were reviewed. A better understanding of the processes that contribute to aging and the effects on chemical messengers remains critical.

References

1. Hayflick L, Moorhead PS. The serial cultivation of human diploid cell strains. Exp Cell Res. 1961;25(3):585–621.
2. Mercado-Sáenz S, Ruiz-Gómez MJ, Morales-Moreno F, Martínez-Morillo M. Cellular aging: theories and technological influence. Braz Arch Biol Technol. 2010;53(6):1319–32.
3. Lennon S, Martin S, Cotter T. Dose-dependent induction of apoptosis in human tumour cell lines by widely diverging stimuli. Cell Prolif. 1991;24(2):203–14.
4. Birben E, Sahiner UM, Sackesen C, Erzurum S, Kalayci O. Oxidative stress and antioxidant defense. World Allergy Organ J. 2012;5(1):9.
5. Orr WC, Sohal RS. Extension of life-span by overexpression of superoxide dismutase and catalase in Drosophila Melanogaster. Science. 1994;263(5150):1128–30.
6. Chung HY, Song SH, Kim HJ, Ikeno Y, Yu BP. Modulation of renal xanthine oxidoreductase in aging: gene expression and reactive oxygen species generation. J Nutr Health Aging. 1998;3(1):19–23.
7. Sawada M, Carlson JC. Changes in superoxide radical and lipid peroxide formation in the brain, heart and liver during the lifetime of the rat. Mech Ageing Dev. 1987;41(1):125–37.
8. Hamilton CA, Brosnan MJ, McIntyre M, Graham D, Dominiczak AF. Superoxide excess in hypertension and aging a common cause of endothelial dysfunction. Hypertension. 2001;37(2):529–34.
9. Patel VP, Chu CT. Nuclear transport, oxidative stress, and neurodegeneration. Int J Clin Exp Pathol. 2011;4(3):215–29.
10. Hoeijmakers JH. DNA damage, aging, and cancer. N Engl J Med. 2009;361(15):1475–85.
11. Douki T, Reynaud-Angelin A, Cadet J, Sage E. Bipyrimidine photoproducts rather than oxidative lesions are the main type of DNA damage involved in the genotoxic effect of solar UVA radiation. Biochemistry. 2003;42(30):9221–6.
12. Cadet J, Delatour T, Douki T, et al. Hydroxyl radicals and DNA base damage. Mutat Res. 1999;424(1):9–21.
13. Freitas AA, de Magalhaes JP. A review and appraisal of the DNA damage theory of ageing. Mutat Res. 2011;728(1):12–22.
14. Lu T, Pan Y, Kao S-Y, et al. Gene regulation and DNA damage in the ageing human brain. Nature. 2004;429(6994):883–91.
15. Cong Y-S, Wright WE, Shay JW. Human telomerase and its regulation. Microbiol Mol Biol Rev. 2002;66(3):407–25.

16. Flores I, Cayuela ML, Blasco MA. Effects of telomerase and telomere length on epidermal stem cell behavior. Science. 2005;309(5738):1253–6.
17. Cawthon RM, Smith KR, O'Brien E, Sivatchenko A, Kerber RA. Association between telomere length in blood and mortality in people aged 60 years or older. Lancet. 2003;361(9355):393–5.
18. Blasco MA. Telomeres and human disease: ageing, cancer and beyond. Nat Rev Genet. 2005;6(8):611–22.
19. Callaway E. Telomerase reverses ageing process. Nature. 2010;28
20. Hanahan D, Weinberg RA. The hallmarks of cancer. Cell. 2000;100(1):57–70.
21. Nyberg L, Bäckman L. Cognitive aging: a view from brain imaging. In: New frontiers in cognitive aging. Oxford: Oxford University Press; 2004. p. 135–60.
22. Leff SE, Gariano R, Creese I. Dopamine receptor turnover rates in rat striatum are age-dependent. Proc Natl Acad Sci. 1984;81(12):3910–4.
23. Wang Y, Chan GL, Holden JE, et al. Age-dependent decline of dopamine D1 receptors in human brain: a PET study. Synapse. 1998;30(1):56–61.
24. Kaasinen V, Kemppainen N, Någren K, Helenius H, Kurki T, Rinne JO. Age-related loss of extrastriatal dopamine D2-like receptors in women. J Neurochem. 2002;81(5):1005–10.
25. Meng SZ, Ozawa Y, Itoh M, Takashima S. Developmental and age-related changes of dopamine transporter, and dopamine D1 and D2 receptors in human basal ganglia. Brain Res. 1999;843(1):136–44.
26. Wong DF, Wagner HN, Dannals RF, et al. Effects of age on dopamine and serotonin receptors measured by positron tomography in the living human brain. Science. 1984;226(4681):1393–6.
27. Møller M, Jakobsen S, Gjedde A. Parametric and regional maps of free serotonin 5HT1A receptor sites in human brain as function of age in healthy humans. Neuropsychopharmacology. 2007;32(8):1707–14.
28. Yamamoto M, Suhara T, Okubo Y, et al. Age-related decline of serotonin transporters in living human brain of healthy males. Life Sci. 2002;71(7):751–7.
29. McEntee WJ, Crook TH. Glutamate: its role in learning, memory, and the aging brain. Psychopharmacology. 1993;111(4):391–401.
30. Doble A. The role of excitotoxicity in neurodegenerative disease: implications for therapy. Pharmacol Ther. 1999;81(3):163–221.
31. Sailasuta N, Ernst T, Chang L. Regional variations and the effects of age and gender on glutamate concentrations in the human brain. Magn Reson Imaging. 2008;26(5):667–75.
32. Chang L, Jiang CS, Ernst T. Effects of age and sex on brain glutamate and other metabolites. Magn Reson Imaging. 2009;27(1):142–5.
33. Molinuevo JL, Lladó A, Rami L. Memantine: targeting glutamate excitotoxicity in Alzheimer's disease and other dementias. Am J Alzheimers Dis Other Demen. 2005;20(2):77–85.
34. Bormann J. The 'ABC' of GABA receptors. Trends Pharmacol Sci. 2000;21(1):16–9.
35. Petroff OA. Book review: GABA and glutamate in the human brain. Neuroscientist. 2002;8(6):562–73.
36. Lanctôt KL, Herrmann N, Mazzotta P, Khan LR, Ingber N. GABAergic function in Alzheimer's disease: evidence for dysfunction and potential as a therapeutic target for the treatment of behavioural and psychological symptoms of dementia. Can J Psychiatr. 2004;49(7):439–53.
37. Mravec B, Lejavova K, Cubinkova V. Locus (coeruleus) minoris resistentiae in pathogenesis of Alzheimer's disease. Curr Alzheimer Res. 2014;11(10):992–1001.
38. Wilson RS, Nag S, Boyle PA, et al. Neural reserve, neuronal density in the locus ceruleus, and cognitive decline. Neurology. 2013;80(13):1202–8.
39. Javier Meana J, Barturen F, Asier Garro M, García-Sevilla JA, Fontán A, Zarranz JJ. Decreased density of presynaptic α2-Adrenoceptors in postmortem brains of patients with Alzheimer's disease. J Neurochem. 1992;58(5):1896–904.
40. Atri A, Sherman S, Norman KA, et al. Blockade of central cholinergic receptors impairs new learning and increases proactive interference in a word paired-associate memory task. Behav Neurosci. 2004;118(1):223.
41. Hasselmo ME, McGaughy J. High acetylcholine levels set circuit dynamics for attention and encoding and low acetylcholine levels set dynamics for consolidation. Prog Brain Res. 2004;145:207–31.
42. Green A, Ellis KA, Ellis J, et al. Muscarinic and nicotinic receptor modulation of object and spatial n-back working memory in humans. Pharmacol Biochem Behav. 2005;81(3):575–84.
43. Buccafusco JJ, Letchworth SR, Bencherif M, Lippiello PM. Long-lasting cognitive improvement with nicotinic receptor agonists: mechanisms of pharmacokinetic–pharmacodynamic discordance. Trends Pharmacol Sci. 2005;26(7):352–60.

44. Whitehouse PJ, Martino AM, Antuono PG, et al. Nicotinic acetylcholine binding sites in Alzheimer's disease. Brain Res. 1986;371(1):146–51.
45. Nordberg A. Nicotinic receptor abnormalities of Alzheimer's disease: therapeutic implications. Biol Psychiatry. 2001;49(3):200–10.
46. Maelicke A, Albuquerque EX. Allosteric modulation of nicotinic acetylcholine receptors as a treatment strategy for Alzheimer's disease. Eur J Pharmacol. 2000;393(1):165–70.
47. Levin ED. Nicotinic receptor subtypes and cognitive function. Dev Neurobiol. 2002;53(4):633–40.

8 Anatomy and Physiology

Caitlin Snow, Katherine Rice Goettsche, and Jimmy Avari

Age-associated anatomical and physiological changes occur across all organ systems, at varying rates according to differences among individuals' genetic makeup and environmental exposures. The precise effects of usual aging have been challenging to characterize. This is because long-term studies are limited by the high mortality rate in old age, the heterogeneity of the older patient population results in high variability of outcomes, and confounding factors make it difficult to determine which changes are a result of usual aging unrelated to a disease process or other extrinsic factors [1]. Although a comprehensive narrative has yet to emerge, many age-related physiologic changes have been identified. These changes have important pharmacokinetic and pharmacodynamic implications that are reviewed in a later chapter. This section reviews the impact of age on the major organ systems.

Body Composition and Musculoskeletal System

With advancing age, there are alterations in body composition that include a decrease in lean body mass and total body water and an increase in total body fat [2]. Adipose tissue is redistributed centrally with a loss of fat subcutaneously, making older people more sensitive to extremes of ambient temperature [3]. The increased fat-to-water ratio carries clinical significance because fat-soluble drugs, such as benzodiazepines, have a larger volume of distribution that may lead to increased half-life and medication effect.

Age-related changes in the musculoskeletal system also impact older adults' functioning. There is a decrease in stature and bone mineral density, and fat accumulates in the bone marrow [4]. Additionally, cartilage becomes brittle, and tendons and ligaments weaken and stiffen [5]. Together these changes increase the risk of developing osteoarthritis, which is a common cause of chronic disability in older adults.

Skin

Aging of the skin is more influenced by environmental exposures (e.g., photoaging) than by intrinsic processes and is primarily caused by oxidative degeneration [6]. Age-related physiologic changes include a loss of subcutaneous fat, diminished capillarity, a decreased number of sebaceous and eccrine glands, and reduced nutrient transfer across the dermal-epidermal junction. This causes the skin to atrophy and become xerotic, and the barrier and thermoregulation functions of skin are impaired [3]. Composition changes, including the fragmentation of elastin and accumulation of collagen, result in diminished elasticity and wrinkling of the skin. Furthermore, vitamin D synthesis is impaired, and healing occurs at a slower rate [7].

R. R. Tampi et al. (eds.), *Psychiatric Disorders Late in Life*, https://doi.org/10.1007/978-3-319-73078-3_8

Cardiovascular System

A host of age-related structural and functional changes occurs in the cardiovascular system that results in a diminished cardiac output in response to increased work demands [8]. These changes can manifest as nonspecific symptoms such as low energy, fatigability, and light-headedness, and predispose older adults to developing cardiovascular disease, a known risk factor for depression and anxiety.

Age-related changes contribute to both a lower cardiac output and a lower cardiac reserve. The ventricular myocardium thickens, and the size of ventricular cavities decreases, resulting in a lower volume of blood pumped per contraction [9]. The responsiveness of adrenergic receptors is diminished, and the number of sinus node cells is decreased, resulting in a lower intrinsic and maximal heart rate [10]. Blood vessels thicken and become less distensible, and blood vessel lumens narrow, resulting in slow elevation in blood pressure [11]. Additionally, there is an accumulation of degenerative products such as lipids, collagen, and calcium deposits, thereby increasing the risk of atherosclerotic disease [3].

Respiratory System

Age-related anatomic changes and functional decline occur throughout the respiratory system in an analogous fashion to the aging of the cardiovascular system but at a more rapid rate [3]. These changes contribute to an increased work of breathing and a diminished respiratory reserve. There is a loss of elastic and parenchymal tissue in the lung, and pulmonary vasculature stiffens. This results in a decrease in static elastic recoil ability and a diminished surface area for gas exchange [12]. In addition, alveolar ducts and bronchioles dilate, cough reflexes are depressed, mucociliary clearance ability is impaired, and there is a diminished ventilatory response to hypoxemia and hypercapnia with age [13].

Age-related changes outside of the lung also contribute to diminished airway expansion. The chest wall stiffens and becomes less compliant, respiratory smooth muscle strength declines, and the diaphragm flattens and loses function over time [14].

Pulmonary function tests reveal age-associated changes in the respiratory system. Total lung capacity does not change with age, but residual volume increases due to a loss of expiratory muscle strength. There is a decrease in vital capacity, functional reserve capacity, expiratory reserve volume, forced vital capacity, and forced expiratory volume. Closing volume and ventilation-perfusion mismatch increase, and there is a larger region of alveolar dead space. Pulmonary diffusing capacity and gas exchange progressively decrease with age [14].

Gastrointestinal System

As individuals age, changes occur throughout the gastrointestinal tract that have functional significance. The epithelial lining of the oral mucosa thins and the gums recede, making older adults more susceptible to root caries and tooth loss. Saliva production decreases with age, resulting in dry mouth that can impact chewing and swallowing. This can lead to incomplete mastication and an increased risk of inadequate nutritional intake or aspiration. Esophageal function is largely preserved with age, but there is a decrease in the amplitude of peristalsis and a decline in the number of myenteric ganglion cells [3].

Anatomic and physiologic changes throughout the stomach and colon can lead to changes in basic digestive functions such as motility, secretion, digestion, and absorption [15]. The stomach secretes lower levels of gastric acid, serum gastrin levels increase, and intrinsic factor levels decrease. There is a loss of microvilli of the brush border and diminished enzymatic activity in the colon [3]. Transit through the gastrointestinal tract may be slower, leading to increased sensitivity to irritants and risk of constipation. However, studies implicating normal aging as a cause of dysmotility in the elderly are inconclusive due to abundant confounding factors [16].

Hepatobiliary System

Age-related hepatic changes include a decrease in hepatic mass and perfusion, diminished function of enzymes of drug metabolism, a decline in detoxification and inflammatory functions, and reduced rate of hepatic regeneration following injury [17]. Hepatic mass is estimated to decrease between 20% and 40% across the human lifespan [18], and hepatic blood flow is estimated to decrease by 40–60% [19].

Many liver functions decline with age. There is a progressive decline of the cytochrome P-450 system beginning in the fifth decade of life, impacting the clearance of many drugs [20]. Low-density lipoprotein metabolism decreases, contributing to high cholesterol levels. Studies regarding the effect of aging on albumin synthesis in the liver have been inconsistent. However, albumin has been shown to decrease with age, which is significant because hypoalbuminemia impacts the clearance of highly protein-bound drugs and low levels have been correlated with high mortality in a nursing home patient population [20]. Of note, some hepatic functions are unaffected, and standard liver function tests are only minimally affected with age [21].

There are some age-related changes in biliary function, including decreased bile acid flow and secretion. In addition, bile has a higher lithogenic index thereby increasing the risk of gallstone formation [22].

Renal System

The kidney undergoes a progressive age-related decline in structure and function. There is a decrease in total renal mass, with dominant cortical losses and relative sparing of the medulla. Renal blood flow similarly decreases with age by approximately 10% per decade after the fourth decade. The reduction in renal perfusion exceeds the reduction in renal mass, suggesting that limited blood flow is a primary factor in, and not a consequence of, the involution of the kidney [23].

Renal vasculature and limited blood supply is similarly implicated in the age-related decline of kidney function on a microanatomical level. Senescence of nephrons, the basic structural and functional units of the kidney, is primarily characterized by diffuse nephrosclerosis that is the result of ischemic injury. Glomeruli, the networks of capillaries that function as the initial filtering component of the nephron, decrease in number and undergo morphological changes that are characterized by diminished lobulation and an increased incidence of glomerulosclerosis. The glomerular basement membrane (GBM) folds and thickens. Furthermore, multiple studies have demonstrated an age-associated increase in the permeability of the GBM, which is accompanied by a rise in microalbuminuria and proteinuria [24, 25].

These structural changes result in diminished function of the aging kidney. Functional losses include a reduction of the glomerular filtration rate, impaired excretion and reabsorption, and a decline in the renal vasculature's ability to autoregulate. The estimated glomerular filtration rate (eGFR) is the rate at which blood passes through the glomeruli each minute and is the standard lab value for measuring overall kidney function. Values of glomerular filtration rate in healthy adults are on average 140 mL/min/1.73 m^2 until age 40 and then drop by approximately 8 mL/min/1.73 m^2 per decade [25, 26]. Glomeruli receive blood supply from an afferent arteriole and drain into an efferent arteriole, which supports the process of ultrafiltration. With ischemic injury of age, afferent and efferent arterioles atrophy. Additionally, changes in the activity of key vasoactive mediators, such as those in the renin-angiotensin-aldosterone and nitric oxide systems, contribute to the age-related physiological changes in the kidney [25]. There is an impaired responsiveness to vasoactive stimuli, thereby diminishing the ability of the vasculature to autoregulate.

Senescence of the kidney carries important clinical considerations when caring for older adults due to increased potential for toxic levels of renally excreted drugs. Specific to psychiatry, frequently used drugs that are primarily excreted by the kidneys include lithium, bupropion, and venlafaxine.

Genitourinary System

Age-related changes in the genitourinary system contribute to the risk of urinary issues and a decline of reproductive ability in older adults. Impaired bladder contractility is thought to be due to myogenic and neurogenic factors [27].

The detrusor muscle weakens due to decreased autonomic innervation of the bladder [28]. The result is decreased urinary flow rates and increased post-void residual [1]. In addition, studies in women have demonstrated that the urethra atrophies and there is decreased urethral closure pressure, which is thought to be due to lower levels of estrogen [1].

Age-related changes impact reproductive ability. In men, testosterone levels decrease over time due to increased levels of sex hormone-binding globulin with age, mean testicular volume declines, and there is a decrease in the number of germ cells, Sertoli cells, and Leydig cells [3]. Sperm production decreases, and sperm have an increased frequency of chromosomal abnormalities. Age-related prostate gland enlargement is caused by hyperplasia of basal cells and stromal cells and can manifest as urinary problems [29].

In women aging of the ovary begins in utero, after which there is a steady decline in potential germ cells. Estrogen and progesterone production decreases progressively. Menopause occurs at the average age of 51 when there are inadequate hormone levels to support the negative-feedback loop between the pituitary and the gonads. Lower hormone levels cause atrophy of the breasts and genitalia [3]. Of note, many urinary and sexual problems are caused by problems that are not directly related to the genitourinary system, such as medication side effects and comorbidities.

Sensory System

As individuals age, there is a decline of all five senses, which carries significant implications for health and quality of life. Vision diminishes as a result of many anatomic changes including weakening of the ciliary muscle, decreased lens curvature, increased pupil and blood vessel rigidity, and atrophy of the conjunctiva [30]. Older adults experience a loss of accommodation and diminished ability to adapt to changes in light. Anatomical changes in the ear lead to hearing loss across all frequencies, but age is particularly associated with high-frequency sensorineural hearing loss. Presbycusis, or age-related hearing loss, occurs due to a number of factors that primarily impact the inner ear. Olfactory and taste senses also deteriorate. Finally, touch sensation diminishes with age, with functional implications for articulation of speech, handgrip, and postural stability [31].

Conclusion

Age-associated anatomic and physiologic changes impact all organ systems. These changes contribute to functional decline and risk of illness. Often therapeutic and pharmacologic modifications must be made in order to safely treat older patients. Further research is essential to better understand the impact of age on the various organ systems.

References

1. DuBeau CE. The aging lower urinary tract. J Urol. 2006;175(3):S11–5.
2. Fulop T Jr, Worum I, Csongor J, et al. Body composition in elderly people: determination of body composition by multiisotope method and the elimination kinetics of these isotopes in healthy elderly subjects. Gerontology. 1985;31(1):6–14.
3. Leventhal EA, Burns EA. The biology of aging. In: Sadavoy J, Jarvik LF, Grossberg GT, et al., editors. Comprehensive textbook of geriatric psychiatry. 3rd ed. New York, NY: W.W. Norton & Company; 2004. p. 105–30.
4. Tchkonia T, Morbeck DE, Zglinicki T, et al. Fat tissue, aging, and cellular senescence. Aging Cell. 2010;9(5):667–84.
5. Loeser RF. Age-related changes in the musculoskeletal system and the development of osteoarthritis. Clin Geriatr Med. 2010;26(3):371–86.
6. Kammeyer A, Luiten RM. Oxidation events and skin aging. Ageing Res Rev. 2015;21:16–29.
7. Ashcroft GS, Mills SJ, Ashworth JJ. Ageing and wound healing. Biogerontology. 2002;3:337–45.
8. Folkow B, Svanborg A. Physiology of cardiovascular aging. Physiol Rev. 1993;73:725–64.
9. Van de Veire NR, De Backer J, Ascoop AK, et al. Echocardiographically estimated left ventricular end-diastolic and right ventricular systolic pressure in normotensive healthy individuals. Int J Cardiovasc Imaging. 2006;22(5):633–41.
10. Stratton JR, Cerqueira MD, Schwartz RS, et al. Differences in cardiovascular responses to isopro-

terenol in relation to age and exercise training in healthy men. Circulation. 1992;86(2):504–12.
11. Kitzman DW, Scholz DG, Hagen PT, et al. Age-related changes in normal human hearts during the first 10 decades of life. Part II (maturity): a quantitative anatomic study of 765 specimens from subjects 20 to 99 years old. Mayo Clin Proc. 1988;63(2):137–46.
12. Taylor BJ, Johnson BD. The pulmonary circulation and exercise responses in the elderly. Semin Respir Crit Care Med. 2010;31(5):528–38.
13. Kronenberg RS, Drage CW. Attenuation of the ventilatory and heart rate responses to hypoxia and hypercapnia with aging in normal men. J Clin Invest. 1973;52(8):1812–9.
14. Lalley P. The aging respiratory system—pulmonary structure, function and neural control. Respir Physiol Neurobiol. 2013;187(3):199–210.
15. Grassi M, Petraccia L, Mennuni G, et al. Changes, functional disorders, and diseases in the gastrointestinal tract of elderly. Nutr Hosp. 2011;26(4):659–68.
16. O'Mahony D, O'Leary P, Quigley EM. Aging and intestinal motility: a review of factors that affect intestinal motility in the aged. Drugs Aging. 2002;19(7):515–27.
17. Schmucker DL, Sanchez H. Liver regeneration and aging: a current perspective. Curr Gerontol Geriatr Res. 2011;2001:8. https://doi.org/10.1155/2011/526379.
18. Schmucker D. Age-related changes in liver structure and function: implications for disease? Exp Gerontol. 2005;40(8–9):650–9.
19. Wynne HA, Cope LH, Mutch E, et al. The effect of age upon liver volume and apparent liver blood flow in healthy man. Hepatology. 1989;9(2):297–301.
20. Anantharaju A, Feller A, Chedid A. Aging Liver. A review. *Gerontology*. 2002;48(6):343–53.
21. Woodhouse K, Wynne HA. Age-related changes in hepatic function. Implications for drug therapy. Drugs Aging. 1992;2(3):243–55.
22. Desai AK, Morley JE. The aging body and brain. In: Agronin ME, Maletta GJ, editors. Principles and practice of geriatric psychiatry, vol. 1. 2nd ed. Philadelphia, PA: Lippincott Williams & Wilkins; 2011. p. 4–11.
23. Hollenberg NK, Adams DF, Solomon HS, et al. Senescence and the renal vasculature in normal man. Circ Res. 1974;34:309–16.
24. Bolton WK, Benton FR, Maclay JG, et al. Spontaneous glomerular sclerosis in aging Sprague-Dawley rates. Am J Pathol. 1976;85:227–302.
25. Weinstein JR, Anderson S. The aging kidney: physiological changes. Adv Chronic Kidney Dis. 2010;17(4):302–7.
26. Davies DF, Shock NW. Age changes in glomerular filtration rate, effective renal plasma flow, and tubular excretory capacity in adult males. J Clin Invest. 1950;29:496–507.
27. Tadic SD, Griffiths D, Schaefer W, et al. Brain activity underlying impaired continence control in older women with overactive bladder. Neurourol Urodyn. 2012;31(5):652–8.
28. Gilpin SA, Gilpin CJ, Dixon JS, et al. The effect of age on the autonomic innervation of the urinary bladder. Br J Urol. 1986;58(4):378–81.
29. Gunes S, Hekim GN, Arsian MA, et al. Effects of aging on the male reproductive system. J Assist Reprod Genet. 2016;33(4):441–54.
30. Kaiser RM. Physiological and clinical considerations of geriatric patient care. In: Steffens DC, Blazer DG, Thakur ME, editors. The American Psychiatric Publishing textbook of geriatric psychiatry. 5th ed. Arlington, VA: American Psychiatric Publishing; 2015. p. 2.
31. Wickremaratchi MM, Llewelyn JG. Effects of ageing on touch. Postgrad Med J. 2006;82(967):301–4.

Part III

Diagnostic Methods

9 Interviewing and History Taking

Lisa L. Boyle and Ali Abbas Asghar-Ali

A complete assessment of an elderly person is multifaceted and includes the elements of an assessment of an adult with special attention to issues related to aging. Older individuals can be expected to have more complex histories and problems that require an interdisciplinary biopsychosocial approach to assessment and management. To help providers with the biopsychosocial assessment of older adults and facilitate tracking of complex data and interrelationships, the Wisconsin Star Method (Figure 9-1) adopts an approach to visually map the individual's medical factors, medications, behavioral or psychiatric factors, social factors, and personal factors [1, 2].

The Wisconsin Star Method can help facilitate the provider or interdisciplinary team's approach to gathering data during interview and history taking while keeping the data organized and accessible. The various points of the star are filled in to help provide a better understanding of the patient and facilitate visual mapping of potential interactions across the five domains to inform the biopsychosocial formulation and subsequent treatment planning for complex geriatric patients. Generally, the personal arm of the star tends to need more deliberate attention as it is less likely to be captured within traditional electronic medical records. The personal arm of the star is essential for the provider to understand the personal meaning of the problem for the patient. It covers areas such as the patient's values, loyalties, personality traits, and coping. Generally, understanding the problem and developing an acceptable treatment plan for the patient requires consideration of the personal arm of the star. Additional templates and supporting materials to adopt the Wisconsin Star Method in geriatric assessment are available for free public use [2].

Older adults' medical and treatment histories tend to have higher degrees of multimorbidities and polypharmacy [3], resulting in more complexity. Older adults are more at risk for developing medical ailments that can cause or worsen cognitive function or psychiatric symptoms. Moreover, individuals with severe and persistent mental illness who are aging also have high medical comorbidity, premature disability with higher rates of institutionalization, and higher use of emergency services [4]. These challenges can be due to long-standing problems with self-care and lack of access to preventative health services [4]. It is therefore important for a geriatric psychiatric evaluation to include a thorough review of past medical history in addition to a medical evaluation, along with an assessment of its impact on the individual. Common areas to which one needs to be especially vigilant include assessment of geriatric syndromes such as cognitive impairment, sensory impairments such as vision and hearing loss, gait disturbance and falls, and iatrogenic effects. It is important to remember that older adults have higher risk for delirium [5].

R. R. Tampi et al. (eds.), *Psychiatric Disorders Late in Life*, https://doi.org/10.1007/978-3-319-73078-3_9

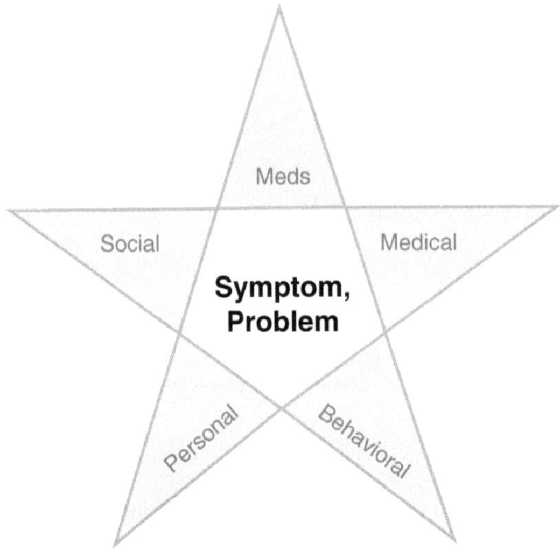

FIGURE 9-1. The Wisconsin Star Method [1, 2] (Reproduced with permission from T. Howell. Disclaimer: The Wisconsin Star Method is published in the public domain and as such may not be copyrighted, trademarked, or patented. Permission is granted to use, reproduce, and/or adapt the Wisconsin Star Method provided this disclaimer is included in any and all such materials, including the following acknowledgment: The Madison Veterans Administration Hospital, the University of Wisconsin-Madison School of Medicine and Public Health, the Division of Mental Health and Substance Abuse Services of the Wisconsin Department of Health Services, NAMI Wisconsin, and members of the Wisconsin Department of Geriatric Psychiatry Initiative have provided in-kind support for the development of the Wisconsin Star Method)

As well, providers working with older adults can expect a high degree of heterogeneity in their patients as various factors, stemming from the interplay of genetic and environmental factors and lived experiences, can impact how an individual copes with emotional problems or psychiatric illness throughout her or his life. One should assess the older adult's coping mechanisms, personal values, and goals to help inform what treatment approaches to consider. An assessment of psychosocial domains over the course of the patient's life is essential. Assessing and affirming a person's relevant cultural aspects during the interview helps build rapport and allows for a better biopsychosocial formulation. The *Diagnostic and Statistical Manual of Mental Disorders*, fifth edition (DSM-5), contains guidelines for a cultural formulation interview with a special supplementary module that accounts for the needs of older adults [6]. Briefly, the supplementary module contains the following categories that can help the clinician obtain a thorough understanding of the geriatric person: (1) conceptions of aging and cultural identity, (2) conceptions of aging in relationship to illness attributions and coping, (3) influence of comorbid medical problems and treatments, (4) quality and nature of social supports and caregiving, (5) additional age-related transitions, and (6) positive and negative attitudes toward aging and clinician-patient relationship. The questions in these categories can be implemented throughout the evaluation process.

Moreover, the functional assessment, along with social support network, is an essential component of the geriatric psychiatry evaluation. Knowledge of the older adult's residential setting along with functional status and supports available can provide a better understanding of whether current demands on the older adult match her or his capabilities and can inform what additional social or environmental supports may be needed to promote well-being. Additional emphasis on the patient's perceived quality of life, optimal residential setting, and evaluation of long-term care needs is also part of a comprehensive assessment. The components of the interview and history taking are provided in Table 9-1.

TABLE 9-1. Elements of interviewing and history taking

History of present illness
Psychiatric and substance use history
Medical history
Medications
Family history
Developmental history
Social history

Considerations in Working with Older Adults

Older adults have higher risk for sensory impairments as they age [7]. It is important to assess for visual or hearing impairment that can affect the person's ability to engage in the interview. Using corrective lenses, hearing aids, and, if needed, amplifiers can ensure that accurate information is obtained. Also, normal age-associated cognitive changes result in slower processing of information and psychomotor speed [8]. This can present as benign word-finding delays. The individual who is interviewing an older adult needs to be aware of these differences compared to younger patients and convey patience to the older adult whom he or she is interviewing. It is helpful to provide additional time for completion of the geriatric assessment. Also, conducting the interview in a quiet room can help to minimize distractions.

Stigma associated with mental illness is a significant barrier among older Americans. Negative attitudes held by society and the individual themselves can impact a person's willingness to share information or seek help. Accordingly, older patients may be more hesitant to acknowledge or provide information regarding psychiatric symptoms and therefore require more sensitivity when eliciting symptoms. Older adults underutilize mental health services compared with other age groups, are more likely to receive mental health care in primary care settings, and tend to engage in mental health treatment if integrated into primary care [9]. Primary care providers especially may have to carve out longer appointment times or employ a collaborative care team approach to help support meeting the needs of their geriatric patients.

The Role of Collateral Informants

In geriatric assessment, the inclusion of collateral informants, who may be a family member, paid caregiver, or residence staff member, will help the interdisciplinary geriatric team to gather a complete picture of the person's history and current condition, especially in situations in which the older adult is unable to provide the information due to cognitive impairment. It is advisable to meet separately with the older individual prior to including an informant to build rapport, promote the patient's autonomy, and provide an opportunity to address concerns in a confidential setting. Providing protected time and space with the older adult alone at some time during the assessment provides the patient an opportunity to respond to questions about sensitive issues such as potential suicidal ideation, elder mistreatment, or past trauma history, without fear or undue influence from others. There may be times when the provider will have to set firm boundaries if, at any time during the encounter, it becomes apparent that a family member, caregiver, or other support person is dominating the interview or acting in a way that is dismissive of the older adult or the older adult does not appear comfortable speaking up. In these situations, the provider should request that the support person step out so that the provider can continue the encounter alone with the older adult.

Along these lines, it can be helpful to also allow collateral informants an opportunity to share their concerns and observations privately in case there are similar safety or sensitive concerns. Some family or caregivers may not feel comfortable speaking of their concerns otherwise for fear of upsetting the older adult. Ideally, an interdisciplinary team would increase opportunities for open communication and support of the older adult and their family or caregivers. The DSM-5 supplementary modules to the core cultural formulation interview have one designed for caregivers [6]. It allows for ascertaining the cultural context of caregiving by addressing the following categories: (1) nature of relationship, (2) caregiving activities and cultural perceptions of caregiving, (3) social context of caregiving, and (4) clinical support for caregiving.

History of Present Illness

Obtaining a thorough history is the first and most important aspect of the assessment. Though many older people have intact cognition, others may not. In either situation, remember to involve a collateral informant when able.

When eliciting the history, it can be helpful to hear from the older adult patient her or his understanding of the purpose of the visit. Empathic listening can help facilitate developing rapport and trust during the encounter. Generally, providing some time in the beginning to let the patient speak without interruption can give the provider a sense of what the patient perceives as her or his most pressing concerns. Sometimes the older adult patient may not be aware of the reason for the visit, and one can reorient the individual about the purpose to determine if it helps jog her or his memory or if she or he has some insight about the concerns. However, another approach to help facilitate rapport when it becomes clear that the individual has little insight or concerns about the referring problem can be to explore personal and social history before delving into more sensitive issues.

Ideally, a history of present illness will provide a clear course of the symptoms (onset and frequency) and their relationship with other health, medication, personal, and social factors. Taking a systematic approach to explore the presenting problem or symptoms includes an exploration of timeline and precipitating, aggravating, or potentially protective factors or stressors. This approach should determine whether and how the symptoms impact daily quality of life and functioning to meet criteria for established psychiatric disorders. Some conditions like Alzheimer's disease tend to follow an insidious and gradually progressive course, whereas other conditions, like depression, are more likely to be episodic. The DSM-5 provides an established approach to diagnosis of mental disorders and can help guide the types of symptoms to explore during interview [10].

Moreover, due to higher risk for medical comorbidities and medication use in older adults, this approach helps to also inform the provider whether the problem is secondary to another medical condition, medication or substance use. For instance, the presence of delirium or medical/iatrogenic conditions could be a source of an acute condition. Older adults are at much greater risk for developing delirium [5], and even relatively minor metabolic or infectious conditions can precipitate alterations in mental status or precipitate psychiatric sequelae. Given the longevity of many symptoms and the presence of more than one medical and psychiatric condition, careful delineation of the multiple complaints is necessary to understand the different syndromes and their potential interplay. Additionally, some conditions like neurocognitive disorders can be associated with changes in personality, so it can be helpful to determine premorbid personality characteristics and whether there have been any changes.

In general, providers must pay attention to safety concerns such as whether the older adult has been experiencing hopelessness, passive death ideation, or suicidal ideation. There are different assessment tools that have been validated to identify older adults who are at risk and aid providers to help stratify suicide risk between passive and more active suicidal ideation and behaviors [11]. Further discussion of suicide screens can be found in Chap. 12. Assessing access to lethal means for suicide (e.g., access to firearms) is important. Additionally, use of alcohol or other psychoactive drugs that can be associated with impulsivity and disinhibition, presence of psychotic symptoms or violent thoughts, or homicidal ideation is part of the comprehensive geriatric psychiatry assessment.

Psychiatric and Substance Use History

While most psychiatric illnesses present prior to the age of 60 years, older individuals may develop psychiatric illnesses later in life [12]. In either case, medical/iatrogenic contributors should first be ruled out as the cause of the psychiatric symptoms. When gathering the psychiatric history, collect as much information about the onset of symptoms, the frequency and duration of symptoms, past treatments and response (psychopharmacological, other biologic treatments like electroconvulsive treatment, as well as nonpharmacological approaches like psychotherapy), past hospitalizations, and past suicidal and aggressive behaviors.

Though alcohol and substance use is not as frequent among older persons than in the younger population, the rates of use are increasing as the baby boomer generation ages. The National Survey on Drug Use and Health (NSDUH) revealed from 2005 to 2014 increase in alcohol use disorders in older adults, including in females [13]. Providers should keep in mind that at least one in four older adults is prescribed a psychoactive medication with abuse potential and that these numbers are expected to increase [14]. Given the substantial number of people affected by substance use in the geriatric population, screening for these conditions is essential. Screening instruments validated in older adults and additional assessment approaches for alcohol and substance use disorders are reviewed in Chap. 20.

Establishing a timeline of lifetime exposure to alcohol, drug, or other psychoactive medications with potential for misuse and relationship with behavioral or psychiatric symptoms and functioning can help inform potential substance-induced psychiatric diagnoses, as substance use problems can contribute to secondary anxiety, mood, psychotic, and neurocognitive disorders.

Medical History

Older adults have more comorbid multiple medical illnesses, and these illnesses can directly result in neuropsychiatric symptoms or exacerbate previously existing psychiatric disorders. As well, psychiatric disorders can increase risk for medical or neurologic diseases or complicate treatment for these conditions. More detailed review of the associations among medical and neurologic disorders and behavioral or psychiatric conditions in later life can be found in Chaps. 32–34.

Special attention should be paid to acute changes in medical illnesses that can result in delirium. Depending on the practice setting (i.e., intensive care unit, medical or surgical acute hospitalization, or outpatient clinic), one could consider implementing different delirium screens and assessment tools as part of an evaluation [15]. An assessment of pain and treatments received for pain is essential as approximately 60–75% of older adults have complaints of chronic pain, and persistent pain has been associated with higher rates of depression, sleep disturbance, and suicidal ideation [16]. Also, many older adults with chronic pain are prescribed psychoactive medications.

TABLE 9-2. Common geriatric syndromes

Apathy
Cognitive impairment (delirium, dementia)
Falls
Frailty
Incontinence
Malnutrition
Mood disturbance
Pain
Sensory impairment
Sleep disturbance
Polypharmacy and inappropriate prescribing
Pressure sores

Table 9-2 highlights common geriatric syndromes that can either contribute to behavioral or psychiatric problems or can be complications of psychiatric disorders or its management. Screening for these is part of a comprehensive geriatric assessment [17].

The American Geriatrics Society has published a Geriatrics Evaluation and Management Tools (GEMS) mobile app to aid providers caring for older adults to manage several geriatric syndromes, including assessment and management of behavioral disturbances in dementia, delirium, and depression, among several others [18].

Medications

Medication reconciliation is of much greater importance in older adults since they are prescribed more medications than younger adults and they are more prone to adverse side effects, cognitive and functional impairments, poorer health outcomes, and higher costs [19]. Providers should be aware of the 2015 American Geriatrics Society's Beers Criteria [20]. The Beers Criteria provide guidelines for potentially inappropriate medications to be avoided in older adults in general and in older adults with certain diseases and syndromes in which drugs can exacerbate the disease or syndrome. Also, it provides guidelines for medications that are to be used with caution among older adults or for which dose adjustment is required based on kidney function and medications that can result in drug-drug interactions. A review of potential psychoactive effects of various medications is beyond the scope of this chapter; however, a thorough review of issues related to pharmacology and psychopharmacology can be found in Chap. 25.

The medication reconciliation should include assessment of over-the-counter medications and supplements as well as any "borrowed" medications. Asking the older adult to bring their medication bottles and reviewing how he or she takes one's medications can enhance medication reconciliation. During discussion of medication use, it may become apparent that the older adult is experiencing cognitive or other challenges with self-administering her or his medications, and this can be an opportunity to address barriers. Exploration of adopted strategies (e.g., charting, pillboxes) or willingness to try different memory-cuing approaches can help facilitate adherence. Some older adults rely on family or other caregivers such as visiting nurses or residential facility nurses to help with administration of their medications, and in such circumstances, any recommended changes must be shared with caregivers. In general, it is standard practice to provide all changes to medications in writing along with possible, common, or concerning side effects.

Family History

A family psychiatric history provides essential information regarding genetic vulnerability for certain illnesses. If there is a history of psychiatric illness in family members, asking about medications that have been helpful to family members is important as the older adult may also respond to the same medication. A family member's illness course and history of suicidal behaviors may provide additional insights and inform risks to help care for the older adult. People with family psychiatric history will likely present at a younger age compared to those who do not have a family history. Some disorders, like Alzheimer's disease, more commonly present later in life and establishing a family history of Alzheimer's disease or dementia, can help inform risk. Though many seniors may present for the first time with psychiatric symptoms at an older age, they may have been experiencing symptoms for several years.

Developmental History

Depending on the person's cognitive function, obtaining a developmental history may be challenging as children and spouses may not have as much information about an older person's early developmental experiences. Nonetheless, childhood experiences, years of schooling, any perceived or formally diagnosed history of learning disability or ADHD during early schooling, relationships with parents, and exposure to abuse, neglect, or trauma are all necessary to understand a person's psychological strengths and vulnerabilities. This information can help a clinician better appreciate the patient's perspectives and treatment goals.

Social History

The social history is a varied collection of information related to the older person's social circumstances and well-being. The elements of the social history can be found in Table 9-3. The evaluation of an older adult's late-life development is essential, and a more detailed review of common challenges such as bereavement and retirement can be found in Chap. 1.

Ultimately the social history should forge an understanding of the person as a whole. Paired with an assessment of personality traits, strengths, and coping strategies, it creates a psychosocial context for the biologically related complaints and conditions. Frequently, barriers to implementation of behavioral changes and adherence to treatment recommendations can be understood in the context of an individual's psychosocial history (e.g., an older adult not taking prescribed medications due to severe financial

Table 9-3. Social history

Relationships (e.g., marital status, children, sexual orientation, support network)
Living arrangements (to include caregiving supports and transportation)
Work history (including retirement)
Financial status
Affiliations with social organizations, religious/spiritual practices
Recreational activities
Losses (family, friends, possessions, functional ability) or recent transitions
Legal issues (e.g., driving infractions, divorce)
Advance directives and preferences for future care needs

barriers, an older adult not engaging in behavioral therapy if the recommended treatments do not align with her or his personal values or motivation for change).

When attempting to engage with a patient and establish rapport, exploring what the older adult finds meaningful can provide a foundation to develop and negotiate an approach to treatment that the patient finds acceptable. Kunik proposed asking geriatric patients five questions during the clinical assessment to help assess what gives the patient meaning in life and purpose: (1) What gives your life purpose or meaning currently?, (2) What brings you enjoyment or pleasure in life?, (3) What are the most important relationships in your life right now?, (4) What role does religion or spirituality play in your life?, and (5) What are your current life goals [21]?

Caregiver and Family Considerations

Although formally, the older adult is the geriatric provider's patient, when older adults have caregivers or involved family, optimal care and interventions will address family and caregivers' needs in therapeutic interventions. Therefore, as part of a comprehensive geropsychiatric assessment, the provider will need to assess also the caregiver or family for possible depression, stress, or unmet needs. Assessment of the older adult's family can help providers better understand long-established family dynamics, communication, and conflict management tendencies that may impact the care of the older adult, potentially pose barriers to implementation of interventions, or help resolve conflict [22]. Several caregiver assessment tools are available [23]. The Zarit Caregiver Burden Interview's 12-item short-version and 4-item screen have been validated to identify caregivers of older adults at risk [24]. More details regarding the role of caregivers and family supports and potential needs can be found in Chap. 4.

Routine screening for caregiver distress can help providers facilitate referrals for supportive services for caregivers or family members, including referrals to their primary care providers, social work consults to link with additional in-home or community supports, or referrals for psychotherapy and counseling. The National Alliance for the Mentally Ill (NAMI, www.nami.org) provides support to family members and caregivers for those with mental illness, while the Alzheimer's Association (www.alz.org) provides support for family members and caregivers for those with dementia.

Conclusion

A comprehensive interview of an older adult is essential to inform appropriate diagnosis and treatment. It is essential to establish rapport and address any potential barriers that could interfere with the interview. Providing a quiet space to minimize distractions, along with an adequate amount of time to complete the assessment, is essential for success. In addition to being aware of normal age-associated changes in information processing and psychomotor speed as well as higher risks for cognitive and sensory impairments that can impact the quality of the interview, providers need to be able to gather complex histories that encompass interactive psychiatric, psychological, medical, and social histories over the life span. Obtaining additional history from collateral informants can provide further information, especially in cases when the older adult has cognitive impairment. However, providers need to be sensitive to issues related to autonomy and confidentiality and managing potential patient and family or caregiver dynamics during the encounter. Finally, in many situations when working with an older adult, the provider will be caring not just for the older adult patient, but also providing support for her or his caregiver or family. It is helpful to remember to assess for possible caregiver depression, stress, or unmet needs to minimize potential barriers to care and optimally care for the older adult.

References

1. Howell T. The Wisconsin star method: understanding and addressing complexity in geriatrics. In: Malone ML, Capezuti E, Palmer RM, editors. Geriatrics models of care: bringing "best practices" to an aging America. 1st ed. Switzerland: Springer International Publishing; 2015. p. 87–94.
2. The Wisconsin Geriatric Psychiatry Initiative. WI STAR Method. https://wgpi.wisc.edu/wisconsin-star-method/. Accessed 4 Sept 2017.
3. Forester BP, Gatchel JR. Medical co-morbidity, brain disease, and the future of geriatric psychiatry. Am J Geriatr Psychiatry. 2014;22:1061–5. https://doi.org/10.1016/j.jagp.2014.08.007.
4. Bartels SJ, Pratt SI, Mueser KT, et al. Long-term outcomes of a randomized trial of integrated skills training and preventive healthcare for older adults with serious mental illness. Am J Geriatr Psychiatry. 2014;22:1251–61. https://doi.org/10.1016/j.jagp.2013.04.013.
5. Inouye SK, Westendorp RGJ, Saczynski JS. Delirium in elderly people. Lancet. 2014;383:911–22. https://doi.org/10.1016/S0140-6736(13)60688-1.
6. American Psychiatric Association. Diagnostic and statistical manual of mental disorders. 5th ed. Washington, DC: American Psychiatric Association; 2013. https://doi.org/10.1176/appi.books.9780890425596. CulturalFormulation. Accessed 4 Sept 2017.
7. Swenor B, Guralnik JM, Ferrucci L, Swenor B, Guralnik JM, Ferrucci L, Bonnielin S, et al. Demography and epidemiology. In: Halter JB, Ouslander JG, Studenski S, High KP, Asthana S, Supiano MA, Ritchie C, Halter JB, Ouslander JG, Studenski S, High KP, Asthana S, Supiano MA, Eds RC, Halter JB, et al., editors. Hazzard's geriatric medicine and gerontology. 7e New York, NY: McGraw-Hill; 2008. http://accessmedicine.mhmedical.com.ezproxy.library.wisc.edu/content.aspx?bookid=1923&ionid=144516968. Accessed 4 Sept 2017.
8. Harada CN, Natelson Love MC, Triebeld K. Normal cognitive aging. Clin Geriatr Med. 2013;29:737–52. https://doi.org/10.1016/j.cger.2013.07.002.
9. Bartels SJ, Coakley EH, Zubritsky C, et al. Improving access to geriatric mental health services: a randomized trial comparing treatment engagement with integrated versus enhanced referral Care for Depression, anxiety, and at-risk alcohol use. Am J Psychiatry. 2004;161:1455–62.
10. American Psychiatric Association. Diagnostic and statistical manual of mental disorders. 5th ed. Washington, DC: American Psychiatric Association; 2013. http://dsm.psychiatryonline.org/doi/full/10.5555/appi.books.9780890425596.ion2. Accessed 4 Sept 2017.
11. Raue PJ, Ghesquiere AR, Bruce ML. Suicide risk in primary care: Identification and Management in Older Adults. Curr Psychiatry Rep. 2014;16:466–73. https://doi.org/10.1007/s11920-014-0466-8.
12. Kessler RC, Amminger GP, Aguilar-Gaxiola S, et al. Age of onset of mental disorders: a review of recent literature. Curr Opin Psychiatry. 2007;20:359–64. https://doi.org/10.1097/YCO.0b013e32816ebc8c.
13. Han BH, Moore AA, Sherman S, et al. Demographic trends of binge alcohol use and alcohol use disorders among older adults in the United States, 2005-2014. Drug Alcohol Depend. 2017;170:198–207. https://doi.org/10.1016/j.drugalcdep.2016.11.003.
14. Simoni-Wastila L, Yang HK. Psychoactive drug abuse in older adults. Am J Geriatr Pharmacotherapy. 2006;4:380–94. https://doi.org/10.1016/j.amjopharm.2006.10.002.
15. Martins S, Simoes M, Fernandes L. Elderly delirium assessment tools review. Curr Psychiatr Rev. 2012;8:168–74. https://doi.org/10.2174/1573400511208020168.
16. Molton IR, Terrill AL. Overview of persistent pain in older adults. Am Psychol. 2014;69:197–207. https://doi.org/10.1037/a0035794.
17. Tran HT, Leonard SD. Geriatric assessment for primary care providers. Prim Care Clin Office Pract. 2017;44:399–411. https://doi.org/10.1016/j.pop.2017.05.001.
18. American Geriatrics Society Geriatrics Evaluation and Management Tools (GEMS) App. https://geriatricscareonline.org/ProductAbstract/ags-geriatrics-evaluation-management-tools-gems-app/B025/. Accessed 4 Sept 2017.
19. Maher RL, Hanlon JT, Hajjar ER. Clinical consequences of Polypharmacy in elderly. Expert Opin Drug Saf. 2014;13:57–65. https://doi.org/10.1517/14740338.2013.827660.
20. By the American Geriatrics Society 2015 Beers Criteria Update Expert Panel. American Geriatrics Society 2015 updated beers criteria for potentially inappropriate medication use in older adults. J

Am Geriatr Soc. 2015;63:2227–46. https://doi.org/10.1111/jgs.13702.
21. Kunik ME. Addressing purpose in life and meaning in the clinical setting. Am J Geriatr Psychiatry. 2016;24:715–6. https://doi.org/10.1016/j.jagp.2016.04.006.
22. King DA, Quill T. Working with families in palliative care: one size does not fit all. J Palliative Medicine. 2006;9:704–15. https://doi.org/10.1089/jpm.2006.9.704.
23. Van Durme T, Macq J, Jeanmart C, et al. Tools for measuring the impact of informal caregiving of the elderly: a literature review. Int J Nurs Stud. 2012;49:490–504. https://doi.org/10.1016/j.ijnurstu.2011.10.011.
24. Bedard M, Molloy W, Squire L, et al. The Zarit burden interview: a new short version and screening version. Gerontologist. 2001;41:652–7. https://doi.org/10.1093/geront/41.5.652.

Check for updates

10 Mental Status Examination

Ali Abbas Asghar-Ali and Lisa L. Boyle

The mental status exam is an assessment of the mental and emotional state of the person during the meeting. Like the physical exam, it plays a central role in the evaluation and understanding of a patient. Accordingly, it must be a part of a complete examination. While many aspects of the mental status exam will be similar across all age groups, when examining an older adult, the provider should be aware of some potential differences. Benign age-associated information processing and psychomotor slowing may erroneously lead an examiner to attribute observed changes in these areas to pathologic etiologies if one is not aware of these normal cognitive aging changes. Additionally, hearing or visual impairments, which occur more frequently as people age, may lead to an examiner to observe that a patient appears aloof, confused, or distracted which can lead to a broad differential diagnosis. However, it is important the examiner be able to recognize sensory impairment contributing to these findings on exam to facilitate appropriate management.

While some aspects of the mental status exam will require specific questions, most elements can be assessed over the course of the interview. We will review each of the items in a mental status exam below.

Mental Status Examination [1, 2]

Appearance

Pay attention to the person's grooming, dress, and physical features. Include features that are notable or contribute to an understanding of the person. For example, an elderly patient with depressive illness who is not eating and not attentive to his personal hygiene may present as "Dressed in soiled clothing, shirt unbuttoned; unshaven and hair in disarray; cachectic w/visible temporal wasting."

Behavior and Attitude

This describes the manner in which the person interacts with the clinician, e.g., "forthcoming and polite" or "guarded and distant."

Motor Activity

In younger adults, this may often be limited to a description of the degree of activity, i.e., retarded or increased (e.g., fidgety, pacing, twitching). However, in the elderly, there is an increased risk for neurologic changes that may manifest with motor findings. In the geriatric person, include

R. R. Tampi et al. (eds.), *Psychiatric Disorders Late in Life*, https://doi.org/10.1007/978-3-319-73078-3_10

a comment about tremors, hyperkinetic motor movements (dyskinesias), and gait. These are important in assessing medication side effects, concurrent neurologic illnesses, and safety. Further review of this topic can be found in Chap. 4E.

Speech

Speech can reveal both an emotional state and also neurologic findings. Document the rate, volume, tone (e.g., monotone), and spontaneity. For example, an older adult with dementia may have pronounced word-finding difficulties or exhibit paraphasic errors in speech. Further review of this topic can be found in Chap. 4E.

Mood

Mood is generally considered to be the internal state of a person that is sustained over time. It is often documented in the patient's words, though it does not always have to be explicitly elicited and may come up spontaneously in the interview.

Affect

Affect is a description of the person's physical manifestations of their emotional state. Affect is defined by six features: (1) general description (e.g., euthymic, elevated, dysphoric), (2) range (flat, blunted, constricted, full), (3) stability (stable vs. labile), (4) appropriateness (degree to which affect matches the content of the thoughts being conveyed), (5) intensity (the depth or degree of the emotions), and (6) congruency (whether the affect is congruent or incongruent with the stated mood). A person in the midst of a depressive episode may present as "Dysthymic, blunted, stable, appropriate, increased intensity, congruent with mood."

Though Process

Thought process is usually described using one of the following terms: (1) goal directed (thoughts flow coherently from one point to another), (2) circumstantial (thoughts are often convoluted and meandering though ultimately answer the posed question; may be seen in persons with mild cognitive impairment), (3) flight of ideas (rapidly shifting, connected thoughts in the context of pressured speech; commonly seen in persons experiencing mania), (4) loosening of associations (fragmented thoughts with no discernible connections between thoughts; commonly seen in persons experiencing psychosis or moderate degrees of neurocognitive compromise), or (5) word salad (individual words seemingly unconnected; rare and if observed, it is typically in context of delirium or significant language impairment).

Thought Content

Suicidality, homicidality, and disturbances in thoughts (delusions and obsessions) are recorded in this section.

For suicidality, it is best to ask these questions directly but with empathy as many people experience great shame in disclosing suicidal thoughts. First assess whether suicidal thoughts are present. If present, these may be passive, i.e., believing that one would be better off dead, or active, i.e., a desire to end one's life. If suicidality is present, assess for a plan for harming or killing herself or himself and access to the means of executing the plan. For example, the plan may be shoot herself or himself, and the patient has access to a loaded gun at home. Finally, assess for intent to enact the plan. You may ask "have you ever shot yourself," or "how close have you come to shooting yourself." Developing a suicide safety plan which includes means restriction with the older adult is critically important. Conti et al. have provided a step-by-step manual for safety planning with older adults [3]. Various suicide screening tools have been developed [4], and adopting such tools can be helpful as part of the geropsychiatric assessment [5]. Chapter 4D will review suicide screens in older adults.

Delusions in the elderly occur most commonly in those experiencing psychotic features as a part of a major depressive disorder in which case the delusions are often nihilistic or as a part of neuropsychiatric symptoms due to a major neurocognitive disorder. In the latter situation, phantom boarder, delusions of jealousy, and persecutory delusions are most common.

Perceptions

Hallucinations and illusions are recorded in this section of the mental status exam. Hallucinations in the elderly, especially visual hallucinations, are concerning for delirium. Dementia with Lewy bodies is also often known to manifest with visual hallucinations. Additional types of hallucinations can be olfactory and tactile.

Judgment

Judgment refers to the older adult's ability to make informed decisions about their life, including health and finances. As noted with other elements of the mental status exam, judgment should be assessed throughout the interview. Additional collateral data may need to be collected to objectively determine judgment.

Insight

Insight is defined as the degree of the patient's understanding of his or her condition (illnesses and their impact).

Both judgment and insight can be impaired by alterations in mood, thought processes or content (as seen in psychotic disorders), and cognition. When there is concern for impairment in judgment, or insight, the physician should assess the reason for the impairment and whether the patient has decisional capacity to manage her or his healthcare.

Cognition

For many younger patients, cognition is not evaluated formally beyond whether the patient appears to be alert and able to provide reliable history. Commonly, providers will screen for orientation at the most basic level. However, for the older adult, it is important to systematically establish cognitive functioning.

In brief, the cognitive domains include alertness, attention, orientation, executive function, abstraction, memory, language, and visuospatial processing. Additionally, providers should be aware that sensory impairments (e.g., hearing or vision loss) can impact performance on cognitive tests and consider these impairments in their interpretation of findings. The approach to cognitive screening will be reviewed in Chap. 4D.

Conclusion

The mental status exam in an older adult generally follows the same approach one would take with a younger adult with the exception that the examiner needs to be sensitive to potential cognitive and sensory changes and provide accommodations if needed. Additionally, due to higher prevalence and risk of neurocognitive disorders in older adults, assessment of the cognitive part of the mental status exam needs to be more comprehensive.

References

1. Cole SA, Bird J. Mental Status. In: Cole SA, Bird J, editors. The medical interview: the 3 function approach. 3rd ed. Philadelphia, PA: Elsevier Saunders; 2014. p. 93–7.
2. Shea SC. The mental status: how to perform and document it effectively. In: Shea SC, editor. Psychiatric interviewing: the art of understanding. 3rd ed. New York, NY: Elsevier; 2017. p. 662–81.
3. https://www.mirecc.va.gov/VISN16/new_and_featured_products.asp. Accessed 28 Sept 2017.
4. O'Connor E, Gaynes B, Burda BU, Williams C, Whitlock EP. Screening for suicide risk in primary care: a systematic evidence review for the U.S. preventive services task force. Evidence synthesis no. 103. AHRQ publication no. 13–05188-EF-1. Agency for Healthcare Research and Quality: Rockville, MD; 2013.
5. Raue PJ, Ghesquiere AR, Bruce ML. Suicide risk in primary care: identification and Management in Older Adults. Curr Psychiatry Rep. 2014;16:466–73. https://doi.org/10.1007/s11920-014-0466-8.

11
Functional Assessment

Lisa L. Boyle

The provider should assess functioning as part of a comprehensive geropsychiatric assessment and consider reviewing functional status with older patients at follow-up appointments and at minimum, annually. In general, late-life developmental challenges such as retirement or loss of a spouse or elderly friends can pose challenges when assessing impact of psychiatric symptoms on social and occupational functioning. However, it can be helpful to establish current day-to-day functioning and compare with premorbid functioning. One can ask about the context of retirement to help determine whether the transition to retirement was volitional or caused by mental or physical health problems. Additionally, for isolated elderly who live alone or lack access to easy transportation, assessment of social functioning can be challenging.

There are well-established approaches to assessing daily functioning, and the most commonly used are the Katz Index for Independence in Activities of Daily Living (ADL) [1] and the Lawton Instrumental Activities of Daily Living (IADL) Scale [2].

ADL refers to activities that focus on basic personal care, compared with IADL referring to more complicated and cognitive tasks to support independent living. ADL and IADL should be assessed in the context of both psychiatric and medical history taking. For instance, it is helpful to gather self-report from the older adult about one's functioning. Unfortunately, older adults with neurocognitive disorders and limited insight may overestimate their ability to care for one self independently, and this may not come to light unless collateral information is available. Therefore, comparing self-report with report from a collateral informant, when available, is advisable. Also, it can be helpful to obtain opinions whether any impairment in her or his ability to perform ADL or IADL functions is due to cognitive, psychological (e.g., from amotivational symptoms of depression or avoidance due to anxiety), or physical or sensory impairment challenges.

The Katz ADL scale [1] assesses six areas of functioning, including bathing, dressing, toileting, transferring, continence, and feeding, and whether the individual can perform these independently. Scores range from 0 to 6, with scores of 2 or less revealing severe functional impairment, compared with scores of 3–4 revealing moderate impairment, and scores of 6 indicating full functioning.

The Lawton IADL scale [2] assesses more complex functioning and surveys eight areas, including ability to use the telephone, shopping, food preparation, housekeeping, laundry, mode of transportation, responsibility for own medications, and ability to handle finances. Given potential for cultural or gender differences, it can help to establish whether the older adult ever historically participated in the tasks (e.g., food preparation, housekeeping) to determine whether he or she has experienced a decline in functioning. Scores range from 0 to 8, with lower scores associated with

R. R. Tampi et al. (eds.), *Psychiatric Disorders Late in Life*, https://doi.org/10.1007/978-3-319-73078-3_11

lower functioning and higher degrees of dependency and higher scores associated with higher functioning and higher degrees of independence.

An additional tool to screen for risk for physical disability includes the Short Physical Performance Battery Protocol (SPPB). The SPPB consists of a brief series of three tests that include balance (side-by-side, semi-tandem standing, and tandem stand) (score range 0–4), walking speed (score range 0–4), and chair stand test (score range 0–4). It results in a composite score (range 0–12) that stratifies physical disability and has been associated with disability, nursing home placement, and mortality [3, 4]. Scores <10 have been shown to identify seniors at risk for all-cause mortality [5].

Frailty is a geriatric syndrome that is associated with muscle weakness, fatigue, slowed walking, and reduced weight and physical activity and associated with poorer outcomes such as falls, slower recovery times, and increased dependency, disability, and mortality [6]. The Vulnerable Elders Survey (VES-13) provides a risk assessment for frailty [7]. The VES-13 screens age, perceived health status, and difficulty performing physical activities such as stopping, crouching, or kneeling, lifting or carrying objects as heavy as ten pounds, reaching or extending arms above shoulder level, writing or handling and grasping small objects, walking a quarter of a mile, and heavy housework such as scrubbing floors or washing windows. Also, it asks about whether impairments from health or physical conditions interfere with five functional tasks (shopping, managing finances, walking across a room, doing light housework, and bathing or showering). Positive screens can inform degree of vulnerability risk and guide additional assessment including possible referrals to nutrition, physical, or occupational therapy to optimize nutrition and strength.

In situations when individual or collateral self-report does not align or there is discrepancy between the examination and reported functioning, providers may need additional objective information to augment the assessment of an older adult. Commonly, this occurs in situations of suspected cognitive impairment. It can be helpful to refer to neuropsychology, speech, occupational therapy, physical therapy, audiology, or nutritional services to complete additional cognitive or functional assessments. Referral for behind-the-wheel driving assessment may be helpful [8].

Conclusion

The geriatric mental health provider needs to be well-versed with various approaches to assess functioning in her or his older adult patient. Beyond self-report, obtaining additional collateral informant report and objective bedside assessment can help supplement understanding of an older adult's functional impairments, risk for disability and poor health outcomes, and potential targets for intervention. Additionally, one can consider further referral to neuropsychology, speech, occupational therapy, physical therapy, audiology, or nutritional services for additional evaluation and management.

References

1. Katz S, Ford AB, Moskowitz RW, et al. Studies of illness in the aged. The index of ADL: a standardized measure of biological and psychosocial function. JAMA. 1963;185:914–9.
2. Lawton MP, Brody EM. Assessment of older people: self-maintaining and instrumental activities of daily living. Gerontologist. 1969;9:179–86.
3. Guralnik JM, Simonsick EM, Ferrucci L, et al. A short physical performance battery assessing lower extremity function: association with self-reported disability and prediction of mortality and nursing home admission. J Gerontol. 1994;49:M85–94. https://doi-org.ezproxy.library.wisc.edu/10.1093/geronj/49.2.M85.
4. Corsonello A, Lattanzio F, Pedone C, et al. Prognostic significance of the short physical performance battery in older patients discharged from acute care hospitals. Rejuvenation Res. 2012;15:41–8. https://doi.org/10.1089/rej.2011.1215.
5. Pavasini R, Guralnik J, Brown JC, et al. Short physical performance battery and all-cause mortality: systematic review and meta-analysis. BMC Med. 2016;14:215–23. https://doi.org/10.1186/s12916-016-0763-7.
6. Fried LP, Tangen CM, Walston J, et al. Frailty in older adults: evidence for a phenotype. J Gerontol A Biol Sci Med Sci. 2001;56:M146–56.
7. Saliba D, Elliott M, Rubenstein LZ, et al. The vulnerable elders survey: a tool for identifying vulnerable older people in the community. J Am Geriatr Soc. 2001;49:1691–9. https://doi.org/10.1046/j.1532-5415.2001.49281.x.
8. Pomidor A, editor. Clinician's guide to assessing and counseling older drivers. 3rd ed. New York: The American Geriatrics Society; 2015. https://geriatricscareonline.org/ProductAbstract/clinicians-guide-to-assessing-and-counseling-older-drivers-3rd-edition/B022. Accessed 4 Sept 2017.

12 Psychological and Neuropsychological Testing

Lisa L. Boyle

Geriatric mental health providers have several tools available to help characterize older adults' personality traits, along with screens for depression, suicidal ideation, anxiety, trauma, and bipolar disorder. Some of these tools also can be helpful to track treatment response. This section will review additional diagnostic tools that can be used to supplement the geriatric mental health provider's history taking and exam. Regardless of the tools used, it is important that providers understand the patient's cognitive functioning to validly interpret the results. Normal age-associated cognitive changes and commonly used cognitive assessment tools to help identify abnormal changes consistent with dementia during bedside testing will be reviewed. Some patients may need further, more detailed psychometric assessment, and especially in situations when there is diagnostic uncertainty, comorbid mood or other psychiatric conditions that may confound cognitive assessment, or lack of treatment response, patients can be referred to neuropsychology.

Personality and Psychological Assessment

In concert with understanding an older adult's development and social history, an understanding of an individual's personal strengths and values, characterological or personality traits, and coping strategies when faced with loss or stress is invaluable. Generally, collection of this data may take some time and may not be apparent in the initial evaluation but unfold as the therapeutic relationship builds. These data usually will not be readily apparent from chart review of traditional medical records. If using the Wisconsin Star Method [1], this information would be recorded under the personal arm of the star and is essential to help inform potential therapy approaches.

The NEO Five-Factor Inventory [2] is a tool that has been developed that assesses five different personality characteristics: neuroticism (vs. emotional stability), extraversion (vs. introversion), openness to experience (vs. closedness), agreeableness (vs. antagonism), and conscientiousness (vs. irresponsibility). It is self-administered and has been used in older adults. Certain personality traits have been found to be associated with increased health services utilization [3]. Also, certain personality traits, such as higher conscientiousness, may be protective and have been associated with lower mortality risk [4], while higher neuroticism in older adults has been associated with higher risk for medication nonadherence [5]. Low conscientiousness, low openness to experience, and high neuroticism have been associated with higher risk for developing Alzheimer's disease [6].

Beyond gathering data through unstructured interview or the use of self-administered tools, the geriatric mental health provider may consider

R. R. Tampi et al. (eds.), *Psychiatric Disorders Late in Life*, https://doi.org/10.1007/978-3-319-73078-3_12

asking the patient to undergo further psychological assessment with a psychologist, especially in cases that are atypical in presentation, or if there is diagnostic uncertainty or treatment resistance.

Depression

Patient self-administered screens can be helpful to identify seniors who have depression [7]. The following section will discuss options that are available in the public domain for free use. Two of the most commonly used screens in the clinical setting include the Geriatric Depression Scale (Short Form, GDS) [8] and the Patient Health Questionnaire (PHQ9) [9]. The GDS short form is a 15-item yes-no scale that focuses more on cognitive and non-neurovegetative symptoms of depression. Scores >5 points are considered positive and should be further evaluated.

The PHQ9, an alternative depressive screen also has been validated for use in older adults and has been widely used in primary care and collaborative care practices [7]. It consists of nine questions that assess the frequency of the nine symptoms found in the Diagnostic and Statistical Manual of Mental Disorders 5th Edition (DSM5) [10] criteria for major depression (each individually scored 0–3) and a final question asking how much the endorsed symptoms interfere with functioning (unscored). Total scores range from 0 to 27. Scores above 5 are considered a positive screen for depression, with 5–9 suggestive of mild depression, 10–14 suggestive of moderate depression, 15–19 suggestive of moderately severe depression, and 20 or above suggestive of severe depression. Providers should then follow up with additional interview questions and evaluation to verify the mood diagnosis. Protocols for treatment that utilize tracking PHQ9 response are common in collaborative care models of treatment of late-life depression in primary care settings. The PHQ2 is a shorter screen that asks about the two cardinal symptoms of depression: little interest or pleasure and feeling down, depressed or hopeless. It has also been validated for use in screening older adults for depression [11]. Positive PHQ2 screens should lead to completion of the full PHQ9 screen.

An additional option for a depression self-administered assessment tool is the Center for Epidemiologic Studies Depression (CESD) Scale [12]. The CESD is a 20-item scale that assesses the nine depressive symptoms found in the DSM5 and scores range from 0 to 60.

Generally, geriatric mental health providers need to recognize that evaluation of depression in patients with significant cognitive impairment or depression is challenged by several factors, including potential underreporting due to forgetfulness, reliance on caregiver report, and overlapping neurovegetative symptoms between dementia and depression [13]. Depressive screens may be limited for use in patients with severe cognitive impairment or dementia [14], so providers should assess cognitive status before interpreting results. The Cornell Scale for Depression in Dementia [15] is a validated depression assessment tool for patients with dementia. It consists of two semi-structured interviews (caregiver informant and the patient), takes about 20 min to complete, and has a caregiver-informant section along with a clinical assessment section. Scores are totaled, with <6 considered negative, >10 positive for probable major depression, and scores >18 definite major depression.

Suicide Screens in Older Adults

The US Preventive Services Task Force (USPSTF) found insufficient evidence to recommend routine screening for suicide in primary care [16]; however, when evaluating older adults for behavioral or psychiatric concerns, assessment for suicide risk is necessary. Psychiatric illness is the most robust risk factor for suicide in older adults. Poor health, impaired functioning, pain, loss of independence, and stressful life events have also been recognized, while social connectedness is felt to be a protective factor [17]. Generally, providers should ask about the presence of suicidal ideation, and if present, then evaluate the severity to inform safe treatment planning and disposition. If providers use standardized depression screens in their practice, then positive screens should be coupled with further assessment of suicidal ideation.

Raue and colleagues propose an approach that follows a hierarchical set of questions, starting with questions assessing passive suicide ideation and active suicide ideation; type of method, frequency, and persistence; and survey for life stressors, followed by specific suicide plan, intention to act, reasons for living, and impulse control [18].

The USPSTF assessed various tools such as a three-item screen that consists of "thoughts of death," "wishing you were dead," and "feeling suicidal" within the previous month, which had been used in a primary care population with older adult representation [16].

Heisel and colleagues found that the Geriatric Depression Scale (GDS), using a cutoff of four (sensitivity 0.754, specificity 0.815), along with an adapted version of the GDS consisting of five items from the GDS that included symptoms of feeling life is empty, worthlessness, and hopelessness and two questions about mood (GDS-SI) with cutoff of one, can help identify older adults with suicidal ideation in a primary care setting [19].

Other potential tools to assess for suicide ideation include the Columbia-Suicide Severity Rating Scale [20] and the P4 screener [21], which is a shorter screen that has been developed for use in primary care.

Anxiety, Trauma, and Bipolar Disorders

Assessment of anxiety disorders in older adults can be more challenging due to overlap of some somatic symptoms associated with other medical problems. Generalized anxiety disorder (GAD) is the most common anxiety disorder in late life [22]. Compared with depression, anxiety in older adults and screening tools to identify anxiety disorders in late life have not been as well studied [23]. The GAD-7 is a seven-item tool that maps to DSM criteria for GAD and can be used to screen for GAD, characterize symptom severity, and response to treatment [24]. Its use has been validated in older adults with a suggested lower cutoff of 5 (instead of 10), while the two-item GAD (GAD-2), which consists of the first two items of the GAD-7, should have a lower cutoff of 2 instead of 3 [23]. The 14-item Hamilton Anxiety Rating Scale (HAM-A) has been used to follow treatment response in anxiety intervention trials in older patients with GAD [25].

The DSM-5 re-categorized post-traumatic stress disorder (PTSD) to a new category, trauma- and stressor-related disorders. The self-report PTSD Checklist (PCL) has been used with older adults, and generally a lower cutoff is recommended [26].

Bipolar screening tools have not been developed specifically for older adults [27]. Tools to assess bipolar disorder have largely been validated in younger or mixed-age populations; however, several tools, such as the Young Mania Rating Scale, Montgomery-Asberg Depression Rating Scale, and the Clinical Global Impression-Bipolar Disorder, have been recently included in a multicenter clinical trial of mood stabilizers in late-life mania [28].

Normal Age-Associated Cognitive Changes

Cross-sectional and longitudinal studies of cognitive abilities across the life span support that there are normal age-associated cognitive changes that can be expected in healthy older adults [29]. With that said, there can also be heterogeneity in the degree in which older adults experience decline in their abilities. The geriatric mental health provider needs to be aware of what is likely to be normal benign cognitive changes compared with pathological changes in order to ensure appropriate diagnosis and management of cognitive concerns. Table 12-1 provides an overview of various cognitive domains, whether one can expect age-associated cognitive changes and potential clinical implications of these changes.

Adapted from: Harada CN, Natelson Love MC, Triebeld K. Normal Cognitive Aging. *Clin Geriatr Med.* 2013; 29:737–752. doi:https://doi.org/10.1016/j.cger.2013.07.002

TABLE 12-1. Normal age-associated cognitive changes [29]

Cognitive domain	Abilities	Age-associated changes	Clinical implications
Crystallized intelligence	Overlearned, well-practiced knowledge and skills (e.g., vocabulary, general knowledge)	Stable or gradually improved with age through the sixth or seventh decades	Accumulated wisdom can be a strength for an older adult.
Fluid intelligence	Problem-solving and reasoning in novel, less familiar situations (incorporates executive function, processing speed, memory, psychomotor)	Declines with age	May impact an older adult's ability to novel-problem solve or adapt to new situations as quickly as someone younger.
Processing speed (fluid)	Cognitive processing and motor response speed	Declines with age after third decade	Can impact other neuropsychological test results, older adults may need longer time to process information and complete an assessment or interview.
Attention (fluid)	Concentration, focus Simple attention: – Immediate recall (repeating string of numbers) Complex attention: – Selective attention: ability to focus on task when in distracting environment (conversation in loud restaurant) – Divided attention: focus divided while multitasking	Minimal change on simple attention tasks Complex attention declines with age.	Important to minimize distractions during the assessment. It can be helpful to counsel patients to focus on one task at a time before moving to the next task and avoid multitasking. Counsel family or caregivers to ensure full attention of the older adult when communicating.
Memory (fluid)	Ability to recall information Declarative (explicit) memory: – Conscious recall of events/ facts – Two types: 1. Semantic memory (fund of knowledge, such as meaning of words) 2. Episodic memory (autobiographical or personal memory)	Episodic memory declines over the life span. Semantic memory declines in later life.	Age-associated memory decline can be multifactorial (e.g., changes in processing speed, ability to disregard unrelated info, or utilizing less pro-memory/learning strategies). Some memory stages affected by aging
	Nondeclarative (implicit) memory: – Unconscious recall (outside of awareness) – Procedural memory (motor and cognitive, e.g., riding a bicycle)	Remains unchanged with age	– Decreased rate for encoding new memories with age – Preserved ability to retain newly learned information with age – Decreased access to stored memories (retrieval) with age
Language (crystallized > fluid)	Vocabulary	Stable/improves across life span	Words "on the tip of the tongue" more common in older adults
	Confrontation naming (e.g., object naming)	Initially stable but declines in later life (>70)	May take a little longer for older adults to express themselves in an interview
	Verbal fluency (e.g., categorical or letter naming)	Decreases with age	

Table 12-1 (continued)

Cognitive domain	Abilities	Age-associated changes	Clinical implications
Visuospatial construction (both crystallized and fluid)	Ability to conceptualize 2D/3D space		Abnormalities in visuospatial perception (e.g., fender benders or difficulties parking the car) should signal further work-up for etiology.
	Visual construction – Ability to assimilate parts to construct a comprehensive whole	Decreases with age	
	Visual spatial – Object perception: identify objects (e.g., familiar faces) – Spatial perception: how objects physically relate in space with each other	Stable with age	
Executive function (fluid)	Heterogeneous set of cognitive skills that facilitate independent functioning – Self-monitoring – Planning – Organization – Reasoning – Set-shifting/mental flexibility – Problem-solving	Aging (>70 years old) has been associated with decreases in: – Abstraction – Mental flexibility – Response inhibition – Slower if executive function task tied to motor speed – Inductive reasoning (starting >45 years old) – Reasoning for novel situations stable across life span – Recognizing similarities – Proverb interpretation – Reasoning for familiar situations	Executive dysfunction increases risk for inability to manage self-care, associated with decline in instrumental activities of daily living (IADL) [30].

Cognitive Screening

The USPSTF guidelines report that there is not enough evidence to support screening for cognitive impairment in community-dwelling populations 65 years and over [31]. However, if the geriatric mental health or primary care provider has clinical suspicion or if there are caregiver or patient concerns, further assessment is warranted.

Additionally, late-onset psychiatric disorders have high associations with neurocognitive disorders, so at-risk populations of older adults who present with behavioral or psychiatric concerns should have at minimum a brief cognitive assessment. Older adults with chronic mood disorders (i.e., depressive or bipolar disorder) or other psychiatric disorders (i.e., schizophrenia or PTSD) may be at higher risk for developing cognitive disorders later in life and should be considered for screening and baseline cognitive assessment.

There are a variety of cognitive screens that can be used in the office or inpatient setting. The Alzheimer's Association, in collaboration with a panel of dementia experts, has developed online resources for providers to use for cognitive assessment as part of the Medicare's Annual Wellness Visit in primary care [32]. They recognize that there is no "gold standard" tool for detection of cognitive impairment and recommend objective cognitive assessment. They include three options of validated patient-assessment cognitive screens, the mini-cog, the Memory Impairment Screen, and the General Practitioner Assessment of Cognition (GPCOG). All of these screens are brief (<5 min), validated, and comparable or superior to the MMSE for detection of dementia. They also include three options for informant-based cognitive screens: the short form of the Informant Questionnaire for Cognitive Decline in the Elderly (short-IQCODE), the 8-Item Informant Interview to Differentiate Aging and Dementia (AD8), and the GPCOG.

Commonly used bedside cognitive screens are listed in Table 12-2. This table is not considered all-inclusive.

When adopting a cognitive screen, it is essential to be familiar with what the screen was designed to detect (e.g., cortical dementia such as Alzheimer's disease vs. other subcortical types of dementia). An example of a bedside assessment tool that can help distinguish frontal type dementia from mild Alzheimer's disease is the Frontal Assessment Battery, with a cutoff of ≤12 suggestive of frontal dysexecutive type dementia (sensitivity 77%, specificity 87%) [39].

Scales, such as the Functional Assessment Staging Test (FAST) [40] and the Clinical Dementia Rating (CDR) Scale [41, 42], that characterize global assessment of functioning in dementia patients can be useful. The data collected from semi-structured interview of the patient and informant caregivers are used to complete these scales. The FAST has seven stages to characterize the course of Alzheimer's disease, ranging from no functional difficulties (stage 1) to severe impairments such as speaking less than

TABLE 12-2. Common cognitive screens

A.

	Mini-cog [33]	Mini-Mental State Exam (MMSE) [34]
Neurocognitive domains	Memory, executive function, perceptual-motor function	Orientation, memory, attention, language, and perceptual-motor function
Administration time	Approximately 3 min	Approximately 5–10 min
Materials required	Test and pen	Test and instructions, pen
Scoring	0–5, abnormal score <3 for dementia, can use cutoff of <4 if need higher sensitivity to refer patients for further assessment	0–30, abnormal score <24 for cognitive impairment, adjustments in score cutoff depending on age and education
Test characteristics	76% sensitivity and 89% specificity for dementia	Variable sensitivity and specificity data have been reported, depending on sample population and criteria
Additional considerations	Less associated with education, has been validated for use in primary care populations with different cultures and languages	Copyrighted, available for a fee. Designed to distinguish organic from functional cognitive impairment. Less useful to identify frontal executive dysfunction. Generally, well-established expectations for MMSE score decline and AD progression

B.

	Montreal Cognitive Assessment (MoCA) [35]	Saint Louis University Mental Status Exam (SLUMS) [37]
Neurocognitive domains	Orientation, memory, attention, executive function, language, and perceptual-motor function	Orientation, memory, attention, executive function, and language
Administration time	Approximately 10 min	Approximately 7 min
Materials required	Test and instructions, watch with second hand, pen	Test, watch with a second hand, pen

TABLE 12-2 (continued)

A.	Mini-cog [33]	Mini-Mental State Exam (MMSE) [34]
Scoring	0–30, add 1 point if high school education or less, <26 is abnormal for mild cognitive impairment or Alzheimer's disease	0–30, *Mild neurocognitive disorder:* 20–24 is abnormal for less than high school education; 21–26 is abnormal for high school *Dementia:* <20 for less than high school education; <21 for high school
Test characteristics	90% sensitivity for mild cognitive impairment and 100% for Alzheimer's disease; 87% specificity	*Mild neurocognitive disorder:* 92% sensitivity and 81% specificity for less than high school education; 95% sensitivity and 76% specificity for high school *Dementia:* 100% and 98% for less than high school education; 98% and 100% for dementia
Additional considerations	Free public use [36], multiple versions available (three English versions, several other languages, blind)	Free public use [38], only one version available

six words and inability to walk or sit without assistance (stage 7). The CDR is a 5-point scale that characterizes memory, orientation, judgment/problem-solving, community affairs, home and hobbies, and personal care. Scores range from 0 (normal) to 3 (severe dementia) and, like the FAST, can be used to track dementia progression.

Behavioral and psychological symptoms of dementia (BPSD) are nearly universal in dementia patients [43]. One of the most commonly used BPSD tools is the Neuropsychiatric Inventory (NPI) [44], and there is an abbreviated version, the NPI-Questionnaire (NPI-Q) [45] that can be used in clinical practice. The NPI assesses 12 neuropsychiatric symptoms, such as depression, apathy, motor disturbance, and nighttime behaviors. The shorter NPI-Q can be completed either by self-administration by a reliable informant or by the clinician based on informant interview. It assesses the 12 NPI domains as either present or absent. When symptoms are present, it then assesses severity (1–3, mild-severe) and degree of caregiver distress (0–5, not distressing—extreme or very severe distress).

Brief cognitive screens are not diagnostic tools but rather should be used in conjunction with a full examination and medical and neurologic work-up to assess for presence of a neurocognitive disorder. Patients may later be referred for formal neuropsychological testing that provides more definitive cognitive testing and can help establish diagnoses, though not every patient with cognitive complaints will need formal neuropsychological testing.

Neuropsychological Testing

As mentioned previously, the geriatric mental health provider may seek out additional neuropsychological assessment when there is diagnostic uncertainty, such as in a patient with cognitive complaints in the setting of major depression. Objective testing can help distinguish cognitive performance patterns that may be more consistent with depression than neurocognitive disorder. Additionally, one could consider referral when patients present with atypical features, such as early-onset Alzheimer's disease or to help differentiate dementia etiology (e.g., frontal temporal dementia from Alzheimer's disease) after the usual clinical assessment is not definitive. It can be helpful to consider also for patients with milder or early symptoms in which bedside cognitive screens may not yet pick up mild impairments but for whom the provider has clinical suspicion for neurocognitive disorder.

Neuropsychological testing also can help with treatment planning. Patients and their family can develop a better understanding of relative cognitive strengths and weaknesses to guide management strategies, such as whether to employ memory cuing or other environmental or communication strategies. Objective psychometrics also can help monitor progression of dementia or response to treatment (e.g., improvement in cognitive testing after successful treatment of depression). Neuropsychologists also may be asked to evaluate decision-making capacity or need for guardianship.

During a neuropsychological evaluation, the neuropsychologist interviews the patient and available informant (usually family member or caregiver). The neuropsychologist frequently incorporates the referral source; psychosocial, developmental, medical, and psychiatric histories; current social supports and current environmental demands; and significant other interviews into the assessment and complete mental status exam [46]. Evaluations include either the neuropsychologist or psychometrician assisting with the case, administration of measures assessing mood and affect, objective personality tests, and neuropsychological tests. Additional behavioral assessments, functional assessments, projective personality tests, and review of school and work records can also be considered [46].

Table 12-3 reviews specific cognitive domains frequently examined during neuropsychological assessments and common neuropsychological tests that may be utilized. It is not meant to be all-inclusive.

Table 12-3. Cognitive domains and examples of neuropsychological tests [47, 48]

Cognitive domain	Neuropsychological test(s) examples
Intelligence/intellectual function	*Premorbid intelligence*: Wechsler Adult Intelligence Scale-4th Edition (WAIS-IV) Vocabulary subtest; revised Wechsler Test of Adult Reading (WTAR), Test of Premorbid Functioning (TOPF) *Intellectual functioning*: WAIS-IV
Academic achievement	Woodcock-Johnson Achievement Test
Attention	*Simple auditory attention*: WAIS-IV Digit Span forward trials *Simple visual attention*: Trail Making Test A (Trails A)
Executive functions	*Processing speed*: Trails A; Symbol Digit Modalities Test (SDMT) *Simple auditory working memory*: WAIS-IV Digit span backwards trials; Serial 7's *Phonemic fluency*: Letter-cued verbal fluency *Simple visuospatial planning and Organization*: Clock drawing to request *Abstract verbal reasoning*: WAIS-IV Similarities subtest; Delis-Kaplan Executive Function System (D-KEFS) Proverbs Test *Impulse control*: D-KEFS Color-Word Inhibition Test; (original) Stroop Test *Mental flexibility/set-shifting*: Trail making test B (Trails B); D-KEFS Category Switching Accuracy *Complex problem-solving skills*: D-KEFS Tower Test; Wisconsin Card Sorting Test (WCST)
Language	*Basic receptive and expressive language skills*: Western Aphasia Battery-Revised (WAB-R); Boston Aphasia Diagnostic Examination III *Aural comprehension*: Ability to understand test instructions, by observation; Token Test *Object naming*: Boston Naming Test (BNT) *Word fluency*: Controlled Oral Word Association Test (name words beginning with specific letter within set time) *Semantic fluency*: Category-cued verbal fluency
Verbal learning and memory	*Verbal learning and memory of structured information (i.e., stories)*: Wechsler Memory Scale-4th Edition (WMS-IV) Logical Memory subtest *Verbal learning and memory of unstructured information (i.e., a word list)*: Hopkins Verbal Learning Test-Revised (HVLT-R); California Verbal Learning Test-2nd Edition (CVLT-II); Rey Verbal Learning Test
Visual learning and memory	WMS—Visual Memory Index; Rey Complex Figure Test (RCFT)
Visuoconstruction skills	WAIS-IV Block Design subset; Clock drawing to copy
Motor skills	*Fine motor speed*: Finger-tapping test *Fine motor coordination and speed*: Grooved Pegboard Test

Conclusion

Self- and provider-administered tools to help screen older adults at risk who need further assessment and to help providers track symptom severity and response to treatment for common psychiatric disorders in older adults are useful and can be implemented easily into routine practice. Normal age-associated cognitive changes affect several cognitive domains, and the geriatric psychiatrist needs to be familiar with these changes and how they can impact the approach to assessment compared with a younger adult. Objective cognitive screens have a role in routine geriatric psychiatry assessment, and there are several options to choose from. Though not every patient will require neuropsychology consultation, it can be useful for patients when there is diagnostic uncertainty and atypical presentations or to help inform treatment response and planning.

References

1. Howell T. The Wisconsin star method: understanding and addressing complexity in geriatrics. In: Malone ML, Capezuti E, Palmer RM, editors. Geriatrics models of care: bringing "Best Practices" to an aging America. 1st ed. Switzerland: Springer International Publishing; 2015. p. 87–94.
2. Costa PT, RR MC. Revised NEO Personality Inventory (NEO PI-R) and NEO Five-Factor Inventory (NEO FFI): professional manual. Odessa, FL: Psychological Assessment Resources; 1992.
3. Friedman B, Veazie PJ, Chapman BP, et al. Is personality associated with health care use by older adults? Milbank Q. 2013;91:491–527. https://doi.org/10.1111/1468-0009.12024.
4. Turiano NA, Chapman BP, Gruenewald TL, et al. Personality and the leading behavioral contributors of mortality. Health Psychol. 2015;34:51–60. https://doi.org/10.1037/hea0000038.
5. Jerant A, Chapman B, Duberstein P, et al. Personality and medication non-adherence among older adults enrolled in a six-year trial. Br J Health Psychol. 2011;16:151–69. https://doi.org/10.1348/135910710X524219.
6. Duberstein PR, Chapman BP, Tindle HA, et al. Personality and risk for Alzheimer's disease in adults 72 years of age and older: a 6-year follow-up. Psychol Aging. 2011;26:351–62. https://doi.org/10.1037/a0021377.
7. Smith M, Haedtke C, Shibley D. Late life depression detection: an evidence-based guideline. J Gerontol Nurs. 2015;41(2):18–25. https://doi.org/10.3928/00989134-20150115-99.
8. https://web.stanford.edu/~yesavage/GDS.html. Accessed 23 Sept 2017.
9. http://aims.uw.edu/resource-library/phq-9-depression-scale. Accessed 23 Sept 2017.
10. American Psychiatric Association. Diagnostic and Statistical Manual of Mental Disorders. 5th ed. Washington, DC: American Psychiatric Association; 2013.
11. Li MM, Friedman B, Conwell Y, et al. Validity of the patient health questionnaire 2 (phq-2) in identifying major depression in older people. J Am Geriatr Soc. 2007;55:596–602.
12. http://cesd-r.com/cesdr/. Accessed 23 Sept 2017.
13. Brown EL, Raue P, Halpert KD, et al. Evidence-based guideline detection of depression in older adults with dementia. J Gerontol Nurs. 2009;35(2):11–5.
14. Boyle LL, Richardson TM, He H, et al. How do the Phq-2, the Phq-9 perform in aging services clients with cognitive impairment? Int J Geriatr Psychiatry. 2011;26(9):952–60. https://doi.org/10.1002/gps.2632.
15. http://www.scalesandmeasures.net/files/files/The%20Cornell%20Scale%20for%20Depression%20in%20Dementia.pdf. Accessed 23 Sept 2017.
16. O'Connor E, Gaynes B, Burda BU, et al. Screening for suicide risk in primary care: a systematic evidence review for the U.S. Preventive Services Task Force. Evidence Synthesis No. 103. AHRQ Publication No. 13–05188-EF-1. Agency for Healthcare Research and Quality: Rockville, MD; 2013.
17. Conwell Y, Van Orden K, Caine ED. Suicide in Older Adults. Psychiatr Clin North Am. 2011;34:451–68. https://doi.org/10.1016/j.psc.2011.02.002.
18. Raue PJ, Ghesquiere AR, Bruce ML. Suicide risk in primary care: identification and management in older adults. Curr Psychiatry Rep. 2014;16:466–73. https://doi.org/10.1007/s11920-014-0466-8.
19. Heisel MJ, Duberstein PR, Lyness JM, et al. Screening for suicide ideation among older primary care patients. J Am Board Fam Med. 2010;23:260–9. https://doi.org/10.3122/jabfm.2010.02.080163.
20. http://cssrs.columbia.edu/. Accessed 24 Sept 2017.
21. Dube P, Kurt K, Bair MJ, et al. The P4 screener: evaluation of a brief measure for assessing potential suicide risk in 2 randomized effec-

tiveness trials of primary care and oncology patients. Prim Care Companion J Clin Psychiatry. 2010;12(6):PCC.10m00978. https://doi.org/10.4088/PCC.10m00978blu.
22. Lenze EJ, Wetherell JL. A lifespan view of anxiety disorders. Dialogues Clin Neurosci. 2011;13:381–99.
23. Wild B, Eckl A, Herzog W, et al. Assessing generalized anxiety disorder in elderly people using the GAD-7 and GAD-2 scales: results of a validation study. Am J Geriatr Psychiatry. 2014;22:1029–38. https://doi.org/10.1016/j.jagp.2013.01.076.
24. Spitzer RL, Kroenke K, Williams JB, et al. A brief measure for assessing generalized anxiety disorder: the GAD-7. Arch Intern Med. 2006;166:1092–7.
25. Wetherell JL, Ayers CR, Sorrell JT, et al. Modular psychotherapy for anxiety in older primary care patients. Am J Geriatr Psychiatry. 2009;17:483–92. https://doi.org/10.1097/JGP.0b013e3181a31fb5.
26. https://www.ptsd.va.gov/professional/treatment/older/assessment_tx_older_adults.asp. Accessed 24 Sept 2017.
27. Sajatovic M, Chen PJ. Geriatric bipolar disorder: epidemiology, clinical features, assessment, and diagnosis. Philadelphia: Wolters Kluwer Health. UpToDate: Feb 2012; updated on August 2016 www.uptodate.com. Accessed 24 Sept 2017.
28. Marino P, Schulberg HC, Gildengers AG, et al. Assessing bipolar disorder in the older adult: the GERI-BD toolbox. Int J Geriatr Psychiatry. 2017. https://doi.org/10.1002/gps.4738.
29. Harada CN, Natelson Love MC, Triebeld K. Normal cognitive aging. Clin Geriatr Med. 2013;29:737–52. https://doi.org/10.1016/j.cger.2013.07.002.
30. Royall DR, Palmer R, Chiodo LK, et al. Declining executive control in normal aging predicts change in fuctional status: the freedom house study. J Am Geriatr Soc. 2004;52:346–52. https://doi.org/10.1111/j.1532-5415.2004.52104.x.
31. Lin JS, O'Connor E, Rossom RC, et al. Screening for cognitive impairment in older adults: a systematic review for the U.S. preventive services task force. Ann Intern Med. 2013;159:601–12. https://doi.org/10.7326/0003-4819-159-9-201311050-00730.
32. Cordell CB, Borson S, Boustani M, et al. Alzheimer's association recommendations for operationalizing the detection of cognitive impairment during the medicare annual wellness visit in a primary care setting. Alzheimers Dementia. 2013;9:141–50.
33. Borson S, Scanlan JM, Chen P, et al. J Am Geriatr Soc. 2003;51:1451–4.
34. Tombaugh TN, McIntyre NJ. The mini-mental state examination: a comprehensive review. J Am Geriatr Soc. 40(40):922–35. https://doi.org/10.1111/j.1532-5415.1992.tb01992.x.
35. Nasreddine ZS, Phillips NA, Bédirian V, et al. The montreal cognitive assessment, MoCA: a brief screening tool for mild cognitive impairment. J Am Geriatr Soc. 53:695–9. https://doi.org/10.1111/j.1532-5415.2005.53221.x.
36. www.mocatest.org. Accessed 3 Sept 2017.
37. Tariq SH, Tumosa N, Chibnall JT, et al. Comparison of the Saint Louis University mental status exam. Am J Geriatr Psychiatry. 2006;14:900–10. https://doi.org/10.1097/01.JGP.0000221510.33817.86.
38. http://medschool.slu.edu/agingsuccessfully/pdfsurveys/slumsexam_05.pdf. Accessed 27 Sept 2017.
39. Dubois B, Slachevsky A, Litvan I, et al. The FAB: a frontal assessment battery at bedside. Neurology. 2000;55:1621–6. https://doi.org/10.1212/WNL.55.11.1621.
40. Reisberg B. Functional assessment staging. Psychopharmacol Bull. 1988;24:653–9.
41. http://knightadrc.wustl.edu/cdr/PDFs/CDR_Table.pdf. Accessed 24 Sept 2017.
42. Morris JC. The Clinical Dementia Rating (CDR): current version and scoring rules. Neurology. 1993;43:2412–4.
43. Lyketsos CG, Carrillo MC, Ryan JM, et al. Neuropsychiatric symptoms in Alzheimer's disease. Alzheimers Dement. 2011;7:532–9.
44. Cummings JL. The neuropsychiatric inventory: assessing psychopathology in dementia patients. Neurology. 1997;48(Suppl 6):S10–6.
45. Kaufer DI, Cummings JL, Ketchel P, et al. Validation of the NPI-Q, a brief clinical form of the neuropsychiatric inventory. J Neuropsychiatry Clin Neurosci. 2000;12:233–9. https://doi.org/10.1176/jnp.12.2.233.
46. Rabin LA, Barr WB, Burton LA. Assessment practices of clinical neuropsychologists in the United States and Canada: A Survey of INS, NAN, and APA division 40 members. Arch Clin Neuropsychol. 2005;20:33–65. https://doi.org/10.1016/j.acn.2004.02.005.
47. http://emedicine.medscape.com/article/317596-overview#a1. Accessed 24 Sept 2017.
48. Morris RG, Brookes RL. Neuropsychological assessment of older adults. In: Goldstein LH, McNeil JE, editors. Clinical neuropsychology: a practical guide to assessment and management for clinicians. United Kingdom: Wiley; 2013. p. 347–74.

13 Neurologic Examination

Lisa L. Boyle

Because of higher risk of neurologic disease, such as dementia, stroke, and movement disorders in the elderly, the neurologic exam is an important part of a geropsychiatric assessment. The level of detail to various sections of the neurologic exam may vary depending on the chief complaint. For instance, it may be a more focused exam with the evaluation of depression, while more comprehensive with the evaluation of depression in a patient with known Parkinson's disease or memory concerns. The components of the neurologic exam will be reviewed in this section. Additional demonstration of how to conduct the neurologic exam is beyond the scope of this chapter; however, resources demonstrating the neurologic exam can be found online [1].

As reviewed in Chap. 6, normal aging is associated with several changes in the brain, including loss of brain volume, reduced white matter density in areas of the brain, and changes in neurotransmitter levels that are involved with cognitive function and movement. Taken altogether, besides normal age-associated cognitive changes such as mild information processing slowing and decline in executive function [2], additional age-associated neurologic signs can be observed in motor and sensory domains as well. These changes include psychomotor slowing, reduced visual acuity and pupil size, reduced upgaze, reduced hearing (i.e., discrimination of spoken language), atrophy of muscles, reduced range of motion in the neck and back, gait changes such as reduced stride length and arm swing, reduced vibration sense and mild Romberg sway, and reduced Achilles reflexes [3–5]. A more detailed review of commonly encountered neurologic conditions and approaches to management in geriatric patients can be found in Chap. 32.

One should consider pairing the neurologic exam with the medical evaluation and focused physical exam when evaluating older adults for behavioral or psychiatric concerns. For example, in a patient whom one may be concerned for cardiovascular and cerebrovascular disease, a focused physical exam that also includes auscultation of the heart and carotid arteries would be helpful to evaluate for possible heart arrhythmia, murmur, or carotid bruit. Additionally, in a patient who presents with mental status changes, further assessment for possible delirium may lead to obtaining chest X-ray, urinalysis, and blood count to evaluate for a possible infectious etiology.

Neurologic Exam [1, 3, 5]

Mental status exam: The mental status exam and neuropsychological assessment were reviewed in Chaps. 10 and 12. Additional neurocognitive assessment can include evaluation of apraxia, anosognosia, hemi-neglect, testing of speech and language (e.g., decreased fluency suggestive of expressive impairment, decreased understanding of language or commands suggestive of receptive impairment), reading and writing, and calculations.

R. R. Tampi et al. (eds.), *Psychiatric Disorders Late in Life*, https://doi.org/10.1007/978-3-319-73078-3_13

Apraxia is the loss of ability to perform complex motor commands and tasks such as zipping a coat or using a fork and knife and can be assessed by asking the patient to pretend to perform tasks using imaginary tools. Anosognosia refers to reduced awareness of deficits. Hemi-neglect results in decreased attention to one side of the body, not caused by primary sensory or motor deficits. It can be evaluated by observing a patient neglecting to move one side of her or his body in the absence of focal weakness. Alternatively, a patient with hemi-neglect may not detect touch on the affected side if presented with stimulus touch bilaterally, but can discriminate touch on the affected side if presented with stimulus touch only on that side. Assessment for hemi-neglect can overlap with sensory and motor portions of the neurologic exam.

Cranial Nerves (CN): There are 12 cranial nerves.

I: Olfactory nerve—Smell and ability to distinguish different odors. The examiner can ask the patient whether he or she has noted a change in ability to smell. If concerned, one could ask the patient to discriminate among different odors. Differential diagnosis of abnormal exam findings includes nasal congestion, tumor, or brain trauma.

II: Optic nerve—Visual acuity and color vision can be tested using an eye chart, while visual fields testing to confrontation can be done by evaluating each eye separately for peripheral discrimination of fingers to confrontation. The funduscopic exam allows the examiner to visualize the health of the optic nerve, retina and papilledema that may be seen with increased intracranial pressure.

The examiner can assess health of both CN II and III (carries parasympathetic nerve fibers and controls pupillary constrictor muscles) by assessing pupillary reaction to bright light. Bright light should cause pupillary constriction in both the eye the light is directly shone into as well as the consensual eye. Afferent pupillary deficits will result in abnormal pupil dilation when direct light is applied to affected eye. By swinging the penlight between both eyes, this difference can become more apparent. Normal accommodation of the pupils results in constriction when asked to focus on an object that moves closer. Differential diagnosis for abnormalities can be related to retinal or optic nerve damage or disease. Older adults are more prone to visual impairment from cataracts which can be found on physical exam. Additionally, visual extinction (visual hemi-neglect) can be demonstrated if patient cannot distinguish stimuli on the affected side when the stimuli are presented simultaneously on both sides, but the patient can distinguish the stimulus if presented one side at a time.

III, Oculomotor; IV, Trochlear; VI, Abducens—These three cranial nerves are involved with controlling movement of the eye. The examiner can assess for smoothness and fullness of eye movements by asking the patient to watch the examiner's finger or pen while they move it in different directions, including testing for accommodation (moving the object from far away to closer to the patient's eyes). Problems with functioning of these nerves can result in complaints of double vision or observed restricted range of motion of the eyes. Progressive supranuclear palsy is an example of a neurologic condition that manifests with abnormal control of extraocular movements, gait, and cognitive and mood disturbances. Nystagmus, a rhythmic oscillating motion of the eyes, may be observed on exam and can be pathological due to alcohol or another drug toxicity.

V: Trigeminal—The trigeminal nerve has both motor and sensory functions, though the sensory function is more prominent. The examiner can assess for whether the patient can clench the jaw. The examiner can check for an abnormal jaw jerk reflex by tapping on the jaw with the mouth slightly open. Presence of a jaw jerk reflex suggests upper motor neuron abnormality in the trigeminal nerve. Dysfunction of the trigeminal nerve is more often picked up by detecting loss of sensation of the face. Both sides of the face should be tested for comparison. Trigeminal neuralgia is a painful condition that results in distressing pain in the distribution of the trigeminal nerve.

VII: Facial—The facial nerve has a larger role for movement of the face when compared to the smaller scope of movement from the trigeminal nerve. The examiner should assess for asymmetry and may observe during the interview asymmetry of the depths of the nasolabial folds as well as decreased spontaneous facial movement.

Additionally, the examiner can ask the patient to perform different movements of the face to assess for asymmetry (e.g., raise eyebrows, close eyes, puff out cheeks, smile). Abnormal facial nerve function may be the result of stroke or Bell palsy. Also, the facial nerve is responsible for taste.

VIII: Auditory (vestibulocochlear)—The auditory nerve facilitates hearing and vestibular function. It can be examined grossly by auditory whisper test and by formal hearing test. Tests using a tuning fork can help to discriminate mechanical conduction from sensorineural deficits. In patients with vertigo, positional vestibular testing such as the Hallpike maneuver can be helpful.

IX, Glossopharyngeal; X, Vagus—These nerves work together for movement of the palate and can be assessed by asking the patient to say "ahhh" while observing the palate and uvula. One should see symmetric elevation of the palate and the uvula at midline. Additionally, one can assess the integrity of these cranial nerves by testing gag reflex.

XI: Spinal accessory—The spinal accessory nerve innervates the sternomastoid and trapezius muscles and can be assessed by asking the patient to turn her or his head from side to side and raise the shoulders. The examiner is assessing for any evidence for asymmetry.

XII: Hypoglossal—The hypoglossal nerve controls the tongue. The examiner can observe for evidence of lower motor nerve lesion by looking for possible atrophy of the tongue muscle or fasciculation. If there is weakness on one side, the tongue will go toward the weak side when the examiner asks the patient to stick out her or his tongue. Additional testing includes asking the patient to move the tongue from one side of the cheek to the other.

CN V, VII, IX, X, and XII are collectively involved with speech articulation. Dysarthric speech (e.g., slurred or altered pronunciation of speech) may result from lesions to these nerves.

Motor: Adults may experience some generalized atrophy of muscles with aging, and the degree can vary depending on physical activity and lifestyle and other health conditions. The examiner should observe the patient's general appearance during the interview. More focused neurologic motor exam consists of visual inspection of muscle groups, palpation for tenderness, assessment of tone, motor sequencing (e.g., rapid alternating movements, fine finger tapping), pronator drift (i.e., asking patient to hold arms raised with eyes closed to assess for drift), and strength testing. Looking for evidence of tremors or involuntary movements or abnormal tone can provide clues of possible movement disorders such as Parkinson's disease or adverse psychotropic medication reactions such as tardive dyskinesia. Additionally, evidence of upper motor neuron lesions includes weakness in the context of increased tone and absence of atrophy and fasciculations, while lower motor neuron lesions include weakness in the context of decreased tone and presence of atrophy and fasciculations. The motor exam should also be interpreted in the context of the findings of the reflexes exam.

Reflexes: The examiner generally uses a reflex hammer to assess deep tendon reflexes. The most commonly tested deep tendon reflexes are biceps, brachioradialis, triceps, patellar, and Achilles tendons. Generally, hyporeflexic responses are concerning for lower motor neuron lesions, while hyperreflexic responses are concerning for upper motor neuron lesions. Additionally, presence of abnormal reflexes such as the Babinski may be seen with upper motor neuron lesions such as stroke, while frontal release signs (e.g., palmomental, grasp, snout, suck) can be associated with dementia and other conditions causing diffuse brain disease affecting the frontal lobes and pyramidal tracts [6].

Coordination: Cerebellar integrity can be assessed with maneuvers such as rapid alternating hand movements and finger-to-nose testing. Additionally, the Romberg maneuver can be employed by asking the patient to stand with feet together and eyes closed. The examiner observes for body sway or loss of balance.

Gait: The assessment of a patient's gait generally can occur naturally at the start of the encounter with the examiner observing how the patient ambulates to the room. The examiner can make observations about the patient's posture, the width of the patient's stance, step height, stride length, and arm swing. The examiner is observing for any evidence of asymmetrical movements or abnormalities such as shuffling gait. Depending on the patient's problem, the examiner may pursue more formal assessment by asking the patient to walk back and forth in the hallway under different conditions (e.g., tandem gait or toe and heel walking). Gait changes can range from shuffling gait seen in Parkinson's disease, antalgic gait from arthritis, ataxic gait from alcoholism, and apraxic gait from normal pressure hydrocephalus, among others.

Sensory: The sensory exam usually involves assessment of the upper and lower limbs for sensation to pinprick, light touch, temperature, and vibration. Additionally, the examiner can assess ability to discriminate positional change by moving the big toe up or down with the patient's eyes closed. As with visual and facial sensation testing, the examiner can apply a similar approach to evaluate for evidence of tactile extinction (hemineglect) in the limbs. Additional cortical sensory testing includes assessment for graphesthesia by tracing a letter or number on a patient's hand with a fingertip while the patient's eyes are closed and asking the patient to identify the letter or number that was traced. Assessment for stereognosis involves asking a patient to recognize objects placed in her or his hands while the patient's eyes are closed.

Electroencephalogram (EEG)

If there are concerns for potential seizures or mental status changes or brain disease, the geriatric psychiatry patient may be referred for additional assessment to include an electroencephalogram (EEG). The EEG records electrical activity of the brain using scalp electrodes. It usually can be completed in approximately 30 min and typically is completed with eyes open and eyes closed while awake. Rarely will a routine EEG detect seizure activity, so a normal study does not exclude the possibility of seizure disorder. Between seizures, more than 50% of epilepsy patients have normal routine EEG [7].

The EEG's electrical activity is described in terms of amplitude (voltage) and frequency (Hz). Characteristic waveforms are delta (<4 Hz), theta (4–7 Hz), alpha (8–14 Hz), and beta (>14 Hz) [7]. Sleep cycle phases have characteristic predominance of different EEG waveforms, with beta waves predominant when awake with eyes open, alpha waves when awake with eyes closed, theta waves when in stage I sleep (drowsy), theta waves with sleep spindles (12–14 Hz, >0.5 s) and K complexes (triphasic waves) when in stage II sleep, <50% delta waves during stage III sleep, and >50% delta waves during stage IV sleep [8, 9]. The EEG during REM sleep is similar to the EEG when awake with eyes open. Table 13-1 highlights common EEG abnormalities.

TABLE 13-1. EEG abnormalities [9–12]

Condition	EEG pattern
Grand mal seizures	Generalized, bilaterally synchronous spike discharges
Petit mal (absence) seizures	Generalized, bilateral 3 Hz spike-wave
Partial seizures	Focal discharges
Herpes simplex encephalitis	Focal or lateralized periodic slow waves
Acute hemispheric pathology (e.g., abscess, hematoma, tumor)	Periodic lateralizing epileptiform discharges (PLEDs)
Delirium tremens or pharmacologic (benzodiazepine, barbiturate)	Fast activity
Metabolic encephalopathy	*Frontal Intermittent Rhythmic Delta Activity* (FIRDA)
Dementia	Normal or diffuse slowing
Creutzfeldt-Jakob disease	Periodic complexes, 1–2 Hz biphasic and triphasic waves

Adapted from: Tampi RR. Laboratory Investigations. In: Tampi, RR and Williamson, D, ed. Fundamentals of Geriatric Psychiatry. New York, NY; 2013: 15–25

Lumbar Puncture for Cerebrospinal Fluid (CSF) Analysis

Although lumbar puncture is not routinely indicated for behavioral or psychiatric complaints that are encountered in geriatric psychiatry practice, there are situations when referral to neurology for a lumbar puncture is indicated [7, 13]. The lumbar puncture is a diagnostic approach to evaluate for concerns of possible central nervous system infection. In situations when a patient develops mental status changes suspicious for possible central nervous system infection (encephalitis, meningitis), the cerebrospinal fluid (CSF) analysis can help distinguish whether an infection is present and, if so, whether the pathogen is bacterial, fungal, or viral to inform appropriate management. Additionally, a lumbar puncture can be used to help diagnose subarachnoid hemorrhage, demyelinating processes like Guillain-Barré or multiple sclerosis, and central nervous system malignancies. Therapeutic lumbar punctures may also be considered for normal pressure hydrocephalus. Imaging guided-lumbar punctures should also be considered with older patients who have degenerative spine disease.

In clinical practice, the evaluation of Alzheimer's disease (AD) does not include CSF analysis as standard of care; however, the identification of CSF biomarkers to help identify prodromal AD is quickly building research data to support an "AD signature" (low Aβ42 and high total tau and phosphorylated tau proteins) in the CSF [14]. Additional research is necessary to validate these findings.

Conclusion

The neurologic assessment is an important component of a comprehensive geropsychiatric evaluation. The comprehensiveness of the neurologic exam will vary depending on the patient's complaint and other comorbidities. This section of the chapter reviewed the approach to the neurologic exam and the use of EEG and lumbar puncture for CSF analysis.

References

1. http://www.neuroexam.com/neuroexam/content2.html. Accessed 4 Sept 2017.
2. Harada CN, Natelson Love MC, Triebeld K. Normal Cognitive Aging. Clin Geriatr Med. 2013;29:737–52. https://doi.org/10.1016/j.cger.2013.07.002.
3. Galvin JE. Mental status and neurologic examination. In: Halter JB, Ouslander JG, Studenski S, High KP, Asthana S, Supiano MA, Ritchie C, editors. Hazzard's geriatric medicine and gerontology. 7th ed. New York, NY: McGraw-Hill. http://accessmedicine.mhmedical.com.ezproxy.library.wisc.edu/content.aspx?bookid=1923&sectionid=144517915. Accessed 4 Sept 2017.
4. Nichols ME, Meador KJ, Loring DW, et al. Age-related changes in the neurologic examination of healthy sexagenarians, octogenarians, and centenarians. J Geriatr Psychiatry Neurol. 1993;6:1–7.
5. Mancall EL. Neurological assessment of the elderly psychiatric patient. In: Agronin ME, Maletta GJ, editors. Principles and practice of geriatric psychiatry. 2nd ed. Philadelphia, PA: Lippincott Williams & Wilkins; 2011. p. 77–92.
6. Walker HK. The suck, snout, palmomental, and grasp reflexes. In: Walker HK, Hall WD, Hurst JW, editors. Clinical methods: the history, physical, and laboratory examinations. 3rd ed. Boston, MA: Butterworths; 1990. p. 363–4.
7. Clarke C, Frackowiak R, Howard R, et al. The language of neurology: symptoms, signs and basic investigations. In: Clarke C, Howard R, Rossor M, Shorvon S, editors. Neurology: a queen square textbook. Oxford, UK: Blackwell Publishing Ltd; 2009. p. 75–107.
8. http://emedicine.medscape.com/article/1140322-overview. Accessed 4 Sept 2017.
9. Tampi RR. Laboratory investigations. In: Tampi RR, Williamson D, editors. Fundamentals of geriatric psychiatry. New York, NY: Nova Science Publishers; 2013. p. 15–25.
10. Aminoff MJ. Electrodiagnostic studies of nervous system disorders: EEG, evoked potentials, and EMG. In: Kasper D, Fauci A, Hauser S, Longo D, Jameson J, Loscalzo J, editors. Harrison's principles of internal medicine. 19th ed. New York, NY: McGraw-Hill; 2014. http://accessmedicine.mhmedical.com.ezproxy.library.wisc.edu/content.aspx?bookid=1130&sectionid=79754895. Accessed 5 Sept 2017.
11. http://emedicine.medscape.com/article/1140075-overview#a4. Accessed 4 Sept 2017.
12. Libenson MH. The abnormal EEG. In: Libenson MH, editor. Practical approach to electroencephalography. Philadelphia, PA: Saunders; 2010. p. 176–203.
13. https://www.uptodate.com/contents/lumbar-puncture-technique-indications-contraindications-and-complications-in-adults?source=search_result&search=lumbar%20puncture&selectedTitle=1~150. Accessed 5 Sept 2017.
14. Blennow K, Dubois B, Faga AM, et al. Clinical utility of cerebrospinal fluid biomarkers in the diagnosis of early Alzheimer's Disease. Alzheimers Dement. 2015;11:58–69. https://doi.org/10.1016/j.jalz.2014.02.004.

14 Clinical Laboratory Testing

Lisa L. Boyle

Older patients with mental illness have higher levels of multimorbidity [1, 2]. Medical comorbidities, in themselves, can increase likelihood of developing behavioral and psychiatric conditions later in life or exacerbate chronic mental conditions as people age. Medical comorbidities also complicate decisions regarding management due to concerns about possible disease-medication interactions that can impact tolerability of different treatments and lead to higher risk for toxicity and delirium. Therefore, when evaluating a patient for a new psychiatric concern, it is helpful to evaluate and manage comorbid medical conditions. Laboratory screening and electrocardiogram (EKG) may be indicated to achieve these tasks.

Additionally, depending on the type of psychiatric medication used in treatment, additional standard drug monitoring may be necessary [3]. Standard laboratory surveillance is standard of care when prescribing atypical antipsychotics and many mood stabilizers (e.g., lithium, valproic acid, carbamazepine). Certain psychotropic medications (e.g., lithium, valproic acid, carbamazepine, tricyclic antidepressants) have well-established drug levels that can be monitored periodically during therapy. Moreover, in situations when providers suspect possible overdose or intoxication, serum alcohol, acetaminophen, salicylate levels, and urine toxicology studies to evaluate for presence or absence of illicit or prescription benzodiazepine, stimulants, or opioids can be obtained.

This chapter will review common laboratory and EKG studies that providers should be familiar with, along with potential significance of abnormal values. Reference ranges vary depending on laboratory, so it is advised that providers refer to the reference ranges provided by the laboratory that is analyzing the sample. Additional review of potential adverse effects of psychiatric medications and review of medical comorbidities in older adults can be found in Chaps. 25 and 33, respectively. Depending on the chief complaint, providers may consider pursuing additional testing as part of work-up, e.g., screening for sexually transmitted diseases like human immunodeficiency virus (HIV) or syphilis for cognitive concerns in older adults with higher-risk exposures. The tables (Tables 14.1, 14.2, 14.3, 14.4, 14.5, 14.6, and 14.7) provided are meant to highlight commonly encountered studies but are not all-inclusive.

R. R. Tampi et al. (eds.), *Psychiatric Disorders Late in Life*, https://doi.org/10.1007/978-3-319-73078-3_14

Table 14-1. Serum chemistry [3, 4]

Name	Potential meaning of abnormal values
Sodium	High: dehydration, renal failure Low: nutritional depletion, syndrome of inappropriate ADH secretion (SIADH) Note: SIADH associated with antidepressants (selective serotonin reuptake inhibitors) is more common in older adults [5]. Also can be seen with some mood stabilizers.
Potassium	High: potassium supplementation, renal failure Low: nutritional depletion Note: Low potassium levels increase risk for arrhythmia in patients with prolonged QTc on EKG [6].
Chloride	High: vomiting, diarrhea, diabetes, hyperventilation, diuretic therapy Low: hypoventilation, respiratory acidosis
Bicarbonate	High: excessive vomiting, hyperaldosteronism, Cushing's syndrome Low: diabetic ketoacidosis, lactic acidosis, alcoholic ketoacidosis, renal failure, diarrhea, Addison's disease, ethylene glycol poisoning or methanol poisoning
Blood urea nitrogen (BUN)	High: dehydration, renal failure, congestive heart failure Low: severe liver disease, malnutrition, overhydration
Creatinine	High: renal failure, congestive heart failure, cirrhosis of the liver, urinary tract obstruction, high-meat diet, severe exercise Low: elderly, small stature, decreased muscle mass, inadequate dietary protein Note: Baseline screening and routine follow-up monitoring of renal function is recommended for patients starting on or maintained on lithium.
BUN-to-creatinine ratio	High: acute renal failure, shock, severe dehydration, renal stones, gastrointestinal bleed Low: low-protein diet, rhabdomyolysis, pregnancy, cirrhosis, syndrome of inappropriate antidiuretic hormone secretion (SIADH) Note: Baseline screening and routine follow-up monitoring of renal function is recommended for patients starting on or maintained on lithium.
Creatinine clearance Cockcroft and Gault equation: $CrCl = (140 - age) \times IBW/(serum\ creatinine \times 72)$ ($\times$ 0.85 for females) Estimate ideal body weight in (kg) Males: IBW = 50 kg + 2.3 kg for each inch over 5 feet Females: IBW = 45.5 kg + 2.3 kg for each inch over 5 feet IBW, ideal body weight	High: strenuous exercise, muscle injury (crushing injuries), burns, carbon monoxide poisoning, hypothyroidism, pregnancy Low: infections, shock, cancer, low blood flow to the kidneys, urinary tract blockage, heart failure, dehydration, cirrhosis of the liver Note: Acute lithium toxicity and chronic lithium use can be associated with acute and chronic renal failure, respectively [7]. Baseline screening and routine follow-up monitoring of renal function is recommended for patients starting on or maintained on lithium.
Glucose	High: diabetes, steroid use Low: starvation, alcohol intake, diabetic medications Note: Atypical antipsychotic use can increase risk for diabetes. Guidelines for routine monitoring for metabolic risk factors while on atypical antipsychotics exist [8].
Calcium	High: hyperparathyroidism, multiple myeloma, vitamin D intoxication Low: hypoparathyroidism, vitamin D deficiency, renal failure, alkalosis, pancreatitis, hypomagnesemia Note: Low calcium levels can increase risk for arrhythmia in patients with prolonged QTc on EKG [6].
Magnesium	High: renal failure, dietary intake, lithium intoxication, hyperparathyroidism Low: malnutrition, alcoholism, diarrhea, loop and thiazide diuretic use, pancreatitis Note: Low magnesium levels can increase risk for arrhythmia in patients with elevated QTc on EKG [6].
Phosphorous	High: hypoparathyroidism, chronic renal failure, osteomalacia, malabsorption Low: hyperparathyroidism, respiratory alkalosis, decreased dietary intake

Adapted from: Tampi RR. Laboratory Investigations. In: Tampi, RR and Williamson, D, ed. Fundamentals of Geriatric Psychiatry. New York, NY; 2013: 15–25

TABLE 14-2. Liver function tests [3, 4]

Name	Potential meaning of abnormal values
Albumin (Alb)	Low: chronic liver disease, such as cirrhosis and nephrotic syndrome
Alanine transaminase (ALT)	High: hepatitis Note: May become elevated with valproic acid therapy [9]
Aspartate transaminase (AST)	High: hepatitis, cardiac failure, muscle injury Note: May become elevated with valproic acid therapy [9]
Alkaline phosphatase (ALP)	High: hepatitis, intrahepatic cholestasis or infiltrative diseases of the liver, growing children, Paget's disease of the bone
Total bilirubin (TBIL)	High: cirrhosis, hepatitis, hemolytic anemia, cholestasis
Direct bilirubin (conjugated bilirubin)	High: gallstones, biliary cancer
Gamma-glutamyl transpeptidase (GGT)	High: liver disease, chronic alcohol use
5′ Nucleotidase (5′NTD)	High: liver disease, chronic alcohol use
Lactate dehydrogenase (LDH)	High: hepatitis, cardiac failure, muscle injury
Ammonia	High: liver disease Note: May become elevated with valproic acid therapy [9]

Adapted from: Tampi RR. Laboratory Investigations. In: Tampi, RR and Williamson, D, ed. Fundamentals of Geriatric Psychiatry. New York, NY; 2013: 15–25

TABLE 14-3. Thyroid function tests [3, 4]

Name	Potential meaning of abnormal values
Thyroid-stimulating hormone (TSH)	High: hypothyroidism 1. Primary: thyroiditis, iatrogenic 2. Secondary: hypopituitarism 3. Tertiary: hypothalamic conditions Low: Grave's disease, thyroid adenoma, toxic multinodular goiter, thyroiditis, postpartum thyroiditis Note: Lithium can lead to hypothyroidism and less commonly hyperthyroidism [10]. Baseline screening and routine follow-up thyroid monitoring is recommended for patients starting on or maintained on lithium. For older adults >70–80 years old, the TSH target may be higher (4–6 mIU/L) than for younger adults [11]. Although subclinical hypothyroidism is associated with depressive and cognitive symptoms, the efficacy of thyroid hormone replacement for subclinical hypothyroidism of TSH < 10mIU/L to improve these symptoms is not known [12].
Total thyroxine (total T_4)	High: Grave's disease, thyroid adenoma, toxic multinodular goiter, thyroiditis, postpartum thyroiditis, amiodarone Low: hypothyroidism 1. Primary: thyroiditis, iatrogenic 2. Secondary: hypopituitarism 3. Tertiary: hypothalamic conditions
Free thyroxine (free T_4)	Same as above in total T_4
Total triiodothyronine (total T_3)	Same as above in total T_4
Free triiodothyronine (free T_3)	Same as above in total T_4
Thyroxine-binding globulin (TBG)	High: results in an increased total thyroxine level and total triiodothyronine without an actual increase in hormonal activity of thyroid hormones
Thyroid hormone uptake (T_3 uptake) (measures unbound thyroxine-binding globulins in the blood)	High: unsaturated TBG increases with decreased levels of thyroid hormones
Free thyroxine index (FTI or T_7) (reliable indicator of thyroid status in the presence of abnormalities in plasma protein binding)	Same as above in total T_4

Adapted from: Tampi RR. Laboratory Investigations. In: Tampi, RR and Williamson, D, ed. Fundamentals of Geriatric Psychiatry. New York, NY; 2013: 15–25

TABLE 14-4. Vitamin B 12, folic acid, methylmalonic acid (MMA) [3, 4, 13, 14]

Name	Potential meaning of abnormal values
Vitamin B 12	Low: malabsorption syndrome, celiac disease or Crohn's disease, malnutrition, pernicious anemia, h/o bariatric surgery, alcoholism, potential medications such as proton pump inhibitors or H2-receptor antagonists Note: In older adults, neuropsychiatric manifestations of low vitamin B12 can be present at low-normal B12 levels and often precede hematological manifestations of B12 deficiency. Consider screening also for MMA in older adults with B12 < 350 pg/mL as MMA usually is elevated before B12 level becomes abnormally low.
Folic acid	Low: malabsorption syndrome, malnutrition, alcohol abuse, malignancies
Methylmalonic acid (MMA)	High: renal insufficiency, intravascular volume depletion, vitamin B12 deficiency Note: Consider screening also for MMA in older adults with B12 < 350 pg/mL as MMA usually is elevated before B12 level becomes abnormally low.
Vitamin D	High: excessive vitamin D dietary supplements Low: rickets, osteomalacia, low vitamin D diet (e.g., milk allergy, lactose intolerance, veganism), inadequate sun exposure, renal disease, fat malabsorption or history of gastric bypass surgery Note: In older adults, vitamin D deficiency has been associated with depression and cognitive impairment [15].

Adapted from: Tampi RR. Laboratory Investigations. In: Tampi, RR and Williamson, D, ed. Fundamentals of Geriatric Psychiatry. New York, NY; 2013: 15–25

TABLE 14-5. Iron studies [3, 4]

Name	Potential meaning of abnormal values
Serum iron	High: iron overload, iron therapy Low: intercurrent illness, chronic disease
Transferrin	High: iron deficiency, estrogen therapy Low: chronic disease
Transferrin saturation	High: iron therapy, iron overload Low: iron deficiency, chronic disease
Ferritin	High: iron overload Low: liver disease, malignancy, iron deficiency Note: Low ferritin may be associated with restless legs syndrome [16].

Adapted from: Tampi RR. Laboratory Investigations. In: Tampi, RR and Williamson, D, ed. Fundamentals of Geriatric Psychiatry. New York, NY; 2013: 15–25

TABLE 14-6. Complete blood count (CBC) and differential [3, 4]

Name	Potential meaning of abnormal values
White blood cells (WBC)	High: bacterial infection, leukemia Low: viral diseases, aplastic anemia
Red blood cells (RBC)	High: polycythemia, smoking and pulmonary disease Low: iron deficiency, internal bleeding, anemias
Hemoglobin (HGB)	High: polycythemia, smoking and pulmonary disease Low: iron deficiency, internal bleeding, anemias
Hematocrit (HCT)	High: polycythemia, smoking and pulmonary disease Low: iron deficiency, internal bleeding, anemia
Mean corpuscular volume (MVC)	High: vitamin B12 deficiency, folic acid deficiency, alcohol abuse Low: iron deficiency anemias, internal bleeding
Mean corpuscular hemoglobin (MCH)	High: lung disease Low: iron deficiency, anemia, excessive bleeding
Platelets	High: leukemias Low: anemias

(Continued)

TABLE 14-6. (Continued)

Name	Potential meaning of abnormal values
Red blood cell distribution width (RDW)	High: iron deficiency anemia, folate and vitamin B12 deficiency, recent hemorrhage Low: anemias
Neutrophils (polymorphonuclear leukocyte, PMN)	High: bacterial infections, cigarette smoking, stress reactions, leukemias Low: viral infections, aplastic anemia, overwhelming infections
Lymphocytes	High: viral infections, leukemias Low: bacterial infections, aplastic anemia
Eosinophils	High: allergies, leukemias, parasitic infestations Low: anemias
Basophils	High: chronic infections, allergies, leukemias Low: anemias
Absolute neutrophil count (ANC)	High: leukemias, infections Low: chemotherapy Note: Patients on clozapine require ANC monitoring due to risk for severe neutropenia [17]
Erythrocyte sedimentation rate (ESR)	High: multiple myeloma, temporal arteritis, polymyalgia rheumatica, systemic lupus erythematosus, rheumatoid arthritis, chronic kidney diseases Low: polycythemia, sickle cell anemia

Adapted from: Tampi RR. Laboratory Investigations. In: Tampi, RR and Williamson, D, ed. Fundamentals of Geriatric Psychiatry. New York, NY; 2013: 15–25

TABLE 14-7 Urine study findings [3, 18, 19]

Name	*Potential meaning of abnormal values*
Urine toxicology	Presence or absence of benzodiazepine, stimulants, opioid, and illicit drugs. Depending on the substance or test used, additional confirmatory studies may be needed.
Urinalysis	Discoloration could indicate infection or blood or myoglobin (rhabdomyolysis); urine dipstick could reveal infection (positive WBC, leukocyte esterase, nitrites, bacteria) or elevated protein or glucose (kidney disease); urine culture and sensitivity to confirm infection
Urine culture	Provides evidence to establish urinary tract infection. Bacterial or fungal growth, along with identified organisms/species and antibiotic sensitivity, helps guide treatment
Urine osmolality	Reduced in diabetes insipidus. Chronic lithium can increase risk for nephrogenic DI [7]. Psychogenic polydipsia

Electrocardiogram (ECG or EKG)

In geriatric psychiatric practice, when starting a new medication that is associated with potential for QTc prolongation (which can increase risk for fatal arrhythmia), providers should obtain a baseline and follow-up EKG, especially in patients with known cardiac disease or risk factors such as co-administered medications with potential for QTc prolongation [20]. Psychiatric medications such as many antipsychotics (e.g., haloperidol, atypical antipsychotics) and some antidepressants (e.g., citalopram, tricyclics) are associated with potential for QTc prolongation [20–22].

Conclusion

Geriatric mental health providers need to be well versed with the use of laboratory and EKG diagnostic tools in the evaluation and management of older adults with behavioral and psychiatric disorders. These approaches can be used as part of the initial work-up or as part of ongoing surveillance and monitoring to ensure safe use of psychotropic medications.

References

1. AMY G, Westphal A, Daws T, et al. A retrospective study of medical comorbidities in psychogeriatric patients. Psychogeriatrics. 2016;16:12–9. https://doi.org/10.1111/psyg.12111.
2. Forester BP, Gatchel JR. Medical co-morbidity, brain disease, and the future of geriatric psychiatry. Am J Geriatr Psychiatry. 2014;22:1061–5. https://doi.org/10.1016/j.jagp.2014.08.007.
3. Smith FA, Hogan C. Laboratory tests and diagnostic procedures. In: Stern TA, Fava M, Wilens TE, Rosenbaum JF, editors. Massachusetts general hospital comprehensive clinical psychiatry. 2nd ed. London, UK: Elsevier; 2016. p. 20–38.
4. Tampi RR. Laboratory investigations. In: Tampi RR, Williamson D, editors. Fundamentals of geriatric psychiatry. New York, NY: Nova Science Publishers; 2013. p. 15–25.
5. Jacob S, Spinier SA. Hyponatremia associated with selective serotonin-reuptake inhibitors in older adults. Ann Pharmacother. 2006;40:1618–22. https://doi.org/10.1345/aph.1G293.
6. Yap YG, Camm AJ. Drug-induced QT prolongation and Torsades de Pointes. Heart. 2003;89:1363–72. https://doi.org/10.1136/heart.89.11.1363.
7. Rej S, Herrmann N, Shulman K. The effects of lithium on renal function in older adults: a systematic review. J Geriatr Psychiatry Neurol. 2012;25:51–61. https://doi.org/10.1177/0891988712436690.
8. American Diabetes Association, American Psychiatric Association, American Association of Clinical Endocrinologists, North American Association for the Study of Obesity. Consensus development conference on antipsychotic drugs and obesity and diabetes. Diabetes Care. 2004;27:596–601. https://doi.org/10.2337/diacare.27.2.596.
9. Nanau RM, Neuman MG. Adverse drug reactions induced by valproic acid. Clin Biochem. 2013;46:1323–38. https://doi.org/10.1016/j.clinbiochem.2013.06.012.
10. Kibirige D, Luzinda K, Ssekitoleko R. Spectrum of lithium induced thyroid abnormalities: a current perspective. Thyroid Res. 2013;6:3. https://doi.org/10.1186/1756-6614-6-3.
11. Jonklaas J, Bianco AC, Bauer AJ, et al. Guidelines for the treatment of hypthyroidism: prepared by the American thyroid association task force on thyroid hormone replacement. Thyroid. 2014;24:1670–751. https://doi.org/10.1089/thy.2014.0028.
12. Lachner C, Steinle NI, Regenold WT. The neuropsychiatry of vitamin B12 deficiency in elderly patients. J Neuropsychiatry Clin Neurosci. 2012; 24:5–15. https://doi.org/10.1176/appi.neuropsych.11020052.
13. Joffe RT, Pearce EN, Hennessey JV, et al. Subclinical hypothyroidism, mood and cognition in older adults: a review. Int J Geriatr Psychiatry. 2013;28:111–8. https://doi.org/10.1002/gps.3796.
14. https://ods.od.nih.gov/factsheets/VitaminD-HealthProfessional/#h8. Accessed 5 Sep 2017.
15. https://www.uptodate.com/contents/treatment-of-restless-legs-syndrome-willis-ekbom-disease-and-periodic-limb-movement-disorder-in-adults?source=search_result&search=ferritin%20and%20rls&selectedTitle=1~150. Accessed 5 Sep 2017.
16. Wilkins CH, Sheline YI, Roe CM, et al. Vitamin D deficiency is associated with low mood and worse cognitive performance in older adults. Am J Geriatr Psychiatry. 2006;14:1032–40. https://doi.org/10.1097/01.JGP.0000240986.74642.7c.
17. https://www.clozapinerems.com/CpmgClozapineUI/rems/pdf/resources/ANC_Table.pdf. Accessed 5 Sep 2017.
18. https://www.uptodate.com/contents/diagnosis-of-polyuria-and-diabetes-insipidus. Accessed 5 Sep 2017.
19. https://www.uptodate.com/contents/urinalysis-in-the-diagnosis-of-kidney-disease?source=search_result&search=urinalysis%20interpretation&selectedTitle=1~150. Accessed 5 Sep 2017.
20. Shah AA, Aftab A, Coverdale J. QTc prolongation with antipsychotics: is routine ecg monitoring recommended? J Psychiatr Pract. 2014;20:196–206. https://doi.org/10.1097/01.pra.0000450319.21859.6d.
21. Dodd S, Malhi GS, Tiller J, et al. A consensus statement for safety monitoring guidelines of treatments for major depressive disorder. Aust N Z J Psychiatry. 2011;45:712–25. https://doi.org/10.3109/00048674.2011.595686.
22. https://www.fda.gov/Drugs/DrugSafety/ucm297391.htm. Accessed 5 Sep 2017.

15 Structural and Functional Imaging

Vimal M. Aga

Introduction

A biomarker can be defined as an objective physiological, biochemical, or anatomical parameter that indicates a normal biological process, a pathological process, or a response to a therapeutic intervention [1]. A recently proposed taxonomy classified biomarkers into biomarkers of risk, biomarkers of trait/diagnosis, biomarkers of state/acuity, biomarkers of stage, biomarkers of treatment response, and biomarkers of prognosis [2]. In neuropsychiatric practice, imaging and cerebrospinal fluid biomarkers are still mostly being used only for diagnostic purposes in patients with neurocognitive disorders, although in the future they will likely be used for other indications as well. This chapter will therefore focus mainly on the current state of *diagnostic* imaging in clinical neuropsychiatry, while other potential roles of imaging biomarkers in clinical practice, such as in determining prognosis and response to treatment, will not be covered.

Indications for the use of imaging in routine clinical practice will be provided first which will lay out the scope of the chapter. A case will then be made for training in imaging modalities that is relevant to psychiatric practice. This will be followed by a discussion of the various structural and functional imaging modalities which have been shown to have diagnostic utility at the individual level. There are also many advanced imaging techniques that are being extensively used in research which do not have a place in routine clinical practice yet, and these will not be discussed in the interest of brevity, with occasional exceptions. Readers who are interested in learning more about imaging techniques used in psychiatric research are referred to this excellent review of the topic [3].

Note that in the remainder of this chapter, the DSM-5 term *major neurocognitive disorder* has been used interchangeably with the more traditional term *dementia* for the sake of continuity. This is not to imply that these are completely overlapping constructs, since the DSM-5 text indicates that *major neurocognitive disorder* is a broader construct than *dementia* and recommends restricting the use of the latter term to indicate only degenerative dementias in older adults where there is substantial decline in at least two cognitive domains. It is essential to note that almost no research that forms the basis for the use of imaging in clinical neuropsychiatric practice has been done using the broader DSM-5 construct of major neurocognitive disorder.

Practical Indications for Imaging in Psychiatry

While imaging has been studied as a diagnostic tool in psychiatric research for decades, imaging studies are seldom ordered and almost never interpreted by the psychiatrist in general clinical practice, with the exception of those working in specialized settings. There are several reasons for this. Imaging did not have a place in the syndromic

R. R. Tampi et al. (eds.), *Psychiatric Disorders Late in Life*, https://doi.org/10.1007/978-3-319-73078-3_15

approach to psychiatric diagnosis adopted by successive iterations of the Diagnostic and Statistical Manual of Mental Disorders (DSM) published by the American Psychiatric Association (APA) until the fifth edition (DSM-5) came out in 2013. While several APA clinical practice guidelines do recommend the use of imaging studies in the diagnostic work-up of psychiatric disorders other than the neurocognitive disorders, the goal in such cases appears to be mainly to exclude "organic" (disorders due to "another medical condition" in DSM-5 [4]) phenocopies of psychiatric disorders, and clear guidelines on practical aspects of ordering and interpreting these expensive studies are still mostly lacking.

An example of this is the 2004 clinical practice guideline for treatment of patients with schizophrenia, which recommends that "*A CT or MRI scan may provide helpful information, particularly in assessing patients with a new onset of psychosis or with an atypical clinical presentation. Although imaging studies cannot establish a diagnosis of schizophrenia, specific findings from a CT or MRI scan (e.g., ventricular enlargement, diminished cortical volume) may enhance the confidence of the diagnosis and provide information that is relevant to treatment planning and prognosis. Given the subtle nature of the neuropathological findings in schizophrenia, MRI is preferred over CT*" [5]. This recommendation for structural neuroimaging in schizophrenia provides no further guidance regarding when brain scans are indicated in "atypical" presentations of schizophrenia at the individual level, or exactly what the referring clinician or the interpreting radiologist might look for in such scans. Specifically, no details are provided regarding the "subtle neuropathological finding(s)" on a brain MRI that would "enhance the confidence of the diagnosis" in the clinic. Ventricular enlargement and diminished cortical volume are nonspecific findings which are especially common in the elderly. The specific biosignature of schizophrenia on neuroimaging is still unclear, even after decades of research in this area, and the widely reported finding of hippocampal atrophy in schizophrenia research has not been consistently replicated [5]. This conundrum applies to the other psychiatric disorders as well. MRI studies of bipolar disorder, for example, have reported modest effect sizes and significant heterogeneity across studies [6].

Functional imaging studies have not fared any better. ^{18}Fluorodeoxyglucose positron emission tomography (^{18}FDG-PET) studies first demonstrated frontal hypometabolism or *hypofrontality* in schizophrenia in the 1980s [7]; more than 30 years later, this has still not translated into a diagnostic biomarker that can be used in routine clinical practice. In bipolar disorder, the anterior and posterior cingulate cortices, precuneus, and cuneus were all implicated in a large quantitative meta-analysis of 55 functional neuroimaging studies, but as in the MRI studies, the results of the ^{18}FDG-PET studies in bipolar disorder are also confounded by clinical and demographic variables such as the subjects' age, mood state at the time of the study, stage of illness, and presence or absence of pharmacological treatments [6, 8].

It was thought that late-onset variants of psychiatric disorders, such as schizophrenia and bipolar disorder, may be distinct from their early onset counterparts by having more of an "organic" etiology. Therefore, the possibility of finding unique structural or functional brain lesions underlying the late-onset disorders was thought to be higher. Unfortunately, no consistent structural or functional lesion has been found to date in late-onset schizophrenia or bipolar disorder, although some of the preliminary results are promising if they can be replicated [9]. For an excellent critique of the search for the "elusive psychiatric lesion," including several methodological problems, the reader is referred to this recent review [10].

In summary, recommending imaging in the clinic in every patient with a young-onset psychiatric disorder cannot be justified based on current evidence, in the absence of a strong clinical suspicion of an "organic" etiology where imaging has known diagnostic value. Unfortunately, current recommendations in clinical practice guidelines for the use of imaging in several psychiatric disorders, such as those mentioned above, may be interpreted as blanket recommendations to order expensive and time-consuming brain scans for every patient with new-onset psychosis or a mood disorder, which will almost certainly result in denied insurance claims for such studies, leaving the patient with a large bill to pay for a study which will contribute minimally, if at all, to the diagnosis and management. Additionally, patients with psychiatric disorders may be unable to tolerate and may even react negatively to the scanning process, which may occasionally place the radiology personnel and expensive scanning equipment at risk. Psychotic patients may interpret the noisy MRI environment as yet more evidence of electronic surveillance, or the injection of a PET tracer may further exacerbate the patient's persecutory delusions of being poisoned, all of which needs to be factored in when referring such patients for imaging studies.

The single most important clinical indication for ordering imaging studies in psychiatric practice is for the diagnostic work-up of the neurocognitive disorders, and several neurocognitive disorders have valid biosignatures on imaging. Patients with neurocognitive disorders usually present to the psychiatrist with behavioral symptoms, while those whose symptoms are predominantly cognitive are usually referred to the neurologist. Concurrent behavioral symptoms occur in the vast majority of community dwelling adults with neurocognitive disorders at some point in time during the course of the illness [11], and are commonly referred to as behavioral and psychological symptoms of dementia (BPSD) or neuropsychiatric symptoms (NPS) of dementia.

Patients with behavioral symptoms can further present in several ways. Patients with known a diagnosis of a major neurocognitive disorder can present to the clinic with new-onset BPSD. In many cases, the underlying disease is not immediately obvious, in which case it behooves the psychiatrist to order further diagnostic work-up to clarify the etiology. Furthermore, as disease-modifying therapies become available in the near future, the current state of nihilism in diagnosing and treating neurocognitive disorders will become increasingly unacceptable, and making an etiological diagnosis will become the critical first step in selecting the appropriate disease-modifying therapy in every patient.

Another group of patients can present with behavioral and psychological symptoms in the context of mild cognitive impairment (MCI, called mild neurocognitive disorder in DSM-5 [4]) or even without any overt cognitive symptoms. A late-onset syndrome consisting of "persistent behavioral changes and mild psychiatric symptoms" in patients with "no serious memory complaints" and "normal activities of daily living" has been called *mild behavioral impairment* (MBI) [12]. MBI was first described in the context of frontotemporal dementia (FTD), the various subtypes of which can present with a psychiatric prodrome which has a substantial phenotypic overlap with the psychiatric disorders. However, it is now recognized that MBI is not restricted to prodromal FTD, but can occur in the other neurodegenerative dementias as well. Even in the original data presented by Taragano in 2003, 45% patients developed frontotemporal dementia, 25% developed dementia of the Alzheimer's type, and 7% developed dementia of the Lewy body type within the 3-year follow-up period, while only 23% did not end up with a dementia [12]. Patients with MBI often receive an erroneous diagnosis of a primary psychiatric disorder early on when cognitive problems are not yet prominent. In a recent blinded, retrospective chart review, the false positive rate for psychiatric disorders was as high as 28% across the various neurodegenerative dementias, being the highest for behavioral-variant FTD (51%), followed by semantic-variant FTD (24%) and Alzheimer's disease (AD) dementia (23%) [13]. The mean time to accurate diagnosis in this study was 33.3 (SD 3.4) months. Such patients usually present to the primary care or psychiatric clinic, and it has been suggested that the psychiatrist's lack of familiarity with interpreting relevant biomarker studies, including imaging studies, contributes to the high misdiagnosis rate in such patients [14]. Accurately diagnosing such patients also has important prognostic implications, since MBI is a bad prognostic marker and such patients have a higher annual rate of conversion to dementia compared to MCI patients without MBI [15].

This has led to the recommendation that patients with *late-onset atypical* psychiatric symptoms should be evaluated for neurocognitive disorders, and in such patients, imaging is essential in making an accurate diagnosis [16]. *Late onset* has been variously defined in this context, such as "patients who present with new onset behavioral, emotional or cognitive changes *after age 40*" (italics mine) [13]. The clinical spectrum of *atypical* psychiatric symptoms in such patients is even broader. The recently proposed provisional research diagnostic criteria for MBI by the Alzheimer's Association International Society to Advance Alzheimer's Research and Treatment (AA-ISTAART) Neuropsychiatric Symptoms Professional Interest Area are a first step toward refining these recommendations [17]. While still overly broad, these criteria define *late onset* as age 50 or above, and psychiatric symptoms are consolidated into five domains, must persist or present intermittently for 6 months (thereby excluding adjustment disorder precipitated by life stressors), and must result in at least minimal impairment in one of the following areas—interpersonal relationships, other aspects of social functioning, or the ability to perform in the workplace without leading to a loss of functional independence. A concurrent diagnosis of MCI is allowed in the AA-ISTAART MBI criteria but is not necessary. These criteria appear to have high sensitivity but low specificity, as they are inadequate for filtering out other late-onset psychiatric disorders that may have a prodrome lasting more than 6 months. The criteria will certainly undergo further revisions but, until then, the clinician should use these criteria to select appropriate candidates for imaging studies to look for biosignatures of neurocognitive disorders within the fairly large cohort of patients whose psychiatric symptoms first appear in mid-life or later. An MBI checklist has been recently developed to assist with the application of these criteria in the clinic [18].

MBI, with or without concurrent MCI, can also confound the clinical presentation of patients with pre-existing psychiatric disorders. Mid- or late-life worsening of a pre-existing stable psychiatric disorder for no apparent reason, or the appearance of behavioral symptoms that are atypical for that psychiatric disorder, e.g., new-onset obsessions later in life in a patient with known young-onset bipolar disorder, often herald the onset of a neurocognitive disorder in such patients. This can either be a superimposed neurodegenerative dementia or a nondegenerative dementia due to risk factors not uncommonly seen in psychiatric patients, such as substance use [19] and cerebrovascular disease [20]. Furthermore, it is well known that patients with chronic psychiatric disorders, such as schizophrenia and bipolar disorder, can develop cognitive impairment, even dementia, later in life [21–23], which appears to be related to the disorder itself [24], but almost nothing is currently known about any specific biomarkers of cognitive decline in such patients. Imaging in such patients should be used only to diagnose those neurocognitive disorders for which there are well-known neuroimaging biosignatures, with the caveat that identical findings due to the pre-existing psychiatric disorder, such as hippocampal atrophy in chronic schizophrenia, may confound interpretation, and therefore fluid biomarkers may be the biomarkers of choice in such patients.

Imaging is also increasingly finding a place in the diagnosis of movement disorders, most of which were hitherto diagnosed based solely on history and clinical examination. The approval of the dopamine transporter scan for the clinical diagnosis of idiopathic Parkinson's disease by the US Food and Drug Administration (FDA) in 2011 has revolutionized this field [25]. While it is certainly not recommended that psychiatrists order imaging studies to diagnose movement disorders, they need to be aware of the applications and limitations of this imaging modality since such patients are often seen in psychiatric practices. Patients on dopamine antagonists often develop drug-induced parkinsonism, and patients with idiopathic Parkinson's disease (and less commonly, those with the atypical parkinsonian syndromes) often develop concurrent neuropsychiatric symptoms [26]. Psychiatrists may therefore be asked by patients, who have already had a dopamine transporter scan done elsewhere, to review their scan and provide a second opinion. Conversely, the psychiatrist may need to refer a patient to a neurologist to determine whether a dopamine transporter scan is indicated.

Finally, clarification of etiology is necessary for accurate coding of neurocognitive disorders in DSM-5 [4]. There are 13 specific etiological subtypes of neurocognitive disorders in DSM-5. Borrowing from the general framework first proposed by the International Working Group (IWG) in 2007 for diagnosing AD [27] and subsequently expanded upon by the National Institute on Aging-Alzheimer's Association (NIA-AA) in 2011 [28], the DSM-5 criteria require clinicians to make a dichotomous "probable" versus "possible" distinction in 5 of the 13 neurocognitive disorders, each of which has a different diagnostic code. Imaging is required to *rule in* the probable neurocognitive disorder in 2 of these 5 disorders (vascular and frontotemporal), while in all the others it is required to *rule out* mixed etiology due to concurrent cerebrovascular disease. Ironically, DSM-5 does not require neuroimaging or cerebrospinal fluid biomarker evidence for the diagnosis of "probable" AD, as the text indicates that these markers are "not yet fully validated."

It should be clear by now that the treating clinician can best integrate clinical, lab, and imaging data meaningfully, thereby improving patient care. Not only is the use of diagnostic biomarkers in memory and movement disorder clinics expected to increase exponentially, but testing for biomarkers is in the not-so-distant future for several other psychiatric disorders as well. The first grants in the ambitious Human Connectome Project were awarded by the U.S. National Institutes of Health in 2010 [29], but 7 years later, the average trainee psychiatrist is unfortunately still receiving minimal training in ordering and interpreting even basic imaging studies, and the practicing psychiatrist is possibly the least "imaging-savvy" amongst all physicians trained in the clinical neurosciences.

The Case for Practice-Relevant Training in Imaging

It is certainly the expectation of accreditation and other agencies tasked with oversight of psychiatric training and practice that psychiatrists will become familiar with ordering appropriate neuroimaging studies relevant to their practice. The Accreditation Council for Graduate Medical Education (ACGME) Program Requirements for Graduate Medical Education in Geriatric Psychiatry (revised 7/1/15) specify that trainees must "demonstrate *proficiency* in the selection and use of clinical laboratory tests, *radiologic and other imaging procedures*… (italics mine)." Third-party payers also acknowledge the psychiatrist's potential in interpreting brain scans. For example, the Center for Medicare and Medicaid Services (CMS) National Coverage Determination (NCD) for PET scans for Dementia and Neurodegenerative Diseases states that the "*reading* of the scan should be done by an expert in nuclear medicine, radiology, neurology, *or psychiatry*…" (italics mine). Unfortunately, in practice, even when trainees have a dedicated neuroradiology rotation as part of their psychiatric training curriculum, they are mostly trained to diagnose neurological conditions such as large-vessel strokes, space occupying lesions, and the demyelinating disorders, but receive relatively little education about the imaging findings that may support a diagnosis of a neurocognitive disorder. It is even more doubtful that any psychiatry training program has a dedicated nuclear medicine rotation as part of the psychiatry residency or geriatric psychiatry fellowship curriculum. It is therefore incumbent upon trainee psychiatrists to make themselves familiar with the common neuroimaging modalities, just as it is incumbent upon the psychiatry residency training directors, and especially geriatric psychiatry fellowship training directors, to collaborate with their radiology and nuclear medicine colleagues to ensure that psychiatry residents and fellows are getting practice-relevant radiology training. As already noted, research in neurocognitive disorders has already moved beyond the study of regional brain structure and function toward multimodal imaging [30] and the study of the human connectome [29], where the connectome has both structural and functional elements and was first defined in 2005 as "a comprehensive structural description of the network of elements and connections forming the human brain" [31]. Therefore, there is an urgent need to incorporate these recent advances into routine psychiatric training and practice in a way that is clinically meaningful [32].

With this background, the common structural, functional, and molecular imaging modalities will now be reviewed in some detail.

Structural Imaging

Structural imaging modalities commonly used in clinical practice are the Computerized Tomography (CT) and Magnetic Resonance Imaging (MRI).

CT remains the imaging modality of choice for acute craniocerebral trauma [33], and geriatric patients who come to the clinic will often have had at least one CT scan of the brain, usually during an emergency room (ER) visit for a fall or a suspected stroke. The technical aspects of CT scanning will not be discussed in detail as these are usually not of relevance to the practicing psychiatrist. However, it is important to note that the use of multidetector computed tomography (MDCT) has shortened the acquisition time greatly, and new generation scanners contain multiple detector arrays or rows perpendicular to the axial CT plane which can generate images within a matter of seconds that can then be processed into high-resolution three-dimensional images [34].

While an MRI is the imaging modality of choice for diagnosing the neurodegenerative disorders in clinical practice, CT scans are the default option for patients who may be agitated, claustrophobic, sensitive to noise, or have MRI-incompatible medical devices. The most common MRI-incompatible medical devices in older individuals are pacing devices. While new pacing devices are designed to be safe in the MRI environment, one should always ask for any implanted medical devices and check for device safety before referring a patient for brain imaging. Every imaging center has an MRI screening checklist for this very purpose. A good online resource for checking device safety can be found at http://www.mrisafety.com/. However, such websites are not a substitute for the expertise of a radiologist, and it is always best to confer with radiology colleagues when questions regarding device safety arise in the clinic. Finally, CT scan should be considered as a viable alternative in patients who cannot afford an MRI because they are either self-paying or their insurance plan will not cover the MRI.

Two safety concerns regarding CT scans require further elaboration. The first is the use of contrast. Note that subtle alterations in the blood-brain barrier in the neurodegenerative [35, 36] and vascular dementias [37] are not enough to allow macroscopic leakage of contrast material, so intravenous (IV) contrast should not be routinely used in both CT and MRI scans to diagnose these disorders. Indications for administration of contrast include disorders that result in gross disruption of the blood-brain barrier, such as inflammatory disorders, infections, and tumors. These disorders may present as rapidly progressive dementias in younger adults. As a general rule of thumb, these disorders are also indications for a neurology referral, since diagnosis and management of these conditions are outside the scope of the typical psychiatric practice. Therefore, if use of contrast appears to be clinically indicated, consultation with a radiologist and preferably, referral to a neurologist must be strongly considered.

All contrast agents used for CT are iodine-based, but the newer contrast media are non-ionic low-osmolality water soluble molecules with a lower risk of allergic and physiologic reactions and toxicity compared to the older ionic high-osmolality contrast media. With the newer contrast media, the risk of acute allergic reactions is about 0.6% overall with serious acute reactions occurring in about 0.04% of cases [38, 39]. High-risk patients are those with a history of asthma, atopic disease, or prior allergy to iodinated contrast media [39]. A test injection of iodinated contrast is *not* recommended for predicting which patients will react to iodinated contrast [40]. Patients with impaired renal function can experience a worsening of their renal function following intravenous (IV) administration of iodinated contrast material (contrast-induced nephropathy). For patients with an estimated glomerular filtration rate (GFR) between 30 and 60 mL/min, a reduced dose of the contrast material is recommended, and for patients with GFR below 30 mL/min, IV iodinated contrast use is best avoided altogether [41]. If contrast administration is imperative in such patients, proper hydration before and after the procedure is essential. Nephrotoxic agents are best avoided for 48 h before and after contrast administration. This is another situation where it is essential to confer with the staff radiologist prior to ordering a contrast CT scan.

The second safety concern with CT is that it utilizes ionizing radiation (x-rays) which can be carcinogenic. Large epidemiologic studies of atomic bomb survivors and nuclear industry workers have demonstrated that there is a linear dose-response curve between radiation exposure and lifetime relative risk of developing a fatal malignancy. These studies have also shown that children are more susceptible to the carcinogenic effects of radiation than adults. CT parameters such as tube current, tube rotation time, peak voltage, pitch, and collimation contribute to the amount of radiation received during a CT scan; in order to maintain image quality, if one parameter is reduced, another needs to be increased [42]. The harm from exposure to radiation, which is what the patient is typically interested in, is a function of the radiation dose, the sensitivity of the scanned body part to radiation, and the patient's age. This has led to the concept of "effective dose," which is the weighted average of the mean absorbed dose to the various body organs and tissues, and is expressed in Sievert (Sv) [43]. The weighting factor is the radiation detriment for the given organ. The average annual ambient environmental radiation in the USA is roughly about 3.00 mSv. Effective dose of radiation from a typical chest radiograph is about 0.1 to 0.2 mSv, but from a typical head CT is 1 to 2 mSv. The estimated risk of fatal malignancy or death from radiation exposure is 0.05 per 1000 individuals for every 1 mSV of effective radiation dose, while the lifetime odds of dying from a motor vehicle accident is 11.9 and from a natural fatal cancer is 212 [44]. The cancer risk for geriatric patients receiving CT scan is even lower, as there is a 1–2 decade lag time between radiation exposure and development of malignancy. For further information on this topic, the reader is referred to the American Association of Medical Physicists Task Group 23 report, which can be accessed online at https://www.aapm.org/pubs/reports/RPT_96.pdf.

MRI is the neuroimaging modality of choice in neurocognitive disorders. The advantage of MRI lies in its superior resolution and soft tissue contrast, as well as the ability to use specialized pulse sequences. Unlike CT, it is important for the referring clinician to have a basic knowledge of the physics of MRI in order to understand pulse sequences. Most contemporary MRI scanners contain a powerful, doughnut-shaped superconducting magnet cooled by liquid helium. At the center of the doughnut, the resultant magnetic field vector (designated B_0) is oriented parallel to the axis of the patient table. B_0 strengths of 1.5 T (T) and 3 T are currently used in clinical practice, while higher strengths (7 T and 11.7 T) are being used in research. In 2015, Siemens introduced the first 7 T MRI scanner for clinical use, but FDA approval has not yet been granted for ultra-high field MR imaging. While there are distinct advantages to using ultra-high field MRI scanning in practice, including the approximately linear increase in the raw signal to noise ratio (SNR) with the increase in the strength of B_0, there are several problems as well, and a longer discussion of this topic can be found elsewhere [45].

The main contribution to the MRI signal comes from water in biological tissues, since hydrogen atoms are abundantly present in water molecules. Hydrogen protons have a native magnetic spin, and the external magnetic field B_0 adds a "wobble" to this spin which is called *precession*. When hydrogen atoms, each containing a single proton with its own native spin, are placed in the strong magnetic field B_0, the spin vectors of all the protons either align with or against the field. More protons align with the field rather than against it, and the sum of all spin vectors within a certain volume of tissue generates the *net magnetization vector* (NMV) which is parallel to the B_0 field. A radiofrequency (RF) wave is then transmitted briefly (hence the use of the word "pulse") at the precessional (Larmor) frequency of the hydrogen proton, which "flips" the NMV away from its original longitudinal direction (z-axis) into the transverse direction perpendicular to the original field (x-axis), thereby forming the *flip angle*. Other MR-active nuclei remain unaffected at the Larmor frequency of the hydrogen proton, since they are precessing at different frequencies which do not resonate with the RF pulse frequency. An RF pulse is defined by the amount of rotation that it generates; thus, if the RF pulse is switched off as soon as the NMV reaches the transverse plane, it is called a 90° pulse because it "flips" the magnetization vector by 90° where the longitudinal magnetization is 0°. The RF magnetic field, called B_1, is applied in a transverse plane. When the RF pulse is switched off, this transverse magnetization starts to return to its original longitudinal direction. *T1 relaxation* is the time taken for the transverse magnetization to revert to the longitudinal direction to 63% of its final value (for a 90° RF pulse), while *T2 decay* is the time taken for the transverse magnetization to reduce to 37% of its original value. Due to inhomogeneities within the magnetic field, T2 decay actually occurs at a faster rate than what would be expected for any given tissue, and this "effective" decay rate is called *T2* (T2-star) decay* [46]. Note that T1 relaxation and T2 decay occur simultaneously but independently of each other. If the effects of both T1 and T2 contrasts are minimized, image contrast is generated due to the difference in the number of protons per unit volume of tissue which is referred to as *proton density* (PD). When "weighting" is applied preferentially to one of these parameters and away from the others, soft tissue contrast is created. As the moving magnetic field cuts across the receiver coil, it generates an electric voltage which is the source of the MRI signal. Alterations in the main magnetic field in any linear direction can be created by "gradient" wire coils, whose primary function is spatial encoding of the signal. There are three gradient wire coils, one in each axis (*x*-coil, *y*-coil, and *z*-coil). Gradient coils are also responsible for most of the noise emanating from an MRI.

There are only two fundamental types of MR sequence families that are used clinically. Spin echo (SE) and its variants use RF pulses as described. Gradient echo (GRE) and its variants use variations of gradients instead of RF pulses, resulting in much faster acquisition times. A "refocusing" pulse eliminates the effect of magnetic inhomogeneities in an SE sequence, so T2* decay can only be seen in GRE sequences, and the T2*-weighting can be increased by manipulating certain parameters [46]. An MRI "pulse sequence" can now be defined as a series of RF pulses, gradient applications, and intervening time periods. Pulse sequences have specific uses and each is tailored to identify specific neuropathology, which is why several pulse sequences are used in every MRI scan. Furthermore, the pulse sequences have names and acronyms, several of which the referring clinician must become familiar with in order to be able to order and interpret MRI scans. To make matters even more confusing, MRI manufacturers use different acronyms for the MRI pulses. For more details regarding the physics of MRI, the interested reader is referred to this standard text [47]. Websites such as http://www.ismrm.org and http://www.users.on.net/~vision/ can be used to obtain more information on the ever-increasing numbers of sequence names. Some common pulse sequences used in neuropsychiatry are discussed later in this section.

There are also safety concerns associated with the use of MRI scans. MRI does not utilize ionizing radiation, so carcinogenesis is not a concern. The relatively long acquisition time relative to CT scan does preclude its use in agitated patients. As with CT scans, there are not many indications for the use of IV contrast material in MRI in psychiatry. Common indications for MRI with IV contrast include rapidly progressive dementia in a younger patient, and suspicion of infection, tumor, demyelination, or vasculitis [48]. IV contrast material for MRI is not iodine-based but instead contains a heavy metal called gadolinium, which is toxic to humans in its elemental form. There are nine gadolinium-based contrast agents (GBCA) currently approved for use by the US FDA, of which two are not approved for contrast-enhanced brain MR imaging [41, 49]. All GBCA are extracellular and do not cross the blood-brain barrier, and all of them selectively shorten T1 relaxation within a lesion compared with healthy tissue, which is the basis for their use in clinical practice. GBCA can be ionic or non-ionic. Allergic reactions to GBCA are rare, with severe life-threatening reaction incidence of 0.001–0.01% [50]. Knowledge of an allergic reaction in a patient to a previous dose of GBCA should prompt pretreatment with steroids for future contrast-enhanced MRI studies. Nephrogenic systemic fibrosis (NSF) is a severe scleroderma-like disease that can develop in patients with renal insufficiency who received GBCA. The first case was first described in 2006 [51], some 18 years after the first GBCA was approved for use by the FDA. The decision to administer a GBCA to a patient with impaired renal function needs to account for the necessity of the MRI study, degree of renal impairment, the specific types of GBCA available, as well as the availability of dialysis, since some GBCA can be cleared by hemodialysis [52]. Consultation with radiologist and nephrologist colleagues can help in the decision-making process.

In 2014, a new concern appeared regarding toxicity from GBCA—gadolinium deposition in neural tissues (globus pallidus, dentate nucleus) after multiple administrations of GBCA [49].

This adverse effect appears to be independent of renal function, and the clinical significance of this is yet to be fully understood.

Formal postgraduate training in interpretation of cross-sectional imaging of the brain entails several years of training. It is neither possible nor expected that non-radiologists will have the same level of expertise. A comprehensive review of brain CT and MRI interpretation is therefore beyond the scope of this chapter. Described next are key elements of brain MRI interpretation and strategies for improving the nonradiologist's interpretive skill.

Clinicians should make it a habit to personally review all of their patients' scans. All images must be reviewed and interpreted independently, and then the interpretation should be compared with the formal radiology read to assess for discrepancies, which is also an efficient way to learn. The same approach should be used each time when reviewing scans. There is no single best approach, but as long as one sticks to the same approach each time, the likelihood of overlooking potentially important findings is decreased. Clinicians must become aware of the "satisfaction of search" phenomenon—identifying a potentially important finding on the MRI scan and subsequently decreasing vigilance for detecting additional abnormalities—as this is well known to lead to oversight of important imaging findings. In reviewing MRI scans, all parts of the imaged anatomy must be assessed for morphology, volume, and *signal change*, where signal change is any inhomogeneity in the intensity of the greyscale and likely represents pathology [53].

There are five MRI pulse sequences standard to most brain MRI protocols: T1, T2, T2*, FLAIR (Fluid Attenuated Inversion Recovery), and diffusion. Each pulse sequence has a particular use, somewhat analogous to the different histologic stains used by the pathologist.

When reviewing the scan, starting with T1-weighted images (T1WI) is useful as it gives a broad overview of the brain anatomy. Grey matter appears grey, white matter appears white, and cerebrospinal fluid (CSF) appears dark in T1WI. Lipid and subacute blood products appear bright on T1WI. T1WI is used for imaging with IV contrast material; structures/lesions that become hyperintense on post-contrast T1WI as compared to pre-contrast T1WI are said to *enhance*.

On T2-weighted imaging (T2WI), CSF appears bright and the white matter appears dark relative to grey matter. Fluid-attenuated inversion recovery (FLAIR) is a variant of T2WI in which an "inversion pulse" has been applied so as to null (darken) the signal arising from normal CSF. T2WI and FLAIR are sensitive for detection of brain edema, which manifests as a bright signal. Many acute brain pathologies generate brain edema (e.g., cerebritis, cerebral abscess, septic emboli, encephalitis, active demyelination, brain tumors), and T2WI and FLAIR are useful in the detection of such pathologies. Also appearing bright on T2WI and FLAIR are sequelae of prior brain injury, including post-ischemic encephalomalacia, post-traumatic encephalomalacia and multiple sclerosis lesions. Chronic microvascular ischemic changes and chronic lacunar infarcts are also well depicted on T2WI and FLAIR. However, T2WI and FLAIR do not have comparable sensitivity in diagnosing all vascular lesions; for example, vascular syndromes involving the thalamus can present with much psychiatric and neurological morbidity [54], but the FLAIR sequence is less sensitive to vascular lesions in the thalamus than T2WI [55]. T2/FLAIR sequence should not be confused with the T1-inversion recovery (T1/IR or T1/FLAIR) sequence that can replace the T1-weighted SE sequence in some protocols as it improves grey-white matter contrast and lesion delineation without significantly increased acquisition time [56]. In the context of the neurocognitive disorders, the T1/IR sequence is especially useful for delineating enlarged perivascular spaces [57]. Other inversion recovery sequences are also used in brain imaging and may be occasionally seen in MRI scans of patients presenting in the psychiatric clinic, such as the short T1-inversion recovery (STIR) sequence for imaging spinal cord lesions in multiple sclerosis [58].

T2*GRE and the related susceptibility-weighted imaging (SWI) are used primarily to detect intracranial blood products. The hemoglobin associated with the extravasated red blood cells in the brain parenchyma follows a sequence of degradation, beginning with oxyhemoglobin and ending with hemosiderin. Hemosiderin remains in the brain parenchyma for decades following extravasation and appears as dark areas on T2*GRE/SWI. On these blood-sensitive sequences, hypertensive microhemorrhages appear as numerous dark spots in the basal ganglia, whereas cerebral amyloid angiopathy appears as numerous dark spots in the peripheral cerebral hemispheres. Due to the much higher detection rate of microhemorrhages with SWI vis-à-vis T2*GRE, the SWI sequence is gradually replacing T2*GRE in clinical dementia imaging protocols [59, 60]. T2*-based MR imaging techniques also include quantitative susceptibility mapping, perfusion-weighted imaging, and blood oxygen level dependent (BOLD) imaging; of these, only BOLD will be discussed briefly later in the section on functional MRI (fMRI).

Diffusion-weighted imaging (DWI) with its accompanying apparent diffusion coefficient (ADC) map is most commonly used to identify acute infarction (ischemic stroke). Acute infarction appears as bright signal on DWI with corresponding dark signal on the ADC map. This combination of DWI and ADC signal change is referred to as "diffusion restriction." These findings are apparent within minutes following stroke symptom onset, whereas it usually requires a couple of hours for infarction to manifest on CT scan. However, a restricted diffusion pattern can also be seen in nonstroke settings. Nine diagnostic patterns of diffusion restriction have been described across various disorders, several of which can present with cognitive impairment, most notably Creutzfeldt-Jakob disease [61].

Particularly relevant to diagnosis of neurodegenerative disorders is the assessment of brain volume and atrophy, which is a key component of any dementia imaging protocol. It is for this reason that 3D magnetization-prepared fast GRE sequences have found a place in the neuroimaging of neurocognitive disorders. Both the inversion recovery spoiled GRE (IR-SPGR) and the magnetization-prepared rapid acquisition GRE (MP-RAGE—Siemens) sequences generate high-resolution 3D T1-weighted images [62]. It is important to be conversant with these acronyms since these sequences are being used in the AD Neuroimaging Initiative (ADNI) research protocols [63]. Consequently, these sequences are now also the MRI sequences of choice for automated volumetric analysis, a topic that is discussed later in the chapter. Newer high-resolution 3D volumetric fast-SE sequences (SPACE/CUBE/VISTA) are also now available with improved tissue contrast and have a number of clinical applications [64].

In addition to the pulse sequence, it is also very important to know which projection planes are best for viewing various brain structures. The *transaxial (axial) plane* provides a good view of the major fissures and cortical sulci, the ventricular system, posterior fossa structures, and the basal ganglia. The central sulcus is the major anatomical landmark in this plane, and various methods have been described for locating it, such as the *precentral knob* [65]. The axial plane is used to evaluate cerebral, basal ganglia, and cerebellar atrophy, as well as white matter signal change, which is critical for diagnosing vascular cognitive impairment. The *sagittal plane* provides the largest field of view, all the way down to the cervical spine. It provides a good view of some important midline structures (corpus callosum, posterior cingulate, precuneus and mammillary bodies, sella, and the pineal gland) and helps estimate cerebellum and brain stem atrophy, which is seen in the atypical parkinsonian syndromes and other disorders. Unless specifically requested, the *coronal plane* is often omitted in routine MRIs, or imaged using a T2-weighted sequence only. The T1-weighted coronal sequence is an essential sequence for evaluating frontal and temporal atrophy, and especially for estimating hippocampal size, symmetry, and gradient, which is critical for diagnosing frontotemporal as well as AD dementia.

A word of caution regarding axial views of the hippocampus. Since the long axis of the hippocampus is slightly oblique to the standard axial slices, posterior sections of the hippocampus will be visible in the more cephalad axial images while the more anterior sections of the hippocampus will appear as one scrolls down to the more caudal images. In order to best visualize the entire hippocampal formation, it is preferable to image the hippocampus parallel to its long axis in the axial plane as well as in a slightly oblique coronal plane that is perpendicular to its long axis [66]. Rather than acquire these separate images, most centers will acquire a single 3D T1W sequence in the sagittal plane, then reconstruct images in the other two planes (or in a plane orthogonal to the hippocampal axis, as discussed).

Once the appropriate brain scan has been done, it is interpreted and typically a *qualitative* report is generated. By and large, radiologists are still practicing what has been termed the "exclusionary approach" when interpreting brain scans in dementia [67]. This involves simply identifying reversible causes of dementia, which usually adds very little information to what is already known clinically. The benefits of this approach become even more questionable when one takes into account the fact that the three most common reversible conditions that can cause dementia and require neuroimaging for diagnosis—normal pressure hydrocephalus, brain tumors, and subdural hemorrhage—together account for only about 2.2% of all dementias [68]. General radiologists also often fail to interpret regional atrophy patterns as characteristic of a particular dementia. In a study performed predominantly in an academic setting, a diagnosis of behavioral-variant frontotemporal dementia (bv-FTD) was considered by the radiologists in only 10% of all cases [69], even though the characteristic atrophy pattern was identified in half the cases. In practice, a majority of neuroimaging studies in dementia patients are reported by general radiologists as "senescent changes, nothing acute" or a variation thereof, which provides neither diagnostic nor prognostic information. This again underscores why the referring clinicians must personally review the scan, as they have the clinical information that provides the context for the scan.

The "inclusionary approach" is strongly recommended instead, with the goal of *ruling in* rather than *ruling out* etiologies [67]. This consists of three steps [70], which can be easily adapted for reading brain scans in any neuropsychiatric disorder. The first step is *excluding reversible lesions*, the second step is *assessing the extent and pattern of brain atrophy*, and the final step involves *assessing signal change*. Assessing atrophy is important as it has been shown to be the major substrate underlying cognitive impairment, even in subcortical ischemic vascular dementia [71] and post-stroke dementia [72, 73]. It remains to be seen whether the association between vascular dementia and cerebral/medial temporal atrophy will persist in patients with DSM-5 vascular neurocognitive disorder, which can be diagnosed in the absence of an amnestic presentation. In the context of neurocognitive disorders, signal change is usually due to small vessel disease [74]. If all three steps are negative, reassessment after a suitable interval or the use of another biomarker is recommended.

Many visual rating scales are now available to rate both generalized and focal cerebral atrophy [53] as well as signal change [75–77]. It is incumbent upon the referring clinician (and the interpreting radiologist) to become familiar with some of the more common scales and to routinely incorporate them into the imaging report. Each scale requires a specific MRI pulse sequence and specific slices for rating. Most of the common visual rating scales have been shown to have satisfactory inter-rater reliability [53]. Not every scale needs to be used in interpreting every scan; rather, clinical judgment must be exercised in selecting the 2–3 rating scales that are the most relevant in each case, based on available history and differential diagnosis. Volumetric or *quantitative* analysis of brain structures using MRI is being increasingly used in clinical practice. Manual segmentation of a region or regions of interest is extremely time consuming and requires considerable neuroanatomical expertise, and therefore does not lend itself well to clinical practice. Fortunately, fully automated atlas-based segmentation tools are now commercially available for routine clinical use. NeuroQuant® was the first FDA-approved software for volumetric analysis of brain structures [78], and the latest version was released in October 2017. It requires the aforementioned high-resolution 3D T1-weighted noncontrast sagittal images for analysis. Mention of this proprietary software should not be viewed as an endorsement of the product. In fact, the institution's MRI vendor may be able to provide a basic open-source software package at minimal cost. Fully automated volumetric analysis software is also available free of charge, such as the plug-ins for the freely available medical image processing, analysis, and visualization (MIPAV) medical image processing software package from the US National Institutes of Health, which runs on any JAVA-based platform [79]. However, visual rating by an experienced rater is still considered to be superior to automated volumetric analysis, and the 2012 European Federation of the Neurological Societies (EFNS) Task Force on neuroimaging in dementia noted that "accepted standards for quantitative analysis are lacking" [80]. This is a rapidly evolving field, however, and the 6-year European AD Consortium-ADNI Harmonized Protocol for manual hippocampal segmentation (HarP) project has already set a new benchmark against which all future automated hippocampal segmentation algorithms, as well as the accuracy of manual tracers, may be validated [81, 82].

All neuroradiology departments have standard MRI protocols for the common neurological disorders, such as strokes, tumors, and demyelinating diseases, but few have a protocol that is appropriate for diagnosing neurocognitive disorders. A standard MRI dementia protocol has been proposed [48], which can be minimally modified to include the following—3D T1 sagittal images with coronal and axial multiplanar reconstructions (MPR) acquired using the NeuroQuant® (or another volumetric analysis) protocol so one can potentially do volumetrics, 3D sagittal T2/FLAIR with axial MPR, axial T2 (Turbo)SE, axial SWI, and axial DWI with ADC map. 3D sequences allow reformatting in any plane. This protocol can be built into the hospital's electronic medical record (EMR) software as a single order set, with additional options for volumetrics and use of IV contrast if needed. Volumetric analysis can also be requested later as needed, as long as the necessary pulse sequence and number of images have been acquired at the time of scan. If CT scanning is the only option for reasons previously discussed, helical CT with reconstructions in the coronal and sagittal planes should be obtained whenever possible in patients with neurocognitive disorders.

The ideal structural neuroimaging report should therefore include a list of the specific visual rating scales used to rate global and regional cerebral atrophy, as well as to rate and localize any signal change, presence or absence of volumetric analysis, presence and localization of any diffusion restriction, mention of any reversible causes of dementia, and a final diagnosis or differential diagnosis regarding the etiology of dementia in that particular patient [48]. If the referring clinician uses an EMR, having a template for the over-read that incorporates some combination of the common visual rating scales can save time and simultaneously ensure that a relatively standardized imaging report is quickly incorporated into the office visit note.

This section has summarized the most common structural neuroimaging modalities. Advanced MRI sequences such as arterial spin labeling (ASL) and diffusion tensor imaging (DTI) tractography are also now being increasingly used in clinical practice but are still not widely available outside of advanced imaging centers, and therefore will not be discussed in detail; DTI tractography will be briefly mentioned later in the section on functional MRI (fMRI) and multimodal imaging.

Functional Imaging

Single photon emission computerized tomography (SPECT) and positron emission tomography (PET) are the two principal functional imaging techniques, both of which are used in neuropsychiatric practice to varying degrees and for different indications. fMRI still remains purely a research tool in neuropsychiatry and, as of now, its clinical application is restricted to a single neurosurgical indication, as discussed later. However, fMRI has made major contributions to neuropsychiatry and will therefore be discussed briefly.

SPECT imaging utilizes standard nuclear medicine cameras and provides an estimate of the regional cerebral blood flow (rCBF). Small lipophilic compounds, such as ^{99}mTc-hexamethylpropyleneamine (^{99}mTc-HMPAO) and ^{99}mTc-ethylcysteine dimer (^{99}mTc-ECD), are typically used as SPECT tracers. A recent review found that there is about a 10% improvement in diagnostic sensitivity with PET scans compared to SPECT scans for separating AD dementia from normal controls, DLB and FTD, while the specificities were comparable; the review also noted that direct PET-to-SPECT comparison studies in neurodegenerative dementias were limited in number and have small numbers of subjects [83]. A recent Cochrane meta-analysis did not recommend the use of rCBF SPECT to differentiate FTD from AD, as it found insufficient evidence in the literature in support of this indication [84]. As PET scanners are becoming relatively ubiquitous in the USA, the use of SPECT scans in the diagnosis of dementia has declined considerably. Families may initially express a preference for SPECT over PET scans for their loved one with dementia, as they can remain in the imaging suite with the patient during a SPECT scan which is standard practice, but this is not routine during a PET scan in order to keep radiation exposure to a minimum. However, diagnostic accuracy has been shown to trump patient and caregiver preference, and most patients do not find either scan more stressful than completing questionnaires at home [85]. Use of SPECT in the diagnosis of the dementias has, therefore, become mostly limited to dopamine transporter scans and myocardial SPECT scans, both of which will be discussed later in the section on molecular imaging.

PET scans do not measure cerebral blood flow; rather, PET tracers are bound to radioactive isotopes, typically ^{18}F or ^{11}C, which target a predefined organ or cell type. The valence number of the isotope indicates the mass of its atomic nucleus. The tracer binds to the target tissue and its decay is measured. ^{18}fluorodeoxyglucose (FDG) is the tracer used most frequently in PET scans for neurocognitive disorders. It is a glucose analogue that is taken up by organs which have high glucose consumption, such as the brain. Ninety-five percent of the energy (adenosine triphosphate or ATP) requirement for brain function comes from glucose metabolism [86], most of which is then used to sustain postsynaptic action potentials [87]. It is important to note that the metabolic signature in neurodegenerative dementias is not simply due to synaptic loss or aging. Neurodegenerative disorders do result in direct synaptic loss early on in the course of the disease, but the magnitude of the reduction in glucose metabolism, called *hypometabolism*, as measured by FDG-PET, is a reflection of not only underlying synaptic loss in the affected areas of the brain but also the result of a true reduction in regional cerebral glucose metabolism [88]. Reduced FDG uptake with age has been most consistently seen in bilateral anterior cingulate, dorsolateral and medial prefrontal and orbitofrontal cortices, and in some regions this can be similar in magnitude to that found in AD [89, 90]. Fortunately, the aging process spares the signature cortical regions that are involved in the common neurodegenerative dementias, which usually makes it possible to differentiate the metabolic signatures of these disorders as distinct from hypometabolism due to normal aging.

The PET radioisotopes are inherently unstable. The time required for half the radioactive nuclei to break down, or *decay*, is the *half-life* of the radioisotope, which is 109.77 min for ^{18}F. Such decay results in the release of a positively charged particle, called a *positron*, which travels through tissue until it collides with an electron. This annihilation event generates a *photon couple* traveling in opposite directions from each other. The PET γ-ray coincidence detectors detect the emission of millions of such photon couples to compute the concentration of tracer decay at each location, which yields a relatively low resolution image [91]. Dedicated PET/CT scanners use low dose radiation CT to obtain co-registered images, which are then fused to the PET images to generate *attenuation maps* to enable *attenuation correction* (photons originating in deeper structures are *attenuated* by the intervening soft tissue and therefore falsely appear to have lower activity than photons released from more superficial tissues). Fused PET/CT images also improve spatial resolution and thereby allow anatomical localization of the lesion. These low radiation CT scans should never be used for diagnostic purposes.

Exposure to radiation is also a concern with PET/CT imaging. The exposure occurs not only from the tracer used, but also from the CT component of the scan in the PET/CT scanner. For PET brain imaging in adults, the dose of FDG recommended is 5–20 mCi. A 10 mCi dose of FDG results in an effective radiation dose of about 4 mSv to the brain; the additional radiation dose from the multidetector CT depends on the scanner model and the technique used [91]. The quality of the CT image can be improved by increasing the CT current and potential, which unfortunately results in higher radiation exposure. It should already be evident by now that the radiation exposure (and therefore, the subsequent risk of cancer) is higher with PET/CT imaging than from just CT imaging of the brain. However, in the context of dementia patients, it is again important to note that most patients are older, and the carcinogenic risk due to radiation exposure declines with increasing age at exposure [92].

Even though FDG-PET scans are not typically done early in the course of the disease in clinical practice, earlier scans may be more useful. One study found that obtaining an FDG-PET at initial clinical evaluation improved the diagnostic accuracy of AD dementia equivalent to a mean of 4.1 (SD 2.7) years of follow-up, and both positive and negative predictive values were higher for FDG-PET vis-à-vis an initial clinical diagnosis [93]. The cost of an FDG-PET scan now is typically less than the cost of one year's worth of unnecessary treatment of an incorrectly diagnosed patient with cholinesterase inhibitors [94], so the earlier the scan is done, the more cost effective it is. In clinical practice however, the use of FDG-PET scans in diagnosing dementia is severely restricted by the Center for Medicare and Medicaid Services (CMS) national coverage determination (NCD) for FDG-PET for Dementia and Neurodegenerative Disease, which was first issued in 2004, and version 3 became effective in 2009. It limits the use of an FDG-PET scan to a single clinical indication differentiating AD dementia from FTD- and only when certain other preconditions are met. These include a "comprehensive clinical evaluation" which should be "conducted by a physician experienced in the diagnosis and assessment of dementia," cognitive screening in the clinic, and checking relevant labs (B12 and thyroid hormone are listed in the document). Presence of cognitive decline of at least 6 months' duration is necessary prior to ordering the scan, along with prior structural brain imaging (CT or MRI), which should have been inconclusive. If a previous FDG-PET or SPECT scan has been obtained for the same indication, another scan is covered only after 1 year and only if the first functional imaging was inconclusive (or if the first functional scan was a SPECT scan that was difficult to interpret due to technological problems). The clinical benefit of a repeat PET/CT must be weighed against the higher radiation exposure risk, keeping the patient's age in mind, as already discussed. In order to operationalize the NCD criteria, nuclear medicine departments across the country have developed checklists, such as the one used at UCLA [95], to assist with determining whether an FDG-PET scan will be covered by CMS in a particular patient. Referring clinicians are strongly encouraged to use such a list and/or consult with their own nuclear medicine department in questionable cases. The referring as well as billing clinicians must be able to demonstrate medical necessity, as set forth in the NCD, upon request by the CMS and/or its agent upon request (*Code of Federal Regulations section 410.32*).

Occasionally, patients will request an FDG-PET scan for diagnostic clarification even when it is clear that the scan will not be covered by CMS. In such cases, if the clinician agrees that the scan is indicated, the issue of out-of-pocket payment for the service should be discussed at the outset. Veterans who use their VA benefits are not bound by the CMS NCD. Therefore, clinicians working for Veterans Administration (VA) clinics and hospitals have the option of using FDG-PET scans for noncovered indications, such as to confirm a clinical diagnosis of DLB or to confirm a diagnosis of AD dementia in atypical cases (e.g., young-onset dementia or nonamnestic AD) even when FTD is not in the differential.

Simultaneous PET and MRI image acquisition was first reported in 2008 using a PET detector ring [96], and fully integrated PET/MRI scanners have been available since 2010 [97]. One clinical advantage of using a dedicated PET/MRI scanner is that most patients with neurocognitive disorders will get an MRI scan of the brain anyway, and obtaining a PET scan at the same time will greatly reduce acquisition time [98]. Another advantage is the lower radiation exposure with PET/MRI imaging vis-à-vis PET/CT imaging. PET/MRI systems are also more suitable for multimodal imaging protocols [99]. Unfortunately, the CMS NCD precludes reimbursement for the simultaneous acquisition of FDG-PET and MRI structural scans in clinical practice. PET/MRI systems are still not widely available and the technology is still evolving. The interested reader is referred to this review [98] for further details.

One vexing problem in PET (and SPECT) scans is the *partial volume effect* (PVE). The small size of brain structures limits an accurate estimate of the tracer concentration. PET and especially SPECT cameras have relatively limited spatial resolution. Therefore, increased tracer concentrations in small areas of the brain can get diluted and *spill out* into the surrounding brain tissue, while increased metabolic activity in the surrounding tissues can *spill in* into the region of interest. Both phenomena lead to a 3D degrading of the final image, and region(s) of interest can therefore appear to have reduced intensity values and appear larger, which is called *partial volume effect*. The spatial resolution of today's PET scanners is about 2–3 mm, which approximates the thickness of the cortical grey matter. Voxel-based image sampling also contributes to the PVE, since the contour of the voxel does not exactly match the contour of the tracer distribution in the brain region of interest, as does patient motion which can be substantial in dementia patients. Cerebral atrophy in dementia further contributes to atrophy-related PVE, as the size of metabolically inactive CSF spaces increases with tissue loss. PVE is a major source of bias in PET and SPECT scans, and different methods of *partial volume correction* have been developed in an effort to resolve this problem [100]. PET/MRI scanners may provide a more accurate partial volume and motion correction than PET/CT scanners [98].

Some procedural issues are also worth considering. Patients should fast for at least 4 h before an FDG-PET scan for neurodegenerative disorders. FDG uptake in the brain is reduced in the presence of hyperglycemia as FDG competes with plasma glucose for intracellular transport, so finger-stick glucose should be checked prior to administration of FDG, and a fasting glucose of less than 150 mg/dL is desirable. This is especially important in patients with dementia, as even mild hyperglycemia can result in an Alzheimer's disease-like pattern leading to an increase in the false positive rate [101, 102]. Use of 5% dextrose should be avoided before and during the scan when the patient is receiving intravenous fluids [103]. The patient should be placed in a low stimulation environment with low lighting and minimal ambient noise. The 2009 Society for Nuclear Medicine Procedure guidelines recommend that the eyes can remain open or closed, as long as either practice is consistent across successive scans for the purpose of comparison. However, in patients with neurodegenerative dementias, an eyes-open study is highly recommended, with the patient staying awake and looking straight ahead following tracer administration and not into the lights. They should be closely monitored in this period to make sure that their eyes do not close and they stay awake (also see ADNI protocol at http://adni.loni.usc.edu/wp-content/uploads/2010/09/PET-Tech_Procedures_Manual_v9.5.pdf). The referring provider should always note whether it was an eyes-open study or not, and the report should ideally mention this fact to alert the referring clinician, who may otherwise make a false positive diagnosis of DLB [104]. In agitated patients, the use of a short acting intravenous benzodiazepine is permitted to obtain the scan, but this should be administered at least 20 min after tracer injection, and the dose should be adjusted for geriatric patients [86].

Similar to MRI scans, FDG-PET and SPECT scans can be analyzed visually or quantitatively. Visual analysis of FDG-PET scans is traditionally done by viewing a series of axial fused CT/PET images. Modern 3D PET/CT scanners can generate over 100 axial slices, which can be challenging to review visually. Nevertheless, visual analysis should always be the first step, preferably using the inverse linear grey scale, the diagnostic accuracy of which is acceptably high [104]. The relative metabolic activity varies for different brain regions, and visual interpretation should take this into account, along with the true reduction in metabolism seen in normal aging as well as the apparent reduction resulting from atrophy of the underlying brain structures, as already discussed. Seven patterns of FDG uptake (FDG-7) have been identified in dementia brain scans on visual analysis, of which four are progressive and three are nonprogressive [105]. In the clinic, a simpler binary classification scheme (FDG-2) can improve the inter-rater agreement substantially [106].

Quantitative analysis should ideally follow visual analysis of PET and SPECT scans, which increases the diagnostic accuracy [107, 108]. Earlier quantitative analyses involved tracing an anatomical region or volume of interest (ROI or VOI). This requires manual tracing of the region(s) of interest based on a priori hypotheses about the topography of the deficit, which is time consuming (large number of ROIs needed to cover the entire brain volume) and results in poor spatial resolution [109]. Relatively newer voxel-based techniques have the advantage of being more data driven and sample the entire brain quickly and effectively at a much higher spatial resolution. The fully automated techniques of voxel-by-voxel analyses most commonly used are the 3D-stereotactic surface projection (3D SSP) metabolic and statistical (z-score) mapping [110] which is part of the NEUROSTAT software library for biomedical image analysis, and statistical parametric mapping [111] which is available as part of the SPM software package. Both are available as free downloads and have been widely used in research, and both require a significant degree of neuroanatomical expertise to interpret the final output. The standardized ROI (SROI) approach blends elements from the ROI and voxel-based approaches. Both the voxel-based and SROI approaches require transformation of individual brain scans to a standard template space, but in the SROI approach, ROIs are predefined in the template space which can then be applied to the patient's transformed brain, thereby covering the entire brain in a matter of seconds which makes this approach easier to interpret, especially for those with limited knowledge of neuroanatomy [104]. NeuroQ™ was the first software for quantification of FDG-PET scans approved by the FDA in 2004, and it is based on the SROI approach.

One final issue that deserves mention is that of intensity normalization, which involves scaling of tracer uptake to a reference brain region or regions defined *a priori* based on theoretical considerations, in order to remove inter-individual differences. Intensity normalization in PET and SPECT scans, hereafter simply referred to as *normalization*, should not be confused with spatial normalization that is used in neuroimaging to fit the native subject scan to a standard atlas or template, as discussed above. The reference region selected for normalization must be relatively spared by the disease under study, must be reliable and easy to localize, and must have stable metabolism in healthy individuals, as well as in those with the disease in question [112]. It should also maximize the contrast in glucose metabolism between patients and healthy controls, and between patients with different neurocognitive disorders [113]. Several reference areas have been used for normalization in FDG-PET scans in persons with dementia, including the sensorimotor strip, cerebellar cortex, pons, the basal ganglia, thalamus, visual cortex, and the cerebral metabolic rate for glucose. There is no perfect reference region for normalization, since most of these regions are affected to some extent in neurodegenerative disorders, especially in advanced AD dementia, which can lead to a substantial overcorrection error. Normalization to the sensorimotor cortex may provide the best discrimination in patients with AD [112], but the sensorimotor cortex has a variable structure [114] and needs to be used with caution as a reference region when tracer uptake in the sensorimotor cortex is anticipated to be less than robust, such as due to frequently co-occurring cerebrovascular disease in AD patients. Using the cerebellum as the reference area for normalization has been shown to effectively discriminate between controls and dementia patients and may be advantageous when there is a question about the diagnosis of dementia [113]. It may be particularly useful in reducing the false positive rate of AD in the presence of mild hyperglycemia [101]. However, while cerebellar and brain stem metabolism increases with age in absolute terms [115], primary involvement of the cerebellum in AD has been reported in some [116], but not all [117, 118] studies. Furthermore, crossed cerebellar diaschisis has been shown in AD [118], where diaschisis is defined as functional impairment in a functionally related region due to a permanent injury in an anatomically remote site [119]. In one study, crossed cerebellar diaschisis was present in about a quarter of AD patients, most of whom had severe dementia [118]. The choice of cerebellum as a reference region for intensity normalization should also be avoided in patients with known or expected cerebellar disease; in neurocognitive disorder patients, this may include patients with a history of alcoholism [120], multisystem atrophy [121], or patients with the C9ORF72 mutation which can involve the cerebellum [122]. Normalization to the pons can be problematic as its relatively small size increases the risk of PVE [113]. Normalization to the cerebral metabolic rate for glucose (CMRglu) can be very useful when differentiating AD dementia from FTD [113], which is also the only

CMS-approved indication for the clinical use of FDG-PET scan in dementia. In practice, more than one reference area can be used sequentially, based on the clinical indication for the scan.

Functional MRI (fMRI) is a relatively new method for studying neural activity that has had tremendous impact, and the use of blood oxygen level dependent (BOLD) fMRI in research has increased exponentially since it was first described [123, 124]. Readers who want to learn more about fMRI history and applications are referred to the 2012 special issue of the journal *NeuroImage*, entitled "Twenty years of functional MRI: The science and the stories." The use of fMRI in clinical practice is still limited only to neurosurgery for presurgical mapping of patients with brain tumors and epilepsy, where it is usually used in conjunction with co-registered DTI tractography and 3D high-resolution T1-weighted volumetric sequences [125]. Three CPT codes related to the use of fMRI for this clinical indication went into effect in 2007 [126], due in part to the stellar efforts by the American Psychological Association [127]. There is no clinical indication yet for ordering an fMRI study in the psychiatric clinic. However, *resting state* fMRI studies have contributed enormously by enhancing our understanding of the functional connectivity networks in the brain which have been the subject of much recent research in psychiatry and neurology, and therefore a nodding acquaintance with this topic is desirable. The BOLD signal is dependent on regional neurovascular coupling and is a surrogate marker for regional neural activity (see [128] for an excellent review). Oxyhemoglobin is diamagnetic but deoxyhemoglobin contains unpaired electrons, which makes it strongly paramagnetic relative to perivascular tissue and leads to perivascular magnetic field perturbations. Neural activity leads to a transient increase in regional blood flow which increases the local oxy/deoxyhemoglobin ratio. The local change in MR signal intensity due to transient changes in oxygen saturation is the basis of the BOLD signal, which can be detected by a fast T2*-weighted GRE sequence [46]. It may be obvious to the discerning reader by now that no special MRI scanner is necessary for routine fMRI studies. However, since the intensity of the BOLD signal increases with the strength of the magnetic field, the introduction of the 3T scanner into clinical practice has been a boon for fMRI studies, and magnetic field strengths of 7T and above are often used in research.

While pre-surgical mapping in neurosurgery is an example of task-evoked fMRI that is used to link structure with function during baseline and activation conditions, the remainder of this section will focus on the resting state fMRI. Resting state activity is measured by asking subjects to lie quietly in the scanner but not fall asleep. Acquisition of the T2*-weighted BOLD signal occurs within a matter of minutes. In this resting state, the BOLD signal can identify low frequency neuronal oscillations (<0.1 Hz) in regional brain activity [129]. These spontaneous fluctuations in the resting state signal correlate temporally and in magnitude (coherence) and are used to map specific resting state networks (RSN), the individual elements of which may or may not be contiguous.

A number of RSN have been defined, including the default mode network (DMN), salience network, and cognitive control network, which are remarkably consistent across subjects and time [130, 131]; of these, the DMN deserves special mention. It was shown as far back as 2001 that, in the resting state, "a default state of brain activity exists" in a network that includes several brain structures, including the medial prefrontal cortex anteriorly, and the precuneus and the posterior cingulate posteriorly [132]. This has become known as the DMN. The DMN is believed to support self-referential thinking. External tasks attenuate but do not abolish DMN activity, and simultaneously activate the task-positive network, which has strong anticorrelation with the DMN [133]. The DMN has been studied the most among all the RSN, both in health and in disease.

Developmentally, the RSN appear to emerge as early as the last trimester of gestation [134], and core patterns become well established by age 12. However, the networks continue to mature well into young adulthood, resulting in increased efficiency [135]. RSN have been studied in major psychiatric disorders, including schizophrenia [136], depression [137], ADHD [138], and neurocognitive disorders [139], but further standardization is necessary for routine clinical use. fMRI may eventually become clinically useful in neuropsychiatry as part of a multimodal imaging strategy that simultaneously looks at the temporal and spatial relationships between several pathologic variables and includes some combination of task-evoked fMRI, resting state fMRI, structural MRI, FDG-PET, amyloid PET, and DTI tractography [30]. Multimodal imaging that also includes electroencephalography and magnetoencephalography is the basis for the Human Connectome Project [29].

Molecular Imaging

When SPECT or PET technology is used to image molecular pathology, it is called molecular imaging. Radiopharmaceuticals are now available that allow elucidation of pathology at the molecular level, such as receptors and proteins. As already mentioned, imaging the dopamine transporter using SPECT is now approved in the United States for differentiating neurodegenerative causes of parkinsonism (with or without cognitive impairment) from other disorders causing tremors, and will be discussed in this section. ^{123}I-metaiodobenzylguanidine (MIBG) myocardial scintigraphy also has practical clinical applications in diagnosing some movement and neurocognitive disorders, and will be discussed in some detail. It is approved for clinical use in some countries but not in the United States as yet. PET ligands that bind to insoluble, fibrillary amyloid arranged in a beta-pleated sheet conformation (as seen in Aβ plaques) have been commercially available for clinical use since 2012, but amyloid PET is also not reimbursed by CMS at this time and, therefore, not yet used in routine clinical practice. However, the decision not to reimburse for amyloid PET may change in the not-too-distant future, so amyloid PET will be also discussed here, albeit briefly. On the other hand, PET imaging in the movement disorders, such as imaging the dopamine terminals using ^{18}F-DOPA to diagnose idiopathic Parkinson's disease (iPD) [140], is still a research tool and will not be discussed further.

The dopamine transporter, located in the presynaptic nigrostriatal nerve terminals, is responsible for the reuptake of dopamine from the synaptic cleft [141]. The quest for the ideal dopamine transporter-selective radiopharmaceutical culminated in the development of ^{123}I-ioflupane (^{123}Iodine-fluoropropyl (FP)-carbomethoxy-3 β-4-iodophenyltropane) or ^{123}I-FP-CIT (DaTSCAN™), and ^{123}I-β-CIT (DOPASCAN™). These target the presynaptic dopamine transporter and thereby detect loss of functional dopaminergic neuron terminals in the striatum, which is useful for differentiating the neurodegenerative parkinsonian syndromes in vivo from healthy individuals, as well as from nondegenerative causes of parkinsonism (vascular parkinsonism, drug-induced parkinsonism, and psychogenic parkinsonism) and essential tremor. While both the ^{123}I-FP-CIT and the ^{123}I-β-CIT scans are commercially available in Europe, only ^{123}I-FP-CIT SPECT was approved by the FDA in the United States under the trade name DaTSCAN™ in 2011, a decade after it was approved for this purpose in Europe [142], and only for a single clinical indication which is to "help differentiate essential tremor from tremor due to parkinsonian syndromes (idiopathic Parkinson's disease, multiple system atrophy and progressive supranuclear palsy)."

The ^{123}I-FP-CIT tracer is taken up symmetrically by the caudate and lentiform nuclei to create the "double comma" sign, which indicates a normal scan. A forward tilt of the head can inadvertently separate the caudate from the putamen, leading to an artefactual "semi-colon sign," which can result in a false positive interpretation [143]. Abnormal ^{123}I-FP-CIT scans can be rated visually using a simple numerical 3-point scale [142]. A 5-point visual scale has also been proposed, in which grade 1 is a "burst striatum" pattern which involves increased background tracer uptake with markedly reduced or no uptake in the basal ganglia bilaterally, and grade 5 is a normal scan [144, 145]. Visual interpretation is heavily dependent on rater experience, but inter-rater reliability between experienced and inexperienced raters has been shown to be good and compares favorably with semiquantitative assessment [146]. Visual analysis is particularly useful in identifying right-left asymmetry across the midline as well as differences in tracer uptake between the striatal subregions [147]. Semiquantitative methods compare specific tracer binding in the striatum to nonspecific binding in reference regions with minimal or absent dopamine transporter density, usually the occipital cortex [141, 148].

This is used to generate the *specific binding ratio* (SBR), defined as the ratio of specific to nonspecific uptake [149]. Semiquantitative analysis is recommended by the EANM for supplementing visual analysis [141], but semiquantitative and subregional analyses are not yet FDA-approved [142]. Fully automated semiquantitative analysis can also be done using proprietary software, such as DaTQUANT™ (GE Healthcare), which uses an automated VOI approach to calculate SBR, putamen/caudate and left-to-right asymmetry ratios, and also removes head-tilt artifacts. As stated previously, the author does not endorse this or any other software for this purpose.

Age-related decline in dopamine transporter density, which occurs at the rate of approximately 6% per decade, can confound interpretation. Age-related decline involves both the caudate and putamen equally and is relatively symmetric [150]. Automated analysis software adjusts for age and gender by comparing patient data with the binding values in gender and age-matched healthy controls. For example, DaTQUANT™ compares specific binding ratios against the normative database from the Parkinson's Progression Markers Initiative (http://www.ppmi-info.org/) [151]. A large European multicenter normative database of ^{123}I-FP-CIT scans in healthy controls has also been created for semiquantitative analysis [152].

Studies have reported about a 95% sensitivity and specificity for the ^{123}I-FP-CIT scan for the diagnosis of iPD [142]. Real-world experience is more variable, but a positive scan in the clinic setting does make it highly likely that the physician will initiate or maintain the patient on antiparkinsonian medications [153]. The ^{123}I-FP-CIT scan does not image α-synuclein deposition directly (more on PET imaging of α-synuclein later), but rather detects brain dopamine depletion due to downstream damage to the nigrostriatal neurons. Therefore, it does not reliably discriminate among all the various parkinsonian disorders in which there is degeneration of dopaminergic striatonigral neurons, including iPD with or without cognitive impairment, DLB, and the atypical parkinsonian syndromes (APS) [142]. However, if performed within 5 years of symptom onset, the "burst striatum" pattern on visual analysis on the ^{123}I-FP-CIT scan has been found to be predictive of APS (multi-system atrophy, progressive supranuclear palsy, and corticobasal degeneration) [144] with a specificity of 90-93% across two studies [144, 145]. Note that histopathological confirmation of the diagnoses was not obtained in these studies, and clinical consensus criteria were considered to be the gold standard. Also, the sensitivity was only about 30-60% across the two studies, which implies that this pattern is not seen in all APS cases but is a valuable diagnostic finding in the clinic when present.

The ^{123}I-FP-CIT scan also does not reliably differentiate among the nondegenerative causes of parkinsonism [142]. Its value in ruling out vascular parkinsonism (VP) is limited to cases where the ^{123}I-FP-CIT scan is normal, as there is considerable overlap in tracer uptake patterns between VP and iPD [154]. Psychiatric providers should note that the ^{123}I-FP-CIT scan is normal in drug-induced parkinsonism (DIP) due to dopamine receptor antagonists, and it can be especially helpful in making an accurate diagnosis when the DIP either unmasks iPD or antedates iPD [155]. Also, the scan is normal in psychogenic parkinsonism, so a positive scan can help rule *in* neurodegenerative causes of parkinsonism in questionable psychogenic parkinsonism cases [155].

Low dopamine transporter uptake by SPECT (or PET) imaging is listed as a *suggestive* feature in the 2005 revised diagnostic criteria for DLB [156]. Making an accurate diagnosis of DLB is important in the clinic because of the low sensitivity of its diagnostic criteria [156]. This was amply demonstrated in a large autopsy-based study using data from the National Alzheimer's Coordinating Center (NACC) that compared the final clinical diagnosis with the neuropathological diagnosis and found that the sensitivity of a clinical diagnosis of DLB was only 32% for pure DLB, although the specificity was over 95% [157]. AD often coexists with DLB, and this study found that the sensitivity of a clinical diagnosis of AD with DLB was even lower at only 12%. Structural neuroimaging does not help differentiate DLB from other neurodegenerative dementias because structural imaging is usually unremarkable in pure DLB and therefore not indicated in clinical practice. There is usually relative preservation of medial temporal lobe structures in DLB compared to AD dementia of comparable severity, which is listed as a *supportive* feature in the 2005 diagnostic guidelines for DLB [80, 156]. Occipital atrophy is also not typically seen [80]. A small 2007 study ($N = 20$) that used neuropathological criteria as the gold standard for diagnosing DLB found that the sensitivity and specificity of the ^{123}I-FP-CIT scan in the diagnosis of DLB were 88% and 100% respectively, a substantial improvement over the initial clinical diagnosis which had a sensitivity and specificity of only 75% and 42% respectively [158]. Ten years later, the same group reported the largest study ($N = 55$) of the usefulness of ^{123}I-FP-CIT scan in the diagnosis of DLB using autopsy confirmation [159]. Subjects were recruited from a tertiary care center and the study found that the ^{123}I-FP-CIT scan had a sensitivity of 80% and specificity of 92% compared with the clinical diagnosis, which had sensitivity of 87% and specificity of 72%. The study also found a normal scan in 10% of patients with autopsy-confirmed DLB due to minimal brainstem involvement. A positive ^{123}I-FP-CIT scan increases the diagnostic confidence of clinicians when there is a clinical diagnosis of possible DLB [160]. In a large recent clinical study which used the clinical evolution of symptoms over 6 months as the gold standard for diagnosing DLB rather than neuropathological criteria, the presence of a positive ^{123}I-FP-CIT scan and parkinsonism and absence of medial temporal atrophy at baseline best identified patients who went on to develop DLB [161]. It is best used in the memory clinic to differentiate DLB from AD dementia, and the European Medicine Agency has already approved the ^{123}I-FP-CIT scan to differentiate probable DLB from AD dementia, but this is not yet an FDA-approved indication in the United States. The scan does not perform so well when used to differentiate DLB from non-AD neurodegenerative dementias, such as FTD [162] or PD dementia [163], and should not be used for this purpose.

Last but not least, the effects of concurrent medications on the ^{123}I-FP-CIT scan are still being clarified. The package insert from GE Healthcare has the following warning—"Drugs that bind to the dopamine transporter with high affinity may interfere with the image obtained following DaTscan administration." Many of these drugs are commonly used psychotropic medications. Practical recommendations are available about when to stop drugs that reduce ^{123}I-FP-CIT uptake by 20% or more [154]. Many patients are already on levodopa or a dopamine agonist at the time of the scan. Fortunately, dopaminergic therapies do not appear to interfere with the scan and, therefore, do not need to be discontinued prior to the scan [154]. Of note, selegiline (but not rasagiline) is listed in the prescribing information from GE Healthcare as a drug that may potentially interfere with the scan, but it is not included in the aforementioned list of drugs that reduce ^{123}I-FP-CIT uptake by 20% or more [154].

MIBG scintiscans are approved in the USA for the detection and localization of neuroendocrine tumors of neuro-ectodermal origin (neuroblastoma, primary or metastatic pheochromocytoma), and MIBG myocardial scintigraphy was approved in 2013 in the USA under the trade name AdreView™ (GE Healthcare) for the evaluation of patients with NYHA class 2–3 heart failure with a left ventricular ejection fraction ≤35%. MIBG myocardial scintigraphy for detection of the Lewy body disorders was developed in Japan. In the Lewy body disorders (iPD with or without dementia, DLB), the autonomic nervous system, including the sympathetic nerve fibers in the cardiac plexus, becomes pathologically involved, which is not the case in essential tremor, APS, or other neurodegenerative dementias [164]. MIBG itself is an inactive physiologic analogue of norepinephrine and competes with it for uptake by the norepinephrine transporter in functionally intact postganglionic sympathetic nerve terminals, where it is then stored in vesicles. Unlike norepinephrine, it is not metabolized and accumulates in intact synaptic vesicles which allows imaging. The MIBG myocardial scan therefore tests for the functional integrity of the cardiac postganglionic sympathetic innervation [165]. Reduction in cardiac MIBG uptake in the Lewy body disorders has been conclusively shown to correlate with loss of sympathetic cardiac axons in an autopsy-based study [166]. MIBG can be tagged with radioactive iodine, either ^{123}I or ^{131}I. ^{123}I is preferred due to its better dosimetry, improved image quality leading to better anatomical localization on SPECT/

CT systems, and lower radiation burden which allows a higher dose to be injected [167]. While ^{123}I has a physical half-life of only 13.13 h, ^{131}I has a physical half-life of 8.04 days, so the latter is more suitable if delayed scans are necessary [167]. Myocardial MIBG uptake can be measured by anterior planar scintigraphic images of the chest (acquisition time of about 5 min) or by SPECT generated 3D images (acquisition time of over 20 min). Even the slightest patient motion can degrade the SPECT images. For standard clinical use, use of planar scintigraphic images may be adequate [167]. Images can be taken early (usually 30 min post-injection of ^{123}I-MIBG) or late (usually 4 h post-injection).

MIBG scintiscans can differentiate between the Lewy body disorders and APS with high sensitivity and specificity. A 2012 meta-analysis of 13 studies found that the pooled sensitivity and specificity to differentiate iPD from APS were 82.6% and 89.2% respectively by the early heart-to-mediastinum (H/M) ratio, and 89.7% and 82.6%, respectively, by the delayed H/M ratio [168]. Among the three disorders commonly included in the APS, multisystem atrophy (MSA) is somewhat unique. Both progressive supranuclear palsy (PSP) and corticobasal degeneration (CBD) are tauopathies. On the other hand, MSA is an α-synucleinopathy, similar to iPD and DLB, but it is *not* a Lewy body disease; in MSA, misfolded α-synuclein inclusions (Papp–Lantos bodies) are found in the cytoplasm of oligodendrocytes which makes it an *oligodendrocyte α-synucleinopathy,* while Lewy bodies are *neuronal aggregates* of α-synuclein [169]. Furthermore, unlike iPD and DLB, MSA involves the central and preganglionic neurons, while the postganglionic sympathetic neurons are usually spared [170]. The same meta-analysis found that the pooled sensitivity and specificity for differentiating iPD from MSA were 90.2% and 81.9% respectively from 10 studies [168].

Low uptake on MIBG myocardial scintigraphy is listed as a *supportive* feature in the 2005 revised diagnostic criteria for DLB [156]. Visual analysis of the scan is possible by experienced readers and its accuracy in differentiating DLB from AD is comparable to a quantitative analysis using either the early [171] or delayed heart-to-mediastinum (H/M) ratio [172]. Both H/M ratios have been shown to be equally useful for diagnosing DLB using a cut-off of 2.1–2.2 [171, 172], since autopsy data shows that even in the early phase, cardiac MIBG uptake is already reduced by almost 91% in the Lewy body disorders [166]. Visual interpretation and use of the early H/M ratio will likely be more useful in clinical practice as it can greatly reduce the scan time, thus increasing the number of patients that can be scanned in a day.

In 2012, Japanese health authorities approved MIBG myocardial scintigraphy as a diagnostic aid for the Lewy body disorders, and their national health insurance agreed to cover it. Its approval for these indications has lagged in the United States, as there are still concerns about how the test performs in real-world situations. At the 2015 International Dementia with Lewy Bodies Conference held at Ft Lauderdale in Florida, a strong case was made for the approval of MIBG myocardial scintigraphy for the diagnosis of DLB. False positive results are the major real-world concern, as myocardial ^{123}I-MIBG uptake declines with age, while the presence of incidental Lewy bodies in neurologically normal individuals increases with age [173]. Moreover, strict exclusion criteria have been used in most studies. In a 2015 multicenter Japanese study, a very large number of patients were excluded, including patients with medical disorders and those receiving pharmacological treatments [172]. This obviously greatly limits the generalizability of the scan to real-world clinical situations. In order to overcome this criticism, use of MIBG myocardial scintigraphy to diagnose DLB in real-world clinic situations was evaluated in a small European study [174]. Patients with comorbid medical illnesses and those receiving pharmacological treatments were included. The mean follow-up period was 17 ± 14 months (range 6–57 months) and the final clinical (not histopathological) diagnosis was used as the gold standard; autopsy confirmation of neuropathology was available for only one patient. Using the delayed H/M ratio cut-off of 1.68, 95% of the 20 patients with clinically ambiguous diagnoses (DLB versus AD) were correctly classified, with sensitivity and specificity values of 100% and 75% respectively. Only gender and age were found to be confounders in this study—MIBG uptake declined with increasing age and was lower in men. However, the sample size was small ($N = 20$), and demonstration of higher specificity in larger clinical replications may be necessary before approval for clinical use is granted in the United States.

To summarize, neither the ^{123}I-FP-CIT scan nor the MIBG scintiscan can directly image α-synuclein in vivo, and both have somewhat overlapping but still relatively distinct indications. The ^{123}I-FP-CIT scan is used to image striatal dopamine depletion due to degeneration of the nigrostriatal neurons, and therefore does not distinguish between the neurodegenerative causes of parkinsonism, with or without cognitive impairment, unless brain stem involvement is minimal as can happen in some cases of DLB where one can find a false-negative scan. It differentiates between the neurodegenerative and non-neurodegenerative causes of parkinsonism with some exceptions, as previously noted. MIBG scintiscan, on the other hand, detects cardiac norepinephrine depletion due to Lewy body involvement of the postganglionic sympathetic innervation, and therefore differentiates the Lewy body disorders from non-Lewy body disorders that result in parkinsonism and/or cognitive impairment. Combinations of imaging modalities may be more advantageous than any one individually. Given that MSA, PSP, and CBD (but not iPD) have signature findings on structural imaging, the combination of a brain MRI scan and an ^{123}I-FP-CIT scan may be the best way to work up APS patients in the clinic [175]. Similarly, the combination of ^{123}I-FP-CIT scan and MIBG SPECT may more accurately differentiate between DLB and AD patients, vis-à-vis either modality alone [176]. However, in clinical practice, it is hard to justify doing two scans for one indication. Comparing these imaging modalities across studies is problematic due to differences in technique, but a recent small study that directly compared both these imaging modalities found that the ^{123}I-FP-CIT scan had an advantage over delayed MIBG SPECT in differentiating DLB from AD patients (area under curve was 0.969 for ^{123}I-FP-CIT scan and 0.787 for MIBG SPECT) [177]. Autopsy confirmation of the diagnoses was not available in this study, and larger studies with autopsy confirmation are needed to resolve this issue.

Amyloid PET is the final molecular imaging modality covered in this chapter. It is not yet approved for reimbursement for routine clinical use by CMS, although that may change, as noted above. Regardless, research on the use of amyloid PET imaging has exploded in the last several years, and patients who have had amyloid PET scans done in research settings are already appearing in clinical practices nationwide. Therefore, clinicians must have some working knowledge of amyloid PET imaging.

The revised model of AD dynamic biomarkers postulates that amyloid PET positivity precedes brain atrophy as detected by a structural MRI, and hypometabolism as detected by FDG-PET; these, in turn, precede clinical symptoms and functional decline in AD [178]. A positive amyloid PET scan is one of the biomarkers included in the 2007 IWG [27] and 2011 NIA-AA diagnostic criteria for AD [28]. In order to better understand amyloid PET, a brief discussion of AD neuropathology is in order. Amyloid precursor protein (APP) is a transmembrane glycoprotein which is cleaved by β- and γ-secretases to generate the amyloid-beta (Aβ) peptide with 36-43 amino acid residues. There is also a parallel non-amyloidogenic pathway of APP cleavage mediated by α-secretase which does not result in AD. Of the Aβ peptides, the most common isoforms are $A\beta_{1-40}$ and $A\beta_{1-42}$. The former is more abundant but the latter is more pathogenic, as it self-aggregates more readily, forming dimers, oligomers (both soluble and dispersible), and eventually senile plaques composed of insoluble amyloid fibrils arranged in β-pleated sheets which result in neuronal injury [179, 180]. Senile plaques can be further categorized into diffuse and dense-core plaques, based on their staining with histologic stains, such as Thioflavin-S and Congo Red [181]. Diffuse plaques are Thioflavin-S negative and are commonly found in the brains of older individuals. Dense-core plaques contain a dense core of $A\beta_{1-42}$ and become associated with microglia and dystrophic neuronal processes called *dystrophic neurites*, and these plaques are then known as *neuritic plaques* [181, 182]. Currently available amyloid tracers bind weakly to diffuse plaques but have a high affinity for neuritic plaques, which are thought to be characteristic of AD pathology [183]. However, even the association between neuritic plaques and AD becomes weaker with increasing age, and begins to approximate the association of diffuse plaques with AD by age 95 [184]. It is important to note that the current amyloid tracers can only image fibrillary amyloid burden in the brain, which by itself is not diagnostic of AD. A positive amyloid PET scan cannot conclusively *rule in* AD and has to be interpreted with reference to the patient's clinical history, age, and Apo E ε4 status. A recent meta-analysis found that amyloid positivity decreased with age in those clinically diagnosed with AD, especially in Apo E ε4 non-carriers, while in Apo E ε4 carriers, the prevalence of amyloid positivity remained around 90% regardless of age [185]. Histopathological confirmation of AD diagnosis was not available in this meta-analysis. Regardless, the meta-analysis does suggest that the single clinical indication for Apo E genotyping in an older individual with a clinical diagnosis of AD dementia may therefore be for the purpose of accurately interpreting an amyloid PET scan. AD cannot be conclusively *ruled out* from a negative amyloid PET scan either. In a recent study where subjects were recruited from four research centers, the rate of amyloid-negative AD ranged from 9% to 21%, the majority of whom had a normal CSF $A\beta_{42}$ level but half had elevated CSF tau and phospho-tau levels, indicating the presence of neurodegeneration with or without neurofibrillary tangles; note again that the final diagnosis was based on clinical follow-up, and autopsy confirmation was only obtained in three cases in this study [186].

Amyloid tracers have a fascinating history. They were developed from histological dyes that were modified to develop ligands that not only bind with high affinity to the β-pleated sheet configuration of amyloid plaques, but also easily cross the blood-brain barrier to enter the brain, thereby allowing PET imaging in vivo. After over a decade of work and experimentation with over 300 compounds, the problem of poor brain entry was finally resolved with the creation of the ^{11}C-labeled compound called BTA-1 by Drs. William Klunk and Chester Mathis. Since they were both working at the University of Pittsburgh, BTA-1 became known as Pittsburgh Compound A (PiA) during the preliminary meetings between Klunk, Mathis and the PET researchers from Uppsala University where the clinical trials were conducted [187]. However, before human trials could be started, it was decided to replace PiA with another compound, ^{11}C-6-OH-arylbenzothiazole, due to the latter's superior clearance from the brain, and this subsequently came to be known as Pittsburgh Compound B (PiB). PiB is a charge-neutral benzothiazole analogue of the histologic dye Thioflavin-T. The first human study using PiB (16 patients with mild AD and 9 controls) was published in 2004 [188], and it has since been extensively used in research all over the world. However, it was unsuitable for clinical practice due to the short half-life of ^{11}C of only 20 min, which would require an on-site cyclotron [189]. This problem was resolved with the creation of a number of ^{18}F-labeled ligands based on the parent PiB compound, which are commercially viable due to the longer 110-minute half-life of ^{18}F. The first study using an ^{18}F-labeled amyloid tracer was published in 2008 [190]. As of August 2016, three tracers had been approved by the FDA for amyloid PET imaging in the USA—^{18}F-Florbetapir (AMYViD; Avid) in 2012, ^{18}F-Flutemetamol (Vizamyl; GE Healthcare) in 2013, and ^{18}F-Florbetaben (Neuraceq; Piramal) in 2014. While ^{11}C-PiB binds to the grey matter with a high degree of specificity, ^{18}F-labeled amyloid tracers have a relatively higher degree of off-target white matter uptake approximating or even exceeding uptake by the cortical grey ribbon, although tracer uptake and retention by grey versus white matter varies somewhat between the commercially available tracers. Blurring of the normal grey matter-white matter demarcation in amyloid PET scans using one of these ^{18}F-labeled tracers indicates a positive amyloid PET scan [182, 191].

In order to provide guidance for the appropriate use of amyloid PET in clinical practice, the Alzheimer's Association and the Society of Nuclear Medicine and Molecular Imaging convened the Amyloid Imaging Taskforce (AIT) which published appropriate use criteria (AUC) in 2013 [189]. The group noted 97-100% classification concordance between the ^{18}F-radioligands vis-à-vis ^{11}C-labeled PiB. The AUC include three clinical scenarios where use of amyloid PET is appropriate: patients with persistent or progressive unexplained MCI, patients who satisfy the core clinical criteria for AD but have an atypical clinical course or etiologically mixed presentation, and patients with atypically young-onset dementia. The AIT also listed seven situations where the use of amyloid PET is inappropriate. It was proposed that all scans be "performed under the supervision of and interpreted by a physician certified in nuclear medicine or nuclear radiology" and that such physicians have "must have adequate specific training in amyloid PET interpretation." The scan should be appropriately used "only by a dementia expert as a single piece of information to support or oppose a clinical diagnosis of Alzheimer disease dementia or pre-dementia in a patient in whom cognitive impairment has been objectively verified, in whom there is substantial uncertainty as to the underlying pathology, and for whom greater diagnostic certainty would change management" [192]. In a companion article, the credentials of the dementia expert were clarified as a physician who self-identifies training and board-certification "in neurology, *psychiatry* (italics mine), or geriatric medicine who devotes a substantial proportion (>=25%) of patient contact time to the evaluation and care of adults with acquired cognitive impairment or dementia" [192]. The first practice guideline for amyloid PET imaging of the brain was released by the Society of Nuclear Medicine and Molecular Imaging in August 2016 [191]. Visual interpretation of the scans is recommended by the guideline, but it is also noted that semiquantitative techniques "may be helpful." The cerebellar grey matter is typically used as a reference region for visual and semiquantitative interpretation of amyloid PET scans, except in very advanced AD patients and patients with familial AD where cerebellar plaques may be present; in such cases, the pons can be used as an alternate reference region [182, 191]. The pros and cons of using these reference regions have been discussed previously in the section on FDG-PET.

The 2013 CMS NCD on amyloid PET imaging in dementia and neurodegenerative disease concluded that "...evidence is insufficient to conclude that the use of PET amyloid-beta imaging is reasonable and necessary for the diagnosis or treatment of illness or injury." CMS currently only allows coverage of a single amyloid PET scan per patient through the Coverage with Evidence Development (CED) process [193]. The Imaging Dementia–Evidence for Amyloid Scanning (IDEAS) Study got under way in 2016 and may change the status quo [194]. The study, led by the Alzheimer's Association and managed by the American College of Radiology and the American College of Radiology Imaging Network, plans to recruit 19,000 Medicare beneficiaries over 4 years, "to demonstrate that awareness of the results of amyloid PET imaging can assist physicians in making more informed decisions about clinical management" [194]. Board-certified neurologists, *psychiatrists* (italics mine), and geriatric medicine physicians can enroll as referring providers on the study website (www.Ideas-Study.org). Clinical use of amyloid PET has some limitations, however. According to the revised AD biomarker model, amyloid deposition has already plateaued by the time the earliest symptoms of AD dementia become evident [178]. Therefore, using predetermined amyloid thresholds on PET as inclusion criteria for disease-modifying therapy trials in AD appears to be justified, since an early and reliable diagnosis of AD cases is critical for the evaluation of the therapy; recall that, in the bapineuzumab trials, 36% of APOE ε4 noncarriers were found to have a negative PiB-PET scan at baseline [195]. The situation in clinical practice is somewhat different. Due to poor clinicopathological correlation in the dementias [196], the clinical question is usually a broader one of whether a patient has dementia due to AD or another etiology, rather than a narrower one of whether a patient has AD dementia or no dementia at all. FDG-PET is much more suitable for addressing the broader question than amyloid PET. Also, the 2015 meta-analysis [185] suggests that amyloid PET may be most useful for *ruling in* AD dementia in young-onset cases, which is also one of the three clinical indications for amyloid PET in the AUC, but young-onset (non-Medicare) patients are unfortunately excluded from the IDEAS study.

Finally, as far as molecular imaging of other proteins involved in neurodegenerative dementias is concerned, there is active research going on presently on PET imaging of tau deposits in the brain, which is a neuronal injury biomarker [197], but it is likely several years away from entering routine clinical practice. The NIH-supported ADNI-3 is a 5-year study that started recruiting subjects in 2016 and includes tau PET [198]. With the advent of amyloid and tau PET, a completely new A/T/N classification scheme for AD has been proposed, in which A indicates an Aβ biomarker, T indicates a tau pathology biomarker, and N indicates a biomarker of neurodegeneration or neuronal injury, each of which is then rated in a binary fashion as + or - [199]. PET tracers that can be used to directly image α-synuclein in vivo are being studied as well [200], but development of a commercially useful tracer is still many years away. Transactive response DNA binding protein 43 kDa (TDP-43) is a protein that is implicated in the pathogenesis of amyotrophic lateral sclerosis (ALS), chronic traumatic encephalopathy, and some types of frontotemporal lobar degenerations, among other disorders. Research into developing a PET tracer that can be used to image TDP-43 in vivo is just getting under way with initial funding from the ALS Association.

Practical Aspects of Archiving and Viewing Imaging Studies

Almost all radiology facilities across the USA now use a Picture Archiving and Communication System (PACS), which allows electronic storage and retrieval of digital images in the Digital Imaging and Communications in Medicine (DICOM) format. A clinical PACS allows images to be acquired via the modality acquisition computer. The images are then routed to a PACS server via a DICOM gateway. These can be then accessed from different diagnostic workstations within the intranet. Different modes of image distribution are used, which depend upon whether the imaging department is organized by organ system or by imaging modality [201]. The PACS typically interfaces with and is integrated with a dedicated Radiology Information System (RIS), which handles not only the diagnostic reports but also workflow management and billing [202]. Larger medical centers now have multiple PACS archives which are integrated with the EMR. Web-based technology allows the images in the PACS archives to be displayed on practically any web browser. The web server accesses and processes the DICOM images into JPEG or GIF format before sending them to the browser [201]. Web-based medical imaging systems allow the clinician to view the images even from remote locations.

Hospitals have established virtual private networks (VPN) which allow digital images to be electronically "pushed" between hospitals in the network. This greatly reduces the need for requesting images on portable media, and not only allows viewing of the images usually within just a few hours of the request, but has also resolved the problems of corrupted media, confidential storage, and eventual safe disposal of the media. Every patient should be questioned regarding any prior head imaging studies. In patients where structural imaging has already been done, the clinician should never obtain just the original diagnostic report and "cut and paste" it into the clinic note, but make every effort to obtain the scan for personal review, preferably via the hospital's VPN. The hospital's medical imaging library will typically assist with this process, and front-office staff can be easily trained to automatically obtain any prior scans prior to the patient's first clinic visit.

Real-time access to a web-based image system is imperative not only for the referring psychiatrist to be able to view the scans, whether done locally or obtained from a remote location via the VPN, but also to show the images to patients during an office visit. This not only helps educate patients and families about the disease but is also a remarkably effective way to build rapport. Patients will sometimes ask for copies of their scans and the hospital's imaging department should be encouraged to provide copies of scans done locally. At times, patients and families will even take pictures of the scans in the office with their cellphone cameras, and this should not be discouraged as long as other patients' confidentiality is not being inadvertently violated (e.g., care must be taken to close another patient's medical record tab that may be lurking in the corner of the EMR).

Conclusion

While imaging and fluid (blood and CSF) biomarkers do not yet have a role to play in diagnosing psychiatric disorders in the clinic with the exception of neurocognitive disorders, their role in diagnosing primary psychiatric disorders is expected to greatly increase within the next decade. On the other hand, imaging biomarkers have already arrived in the memory and movement disorders clinics, and the various imaging modalities that have been discussed occupy an important place in the diagnostic work-up of these patients. Specific biosignatures of the common neurocognitive and movement disorders have been validated but have not been covered in this chapter as these details will be provided elsewhere in the textbook.

With the burgeoning elderly population in the USA, especially the "oldest-old" who are above the age of 85 [203], there continues to be an exponential increase in the numbers of dementia patients in the country and an increasing shortage of specialists trained in geriatric neurology, geriatric psychiatry, or geriatric medicine to take care of them. It is projected that, by the year 2050, 13.8 million people in the USA will suffer just from AD dementia [204]. Primary care physicians, adult psychiatrists, general neurologists and physician extenders have therefore become front-line providers of dementia care by default, but many of these providers feel ill-equipped to provide such care [205]. Like their neurology and neurosurgery colleagues, psychiatrists potentially have, or can develop with some effort and training, considerable expertise in the imaging modalities that are relevant to their clinical practice. Even if psychiatrists are not comfortable ordering imaging studies, they will increasingly see patients who have had scans done elsewhere and will want to review these with their treating psychiatrist. Adequate practical training in ordering and interpreting imaging studies is therefore critical for providing psychiatrists with the tools they will need in order to provide the best possible care to patients and their families.

Acknowledgments The author gratefully acknowledges the contribution of Dr. David Pettersson, Assistant Professor in Neuroradiology, and Dr. Lisa Silbert, Associate Professor in Neurology and Director of the Neuroimaging Lab at the Layton Aging and Alzheimer's Disease Center, Oregon Health & Science University, Portland, Oregon, who reviewed the final draft of this chapter and provided valuable feedback.

References

1. Jack CR Jr, Holtzman DM. Biomarker modeling of Alzheimer's disease. Neuron. 2013;80(6): 1347–58.
2. Davis J, Maes M, Andreazza A, McGrath JJ, Tye SJ, Berk M. Towards a classification of biomarkers of neuropsychiatric disease: from encompass to compass. Mol Psychiatry. 2015;20(2):152–3.
3. Hoptman MJ, Gunning-Dixon FM, Murphy CF, Lim KO, Alexopoulos GS. Structural neuroimaging research methods in geriatric depression. Am J Geriatr Psychiatry. 2006;14(10):812–22.
4. American Psychiatric A, American Psychiatric Association DSMTF. Diagnostic and statistical manual of mental disorders: DSM-5. 5th ed. Washington, D.C.: American Psychiatric Association; 2013.
5. Honea R, Crow TJ, Passingham D, Mackay CE. Regional deficits in brain volume in schizophrenia: a meta-analysis of voxel-based morphometry studies. Am J Psychiatry. 2005;162(12):2233–45.
6. Arnone D, Cavanagh J, Gerber D, Lawrie SM, Ebmeier KP, McIntosh AM. Magnetic resonance imaging studies in bipolar disorder and schizophrenia: meta-analysis. Br J Psychiatry J Ment Sci. 2009;195(3):194–201.
7. Buchsbaum MS, Ingvar DH, Kessler R, et al. Cerebral glucography with positron tomography. Use in normal subjects and in patients with schizophrenia. Arch Gen Psychiatry. 1982;39(3):251–9.
8. Kupferschmidt DA, Zakzanis KK. Toward a functional neuroanatomical signature of bipolar disorder: quantitative evidence from the neuroimaging literature. Psychiatry Res. 2011;193(2):71–9.
9. Hahn C, Lim HK, Lee CU. Neuroimaging findings in late-onset schizophrenia and bipolar disorder. J Geriatr Psychiatry Neurol. 2014;27(1):56–62.
10. Weinberger DR, Radulescu E. Finding the elusive psychiatric "lesion" with 21st-century Neuroanatomy: a note of caution. Am J Psychiatry. 2016;173(1):27–33.
11. Borsje P, Wetzels RB, Lucassen PL, Pot AM, Koopmans RT. The course of neuropsychiatric symptoms in community-dwelling patients with dementia: a systematic review. Int Psychogeriatr. 2015;27(3):385–405.

12. Taragano F, Allegri R. Mild behavioral impairment: the early diagnosis. Paper presented at: International Psychogeriatrics. 2003.
13. Woolley JD, Khan BK, Murthy NK, Miller BL, Rankin KP. The diagnostic challenge of psychiatric symptoms in neurodegenerative disease: rates of and risk factors for prior psychiatric diagnosis in patients with early neurodegenerative disease. J Clin Psychiatry. 2011;72(2):126–33.
14. Lanata SC, Miller BL. The behavioural variant frontotemporal dementia (bvFTD) syndrome in psychiatry. J Neurol Neurosurg Psychiatry. 2016;87(5):501–11.
15. Rosenberg PB, Mielke MM, Appleby BS, Oh ES, Geda YE, Lyketsos CG. The association of neuropsychiatric symptoms in MCI with incident dementia and Alzheimer disease. Am J Geriatr Psychiatry. 2013;21(7):685–95.
16. Ducharme S, Price BH, Larvie M, Dougherty DD, Dickerson BC. Clinical approach to the differential diagnosis between behavioral variant Frontotemporal dementia and primary psychiatric disorders. Am J Psychiatry. 2015;172(9):827–37.
17. Ismail Z, Smith EE, Geda Y, et al. Neuropsychiatric symptoms as early manifestations of emergent dementia: provisional diagnostic criteria for mild behavioral impairment. Alzheimers Dement. 2016;12(2):195–202.
18. Ismail Z, Aguera-Ortiz L, Brodaty H, et al. The mild behavioral impairment checklist (MBI-C): a rating scale for neuropsychiatric symptoms in pre-dementia populations. J Alzheimers Dis. 2017;56(3):929–38.
19. Winklbaur B, Ebner N, Sachs G, Thau K, Fischer G. Substance abuse in patients with schizophrenia. Dialogues Clin Neurosci. 2006;8(1):37–43.
20. Fan Z, Wu Y, Shen J, Ji T, Zhan R. Schizophrenia and the risk of cardiovascular diseases: a meta-analysis of thirteen cohort studies. J Psychiatr Res. 2013;47(11):1549–56.
21. Ribe AR, Laursen TM, Charles M, et al. Long-term risk of dementia in persons with schizophrenia: a Danish population-based cohort study. JAMA Psychiat. 2015;72(11):1095–101.
22. Arts B, Jabben N, Krabbendam L, van Os J. Meta-analyses of cognitive functioning in euthymic bipolar patients and their first-degree relatives. Psychol Med. 2008;38(6):771–85.
23. Almeida OP, McCaul K, Hankey GJ, Yeap BB, Golledge J, Flicker L. Risk of dementia and death in community-dwelling older men with bipolar disorder. Br J Psychiatry J Ment Sci. 2016;209(2):121–6.
24. Forlenza OV, Aprahamian I, Radanovic M, et al. Cognitive impairment in late-life bipolar disorder is not associated with Alzheimer's disease pathological signature in the cerebrospinal fluid. Bipolar Disord. 2016;18(1):63–70.
25. Marshall V, Grosset D. Role of dopamine transporter imaging in routine clinical practice. Mov Disord. 2003;18(12):1415–23.
26. Todorova A, Jenner P, Ray Chaudhuri K. Non-motor Parkinson's: integral to motor Parkinson's, yet often neglected. Pract Neurol. 2014;14(5):310–22.
27. Dubois B, Feldman HH, Jacova C, et al. Research criteria for the diagnosis of Alzheimer's disease: revising the NINCDS-ADRDA criteria. Lancet Neurol. 2007;6(8):734–46.
28. McKhann GM, Knopman DS, Chertkow H, et al. The diagnosis of dementia due to Alzheimer's disease: recommendations from the National Institute on Aging-Alzheimer's Association workgroups on diagnostic guidelines for Alzheimer's disease. Alzheimers Dement. 2011;7(3):263–9.
29. Van Essen DC, Ugurbil K, Auerbach E, et al. The human Connectome project: a data acquisition perspective. NeuroImage. 2012;62(4):2222–31.
30. Teipel S, Drzezga A, Grothe MJ, et al. Multimodal imaging in Alzheimer's disease: validity and usefulness for early detection. Lancet Neurol. 2015;14(10):1037–53.
31. Sporns O, Tononi G, Kotter R. The human connectome: a structural description of the human brain. PLoS Comput Biol. 2005;1(4):e42.
32. Yaffe K. Moving beyond dualism to advance geriatric neuropsychiatry. Am J Geriatr Psychiatry. 2016;24(5):339–41.
33. Gean AD, Kates RS, Lee S. Neuroimaging in head injury. New Horiz. 1995;3(3):549–61.
34. Parizel PM, Van Goethem JW, Ozsarlak O, Maes M, Phillips CD. New developments in the neuroradiological diagnosis of craniocerebral trauma. Eur Radiol. 2005;15(3):569–81.
35. Chakraborty A, de Wit NM, van der Flier WM, de Vries HE. The blood brain barrier in Alzheimer's disease. Vasc Pharmacol. 2016;89:12–8.
36. Bowman GL, Kaye JA, Moore M, Waichunas D, Carlson NE, Quinn JF. Blood-brain barrier impairment in Alzheimer disease: stability and functional significance. Neurology. 2007;68(21):1809–14.
37. Zhang CE, Wong SM, van de Haar HJ, et al. Blood-brain barrier leakage is more widespread in patients with cerebral small vessel disease. Neurology. 2017;88(5):426–32.
38. Wang CL, Cohan RH, Ellis JH, Caoili EM, Wang G, Francis IR. Frequency, outcome, and appropriateness of treatment of nonionic iodinated contrast media reactions. AJR Am J Roentgenol. 2008;191(2):409–15.

39. Katayama H, Yamaguchi K, Kozuka T, Takashima T, Seez P, Matsuura K. Adverse reactions to ionic and nonionic contrast media. A report from the Japanese committee on the safety of contrast media. Radiology. 1990;175(3):621–8.
40. Meth MJ, Maibach HI. Current understanding of contrast media reactions and implications for clinical management. Drug Saf. 2006;29(2):133–41.
41. Kanal E, Maravilla K, Rowley HA. Gadolinium contrast agents for CNS imaging: current concepts and clinical evidence. AJNR Am J Neuroradiol. 2014;35(12):2215–26.
42. Saba L. Imaging in neurodegenerative disorders. 1st ed. Oxford: Oxford University Press; 2015.
43. McCollough CH, Schueler BA. Calculation of effective dose. Med Phys. 2000;27(5):828–37.
44. Gerber TC, Carr JJ, Arai AE, et al. Ionizing radiation in cardiac imaging: a science advisory from the American Heart Association Committee on cardiac imaging of the council on clinical cardiology and committee on cardiovascular imaging and intervention of the council on cardiovascular radiology and intervention. Circulation. 2009;119(7):1056–65.
45. Balchandani P, Naidich TP. Ultra-high-field MR neuroimaging. AJNR Am J Neuroradiol. 2015;36(7):1204–15.
46. Chavhan GB, Babyn PS, Thomas B, Shroff MM, Haacke EM. Principles, techniques, and applications of T2*-based MR imaging and its special applications. Radiographics. 2009;29(5):1433–49.
47. Westbrook C, Roth CK, Talbot J. MRI in practice. 3rd ed. Malden, MA: Blackwell Pub; 2005.
48. Barkhof F. Neuroimaging in dementia. Heidelberg, New York: Springer; 2011.
49. Ramalho J, Semelka RC, Ramalho M, Nunes RH, AlObaidy M, Castillo M. Gadolinium-based contrast agent accumulation and toxicity: an update. AJNR Am J Neuroradiol. 2016;37(7):1192–8.
50. Runge VM. Safety of magnetic resonance contrast media. Top Magn Reson Imaging. 2001;12(4):309–14.
51. Marckmann P, Skov L, Rossen K, et al. Nephrogenic systemic fibrosis: suspected causative role of gadodiamide used for contrast-enhanced magnetic resonance imaging. J Am Soc Nephrol. 2006;17(9):2359–62.
52. Choyke PL, Girton ME, Vaughan EM, Frank JA, Austin HA 3rd. Clearance of gadolinium chelates by hemodialysis: an in vitro study. J Magn Reson Imaging. 1995;5(4):470–2.
53. Harper L, Barkhof F, Fox NC, Schott JM. Using visual rating to diagnose dementia: a critical evaluation of MRI atrophy scales. J Neurol Neurosurg Psychiatry. 2015;86(11):1225–33.
54. Schmahmann JD. Vascular syndromes of the thalamus. Stroke. 2003;34(9):2264–78.
55. Bastos Leite AJ, van Straaten EC, Scheltens P, Lycklama G, Barkhof F. Thalamic lesions in vascular dementia: low sensitivity of fluid-attenuated inversion recovery (FLAIR) imaging. Stroke. 2004;35(2):415–9.
56. Al-Saeed O, Ismail M, Athyal RP, Rudwan M, Khafajee S. T1-weighted fluid-attenuated inversion recovery and T1-weighted fast spin-echo contrast-enhanced imaging: a comparison in 20 patients with brain lesions. J Med Imaging Radiat Oncol. 2009;53(4):366–72.
57. Patankar TF, Mitra D, Varma A, Snowden J, Neary D, Jackson A. Dilatation of the Virchow-Robin space is a sensitive indicator of cerebral microvascular disease: study in elderly patients with dementia. AJNR Am J Neuroradiol. 2005;26(6):1512–20.
58. Traboulsee A, Simon JH, Stone L, et al. Revised recommendations of the consortium of MS centers task force for a standardized MRI protocol and clinical guidelines for the diagnosis and follow-up of multiple sclerosis. AJNR Am J Neuroradiol. 2016;37(3):394–401.
59. Shams S, Martola J, Cavallin L, et al. SWI or T2*: which MRI sequence to use in the detection of cerebral microbleeds? The Karolinska imaging dementia study. AJNR Am J Neuroradiol. 2015;36(6):1089–95.
60. Robinson RJ, Bhuta S. Susceptibility-weighted imaging of the brain: current utility and potential applications. J Neuroimaging. 2011;21(4):e189–204.
61. Finelli PF. Diagnostic approach to restricted-diffusion patterns on MR imaging. Neurology. 2012;2(4):287–93.
62. Deichmann R, Good CD, Josephs O, Ashburner J, Turner R. Optimization of 3-D MP-RAGE sequences for structural brain imaging. NeuroImage. 2000;12(1):112–27.
63. Jack CR Jr, Bernstein MA, Fox NC, et al. The Alzheimer's disease neuroimaging initiative (ADNI): MRI methods. J Magn Reson Imaging. 2008;27(4):685–91.
64. Mugler JP 3rd. Optimized three-dimensional fast-spin-echo MRI. J Magn Reson Imaging. 2014;39(4):745–67.
65. Yousry TA, Schmid UD, Alkadhi H, et al. Localization of the motor hand area to a knob on the precentral gyrus. A new landmark. *Brain*. 1997;120(Pt 1):141–57.
66. Szabo K, Forster A, Gass A. Conventional and diffusion-weighted MRI of the hippocampus. Front Neurol Neurosci. 2014;34:71–84.

67. Scheltens PH. Structural neuroimaging of Alzheimer's disease and other dementias. Aging (Milano). 2001;13(3):203–9.
68. Clarfield AM. The decreasing prevalence of reversible dementias: an updated meta-analysis. Arch Intern Med. 2003;163(18):2219–29.
69. Suarez J, Tartaglia MC, Vitali P, et al. Characterizing radiology reports in patients with frontotemporal dementia. Neurology. 2009;73(13):1073–4.
70. Harper L, Barkhof F, Scheltens P, Schott JM, Fox NC. An algorithmic approach to structural imaging in dementia. J Neurol Neurosurg Psychiatry. 2014;85(6):692–8.
71. Logue MW, Posner H, Green RC, et al. Magnetic resonance imaging-measured atrophy and its relationship to cognitive functioning in vascular dementia and Alzheimer's disease patients. Alzheimers Dement. 2011;7(5):493–500.
72. Arba F, Quinn T, Hankey GJ, Ali M, Lees KR, Inzitari D. Cerebral small vessel disease, medial temporal lobe atrophy and cognitive status in patients with ischaemic stroke and transient ischaemic attack. Eur J Neurol. 2017;24(2):276–82.
73. Firbank MJ, Burton EJ, Barber R, et al. Medial temporal atrophy rather than white matter hyperintensities predict cognitive decline in stroke survivors. Neurobiol Aging. 2007;28(11):1664–9.
74. Wardlaw JM, Smith EE, Biessels GJ, et al. Neuroimaging standards for research into small vessel disease and its contribution to ageing and neurodegeneration. Lancet Neurol. 2013;12(8):822–38.
75. Scheltens P, Barkhof F, Leys D, et al. A semiquantitative rating scale for the assessment of signal hyperintensities on magnetic resonance imaging. J Neurol Sci. 1993;114(1):7–12.
76. Fazekas F, Chawluk JB, Alavi A, Hurtig HI, Zimmerman RA. MR signal abnormalities at 1.5 T in Alzheimer's dementia and normal aging. AJR Am J Roentgenol. 1987;149(2):351–6.
77. Wahlund LO, Barkhof F, Fazekas F, et al. A new rating scale for age-related white matter changes applicable to MRI and CT. Stroke. 2001;32(6):1318–22.
78. Brewer JB. Fully-automated volumetric MRI with normative ranges: translation to clinical practice. Behav Neurol. 2009;21(1):21–8.
79. Bazin PL, Cuzzocreo JL, Yassa MA, et al. Volumetric neuroimage analysis extensions for the MIPAV software package. J Neurosci Methods. 2007;165(1):111–21.
80. Filippi M, Agosta F, Barkhof F, et al. EFNS task force: the use of neuroimaging in the diagnosis of dementia. Eur J Neurol. 2012;19(12):e131–40, 1487–1501.
81. Frisoni GB, Jack CR. HarP: the EADC-ADNI harmonized protocol for manual hippocampal segmentation. A standard of reference from a global working group. Alzheimers Dement. 2015;11(2):107–10.
82. Bocchetta M, Boccardi M, Ganzola R, et al. Harmonized benchmark labels of the hippocampus on magnetic resonance: the EADC-ADNI project. Alzheimers Dement. 2015;11(2):151–160.e155.
83. Davison CM, O'Brien JT. A comparison of FDG-PET and blood flow SPECT in the diagnosis of neurodegenerative dementias: a systematic review. Int J Geriatr Psychiatry. 2014;29(6):551–61.
84. Archer HA, Smailagic N, John C, et al. Regional cerebral blood flow single photon emission computed tomography for detection of Frontotemporal dementia in people with suspected dementia. Cochrane Database Syst Rev. 2015;6:CD010896.
85. Bamford C, Olsen K, Davison C, et al. Is there a preference for PET or SPECT brain imaging in diagnosing dementia? The views of people with dementia, carers, and healthy controls. Int Psychogeriatr. 2016;28(1):123–31.
86. Varrone A, Asenbaum S, Vander Borght T, et al. EANM procedure guidelines for PET brain imaging using [18F]FDG, version 2. Eur J Nucl Med Mol Imaging. 2009;36(12):2103–10.
87. Attwell D, Iadecola C. The neural basis of functional brain imaging signals. Trends Neurosci. 2002;25(12):621–5.
88. Meltzer CC, Zubieta JK, Brandt J, Tune LE, Mayberg HS, Frost JJ. Regional hypometabolism in Alzheimer's disease as measured by positron emission tomography after correction for effects of partial volume averaging. Neurology. 1996;47(2):454–61.
89. Pardo JV, Lee JT, Sheikh SA, et al. Where the brain grows old: decline in anterior cingulate and medial prefrontal function with normal aging. NeuroImage. 2007;35(3):1231–7.
90. Berti V, Mosconi L, Pupi A. Brain: normal variations and benign findings in fluorodeoxyglucose-PET/computed tomography imaging. PET Clin. 2014;9(2):129–40.
91. Lameka K, Farwell MD, Ichise M. Positron emission tomography. Handb Clin Neurol. 2016;135:209–27.
92. Huang B, Law MW, Khong PL. Whole-body PET/CT scanning: estimation of radiation dose and cancer risk. Radiology. 2009;251(1):166–74.
93. Jagust W, Reed B, Mungas D, Ellis W, Decarli C. What does fluorodeoxyglucose PET imaging add to a clinical diagnosis of dementia? Neurology. 2007;69(9):871–7.

94. Silverman DH, Small GW, Phelps ME. Clinical value of neuroimaging in the diagnosis of dementia. Sensitivity and specificity of regional cerebral metabolic and other parameters for early identification of Alzheimer's disease. Clin Positron Imaging. 1999;2(3):119–30.
95. Torosyan N, Silverman DH. Neuronuclear imaging in the evaluation of dementia and mild decline in cognition. Semin Nucl Med. 2012;42(6):415–22.
96. Schlemmer H-PW, Pichler BJ, Schmand M, et al. Simultaneous MR/PET imaging of the human brain: feasibility study. Radiology. 2008;248(3):1028–35.
97. Drzezga A, Souvatzoglou M, Eiber M, et al. First clinical experience with integrated whole-body PET/MR: comparison to PET/CT in patients with oncologic diagnoses. J Nucl Med. 2012;53(6):845–55.
98. Catana C, Drzezga A, Heiss WD, Rosen BR. PET/MRI for neurologic applications. J Nucl Med. 2012;53(12):1916–25.
99. Bisdas S, Nagele T, Schlemmer HP, et al. Switching on the lights for real-time multimodality tumor neuroimaging: the integrated positron-emission tomography/MR imaging system. AJNR Am J Neuroradiol. 2010;31(4):610–4.
100. Soret M, Bacharach SL, Buvat I. Partial-volume effect in PET tumor imaging. J Nucl Med. 2007;48(6):932–45.
101. Kawasaki K, Ishii K, Saito Y, Oda K, Kimura Y, Ishiwata K. Influence of mild hyperglycemia on cerebral FDG distribution patterns calculated by statistical parametric mapping. Ann Nucl Med. 2008;22(3):191–200.
102. Ishibashi K, Onishi A, Fujiwara Y, Ishiwata K, Ishii K. Relationship between Alzheimer disease-like pattern of 18F-FDG and fasting plasma glucose levels in cognitively normal volunteers. J Nucl Med. 2015;56(2):229–33.
103. Brown RK, Bohnen NI, Wong KK, Minoshima S, Frey KA. Brain PET in suspected dementia: patterns of altered FDG metabolism. Radiographics. 2014;34(3):684–701.
104. Silverman D. PET in the evaluation of Alzheimer's disease and related disorders. Dordrecht: Springer; 2009.
105. Silverman DH, Small GW, Chang CY, et al. Positron emission tomography in evaluation of dementia: regional brain metabolism and long-term outcome. JAMA. 2001;286(17):2120–7.
106. Yamane T, Ikari Y, Nishio T, et al. Visual-statistical interpretation of (18)F-FDG-PET images for characteristic Alzheimer patterns in a multicenter study: inter-rater concordance and relationship to automated quantitative evaluation. AJNR Am J Neuroradiol. 2014;35(2):244–9.
107. Lehman VT, Carter RE, Claassen DO, et al. Visual assessment versus quantitative three-dimensional stereotactic surface projection fluorodeoxyglucose positron emission tomography for detection of mild cognitive impairment and Alzheimer disease. Clin Nucl Med. 2012;37(8):721–6.
108. Matias-Guiu JA, Cabrera-Martin MN, Perez-Castejon MJ, et al. Visual and statistical analysis of (1)(8)F-FDG PET in primary progressive aphasia. Eur J Nucl Med Mol Imaging. 2015;42(6):916–27.
109. Signorini M, Paulesu E, Friston K, et al. Rapid assessment of regional cerebral metabolic abnormalities in single subjects with quantitative and nonquantitative [18F]FDG PET: a clinical validation of statistical parametric mapping. NeuroImage. 1999;9(1):63–80.
110. Minoshima S, Frey KA, Koeppe RA, Foster NL, Kuhl DE. A diagnostic approach in Alzheimer's disease using three-dimensional stereotactic surface projections of fluorine-18-FDG PET. J Nucl Med. 1995;36(7):1238–48.
111. Ashburner JT, Kiebel SJ, Nichols TE, Penny WD, Friston KJ. Statistical parametric mapping the analysis of functional brain images. Burlington: Elsevier Science; 2011.
112. Yakushev I, Landvogt C, Buchholz HG, et al. Choice of reference area in studies of Alzheimer's disease using positron emission tomography with fluorodeoxyglucose-F18. Psychiatry Res. 2008;164(2):143–53.
113. Dukart J, Mueller K, Horstmann A, et al. Differential effects of global and cerebellar normalization on detection and differentiation of dementia in FDG-PET studies. NeuroImage. 2010;49(2):1490–5.
114. Geyer S, Schleicher A, Zilles K. Areas 3a, 3b, and 1 of human primary somatosensory cortex. NeuroImage. 1999;10(1):63–83.
115. Moeller JR, Ishikawa T, Dhawan V, et al. The metabolic topography of normal aging. J Cereb Blood Flow Metab. 1996;16(3):385–98.
116. Fukutani Y, Cairns NJ, Rossor MN, Lantos PL. Cerebellar pathology in sporadic and familial Alzheimer's disease including APP 717 (Val-->Ile) mutation cases: a morphometric investigation. J Neurol Sci. 1997;149(2):177–84.
117. Kushner M, Tobin M, Alavi A, et al. Cerebellar glucose consumption in normal and pathologic states using fluorine-FDG and PET. J Nucl Med. 1987;28(11):1667–70.

118. Akiyama H, Harrop R, McGeer PL, Peppard R, McGeer EG. Crossed cerebellar and uncrossed basal ganglia and thalamic diaschisis in Alzheimer's disease. Neurology. 1989;39(4):541–8.
119. von Monakow C. Die Lokalisation im Grosshirn und der Abbau der Funktion durch kortikale Herde. Wiesbaden: JF Bergmann; 1914.
120. Ritz L, Segobin S, Lannuzel C, et al. Direct voxel-based comparisons between grey matter shrinkage and glucose hypometabolism in chronic alcoholism. J Cereb Blood Flow Metab. 2016;36(9):1625–40.
121. Akdemir UO, Tokcaer AB, Karakus A, Kapucu LO. Brain 18F-FDG PET imaging in the differential diagnosis of parkinsonism. Clin Nucl Med. 2014;39(3):e220–6.
122. Suarez-Calvet M, Camacho V, Gomez-Anson B, et al. Early cerebellar Hypometabolism in patients with Frontotemporal dementia carrying the C9orf72 expansion. Alzheimer Dis Assoc Disord. 2015;29(4):353–6.
123. Kwong KK, Belliveau JW, Chesler DA, et al. Dynamic magnetic resonance imaging of human brain activity during primary sensory stimulation. Proc Natl Acad Sci U S A. 1992;89(12):5675–9.
124. Ogawa S, Tank DW, Menon R, et al. Intrinsic signal changes accompanying sensory stimulation: functional brain mapping with magnetic resonance imaging. Proc Natl Acad Sci U S A. 1992;89(13): 5951–5.
125. Buchbinder BR. Functional magnetic resonance imaging. Handb Clin Neurol. 2016;135:61–92.
126. Bobholz JA, Rao SM, Saykin AJ, Pliskin N. Clinical use of functional magnetic resonance imaging: reflections on the new CPT codes. Neuropsychol Rev. 2007;17(2):189–91.
127. Official position of the division of clinical neuropsychology (APA division 40) on the role of neuropsychologists in clinical use of fMri: approved by the division 40 executive committee July 28, 2004. Clin Neuropsychol. 2004;18(3):349–51.
128. Buxton RB. Interpreting oxygenation-based neuroimaging signals: the importance and the challenge of understanding brain oxygen metabolism. Front Neuroenerg. 2010;2:8.
129. Fox MD, Raichle ME. Spontaneous fluctuations in brain activity observed with functional magnetic resonance imaging. Nat Rev Neurosci. 2007;8(9):700–11.
130. Damoiseaux JS, Rombouts SA, Barkhof F, et al. Consistent resting-state networks across healthy subjects. Proc Natl Acad Sci U S A. 2006;103(37):13848–53.
131. Biswal BB, Mennes M, Zuo XN, et al. Toward discovery science of human brain function. Proc Natl Acad Sci U S A. 2010;107(10):4734–9.
132. Raichle ME, MacLeod AM, Snyder AZ, Powers WJ, Gusnard DA, Shulman GL. A default mode of brain function. Proc Natl Acad Sci U S A. 2001;98(2):676–82.
133. Broyd SJ, Demanuele C, Debener S, Helps SK, James CJ, Sonuga-Barke EJS. Default-mode brain dysfunction in mental disorders: a systematic review. Neurosci Biobehav Rev. 2009;33(3):279–96.
134. Doria V, Beckmann CF, Arichi T, et al. Emergence of resting state networks in the preterm human brain. Proc Natl Acad Sci U S A. 2010;107(46):20015–20.
135. Jolles DD, van Buchem MA, Crone EA, Rombouts SA. A comprehensive study of whole-brain functional connectivity in children and young adults. Cerebral Cortex. 2011;21(2):385–91.
136. Bassett DS, Nelson BG, Mueller BA, Camchong J, Lim KO. Altered resting state complexity in schizophrenia. NeuroImage. 2012;59(3):2196–207.
137. Kaiser RH, Andrews-Hanna JR, Wager TD, Pizzagalli DA. Large-scale network dysfunction in major depressive disorder: a meta-analysis of resting-state functional connectivity. JAMA Psychiat. 2015;72(6):603–11.
138. Posner J, Park C, Wang Z. Connecting the dots: a review of resting connectivity MRI studies in attention-deficit/hyperactivity disorder. Neuropsychol Rev. 2014;24(1):3–15.
139. Zhou J, Seeley WW. Network dysfunction in Alzheimer's disease and frontotemporal dementia: implications for psychiatry. Biol Psychiatry. 2014;75(7):565–73.
140. Loane C, Politis M. Positron emission tomography neuroimaging in Parkinson's disease. Am J Transl Res. 2011;3(4):323–41.
141. Darcourt J, Booij J, Tatsch K, et al. EANM procedure guidelines for brain neurotransmission SPECT using (123)I-labelled dopamine transporter ligands, version 2. Eur J Nucl Med Mol Imaging. 2010;37(2):443–50.
142. Bajaj N, Hauser RA, Grachev ID. Clinical utility of dopamine transporter single photon emission CT (DaT-SPECT) with (123I) ioflupane in diagnosis of parkinsonian syndromes. J Neurol Neurosurg Psychiatry. 2013;84(11):1288–95.
143. Covington MF, McMillan NA, Avery RJ, Kuo PH. The semicolon sign: dopamine transporter imaging artifact from head tilt. J Nucl Med Technol. 2013;41(2):105–7.

144. Kahraman D, Eggers C, Schicha H, Timmermann L, Schmidt M. Visual assessment of dopaminergic degeneration pattern in 123I-FP-CIT SPECT differentiates patients with atypical parkinsonian syndromes and idiopathic Parkinson's disease. J Neurol. 2012;259(2):251–60.
145. Davidsson A, Georgiopoulos C, Dizdar N, Granerus G, Zachrisson H. Comparison between visual assessment of dopaminergic degeneration pattern and semi-quantitative ratio calculations in patients with Parkinson's disease and atypical Parkinsonian syndromes using DaTSCAN(R) SPECT. Ann Nucl Med. 2014;28(9):851–9.
146. Kahraman D, Eggers C, Holstein A, et al. 123I-FP-CIT SPECT imaging of the dopaminergic state. Visual assessment of dopaminergic degeneration patterns reflects quantitative 2D operator-dependent and 3D operator-independent techniques. Nuklearmedizin. 2012;51(6):244–51.
147. Van Laere K, Varrone A, Booij J, et al. EANM procedure guidelines for brain neurotransmission SPECT/PET using dopamine D2 receptor ligands, version 2. Eur J Nucl Med Mol Imaging. 2010;37(2):434–42.
148. Badiavas K, Molyvda E, Iakovou I, Tsolaki M, Psarrakos K, Karatzas N. SPECT imaging evaluation in movement disorders: far beyond visual assessment. Eur J Nucl Med Mol Imaging. 2011;38(4):764–73.
149. Booij J, Tissingh G, Winogrodzka A, et al. Practical benefit of [123I]FP-CIT SPET in the demonstration of the dopaminergic deficit in Parkinson's disease. Eur J Nucl Med. 1997;24(1):68–71.
150. van Dyck CH, Seibyl JP, Malison RT, et al. Age-related decline in dopamine transporters: analysis of striatal subregions, nonlinear effects, and hemispheric asymmetries. Am J Geriatr Psychiatry. 2002;10(1):36–43.
151. DeSantis J, Sun S. Quantitative assessment of DaTQUANT in diagnosis of DaTscan patients. J Nucl Med. 2013;54(2_MeetingAbstracts):2705.
152. Varrone A, Dickson JC, Tossici-Bolt L, et al. European multicentre database of healthy controls for [123I]FP-CIT SPECT (ENC-DAT): age-related effects, gender differences and evaluation of different methods of analysis. Eur J Nucl Med Mol Imaging. 2013;40(2):213–27.
153. Oravivattanakul S, Benchaya L, Wu G, et al. Dopamine transporter (DaT) scan utilization in a movement disorder center. Mov Disord Clin Pract. 2016;3(1):31–5.
154. Kagi G, Bhatia KP, Tolosa E. The role of DAT-SPECT in movement disorders. J Neurol Neurosurg Psychiatry. 2010;81(1):5–12.
155. Tolosa E, Coelho M, Gallardo M. DAT imaging in drug-induced and psychogenic parkinsonism. Mov Disord. 2003;18(Suppl 7):S28–33.
156. McKeith IG, Dickson DW, Lowe J, et al. Diagnosis and management of dementia with Lewy bodies: third report of the DLB consortium. Neurology. 2005;65(12):1863–72.
157. Nelson PT, Jicha GA, Kryscio RJ, et al. Low sensitivity in clinical diagnoses of dementia with Lewy bodies. J Neurol. 2010;257(3):359–66.
158. Walker Z, Jaros E, Walker RW, et al. Dementia with Lewy bodies: a comparison of clinical diagnosis, FP-CIT single photon emission computed tomography imaging and autopsy. J Neurol Neurosurg Psychiatry. 2007;78(11):1176–81.
159. Thomas AJ, Attems J, Colloby SJ, et al. Autopsy validation of 123I-FP-CIT dopaminergic neuroimaging for the diagnosis of DLB. Neurology. 2017;88(3):276–83.
160. Walker Z, Moreno E, Thomas A, et al. Clinical usefulness of dopamine transporter SPECT imaging with 123I-FP-CIT in patients with possible dementia with Lewy bodies: randomised study. Br J Psychiatry J Ment Sci. 2015;206(2):145–52.
161. Walker Z, Moreno E, Thomas A, et al. Evolution of clinical features in possible DLB depending on FP-CIT SPECT result. Neurology. 2016;87(10):1045–51.
162. Morgan S, Kemp P, Booij J, et al. Differentiation of frontotemporal dementia from dementia with Lewy bodies using FP-CIT SPECT. J Neurol Neurosurg Psychiatry. 2012;83(11):1063–70.
163. O'Brien JT, Colloby S, Fenwick J, et al. Dopamine transporter loss visualized with FP-CIT SPECT in the differential diagnosis of dementia with Lewy bodies. Arch Neurol. 2004;61(6):919–25.
164. Taki J, Yoshita M, Yamada M, Tonami N. Significance of 123I-MIBG scintigraphy as a pathophysiological indicator in the assessment of Parkinson's disease and related disorders: it can be a specific marker for Lewy body disease. Ann Nucl Med. 2004;18(6):453–61.
165. Dae MW. Imaging of myocardial sympathetic innervation with metaiodobenzylguanidine. J Nucl Cardiol. 1994;1(2 Pt 2):S23–30.
166. Takahashi M, Ikemura M, Oka T, et al. Quantitative correlation between cardiac MIBG uptake and remaining axons in the cardiac sympathetic nerve in Lewy body disease. J Neurol Neurosurg Psychiatry. 2015;86(9):939–44.
167. Jost WH, Del Tredici K, Landvogt C, Braune S. Importance of 123I-metaiodobenzylguanidine scintigraphy/single photon emission computed tomography for diagnosis and differ-

ential diagnostics of Parkinson syndromes. Neurodegener Dis. 2010;7(5):341–7.
168. Orimo S, Suzuki M, Inaba A, Mizusawa H. 123I-MIBG myocardial scintigraphy for differentiating Parkinson's disease from other neurodegenerative parkinsonism: a systematic review and meta-analysis. Parkinsonism Relat Disord. 2012;18(5):494–500.
169. Fanciulli A, Wenning GK. Multiple-system atrophy. N Engl J Med. 2015;372(3):249–63.
170. Lucio CG, Vincenzo C, Antonio R, Oscar T, Antonio R, Luigi M. Neurological applications for myocardial MIBG scintigraphy. Nucl Med Rev Cent East Eur. 2013;16(1):35–41.
171. Sakamoto F, Shiraishi S, Tsuda N, et al. 123I-MIBG myocardial scintigraphy for the evaluation of Lewy body disease: are delayed images essential? Is visual assessment useful? Br J Radiol. 2016;89(1064):20160144.
172. Yoshita M, Arai H, Arai H, et al. Diagnostic accuracy of 123I-meta-iodobenzylguanidine myocardial scintigraphy in dementia with Lewy bodies: a multicenter study. PLoS One. 2015;10(3):e0120540.
173. Spiegel J, Mollers MO, Jost WH, et al. FP-CIT and MIBG scintigraphy in early Parkinson's disease. Mov Disord. 2005;20(5):552–61.
174. Slaets S, Van Acker F, Versijpt J, et al. Diagnostic value of MIBG cardiac scintigraphy for differential dementia diagnosis. Int J Geriatr Psychiatry. 2015;30(8):864–9.
175. Mascalchi M, Vella A, Ceravolo R. Movement disorders: role of imaging in diagnosis. J Magn Reson Imaging. 2012;35(2):239–56.
176. Shimizu S, Hirao K, Kanetaka H, et al. Utility of the combination of DAT SPECT and MIBG myocardial scintigraphy in differentiating dementia with Lewy bodies from Alzheimer's disease. Eur J Nucl Med Mol Imaging. 2016;43(1):184–92.
177. Shimizu S, Kanetaka H, Hirao K, et al. Neuroimaging for diagnosing dementia with Lewy bodies: what is the best neuroimaging technique in discriminating dementia with Lewy bodies from Alzheimer's disease? Geriatr Gerontol Int. 2017;17(5):819–24.
178. Jack CR Jr, Knopman DS, Jagust WJ, et al. Tracking pathophysiological processes in Alzheimer's disease: an updated hypothetical model of dynamic biomarkers. Lancet Neurol. 2013;12(2):207–16.
179. Hardy J, Selkoe DJ. The amyloid hypothesis of Alzheimer's disease: progress and problems on the road to therapeutics. Science (New York, NY). 2002;297(5580):353–6.
180. De-Paula VJ, Radanovic M, Diniz BS, Forlenza OV. Alzheimer's disease. Subcell Biochem. 2012;65:329–52.
181. Serrano-Pozo A, Frosch MP, Masliah E, Hyman BT. Neuropathological alterations in Alzheimer disease. Cold Spring Harb Perspect Med. 2011;1(1):a006189.
182. Rowe CC, Villemagne VL. Brain amyloid imaging. J Nucl Med. 2011;52(11):1733–40.
183. Hyman BT, Phelps CH, Beach TG, et al. National Institute on Aging-Alzheimer's Association guidelines for the neuropathologic assessment of Alzheimer's disease. Alzheimers Dement. 2012;8(1):1–13.
184. Savva GM, Wharton SB, Ince PG, Forster G, Matthews FE, Brayne C. Age, neuropathology, and dementia. N Engl J Med. 2009;360(22): 2302–9.
185. Ossenkoppele R, Jansen WJ, Rabinovici GD, et al. Prevalence of amyloid PET positivity in dementia syndromes: a meta-analysis. JAMA. 2015;313(19):1939–49.
186. Chetelat G, Ossenkoppele R, Villemagne VL, et al. Atrophy, hypometabolism and clinical trajectories in patients with amyloid-negative Alzheimer's disease. Brain. 2016;139(Pt 9):2528–39.
187. Klunk WE, Mathis CA. Whatever happened to Pittsburgh compound-a? Alzheimer Dis Assoc Disord. 2008;22(3):198–203.
188. Klunk WE, Engler H, Nordberg A, et al. Imaging brain amyloid in Alzheimer's disease with Pittsburgh compound-B. Ann Neurol. 2004;55(3):306–19.
189. Johnson KA, Minoshima S, Bohnen NI, et al. Update on appropriate use criteria for amyloid PET imaging: dementia experts, mild cognitive impairment, and education. Amyloid imaging task force of the Alzheimer's Association and Society for Nuclear Medicine and Molecular Imaging. Alzheimers Dement. 2013;9(4):e106–9.
190. Rowe CC, Ackerman U, Browne W, et al. Imaging of amyloid Beta in Alzheimer's disease with 18F-BAY94-9172, a novel PET tracer: proof of mechanism. Lancet Neurol. 2008;7(2): 129–35.
191. Minoshima S, Drzezga AE, Barthel H, et al. SNMMI procedure standard/EANM practice guideline for amyloid PET imaging of the brain 1.0. J Nucl Med. 2016;57(8):1316–22.
192. Johnson KA, Minoshima S, Bohnen NI, et al. Update on appropriate use criteria for amyloid PET imaging: dementia experts, mild cognitive impairment, and education. J Nucl Med. 2013;54(7):1011–3.

193. Foster NL, Mottola K, Hoffman JM. Coverage with evidence development: what to consider. JAMA Neurol. 2014;71(4):399–400.
194. IDEAS. Study opens registration. J Nucl Med. 2016;57(1):9N.
195. Salloway S, Sperling R, Fox NC, et al. Two phase 3 trials of bapineuzumab in mild-to-moderate Alzheimer's disease. N Engl J Med. 2014;370(4): 322–33.
196. Mesulam MM, Weintraub S, Rogalski EJ, Wieneke C, Geula C, Bigio EH. Asymmetry and heterogeneity of Alzheimer's and frontotemporal pathology in primary progressive aphasia. Brain. 2014;137(Pt 4):1176–92.
197. Shah M, Catafau AM. Molecular imaging insights into Neurodegeneration: focus on Tau PET radiotracers. J Nucl Med. 2014;55(6):871–4.
198. Weiner MW, Veitch DP, Aisen PS, et al. The Alzheimer's disease neuroimaging initiative 3: continued innovation for clinical trial improvement. Alzheimers Dement. 2017;13(5):561–71.
199. Jack CR Jr, Bennett DA, Blennow K, et al. A/T/N: an unbiased descriptive classification scheme for Alzheimer disease biomarkers. Neurology. 2016;87(5):539–47.
200. Shah M, Seibyl J, Cartier A, Bhatt R, Catafau AM. Molecular imaging insights into neurodegeneration: focus on alpha-synuclein radiotracers. J Nucl Med. 2014;55(9):1397–400.
201. Zhang J, Sun J, Stahl JN. PACS and web-based image distribution and display. Comput Med Imaging Graph. 2003;27(2-3):197–206.
202. Ratib O, Swiernik M, McCoy JM. From PACS to integrated EMR. Comput Med Imaging Graph. 2003;27(2-3):207–15.
203. Global health and aging. Bethesda, Maryland: National Institute of Aging, National Institutes of Health, US. Department of Health and Human Services; 2011.
204. Hebert LE, Weuve J, Scherr PA, Evans DA. Alzheimer disease in the United States (2010–2050) estimated using the 2010 census. Neurology. 2013;80(19):1778–83.
205. Hinton L, Franz CE, Reddy G, Flores Y, Kravitz RL, Barker JC. Practice constraints, behavioral problems, and dementia care: primary care physicians' perspectives. J Gen Intern Med. 2007;22(11):1487–92.

Part IV
Psychiatric Diagnosis

16 Neurocognitive Disorders

Rajesh R. Tampi, Deena J. Tampi, Wynnelena C. Canio, Poorvanshi Alag, Dhweeja Dasarathy, and Joel P. Dey

Mild Neurocognitive Disorder

Abstract
Mild neurocognitive disorder is thought to be an intermediate stage between normal age-associated cognitive changes and major neurocognitive disorder. Individuals with mild neurocognitive disorder have a faster rate of progression to major neurocognitive disorder than age-matched controls. Known risk factors for progression to major neurocognitive disorder include greater cognitive deficits at baseline, the presence of the APOE4 carrier gene, greater brain volume changes, cerebrospinal fluid changes, and the presence of neuropsychiatric symptoms. Current data indicates that the progression of mild neurocognitive disorder to major neurocognitive disorder can be delayed through the use of cognitive and physical training. Unfortunately, studies of pharmacotherapeutic agents do not indicate any benefit for cholinesterase inhibitors, the anti-inflammatory drug rofecoxib, and antioxidants in slowing the progression of mild neurocognitive disorder to major neurocognitive disorder.

Keywords
Mild neurocognitive disorders; Mild cognitive impairment; Assessment; Prevention; Treatments

Introduction

The Diagnostic and Statistical Manual of Mental Disorders, fifth edition (DSM-5), describes mild neurocognitive disorder as a condition characterized by modest cognitive decline from a previous level of performance in one or more cognitive domains [1]. In addition, there are subjective complaints of mild cognitive decline and objective evidence for modest cognitive decline from standardized assessments. However, this cognitive decline does not result in impairments in activities of daily living life. Furthermore, these cognitive deficits do not occur exclusively in the context of a delirium and are not due to another psychiatric disorder. It is also stated in the DSM-5 that the mild neurocognitive disorder can have different etiologies including Alzheimer's disease (AD), vascular disease, frontotemporal lobar degeneration, Lewy body disease, Parkinson's disease, etc. Mild neurocognitive disorder may be associated with clinically significant behavioral disturbances including delusions, hallucinations, mood symptoms, apathy, etc.

Mild neurocognitive disorder was previously referred to as mild cognitive impairment (MCI). The term MCI was first used by Reisberg et al. to describe individuals who were rated as a 3 on the Global Deterioration Scale (GDS) [2–5]. MCI was then used to classify individuals who were rated as a 0.5 on the Clinical Dementia Rating Scale (CDR) [6, 7]. Petersen et al. classified MCI as a distinct diagnostic entity that could be differentiated from dementia (major neurocognitive disorder) [8].

Epidemiology

The prevalence of mild neurocognitive disorder ranges from 12 to 18% among individuals

R. R. Tampi et al. (eds.), *Psychiatric Disorders Late in Life*, https://doi.org/10.1007/978-3-319-73078-3_16

≥60 years in age [9]. The prevalence of mild neurocognitive disorder increases with age [10]. In addition, mild neurocognitive disorder may be more common among men, in those who were never married and in those individuals with APOE epsilon3epsilon4 or epsilon4epsilon4 genotypes. Mild neurocognitive disorder is also noted to be less prevalent among individuals with greater number of years of education.

Neurobiology

The brains of individuals with mild neurocognitive disorder show neuropathologic changes that are intermediate between normal aging and early major neurocognitive disorder which indicates a transitional state [11–13]. Common pathologic findings observed in the brains of individuals with mild neurocognitive disorder include argyrophilic grain disease, hippocampal sclerosis, and vascular lesions. The brains of these individuals show atrophy of the medial temporal lobe, entorhinal cortex, hippocampus, and the posterior cingulate gyrus [14]. Increased beta-amyloid (Aβ) deposition is seen in the lateral frontal and posterior cingulate cortices, medial and the lateral parietal lobes, and the lateral temporal lobe on *a*myloid PET scans [15, 16].

Outcomes

Individuals with mild neurocognitive disorder progress to major neurocognitive disorder at a rate of approximately 10–15% per year [17–21]. These rates are significantly greater than the population incidence rates for major neurocognitive disorder which is 1–2% per year [22]. The risk factors for progression include the severity of cognitive impairment at the time of evaluation, *apolipoprotein E ε4* (APOE4) carrier status, neuropathological changes, functional changes noted in the brain, and changes in the cerebrospinal fluid β-amyloid and tau protein levels [23].

Hippocampal atrophy also predicts the rate of progression of mild neurocognitive disorder to major neurocognitive disorder [24]. In addition, greater ventricular annual percent volume change and greater whole brain annual percent volume change predicts the conversion from mild neurocognitive disorder to major neurocognitive disorder [25, 26]. Individuals with reduced blood flow in the temporoparietal and posterior cingulate association cortices have a faster rate of progression to major neurocognitive disorder [27]. The combination of CSF t-tau/Aβ(1–4) ratio and MRI biomarkers or impairments noted on neuropsychological tests can predict the conversion of mild neurocognitive disorder to major neurocognitive disorder correctly in approximately 64% of the cases [28]. Additionally, the presence of neuropsychiatric symptoms increases the rate of conversion from mild neurocognitive disorder to major neurocognitive disorder [29–33].

Assessment

When individuals present with cognitive difficulties, the first step is to obtain a thorough clinical history from the individual and reliable informants [23, 34]. This should be followed by a mental status examination, quantifying and qualifying of the cognitive difficulties using standardized cognitive tests, and a functional assessment [22]. A formal neuropsychological assessment should be done which evaluates all the major cognitive domains including executive functions, attention, language, memory, and visuospatial skills and assists in differentiating the cognitive changes associated with normal aging, mild neurocognitive disorder, and a major neurocognitive disorder [22]. Cognitive impairment resulting from disorders like depression, medical conditions like hypothyroidism or strokes, substance abuse, or medication side effects should be ruled out [1, 35]. Physical examination, appropriate laboratory tests, and neuroimaging studies aid in understanding the etiologies for cognitive impairment. Biomarkers for beta-amyloid (Aβ) deposition and neuronal injury may aid in diagnostic clarification. The biomarkers for Aβ deposition include the cerebrospinal fluid (CSF) concentrations of Aβ42 and positron emission tomography (PET) amyloid imaging. Biomarkers for neuronal injury include CSF tau/phosphorylated tau proteins, hippocampal/medial temporal atrophy, the rate of atrophy of the whole brain, fluorodeoxyglucose (FDG) PET imaging, and SPECT perfusion imaging studies.

Prevention

Current data indicates that participation in cognitively stimulating activities involving visual and information processing like reading, doing crossword puzzles, and playing games like chess is protective against cognitive decline [17, 21, 24, 36, 37].

Treatments

Non-pharmacological

Longitudinal cohort studies of healthy older adults indicate that involvement in intellectually stimulating activities is associated with a reduced risk of cognitive decline [38]. The systematic literature review by Jean et al. found that cognitive intervention programs do improve memory, mood, and the quality of life [39]. The rate of cognitive decline among older adults was also reduced in a randomized controlled trial of physical activity intervention over a 24-week period [40].

Li et al. in their meta-analysis found that cognitive interventions among individuals with mild neurocognitive disorder improved their overall cognition [41]. Small positive effects were noted on episodic memory, semantic memory, executive functioning, visuospatial ability, attention, processing speed, and general cognition. Moderate benefits on language were also noted in the study. Self-rated anxiety and functional abilities also improved in the intervention group when compared to self-rated memory problem, quality of life, activities of daily living, and depression scores.

Cognitive training was found to improve various aspects of cognition. These include memory, executive functioning, processing speed, attention, fluid intelligence, and subjective cognitive performance in a systematic review of randomized controlled trials (RCTs) and clinical studies among healthy older adults and individuals with mild neurocognitive disorder [42]. However, improvements in everyday life activities were limited even with the cognitive training.

Epidemiological data indicates that Mediterranean diet, physical activity, and moderate alcohol consumption are protective against the development of mild neurocognitive disorder, whereas cigarette smoking promotes the development of mild neurocognitive disorder [43]. Available data indicates that the substitution of vitamin B12, vitamin D, or testosterone for the treatments for hyperhomocysteinemia, subclinical hypothyroidism, or hormone replacement therapy after menopause do not benefit individuals with mild neurocognitive disorder.

Pharmacological

There are no Food and Drug Administration (FDA)-approved medications for the treatment of mild neurocognitive disorder. However, different classes of drugs have been tested to delay the progression of individuals to major neurocognitive disorder [23].

Raschetti et al. in their systematic review found trials for donepezil, rivastigmine, and galantamine that compared these drugs to a placebo among individuals with mild neurocognitive disorder [44]. These trials lasted between 24 weeks and 3 years. The investigators found no benefit for these drugs in reducing the probability of conversion from mild neurocognitive disorder to major neurocognitive disorder when compared to the placebo. Diniz et al. in their meta-analysis found that 15.4% of the individuals assigned to the cholinesterase inhibitor-treated group progressed to major neurocognitive disorder when compared to 20.4% in the placebo group [45].

Thal et al. in a double-blind study investigated whether rofecoxib could delay the progression of mild neurocognitive disorder to major neurocognitive disorder due to AD among individuals ≥65 years in age [46]. These individuals were randomized to receive either rofecoxib 25 mg a day or placebo for up to 4 years [46]. There were no differences between the two groups on cognitive or global functions. Adverse events, serious adverse events, and the number of individuals who discontinued treatment due to adverse events were similar between the two groups. Discontinuation rate due to drug-related adverse events was 8.0% in the rofecoxib group and 5.6% in the placebo group, respectively.

Petersen et al. in their study randomized individuals with mild neurocognitive disorder to receive either 2000 IU of vitamin E a day, 10 mg of done-

TABLE 16-1. Summary of treatment studies for mild neurocognitive disorder [38–42, 44–49]

Interventions	Type of study	Outcomes
Intellectually stimulating activities [38]	Review	The risk of cognitive decline and conversion to major neurocognitive disorder was reduced
Cognitive intervention program [39]	Systematic literature review	There were improvements noted for memory, mood, and quality of life
Physical activity [40]	RCT	The rate of cognitive decline was reduced
Cognitive interventions [41]	Meta-analysis	There were overall improvements noted on cognition and self-rating scales
Cognitive interventions [42]	Systematic review of RCTs	Improvements were noted on cognition but not on function
Cholinesterase inhibitors [44]	Systematic review	There was no reduction noted in the rate of conversion to major neurocognitive disorder
Cholinesterase inhibitors [45]	Meta-analysis	There was no reduction noted in the rate of conversion to major neurocognitive disorder
Rofecoxib [46]	RCT	There was no reduction noted in the rate of conversion to major neurocognitive disorder
Vitamin E, donepezil, or placebo [47]	RCT	There was no reduction noted in the rate of conversion to major neurocognitive disorder
Pharmacotherapy [48]	Systematic review of RCTs	There were no benefits noted for cholinesterase inhibitors in reducing the rate of conversion to major neurocognitive disorder
Antioxidants [49]	Review	There were no benefits noted

pezil a day daily, or a placebo for 3 years [47]. The primary outcome was the development of possible or probable major neurocognitive disorder due to AD. The overall rate of progression of mild neurocognitive disorder to major neurocognitive disorder due to AD was 16% per year. There were no significant differences noted in the probability of progression to major neurocognitive disorder due to AD among the vitamin E group. The investigators found that in the first 12 months of the study, individuals in the donepezil group had a reduced likelihood of progression to major neurocognitive disorder due to AD when compared with the placebo group, $P = 0.04$. The investigators also found that among carriers of one or more APOE4 allele, the benefit of donepezil was evident throughout the 3-year study period, but the rate of progression to major neurocognitive disorder due to AD was no different between the groups.

Cooper et al. in a systematic review of randomized controlled trials (RCTs) found that the use of cholinesterase inhibitors among individuals with mild neurocognitive disorder did not reduce the incidence of major neurocognitive disorder [48]. They found that cognition improved in single trials of a heterogeneous psychological group intervention over 6 months; piribedil, which is a dopamine agonist over 3 months; and donepezil over a 48-week period. Additionally, nicotine improved attention over 6 months. A review on the use of antioxidants among individuals with mild neurocognitive disorder did not reveal any benefits for this class of medications [49].

These studies indicate that pharmacotherapy has not been shown to delay the progression of individuals with mild neurocognitive disorder to major neurocognitive disorder. Table 16-1 provides a summary of treatment studies for mild neurocognitive disorder.

Conclusions

Mild neurocognitive disorder represents an intermediate stage between the normal cognitive changes associated with aging and major neurocognitive disorder. Individuals with mild neurocognitive disorder have been noted to have greater rates of progression to major neurocognitive disorder. Risk factors for progression to major neurocognitive disorder include greater cognitive deficits at baseline, the APOE4 carrier status, greater brain volume and CSF changes, and the presence of neuropsychiatric symptoms. Available data indicates that cognitive and physical training appears to slow the progression of the disease process. Studies of pharmacotherapeutics have not noted any benefit cholinesterase inhibitors, the anti-inflammatory drug rofecoxib, and antioxidants in slowing the progression of mild neurocognitive disorder to major neurocognitive disorder.

Major Neurocognitive Disorder

Abstract
Major neurocognitive disorder is the most common neurodegenerative condition in the world and is also the leading cause of dependence and disability among older adults. Alzheimer's disease is the most common etiology for major neurocognitive disorder. The known risk factors for major neurocognitive disorder include older age, female sex, lower educational status, obesity, smoking, hypertension, diabetes mellitus, and hyperlipidemia. The differential diagnoses for major neurocognitive disorder include both depression and delirium. Research data indicates that approximately a third of the cases of major neurocognitive disorder due to Alzheimer's disease may be preventable by modifying the risk factors including diabetes, depression, smoking, physical inactivity, midlife hypertension, midlife obesity, and low educational status. The Food and Drug Administration (FDA) has approved acetylcholinesterase inhibitors and memantine for use in major neurocognitive disorders due to Alzheimer's disease and the acetylcholinesterase inhibitor rivastigmine for use among individuals with major neurocognitive disorder due to Parkinson's disease.

Keywords
Major neurocognitive disorder; Alzheimer's disease; Vascular disease; Frontotemporal lobar degeneration; Lewy body disease; Parkinson's disease; Acetylcholinesterase inhibitors; Memantine

Introduction

The Diagnostic and Statistical Manual of Mental Disorders, fifth edition (DSM-5), states that major neurocognitive disorder is characterized by a decline from a previous level of performance in one or more cognitive domains including attention, executive functioning, learning, memory, and language [50]. The document also indicates that this cognitive decline is noted by the individual, a knowledgeable informant, or by a clinician caring for the individual. In addition, this decline in cognition is identifiable by either a standardized neuropsychological assessment or by a quantifiable clinical assessment. The DSM-5 also states that this decline in cognition is associated with an impairment in activities of daily living. However, this cognitive decline should not occur in the context of delirium or be secondary to another psychiatric disorder like a major depressive disorder or schizophrenia.

The DSM-5 lists various etiologies for major neurocognitive disorder including Alzheimer's disease, vascular disease, frontotemporal lobar degeneration, Lewy body disease, and Parkinson's disease [50]. The DSM-5 also notes that major neurocognitive disorder may be associated with clinically significant behavioral disturbances including delusions, hallucinations, mood symptoms, and apathy among others. In the DSM-5, major neurocognitive disorder may be classified into mild, moderate, and severe based on the extent of the difficulties that the individual encounters with activities of daily living.

For details regarding the diagnostic criteria for major neurocognitive disorder due to different etiologies, kindly refer to the DSM-5 [50]. New criteria and guidelines to diagnose Alzheimer's disease have been jointly issued by the international workgroups convened by the Alzheimer's Association and the National Institute on Aging (NIA) [51]. Please refer to the Alzheimer's Association webpage to access these new criteria and guidelines.

Epidemiology

At present, it is estimated that approximately 35.6 million people worldwide have major neurocognitive disorders, and this number is going to increase to about 115.4 million by 2050 [52]. Additionally, among older adults worldwide, major neurocognitive disorder is thought to be the leading cause of dependence and disability [53, 54]. In the United States, approximately 14% of individuals in the seventh decade of life have some form of major neurocognitive disorder [55]. This prevalence increases to approximately 37.4% among individuals in ninth decade of life. Alzheimer's disease is the most common etiology for major neurocognitive disorder accounting for approximately 68% of all cases [56]. Approximately five million individuals in the United States 65 years and older have a diagnosis of major neurocognitive disorder due to Alzheimer's disease [56]. It is estimated that by 2050, the number of cases of major neurocognitive disorder due to Alzheimer's disease in the United States will rise to almost fourteen million [56].

Risk Factors

Data indicates that increasing age is the strongest and most consistent risk factor for the development of major neurocognitive disorder [52, 57]. In addition, the prevalence of major neurocognitive disorder is higher in women when compared to men and in the institutional settings when compared to the community [58]. An additional risk factor for major neurocognitive disorder is low levels of formal school education [59]. Higher levels of physical activity are protective from the development of major neurocognitive disorders. Additionally, three or more servings a week of oily fish like salmon, tuna, herring, etc., are associated with lower-risk major neurocognitive disorders. The use of Mediterranean, DASH (Dietary Approaches to Stop Hypertension), and MIND (**M**editerranean-DASH Diet **I**ntervention for **N**eurodegenerative **D**elay) diets are all associated with a lower risk for major neurocognitive disorders [59, 60].

Reduced or no alcohol intake is protective against the development of major neurocognitive disorders [59]. Evidence also indicates that smoking increases the risk for major neurocognitive disorder. However, smoking cessation in later life can still reduce the risk for major neurocognitive disorder. Lower risk of major neurocognitive disorder has been noted in older individuals who engage in cognitively stimulating activities like reading or playing puzzles. Higher levels of social engagement are also associated with a reduced risk for major neurocognitive disorder.

Hypertension, atrial fibrillation, cerebrovascular accidents, high cholesterol in midlife, obesity and high body mass index in midlife, elevated blood glucose, and Type II diabetes increase the risk for major neurocognitive disorders [59, 61]. However, data indicates that elevated blood glucose and Type II diabetes increase the risk for major neurocognitive disorder, independent of other cardio-metabolic risk factors.

Depressive symptoms and clinically significant depression are both mid- and late-life risk factors for the development of major neurocognitive disorders [59]. Additionally, repeated moderate to severe head injuries increase the risk for major neurocognitive disorder. The sustained use ($\geq$36 months) of benzodiazepines, anticholinergics, and antihistamines can increase the risk for major neurocognitive disorder [62–64].

Recent data indicates that the use of estrogen, statins, antihypertensive, and nonsteroidal anti-inflammatory agents can reduce the risk for major neurocognitive disorder, although older data had indicated no such benefit when using these agents [65–69].

In addition, the use of folate, vitamins E and C, and coffee can reduce the risk for the development of major neurocognitive disorder due to Alzheimer's disease [65]. No association has been noted between occupational exposures and the development of major neurocognitive disorder.

Neurobiology

Major Neurocognitive Disorder Due to Alzheimer's Disease

Among individuals with major neurocognitive disorder due to Alzheimer's disease, the important pathophysiological change in the brain is the development of extracellular amyloid plaques and intracellular neurofibrillary tangles [70]. The amyloid plaques consist of beta-amyloid $_{1-42}$ which exhibits greater propensity for aggregation. The amyloid cascade hypothesis describes the sequence of molecular events that results in the formation of amyloidogenic protein from the amyloid precursor protein (APP). Among individuals with major neurocognitive disorder due to Alzheimer's disease, the clearance of beta-amyloid from the brain is also impaired. In addition, amyloidogenesis is accompanied by the inflammation of the brain which often occurs early in the course of the illness.

The major genetic risk factor for major neurocognitive disorder due to Alzheimer's disease is the presence of *apolipoprotein E ε4* genes [71]. The lifetime risk for Alzheimer's disease among individuals who are homozygotes for *apolipoprotein E ε4* genes is more than 50% when compared to the overall risk of 11% for men and 14% for women without the *apolipoprotein E ε4* genes. Evidence indicates that the presence of *apolipoprotein E ε4* genes enhances the accumulation of insoluble beta-amyloid in the brain. Mutations in amyloid precursor proteins and *presenilin 1 and 2 genes* result in the enhanced production of beta-amyloid and tau proteins. It is thought that the deposition of beta-amyloid acts as a trigger for the disease process in Alzheimer's disease.

Major Neurocognitive Disorder Due to Vascular Disease

Atherosclerosis of large and small vessels and diseases like cerebral amyloid angiopathy can cause cortical and subcortical infarcts, micro-infarcts in gray matter, white matter lesions, and large and small cerebral hemorrhages that can result in the development of major neurocognitive disorder [72, 73]. It is postulated that a reduction in cerebral blood flow below a critical level (approximately 40% to 50%) can significantly worsen cognition. The severity of cognitive deficits is directly correlated with the total burden of vascular pathology. Disruption of blood supply to the white matter tracts and gray matter of the brain disrupts neural transmission and brain connectivity and also causes cerebral atrophy. Cerebral autosomal dominant arteriopathy with subcortical infarcts and leukoencephalopathy (CADASIL) caused by a frameshift mutation in the notch gene on chromosome 19 can result in major neurocognitive disorder due to vascular disease [72]. *Apolipoprotein E ε4* (associated with Alzheimer's disease and cardiovascular disease) and *MTHFR rs1801133* (related to homocysteine metabolism) genes have been found to be associated with the development of major neurocognitive disorder due to vascular disease.

Major Neurocognitive Disorder Due to Frontotemporal Lobar Degeneration

Degeneration of the frontal and temporal lobes and associated neuronal loss, gliosis, and microvacuolations results in major neurocognitive disorder due to frontotemporal lobar degeneration [74, 75]. Abnormal accumulation of the tau protein (FTLD-TAU), the microtubule-associated protein tau (MAPT), or the 43-kD TAR DNA-binding protein (TDP-43) (FTLD-TDP) in the brain is the cause for the majority (approximately 90%) of cases of major neurocognitive disorder due to frontotemporal lobar degeneration [74]. Abnormal accumulation of fused in sarcoma (FTLD-FUS) protein in the brain results in a minority of the cases of major neurocognitive disorder due to frontotemporal lobar degeneration. Very rarely, frontotemporal lobar degeneration may be present with ubiquitin-only or p62-only positive inclusions or without any inclusions. In approximately 40% of the cases of major neurocognitive disorder due to frontotemporal lobar degeneration, a family history of major neurocognitive disorder is reported. However, autosomal dominant inheritance only accounts for approximately 10% of cases. In approximately 60% of cases of inherited frontotemporal lobar degeneration, mutations of the *C9orf72, MAPT,* and *GRN* genes are noted. In approximately 25% of cases of familial frontotemporal lobar degeneration, mutations in the *C9orf72* gene are noted. The mutations of *C9orf72* gene are also thought to be the most common genetic cause of major neurocognitive disorder due to frontotemporal lobar degeneration and amyotrophic lateral sclerosis. Approximately 5% to 20% cases of familial frontotemporal lobar degeneration are thought to be due to mutations of the *MAPT* and *GRN* genes.

Major Neurocognitive Disorder Due to Lewy Body Disease

The brains of individuals with major neurocognitive disorder due to Lewy body disease present with cortical and subcortical Lewy bodies [76]. The Lewy bodies are intracellular inclusions that have an eosinophilic core [76]. Major neurocognitive disorder due to Lewy body disease, PD, and multiple system atrophy (MSA) are called synucleinopathies. In the brain of individuals with PD, the Lewy bodies are primarily present in the substantia nigra and the brainstem nuclei. The brains of individuals with major neurocognitive disorder due to Lewy body disease may also present with beta-amyloid deposits and tau neurofibrillary tangles but with a lower density than seen in the brain of individuals with Alzheimer's disease. Additionally, there is neuronal loss in the brains of these individuals [77]. The presence of cortical beta-amyloid and tau-containing neurofibrillary tangles indicates more severe disease state. The majority of cases of major neurocognitive disorder due to Lewy body disease are sporadic. Some sporadic cases may also present with *apolipoprotein E ε4* alleles. However, mutations of the *SNCA* and *LRRK2* genes are seen in rare cases with autosomal dominant inheritance.

Quality of Life and Prognosis

Among individuals with major neurocognitive disorder across all stages of severity of the illness – mild, moderate, and severe – functional abilities appear to be the only consistent factor that affects their quality of life [78]. For individuals with major neurocognitive disorder who live in care institutions, environmental factors and quality of care are important factors affecting their quality of life [78]. For the individuals who are living in a community setting, religious factors appear to be the only factor that appears to affect their quality of life. Cognition appears to have a stronger influence on the quality of life of those individuals who live in care institutions than with those who live in communities.

Death is the final outcome for all individuals with major neurocognitive disorder [79]. The average survival time after a diagnosis for major neurocognitive disorder varies between 3 and 12 years. Among individuals with Alzheimer's disease, those who had the onset of illness before the age of 75 years appear to have a longer life expectancy than those individuals who had onset after 75 years. Among individuals with major neurocognitive disorder due to vascular disease, life expectancy varies between 3 and 5 years. Among individuals with major neurocognitive disorder due to frontotemporal lobar degeneration, death occurs approximately 8 years after the onset of symptoms [74]. For individuals with major neurocognitive due to Lewy body disease, the median survival time is approximately 5 years after the onset of symptoms [80].

Assessment

The first step in the evaluation of individuals with major neurocognitive disorder is to obtain a comprehensive history from the individual and a reliable informant [81]. The salient aspects of the history should include the progress of their present condition, medical history, medication history, substance use history, family and social history, and any impairment in basic or instrumental activities of daily living. The next step is the completion of a thorough mental status examination [81]. Behavioral symptoms are commonly seen among individuals with major neurocognitive disorder. These symptoms can occur at any time during the course of the illness. Common behavioral symptoms include apathy, depression, anxiety, paranoia, and auditory or visual hallucinations. Screening tests such as the Mini-Mental State Examination, the Mini-Cog, the Montreal Cognitive Assessment, or the Saint Louis University Mental Status Examination can assist in evaluating the individual's cognition [82, 83]. Available evidence indicates no superiority for one screening test over the others in differentiating the various subtypes of major neurocognitive disorder. It is also recommended to repeat the cognitive tests on multiple occasions over a period of several months to track cognitive changes [84]. Table 16-2 enumerates the clinical features that can help differentiate the various etiologies for major neurocognitive disorder.

Following the mental status examination, the next step would be to rule out treatable medical or neurological disorders that can cause cognitive and functional decline [84]. Standard laboratory investigations recommended for these individuals include a complete blood count, electrolytes, thyroid-stimulating hormone, fasting glucose, serum vitamin B_{12} and folate levels, rapid plasma reagin for syphilis screening, and screening for human immunodeficiency virus antibodies. Neuroimaging studies like computed tomography (CT) or magnetic resonance imaging (MRI) identify the type and extent of structural brain pathology [85]. Common pathologies

TABLE 16-2. Clinical features of the various etiologies for major neurocognitive disorder [81]

Features	Alzheimer's disease	Vascular disease	Frontotemporal lobar degeneration	Lewy body disease
Symptom onset	Usually has an insidious onset Usually has a senile onset	Often has variable onset May have stepwise progression	May have presenile onset	Usually has an insidious onset May present with a fluctuating course
Cognitive change	Usually presents with decline in memory Usually presents with executive dysfunction late in the illness	Often presents with decline in memory May present with executive dysfunction early in the illness	Usually presents with executive dysfunction early in the illness	Usually presents with memory decline May present with visuospatial deficits May present with executive dysfunction early in the illness
Motor symptoms	Are rare and mainly seen late in illness Usually apraxias are seen in more severe stages of illness	Usually variable presentation depending on the location of the lesions	May present with Parkinsonian symptoms	Usually, Parkinsonian symptoms present within 1 year of cognitive symptoms
Survival time from diagnosis	8–10 years	3–5 years	6–8 years	6–8 years

TABLE 16-3. Neuropsychological profile of the various etiologies for major neurocognitive disorder [86]

Cognitive domains	Alzheimer's disease	Vascular disease	Frontotemporal lobar degeneration	Lewy body disease
Memory				
Registration	+++	+	+/–	+++
Retrieval	+++	+++	+/–	+++
Recognition	+++	+	+/–	+++
Attention and concentration	+++	+++	–	+++
Visuoperceptual deficits	+/–	–	–	+++
Executive dysfunction	+++	+++	+++	+++
Behavioral and psychological disturbances		+/–	+++	+/–
Motor signs/symptoms	+/–	+/–	+/–	+++

– absent, +/– variable, + mild, ++ moderate, +++ significant

noted among individuals with major neurocognitive disorder include cerebral atrophy, ventricular enlargement, and cerebrovascular disease. Positron emission tomography helps distinguish between major neurocognitive disorder due to Alzheimer's disease and frontotemporal lobar degeneration. Amyloid positron emission tomography assists in differentiating major neurocognitive disorder due to Alzheimer's disease from other etiologies for major neurocognitive disorder. Dopamine transporter imaging with iodine-123-b-carbomethoxy-3-b-(4-iodophenyltropane) fluoropropyl single-photon emission computed tomography is often used to evaluate individuals with major neurocognitive disorder due to Lewy body disease.

Among individuals with cognitive disorders, neuropsychological testing can assist in distinguishing cognitive changes associated with normal aging from mild neurocognitive disorder and from major neurocognitive disorder [86]. Neuropsychological testing can further assist in distinguishing between the various etiologies for major neurocognitive disorder, evaluating the types and the severity of behavioral and psychological symptoms associated with major neurocognitive disorders, and evaluating the capacity of the individual to care for their activities of daily living. Table 16-3 enumerates the neuropsychological profile of the various etiologies for major neurocognitive disorder.

Table 16-4. Differential diagnosis for major neurocognitive disorder, delirium, and depression [88]

Clinical features	Major neurocognitive disorder	Delirium	Depression
Onset	Insidious	Acute	Subacute
Reversibility	Not reversible	Reversible	Reversible
Disorientation	+	+++	–
Memory problems	+	+	+/–
Impaired attention	+	+++	+/–
Perceptual disturbances	+/–	+++	+/–
Anhedonia	+/–	+/–	++
Apathy	+/–	+/–	++
Mood disturbances	+/–	+/–	++
Sleep disturbances	+/–	+/–	+/–

+/– may be present, + present, ++ usually present, +++ definitely present

Emerging evidence indicates that biomarkers can assist in the diagnosis and assessment of various etiologies for major neurocognitive disorder [87]. Among individuals with early-onset Alzheimer's disease, reduced levels of cerebrospinal fluid beta-amyloid $_{1-42}$ and elevated levels of p-tau are the most accurate and reproducible chemical biomarkers. Biomarkers also help distinguish between major neurocognitive disorder due to Alzheimer's disease and major neurocognitive disorder due to other etiologies.

The differential diagnosis for major neurocognitive disorder includes delirium and depression. Table 16-4 provides the salient features that can distinguish between these three major conditions seen among older adults [88].

Prevention

Ideally, the prevention strategies for major neurocognitive disorder should focus on targeting many of the risk factors, given its multifactorial etiology [89]. Prevention strategies should emphasize the management of diet, exercise, social activities, and cognitive stimulation. At the present time, the strongest evidence for cognitive benefits is for physical activity and smoking cessation. Aerobic exercise has been shown to support the integrity of neuronal structures and preserve the brain mass [90]. In addition, cognitive activity has been shown to strengthen the function and plasticity of neuronal circuits.

Recent evidence indicates that for Alzheimer's disease, the combined worldwide population-attributable risk for the seven risk factors, diabetes, depression, smoking, physical inactivity, midlife hypertension, midlife obesity, and low educational attainment, is approximately 30% [91]. If we can reduce these risk factors by approximately 10–25%, then it is thought that the number of cases of Alzheimer's disease worldwide can be reduced by three million [92].

Treatments

Acetylcholinesterase inhibitors enhance cholinergic neurotransmission via the inhibition of the enzyme acetylcholinesterase which prevents the breakdown of acetylcholine [93]. The FDA has approved four acetylcholinesterase inhibitors, tacrine, donepezil, rivastigmine, and galantamine, for the treatment of mild to moderate Alzheimer's disease [94]. Tacrine, the first drug in this class, is rarely used due to its hepatotoxicity. The FDA has approved memantine, an uncompetitive N-methyl-d-aspartate antagonist, for use in individuals with moderate to severe Alzheimer's disease. Recent data indicates that among individuals with moderate to severe Alzheimer's disease, the combination of acetylcholinesterase inhibitors and memantine can improve cognition, daily functioning, behaviors, and global clinical status when compared to treatment with individual monotherapies [95, 96].

There are no FDA-approved medications for the management of major neurocognitive disorder due to vascular disease [65]. Kavirajan and Schneider in their meta-analysis only found small benefits in cognition for acetylcholinesterase inhibitors and memantine among individuals with mild to moderate major neurocognitive disorder due to vascular disease [97]. They did not find any benefits from the drugs in relation to behavior or function among these individuals.

Currently there are no FDA-approved medications for the treatment of major neurocognitive disorder due to frontotemporal lobar degeneration [74]. Nardell and Tampi, in their systematic review of the literature, assessed data from nine randomized controlled, double-blinded trials of medications for major neurocognitive disorder due to frontotemporal lobar degeneration [98]. There were two trials of selective serotonin reuptake inhibitor, paroxetine; one trial of trazodone; two trials of stimulants, methylphenidate and dextroamphetamine; one trial of acetylcholinesterase inhibitor, galantamine; two trials of N-methyl-d-aspartate antagonist, memantine; and one of the neuropeptide oxytocin. The investigators found that selective serotonin reuptake inhibitors, trazodone, and the amphetamines may have some efficacy in reducing behavioral symptoms among individuals with major neurocognitive disorder due to frontotemporal lobar degeneration, but none of these medications improved cognition or function among them.

Stinton et al. in their meta-analysis found that donepezil and rivastigmine were beneficial for cognition and psychiatric symptoms among individuals with major neurocognitive disorder due to Lewy body disease and Parkinson's disease [99]. However, rivastigmine, when compared to donepezil, was found to be less tolerated among these individuals. Memantine did not show any benefits when used among individuals with major neurocognitive disorder due to Lewy body disease and Parkinson's disease but was well tolerated. Rivastigmine is currently approved by the FDA for the treatment of mild and moderate stages of major neurocognitive disorder due to Parkinson's disease. Recently, the FDA approved pimavanserin, a 5-HT2A receptor inverse agonist, for the treatment of psychosis in Parkinson's disease that does not appear to worsen motor symptoms for these individuals [100].

Conclusions

Major neurocognitive disorder is the most common neurodegenerative condition in the world. It is also the leading cause of dependence and disability among older adults. Risk factors for major neurocognitive disorder include older age, female sex, lower educational status, obesity, smoking, hypertension, diabetes mellitus, and hyperlipidemia. Available data indicates that approximately one-third of the cases of major neurocognitive disorder due to Alzheimer's disease may be preventable by modifying the risk factors including diabetes, depression, smoking, physical inactivity, midlife hypertension, midlife obesity, and low educational status. Currently acetylcholinesterase inhibitors and memantine are FDA-approved for use in major neurocognitive disorder due to Alzheimer's disease, and the acetylcholinesterase inhibitor rivastigmine is approved for use among individuals with major neurocognitive disorder due to Parkinson's disease.

Behavioral and Psychological Symptoms of Dementia

Abstract
The term behavioral and psychological symptoms of dementia (BPSD) describes a group of different symptoms and behaviors that occur commonly among individuals with dementia. Available data indicates that BPSD often results in greater morbidity among individuals with dementia along with a faster decline in cognition and function. BPSD is also associated with greater caregiver burden, higher rates of institutionalization, poorer quality of life, and greater cost of care for these individuals. Both non-pharmacological and pharmacological strategies have shown benefits in managing BPSD. In this sub-chapter we review the salient aspects of BPSD including epidemiology, neurobiology, assessments, and management strategies.

Keywords
Behavioral and psychological symptoms of dementia; Neuropsychiatric symptoms; Apathy; Agitation; Cerebrovascular adverse events; Death

Introduction

Barucha et al. described behavioral and psychological symptoms of dementia (BPSD) as a heterogeneous range of psychological reactions, psychiatric symptoms, and behaviors that are unsafe and disruptive and impair the care of the individual in a given environment [101].

Available evidence indicates that BPSD occurs in about one-third of community-dwelling individuals with dementia, but its prevalence rises to approximately 80% among individuals residing in skilled nursing facilities [102, 103]. One study showed that BPSD may be seen in approximately 72% of individuals with dementia ≥2 years prior to the actual diagnosis having been made, indicating that these symptoms may be a heralding sign for the onset of a neurocognitive disorder [104]. In this study, the investigators found that about 10 months after the formal diagnosis of dementia is made, the prevalence of BPSD increased to approximately 81% [104]. It has also been noted that BPSD tends to fluctuate during the course of the illness, with agitation being the most persistent symptom [105–107].

Although agitation is the most persistent symptom, apathy has been noted to be the most common BPSD with a prevalence rate ranging between 48 and 92% [108]. Additionally, apathy often occurs early in the course of illness and tends to be stable throughout the course of the illness. Delusions occur in a range of 16% to 70% of the individuals with dementia. Common delusions seen among these individuals include beliefs of theft, infidelity, and misidentification syndromes. Hallucinations occur in between 4 and 76% of individuals with dementia, with visual hallucinations being the most prevalent type of hallucination. The prevalence of anxiety symptoms is between 21 and 60% among individuals with dementia. Mood lability is seen in 40% of individuals with dementia, and it becomes more prevalent as the illness progresses. Depressive symptoms tend to occur in between 30 and 50% of individuals with dementia [109, 110]. Individuals who have a family history of depression appear to be at higher risk for developing a major depressive episode when compared to the individuals without a family history [111]. Disinhibition is seen in approximately 33% of individuals with dementia [108]. Approximately one-quarter of individuals with dementia present with sleep disturbance, and one-fifth of individuals present with weight loss [112, 113]. Inappropriate sexual behavior is seen in between 7 and 25% of individuals with dementia [114].

Neurobiology

BPSD occurs due to the interactions between the various anatomical, functional, and biochemical changes associated with aging, the genetic predisposition of the individual, and premorbid psychological factors [111, 115–134].

Anatomical: The presence of neurotic plaques and neurofibrillary tangles in the frontal and temporal cortices of individuals with dementia has been found to be associated with the development of BPSD [115–118]. Atrophy of the right frontal lobe has been noted for individuals with delusional misidentification symptoms (DMS) [119].

Functional: Dysfunction of the frontal, temporal, and parietal cortices has been noted to be associated with psychotic symptoms among individuals with dementia [120–124].

Biochemical: Psychotic symptoms tend to occur among individuals with higher levels of norepinephrine in the substantia nigra and lower levels of serotonin in the presubiculum [115, 116]. BPSD is also noted to occur among individuals who have sustained damage to their cholinergic neurons in the frontal and temporal cortices and adrenergic and serotonergic systems [125]. Delusional misidentification symptoms (DMS) tend to occur more commonly in individuals who have greater EEG delta power over the right hemisphere [119].

Genetic: Depression among individuals with dementia tends to occur more commonly among individuals who have first-degree relatives with depression [111, 126, 127]. The heritability for psychotic symptoms varies between 30 and 61% [128]. The presence of the APOE4 allele is associated with an earlier age for the onset of psychotic symptoms, and the presence of the APOE2 allele is associated with depressive symptoms [129]. The individuals who are homozygotes for APOE4 allele present with greater disorientation, agitation, and motor symptoms [129]. Anxiety and sleep disorders tend to occur more frequently among individuals with the APOE3 allele [130]. Visual and auditory hallucinations, hyperphagia, and aggression occur more commonly among individuals who have serotonin (5-HT2A) receptor polymorphisms [131, 132]. Evidence also indicates that dopamine receptor polymorphisms are associated with psychosis and aggression among individuals with dementia [133, 134].

Psychological: Those individuals who have higher premorbid levels of neuroticism have higher risk for developing depressive symptoms when they become demented [135, 136].

Outcomes

BPSD is a common reason for individuals with dementia to be referred to specialized care [137]. Greater caregiver burden and the risk for institutionalization are higher when the individual with dementia presents with delusions, aggression, and sleep-wake cycle disturbances [138–141]. BPSD is often associated with greater cognitive decline, worsening of activities of daily living (ADLs), and a worse quality of life among individuals with dementia [102, 142, 143]. Additionally, BPSD is associated with greater direct and indirect costs of caring for those individuals with dementia [144, 145].

Assessment

For any individual who presents with a cognitive disorder, obtaining collateral information from a knowledgeable informant is crucial when assessing individuals with BPSD [146]. This information clarifies the onset of symptoms, associated features like environmental triggers, and the types, frequency, and severity of symptoms. Also, this information helps rule out any psychosocial stressors that may cause or result in relapses or recurrences of symptoms. Comorbid medical conditions like infections, pain syndromes, and metabolic disorders must be carefully evaluated as they may cause or worsen BPSD. Additionally, treating these disorders may reduce BPSD, thus assist with minimizing the use of psychotropic drugs. Standardized tools like the Neuropsychiatric Inventory (NPI), the Behavioral Pathology in Alzheimer's Disease Rating Scale (BEHAVE-AD), the Consortium to Establish a Registry for Alzheimer's Disease-Behavior Rating Scale for Dementia (CERAD-BRSD), and the Neurobehavioral Rating Scale (NRS) assist with quantifying and qualifying BPSD [147]. Additionally, these scales can be used to track the progress of BPSD over time and the patients' responses to treatments.

Management

Both non-pharmacological and pharmacological strategies have been found to be beneficial in the management of BPSD [148]. These strategies are often used in combination to optimize benefits.

Non-pharmacological

Livingston et al. in their systematic review found that educating caregivers and residential care staff and possibly cognitive stimulation therapy appears effective for the management of BPSD [149]. Additionally, specialized dementia units did not show consistent benefits, but wandering was reduced by visually changing the environment and unlocking doors. Brodaty and Arasartnam in their meta-analysis found that the frequency and severity of BPSD and caregiver burden were reduced by non-pharmacological interventions provided by family caregivers [150]. These interventions had effect sizes similar to those associated with pharmacotherapy. Nine to twelve individual sessions, designed to meet the needs of the individual with dementia and their caregivers, which were delivered at their homes using multiple components over a 3–6-month time frame with periodic follow-ups were most successful.

Seitz et al. in their systematic review found that non-pharmacological interventions have some benefits for the management of BPSD [151]. Interventions that were found to be beneficial were exercise, recreational activities, music and other sensory therapies, staff training in behavioral management strategies, mental health consultation, and treatment planning. Many of these studies, however, had methodological limitations, and three-quarters of the studies indicated that significant time commitments from the nursing staff and many resources from outside of the facility were needed for the implementation of these strategies.

Pharmacological Management

Antipsychotics

Ballard et al. in their meta-analysis found that the use of risperidone and olanzapine among individuals with BPSD was associated with significant improvements in aggression when compared to the placebo [152]. Individuals who were treated with risperidone also had significant improvements in psychosis when compared to those individuals who were treated with placebo. Schneider et al. in their meta-analysis found that aripiprazole and risperidone were beneficial for the management of BPSD [153]. Schneider et al. in a randomized double-blind, placebo-controlled trial that used olanzapine, quetiapine, risperidone, or placebo to treat psychosis, aggression, or agitation among outpatients with Alzheimer's disease found no significant differences between the active agents when compared to placebo on the primary efficacy measure which was the time to the discontinuation of treatment for any reason [154]. The placebo group also had a longer time to discontinuation of treatment due to adverse events or intolerability when compared to the group that was given active agents. However, the median time to the discontinuation of treatment, due to a lack of efficacy, favored the olanzapine and risperidone groups when compared to the quetiapine and placebo groups.

Concerns have been raised on the safety of antipsychotic medications when they are used among individuals with dementia, including the risk for cerebrovascular adverse events (CVAEs) and death [155]. In a post hoc analysis of pooled results from 11 RCTs of risperidone and olanzapine among individuals with dementia, Herrmann and Lanctot found an increased incidence of cerebrovascular adverse events among the drug-treated group when compared to the placebo group [156]. Some of these events in the risperidone trial were non-specific events and not really strokes. Additionally, in the risperidone trial, there were more individuals with vascular and mixed dementias when compared to the olanzapine trials. However, two large observational studies of administrative health databases did not show evidence of increased risk of stroke in older adults with dementia who were treated with risperidone and olanzapine when compared to untreated individuals or individuals who were treated with typical antipsychotics [157, 158].

The Food and Drug Administration (FDA) included data from 17 placebo-controlled trials of olanzapine, aripiprazole, risperidone, or quetiapine to report the association between the use of atypical antipsychotics among individuals with BPSD and the increased risk of mortality [155]. On these, 15 trials showed numerical increase in mortality (1.6–1.7-fold) among the drug-treated group when compared to the placebo-treated group. Heart failure or sudden death and infections (mainly pneumonia) were the most common reasons for death in these studies. Based on this data, the FDA asked manufacturers of both atypical and typical antipsychotics to include a boxed warning regarding the risk of death and to clearly state that these drugs are not approved for the treatment of BPSD.

Schneider et al. in their meta-analysis found that among individuals with BPSD who were treated with atypical antipsychotics, the risk of death was greater among the drug-treated group than among the placebo-treated group [159]. Differential risks were not noted for individual drugs, for the severity of dementia, sample selection criteria, or for the type of dementia diagnosis. Wang et al. found that the use of typical antipsychotics was associated with a higher adjusted risk for death than atypical antipsychotics among older adults, irrespective of the presence or absence of dementia diagnosis or nursing home residency [160].

The American Psychiatric Association (APA) practice guideline recommends that before non-emergency treatment with an antipsychotic medication is initiated among individuals with BPSD, the potential risks and benefits from these medications must be evaluated by the clinician [161]. Additionally, these risks and benefits must also be discussed with the patient, their family, and or the surrogate decision maker. The guideline recommends that if the risk and benefit assessment favors the use of an antipsychotic for BPSD, the treatment should be initiated at a low dose and titrated up to the minimum effective dose as tolerated. If the individual experiences a clinically significant adverse effect due to the antipsychotic medication, then the potential risks and benefits of the medication should be reviewed by the clinician, and it must be determined if tapering and discontinuing the medication is necessary. The guideline also recommends that if there is no clinically significant response after a 4-week trial with an adequate dose of the medication, then the medication should be tapered and discontinued.

It is also recommended that among individuals who show benefits, the decision to possibly taper the antipsychotic medication should be discussed with the patient and their surrogate decision maker. Among individuals who show an adequate response to treatment, an attempt to taper and withdraw the medication should be made within 4 months of initiation of the treatment unless the individual experiences a recurrence of symptoms with previous attempts at tapering the antipsychotic medication. Assessment of symptoms should occur at least every month during the taper and for at least 4 months after the medication is discontinued to identify signs of recurrence. If there is a recurrence of symptoms of BPSD, then a reevaluation of the benefits and risks of antipsychotic treatment should be conducted. It is also recommended by the APA that haloperidol should be used as a first-line agent only for delirium and not for BPSD. APA also does not recommend the use of long-acting injectable antipsychotic medications among individuals with BPSD unless it is otherwise indicated for a co-occurring chronic psychotic illness.

Antidepressants

Seitz et al. in their meta-analysis found that sertraline and citalopram, when compared to the placebo, reduced symptoms of agitation in individuals with BPSD [162]. Additionally, two studies did not detect any differences in BPSD when comparing trazodone to haloperidol. The investigators also found that SSRIs and trazodone, when compared to typical antipsychotics, atypical antipsychotics, and placebo, were well tolerated. Henry et al. in their review found eight trials of selective serotonin reuptake inhibitors (SSRIs) and three trials of trazodone which showed benefits in the management of BPSD [163]. The investigators also found that these drugs were well tolerated in 74% of the trials that were reviewed.

Mood Stabilizers

Lonergan et al. found that valproate preparations at low doses were ineffective for managing BPSD, whereas higher doses were associated with unacceptable side effects [164]. Konovalov et al. in their review found that only one study of carbamazepine, out of a total of seven RCTs of mood stabilizers, showed statistically significant benefits for the drug when compared to placebo in the management of BPSD [165]. Adverse effects were more frequent in the drug-treated group when compared to the placebo group in a majority of the studies.

Cognitive Enhancers

Trinh et al. in their meta-analysis found that cholinesterase inhibitors, when compared to the placebo, provided modest improvements in BPSD symptoms [166]. The investigators found no difference in efficacy between the various cholinesterase inhibitors for the management of BPSD. Maidment et al. in their meta-analysis found that memantine provided modest improvements in the symptoms of BPSD when compared to placebo [167]. Additionally, memantine was well tolerated. Sedation was the only adverse event which was higher in the drug-treated group than in the placebo group.

Benzodiazepines

Tampi and Tampi in a systematic review did not find that benzodiazepines produced significant benefits for the management of BPSD [168]. The studies on benzodiazepines had a limited number of participants and were of short duration. Although there were no significant side effects noted in these studies, recent evidence indicating worsening cognition and greater risks for falls with its use makes the prescription of benzodiazepines fairly unsafe in this population.

Melatonin

Jansen et al. in their meta-analysis found that the use of melatonin did not appear to improve cognition among individuals with dementia, irrespective of the dose of the medication used or the duration of treatment [169]. However, melatonin, when compared to the placebo, improved symptoms of BPSD at dosing of 2.5 mg or 3 mg a day and in a duration of 4 weeks to 7 weeks. Melatonin was well tolerated in the included studies with no significant differences between melatonin and the placebo on adverse effects.

Conclusion

BPSD is common among individuals with dementia. Individuals with BPSD have poorer clinical outcomes and have a greater burden of care when compared to individuals without BPSD. Both non-pharmacological and pharmacological interventions have shown benefits in the management of BPSD. Pharmacotherapy is usually reserved for behaviors that do not respond adequately to non-pharmacological approaches. A risk benefit analysis should be done prior to prescribing medications for BPSD as some of these medications can cause significant adverse effects when prescribed to older adults with dementia. Additionally, the close monitoring of risk factors will reduce the risk for serious adverse events including cerebrovascular events and deaths.

Delirium

Abstract
Delirium is a common neuropsychiatric disorder seen among older adults. This condition has multifactorial etiologies and occurs due to the interactions between various predisposing and precipitating factors. If untreated, delirium results in high rates of morbidity and mortality. Among older adults, delirium is often under or misdiagnosed as another psychiatric disorder, namely, depression or mild/major neurocognitive. Available data indicates that more than a third of the cases of delirium can be prevented. It has been noted that both non-pharmacological and pharmacological treatments result in decreased incidence of delirium, reduced severity, shortened duration of the episode, and also reduced hospital length of stay.

Keywords
Delirium; Confusion assessment method; Multicomponent intervention; Prevention; Treatment

Introduction

The Diagnostic and Statistical Manual of Mental Disorders 5 (DSM-5) describes delirium as a condition that presents with a disturbance in attention, awareness, and cognition [170]. It is also stated that these symptoms should not occur due to an underlying neurocognitive disorder or in conjunction with a severely reduced level of arousal such as when one is in a state of coma. In addition, changes in attention, awareness, and cognition should have developed over a short period of time (usually hours to days), represent a change from baseline, and tend to fluctuate in severity during the course of the day. Furthermore, there should be evidence from history, physical examination, or laboratory findings indicating that these symptoms are caused by the direct physiological consequences of another medical condition, substance intoxication, or withdrawal. For details regarding the diagnostic criteria for delirium, kindly refer to the DSM-5 [170].

Epidemiology

Among older adults living in the community, the prevalence of delirium is low at 1–2% [171, 172]. However, it is estimated that in the United States between one-tenth and one-half of all individuals who are 65 years or older in age who require hospitalization have delirium [173]. During admission to hospitals, the incidence rate for delirium among the elderly ranges from 11 to 42% [171, 172]. The incidence of delirium during a hospital stay is over 50% [172, 174]. The incidence of delirium for those who are admitted to intensive care units (ICU) is over 70% [171, 172]. The incidence of postoperative delirium varies between 15 and 60%.

Risk Factors

Among the elderly, delirium develops due to the interaction between various predisposing and precipitating factors [171, 172]. The two most common predisposing factors for delirium among older adults are increasing age and the presence of pre-existing cognitive deficits. Impairment in vision, renal disease, and the presence of severe illness are also additional risk factors [175].

Iatrogenic events, medication adverse effects, dehydration, falls, the use of physical restraints, malnutrition, greater than three medications added to the treatment regimen at a time, the use of urinary catheters, and hospital-acquired infections are common precipitating factors for delirium among older adults [172, 175, 176].

Delirium in older adults may also be precipitated by the use of anticholinergics, antihistamines, benzodiazepines, chemotherapeutic agents, dopamine agonists, opioid analgesics, psychostimulants, and steroids among others [177].

Outcomes

The development of delirium among older adults can result in dehydration, worsening of nutritional status, development of pressure ulcers, aspiration pneumonia, and pulmonary emboli [172]. Older adults who develop delirium also tend to decline in their cognition [172]. It has been noted that these individuals never return to their premorbid level of cognitive functioning. The development of delirium among older adults results in the greater use of nursing care, greater risk for hospitalization, longer hospital stays, higher costs of hospitalization, greater risk for institutionalization, and also higher risk for death [172, 176, 178, 179]. In the United States, the average medical care cost for individuals who develop delirium is more than two and a half times the cost for individuals without delirium [180]. Additionally, Medicare spends $7 billion a year on hospital stays due to delirium with the total healthcare cost due to delirium ranging from $38 billion to $152 billion every year [172, 181].

Assessment

It is estimated that approximately one-third of the cases of delirium among older adults go undiagnosed [178]. Common reasons for this lack of diagnosis are poor awareness of the person's premorbid cognitive and functional status and an ageist attitude toward the older adults where older adults are thought to be generally confused [171]. Additional reasons for limited diagnosis include limited awareness of the clinical features of delirium; the overlap between the clinical features of delirium, depression, and dementia; and inadequate screening for cognitive and functional impairments during routine medical appointments for the elderly [171].

In order to diagnose delirium, all relevant clinical information including a detailed history and cognitive, behavioral, and functional assessments should be included [172, 182]. The history should include details regarding the symptom onset, associated symptoms, medical history, and the name of medications and/or drugs that the individual is using. Cognitive, behavioral, and functional assessments provide details regarding the extent of changes noted on these domains. A focused physical examination and laboratory evaluation ascertain possible medical causes for delirium [171, 172, 183].

Standardized screening tools help identify cases of delirium [182]. Confusion Assessment Method (CAM) is the most commonly used screening tool for delirium among older adults [181]. Additional screening tools include the Confusion Assessment Method for the ICU (CAM-ICU), the Nursing Delirium Screening Scale (Nu-DESC), and the Delirium Detection Score (DDS) [184]. Available data indicates that cognitive screening tools like the Mini-Mental State Examination (MMSE) are often unhelpful for the identification of delirium. [181]. The severity of a delirium episode can be assessed using the Delirium Assessment Scale (DAS), Memorial Delirium Assessment Scale (MDAS), Delirium Rating Scale (DRS), Delirium Rating Scale-Revised-98 (The DRS-R-98), Delirium Severity Scale (DSS), and the Delirium-O-Meter (DOM). [185].

Diagnosing delirium using only the available clinical information may result in limited identification of delirium, as the symptoms of delirium often fluctuate [186]. It is best to make the diagnosis of delirium by utilizing all available clinical information obtained from multiple observation points in conjunction with a reliable screening instrument like the CAM. Then the diagnosis of delirium can be confirmed by using standardized diagnostic criteria like the DSM-5 [170].

Prevention

Available evidence indicates that both non-pharmacological and pharmacological interventions can prevent about one-third of the cases of delirium among older adults [172, 173].

Non-pharmacological

Available data indicates that non-pharmacological management including the multicomponent targeted risk factor intervention (MTI) strategy where there was a standardized protocol for the management of six major risk factors for delirium including cognitive deficits, sleep impairment, ambulatory difficulties, visual deficits, hearing problems, dehydration, proactive geriatric consultation, and in-home rehabilitation appears to reduce the incidence, duration, and severity of delirium in older adults and was well tolerated in this population [187–194].

Pharmacological

Data from two meta-analyses indicates that the use of antipsychotic medications may prevent the onset of delirium among older adults who are status-post surgery [195, 196]. Data indicates that prophylaxis with antipsychotic medications resulted in a reduction in the incidence of delirium with the number needed to treat (NNT) between 4.00 and 12.6. These medications appeared to be well tolerated by older adults. The possible mechanisms by which antipsychotic medications prevent delirium include the modulation of dopaminergic and serotonergic activity. Additionally, the use of antipsychotic medications may reduce agitation or aggression among delirious individuals, thereby reducing the need for physical restraints and additional pharmacological treatments.

Treatments

Available evidence indicates that both non-pharmacological and pharmacological interventions are beneficial in the treatment of delirium among older adults.

Non-pharmacological

Non-pharmacological management strategies including making eye contact, frequent reorientation, and the use of clear verbal instructions when communicating have shown benefit in the treatment of older adults with delirium [172, 183]. Minimizing visual and hearing loss using assistive devices, providing care in a non-stimulating environment which is quiet and has adequate but soft lighting, limiting the use of physical restraints, and minimizing room staff changes appear to benefit individuals with delirium [172, 175, 186].

Additionally, data from four studies (three RCTs and one systematic review) indicates that non-pharmacological management strategies including geriatric psychiatry consultation (GPC) and nurse-led interdisciplinary intervention programs for delirium appear to reduce the severity and duration of delirium among older adults [190, 197–200]. Also, these treatment modalities appear to be well tolerated in older adults. The efficacy of these interventions is possibly related to early identification, management of risk factors, and early rehabilitation of individuals.

Milisen et al. in their systematic review found that strategies to treat delirium among older adults admitted to medical services were ineffective [192]. But, among older individuals admitted for surgery, the treatments appeared to reduce the duration and severity of the delirium episode. The investigators also found that none of the intervention strategies resulted in shorter lengths of hospital stay or reduced mortality rates.

Pharmacological

Among older adults with delirium, pharmacotherapy is used to treat the underlying causes of delirium and in situations where the non-pharmacological interventions have failed [170, 172]. Pharmacotherapy is also utilized in situations where these individuals present with symptoms of agitation, aggression, paranoia, and hallucinations [172].

Data from one meta-analysis [201] and one systematic review [202] indicates that antipsychotic medications appear to reduce the severity and the duration of delirium among older adults. Additionally, these medications appear to be well tolerated among older adults. Modulation of dopaminergic and serotonergic activity is thought to be a possible mechanism by which antipsychotic medications exert their efficacy among individuals with delirium [195, 196].

Data from three studies that evaluated the efficacy of acetylcholinesterase inhibitors for the management of delirium did not find any benefit for these drugs in reducing the duration of delirium or the length of hospital stay [203–205]. Overshott et al. in their meta-analysis concluded that the efficacy for donepezil in the treatment of delirium among older individuals with delirium was lacking from controlled trials [206].

Chakraborti et al. in their study found that melatonin appears to reduce the duration and severity of delirium among older adults who develop delirium status-post surgery [207]. Melatonin was found to be well tolerated in this study. Melatonin appears to exert its efficacy among individuals with delirium by resetting the circadian rhythm.

Lonergan et al. in their meta-analysis found one trial that compared the efficacy of lorazepam to dexmedetomidine, a selective alpha-2-adrenergic receptor agonist for the treatment of delirium, among mechanically ventilated individuals who were admitted to intensive care units [208]. The investigators found that the individuals treated with dexmedetomidine had greater number of delirium- and coma-free days when compared to individuals who were treated with lorazepam, $P = 0.01$. Additionally, the investigators found two studies that showed no benefits for alprazolam when compared to antipsychotics, or for lorazepam when compared to haloperidol, and chlorpromazine for the treatment of delirium. Furthermore, the lorazepam group had more side effects than the haloperidol group. The investigators concluded that there is no data to support the efficacy of benzodiazepines for the treatment of non-alcohol withdrawal-related delirium among hospitalized adults.

The American Psychiatric Association (APA) recommends the use of low-dose haloperidol as a first-line drug for the symptomatic treatment of delirium [209]. The APA also states that atypical antipsychotics may be used as an alternative to haloperidol among individuals who have allergies to haloperidol or are not ideal candidates for the use of typical antipsychotic agents including those individuals with Parkinson's disease, dementia with Lewy bodies, and Parkinson-plus syndromes.

Recent evidence indicates that the use of antipsychotic medications among older adults especially those individuals with dementia is associated with an increased risk for cerebrovascular adverse events (CVAEs) and death [155]. The risk for CVAEs and death appears similar for both atypical and typical antipsychotic agents. Among individuals with dementia, the time frame for which the risk for CVAEs remains elevated is about 20 months, and the risk for death appears to be elevated in the first 30 days and possibly lasts for up to 2 years. Given these serious risks, the use of antipsychotic medications should be carefully monitored among older adults especially those individuals with dementia.

Conclusions

Among older adults, delirium is a common neuropsychiatric disorder. Delirium is often poorly diagnosed among these individuals and is associated with significant morbidity and mortality. The diagnosis of delirium requires a thorough clinical history, a focused physical examination, the evaluation of common laboratory test results, and the use of standardized screening tools like the CAM. The incidence of delirium and its overall severity can be reduced through both non-pharmacological and pharmacological interventions. These interventions may also reduce the duration of delirium and the length of hospital stays. Ideally, both non-pharmacological and pharmacological interventions should be combined for the prevention and treatment of delirium, thereby reducing the overall morbidity and mortality rates for this condition among older adults.

References

1. American Psychiatric Association. Diagnostic and statistical manual of mental disorders. 5th ed. Washington, DC: American Psychiatric Association; 2013. p. 299–320.
2. Reisberg B, Ferris SH, Kluger A, et al. Mild cognitive impairment (MCI): a historical perspective. Int Psychogeriatr. 2008;20(1):18–31.
3. Reisberg B, Ferris SH, de Leon MJ. The Global Deterioration Scale for assessment of primary degenerative dementia. Am J Psychiatry. *1982*;139(9):1136–9.
4. Reisberg B, Ferris SH, de Leon MJ, et al. The stage specific temporal cause of Alzheimer's disease: functional and behavioral concomitants based upon cross-sectional and longitudinal observation. Prog Clin Biol Res. 1989;317:23–41.
5. Flicker C, Ferris SH, Reisberg B. Mild cognitive impairment in the elderly: predictors of dementia. Neurology. *1991*;41(7):1006–9.
6. Morris JC. The Clinical Dementia Rating (CDR): current version and scoring rules. Neurology. *1993*;43(11):2412–4.

7. Morris JC, Storandt M, Miller JP, et al. Mild cognitive impairment represents early-stage Alzheimer's disease. Arch Neurol. *2001*;58(3):397–405.
8. Petersen RC, Stevens JC, Ganguli M, et al. Practice parameter: early detection of dementia: mild cognitive impairment (an evidence-based review). Report of the Quality Standards Subcommittee of the American Academy of Neurology. Neurology. 2001;56(9):1133–42.
9. Petersen RC. Mild cognitive impairment. Continuum. 2016;22(2 Dementia):404–18.
10. Petersen RC, Roberts RO, Knopman DS, et al. Prevalence of mild cognitive impairment is higher in men. The Mayo Clinic Study of Aging. Neurology. 2010;75(10):889–97.
11. Stephan BC, Hunter S, Harris D, et al. The neuropathological profile of mild cognitive impairment (MCI): a systematic review. Mol Psychiatry. *2012*;17(11):1056–76.
12. Bennett DA, Schneider JA, Bienias JL, et al. Mild cognitive impairment is related to Alzheimer's disease pathology and cerebral infarctions. Neurology. 2005;64:834–41.
13. Jicha GA, Parisi JE, Dickson DW, et al. Neuropathologic outcome of mild cognitive impairment following progression to clinical dementia. Arch Neurol. 2006;63(5):674–81.
14. Fennema-Notestine C, McEvoy LK, Hagler DJ, et al. The Alzheimer's disease neuroimaging initiative. Structural neuroimaging in the detection and prognosis of pre-clinical and early AD. Behav Neurol. *2009*;21(1):3–12.
15. Koivunen J, Pirttilä T, Kemppainen N, et al. PET amyloid ligand [11C] PIB uptake and cerebrospinal fluid beta-amyloid in mild cognitive impairment. Dement Geriatr Cogn Disord. *2008*;26(4):378–83.
16. Forsberg A, Engler H, Almkvist O, et al. PET imaging of amyloid deposition in patients with mild cognitive impairment. Neurobiol Aging. *2008*;29(10):1456–65.
17. Petersen RC, Smith GE, Waring SC, et al. Mild cognitive impairment: clinical characterization and outcome. Arch Neurol. *1999*;56(3):303–8.
18. Ganguli M, Dodge HH, Shen C, DeKosky ST. Mild cognitive impairment, amnestic type. An epidemiologic study. Neurology. 2004;63(1):115–21.
19. Ritchie K, Artero S, Touchon J. Classification criteria for mild cognitive impairment: a population-based validation study. Neurology. 2001;56(1):37–42.
20. Larrieu S, Letenneur L, Orgogozo JM, et al. Incidence and outcome of mild cognitive impairment in a population-based prospective cohort. Neurology. 2002;59(10):1594–9.
21. Gauthier S, Reisberg B, Zaudig M, et al. International Psychogeriatric Association Expert Conference on mild cognitive impairment. Lancet. 2006;367(9518):1262–70.
22. Petersen RC, Negash S. Mild cognitive impairment: an overview. CNS Spectr. 2008;13(1):45–53.
23. Petersen RC, Caracciolo B, Brayne C, et al. Mild cognitive impairment: a concept in evolution. J Intern Med. 2014;275(3):214–28.
24. Jack CR, Petersen RC, YC X, et al. Prediction of AD with MRI-based hippocampal volume in mild cognitive impairment. Neurology. 1999;52(7):1397–403.
25. Jack CR, Shiung MM, Weigand SD, et al. Brain atrophy rates predict subsequent clinical conversion in normal elderly and amnestic MCI. Neurology. *2005*;65(8):1227–31.
26. Leung KK, Bartlett JW, Barnes J, et al. Cerebral atrophy in mild cognitive impairment and Alzheimer disease. Rates and acceleration. Neurology. 2013;80(7):648–54.
27. Herholz K. Cerebral glucose metabolism in preclinical and prodromal Alzheimer's disease. Expert Rev Neurother. 2010;10(11):1667–73.
28. Ewers M, Walsh C, Trojanowski JQ, Shaw LM, et al. Prediction of conversion from mild cognitive impairment to Alzheimer's disease dementia based upon biomarkers and neuropsychological test performance. Neurobiol Aging. 2012;33(7):1203–14.
29. Feldman H, Scheltens P, Scarpini E, et al. Behavioral symptoms in mild cognitive impairment. Neurology. 2004;62(7):1199–201.
30. Palmer K, Berger AK, Monastero R, et al. Predictors of progression from mild cognitive impairment to Alzheimer disease. Neurology. 2007;68(19):1596–602.
31. Butters MA, Young JB, Lopez O, et al. Pathways linking late-life depression to persistent cognitive impairment and dementia. Dialogues Clin Neurosci. 2008;10(3):345–57.
32. Robert PH, Berr C, Volteau M, et al. Apathy in patients with mild cognitive impairment and the risk of developing dementia of Alzheimer's disease: a one-year follow-up study. Clin Neurol Neurosurg. 2006;108(8):733–6.
33. Rosenberg PB, Mielke MM, Appleby B, et al. Neuropsychiatric symptoms in MCI subtypes: the importance of executive dysfunction. Int J Geriatr Psychiatry. 2011;26(4):364–72.
34. Daly E, Zaitchik D, Copeland M, et al. Predicting conversion to Alzheimer's disease using standardized clinical information. Arch Neurol. *2000*;57(5):675–80.

35. Petersen RC. Clinical practice. Mild cognitive impairment. N Engl J Med. 2011;364(23):2227–34.
36. Tierney MC, Szalai JP, Snow WG, et al. A prospective study of the clinical utility of ApoE genotype in the prediction of outcome in patients with memory impairment. Neurology. 1996;46(1):149–54.
37. Petersen RC, Smith GE, Ivnik RJ, et al. Apolipoprotein E status as a predictor of the development of Alzheimer's disease in memory-impaired individuals. JAMA. 1995;273(16):1274–8.
38. Massoud F, Belleville S, Bergman H, et al. Mild cognitive impairment and cognitive impairment, no dementia: part B, therapy. Alzheimers Dement. 2007;3(4):283–91.
39. Jean L, Bergeron ME, Thivierge S, Simard M. Cognitive intervention programs for individuals with mild cognitive impairment: systematic review of the literature. Am J Geriatr Psychiatry. 2010;18(4):281–96.
40. Lautenschlager NT, Cox KL, Flicker L, et al. Effect of physical activity on cognitive function in older adults at risk for Alzheimer disease: a randomized trial. JAMA. 2008;300(9):1027–37.
41. Li H, Li J, Li N, et al. Cognitive intervention for persons with mild cognitive impairment: a meta-analysis. Ageing Res Rev. 2011;10(2):285–96.
42. Reijnders J, van Heugten C, van Boxtel M. Cognitive interventions in healthy older adults and people with mild cognitive impairment: a systematic review. Ageing Res Rev. 2013;12(1):263–75.
43. Etgen T, Sander D, Bickel H, Förstl H. Mild cognitive impairment and dementia: the importance of modifiable risk factors. Dtsch Arztebl Int. 2011;108(44):743–50.
44. Raschetti R, Albanese E, Vanacore N, et al. Cholinesterase inhibitors in mild cognitive impairment: a systematic review of randomised trials. PLoS Med. 2007;4(11):e338.
45. Diniz BS, Pinto JA, Gonzaga ML, et al. To treat or not to treat? A meta-analysis of the use of cholinesterase inhibitors in mild cognitive impairment for delaying progression to Alzheimer's disease. Eur Arch Psychiatry Clin Neurosci. 2009;259(4):248–56.
46. Thal LJ, Ferris SH, Kirby L, et al. A randomized, double-blind, study of rofecoxib in patients with mild cognitive impairment. Neuropsychopharmacology. 2005;30(6):1204–15.
47. Petersen RC, Thomas RG, Grundman M, et al. Vitamin E and donepezil for the treatment of mild cognitive impairment. New Engl J Med. 2005;352(23):2379–88.
48. Cooper C, Li R, Lyketsos C, Livingston G. Treatment for mild cognitive impairment: systematic review. Br J Psychiatry. 2013;203(3):255–64.
49. Mecocci P, Polidori MC. Antioxidant clinical trials in mild cognitive impairment and Alzheimer's disease. Biochim Biophys Acta. 2012;1822(5):631–8.
50. American Psychiatric Association. Diagnostic and statistical manual of mental disorders. 5th ed. Arlington, VA: American Psychiatric Publishing; 2013. p. 285–320.
51. New Diagnostic Criteria for Alzheimer's Disease. http://www.alz.org/research/diagnostic_criteria/. Accessed 1 Mar 2017.
52. Prince M, Bryce R, Albanese E, et al. The global prevalence of dementia: a systematic review and metaanalysis. Alzheimers Dement. 2013;9(1):63–75.
53. Sousa RM, Ferri CP, Acosta D, et al. Contribution of chronic diseases to disability in elderly people in countries with low and middle incomes: a 10/66 Dementia Research Group population-based survey. Lancet. 2009;374(9704):1821–30.
54. Sousa RM, Ferri CP, Acosta D, et al. The contribution of chronic diseases to the prevalence of dependence among older people in Latin America, China and India: a 10/66 Dementia Research Group population-based survey. BMC Geriatr. 2010;10:53.
55. Plassman BL, Langa KM, Fisher GG, et al. Prevalence of cognitive impairment without dementia in the United States. Ann Intern Med. 2008;148(6):427–34.
56. Hebert LE, Weuve J, Scherr PA, et al. Alzheimer disease in the United States (2010–2050) estimated using the 2010 census. Neurology. 2013;80(19):1778–83.
57. Hugo J, Ganguli M. Dementia and cognitive impairment: epidemiology, diagnosis, and treatment. Clin Geriatr Med. 2014;30(3):421–42.
58. Fiest KM, Jetté N, Roberts JI, et al. The Prevalence and Incidence of Dementia: a Systematic Review and Meta-analysis. Can J Neurol Sci. 2016;43:S3–S50.
59. Anstey KJ, Eramudugolla R, Hosking DE, et al. Bridging the Translation Gap: from Dementia Risk Assessment to Advice on Risk Reduction. J Prev Alzheimers Dis. 2015;2:189–98.
60. Morris MC, Tangney CC, Wang Y, et al. MIND diet slows cognitive decline with aging. Alzheimers Dement. 2015;11(9):1015–22.
61. Abete P, Della-Morte D, Gargiulo G, et al. Cognitive impairment and cardiovascular diseases

in the elderly. A heart-brain continuum hypothesis. Ageing Res Rev. 2014;18:41–52.
62. Billioti de Gage S, Pariente A, Bégaud BI. there really a link between benzodiazepine use and the risk of dementia? Expert Opin Drug Saf. 2015;14(5):733–47.
63. Gray SL, Anderson ML, Dublin S, et al. Cumulative use of strong anticholinergics and incident dementia: a prospective cohort study. JAMA Intern Med. 2015;175(3):401–7.
64. Tannenbaum C, Paquette A, Hilmer S, et al. A systematic review of amnestic and non-amnestic mild cognitive impairment induced by anticholinergic, antihistamine, GABAergic and opioid drugs. Drugs Aging. 2012;29(8):639–58.
65. Xu W, Tan L, Wang HF, et al. Meta-analysis of modifiable risk factors for Alzheimer's disease. J Neurol Neurosurg Psychiatry. 2015;86(12):1299–306.
66. Henderson VW. Action of estrogens in the aging brain: dementia and cognitive aging. Biochim Biophys Acta. 2010;1800(10):1077–83.
67. Zhou B, Teramukai S, Fukushima M. Prevention and treatment of dementia or Alzheimer's disease by statins: a meta-analysis. Dement Geriatr Cogn Disord. 2007;23(3):194–201.
68. McGuinness B, Todd S, Passmore P, Bullock R. Blood pressure lowering in patients without prior cerebrovascular disease for prevention of cognitive impairment and dementia. Cochrane Database Syst Rev. 2009;7(4):CD004034.
69. Imbimbo BP. An update on the efficacy of non-steroidal anti-inflammatory drugs in Alzheimer's disease. Expert Opin Investig Drugs. 2009;18(8):1147–68.
70. Dá Mesquita S, Ferreira AC, Sousa JC, et al. Insights on the pathophysiology of Alzheimer's disease: the crosstalk between amyloid pathology, neuroinflammation and the peripheral immune system. Neurosci Biobehav Rev. 2016;68: 547–62.
71. Scheltens P, Blennow K, Breteler MM, et al. Alzheimer's disease. Lancet. 2016;388(10043): 505–1.
72. O'Brien JT, Thomas A. Vascular dementia. Lancet. 2015;386(10004):1698–706.
73. Iadecola C. The pathobiology of vascular dementia. Neuron. 2013;80(4):844–66.
74. Bang J, Spina S, Miller BL. Frontotemporal dementia. Lancet. 2015;386(10004):1672–82.
75. Perry DC, Miller BL. Frontotemporal dementia. Semin Neurol. 2013;33(4):336–41.
76. Mayo MC, Bordelon Y. Dementia with Lewy bodies. Semin Neurol. 2014;34(2):182–8.
77. Walker Z, Possin KL, Boeve BF, et al. Lewy body dementias. Lancet. 2015;386(10004):1683–97.
78. Jing W, Willis R, Feng Z. Factors influencing quality of life of elderly people with dementia and care implications: a systematic review. Arch Gerontol Geriatr. 2016;66:23–41.
79. Kua EH, Ho E, Tan HH, et al. The natural history of dementia. Psychogeriatrics. 2014;14(3):196–201.
80. Jellinger KA, Wenning GK, Seppi K. Predictors of survival in dementia with lewy bodies and Parkinson dementia. Neurodegener Dis. 2007;4(6): 428–30.
81. Darrow MDA. practical approach to dementia in the outpatient primary care setting. Prim Care. 2015;42(2):195–204.
82. Tsoi KK, Chan JY, Hirai HW, et al. Cognitive tests to detect dementia: a systematic review and meta-analysis. JAMA Intern Med. 2015;175(9): 1450–8.
83. Feliciano L, Horning SM, Klebe KJ, et al. Utility of the SLUMS as a cognitive screening tool among a nonveteran sample of older adults. Am J Geriatr Psychiatry. 2013;21(7):623–30.
84. Feldman HH, Jacova C, Robillard A, et al. Diagnosis and treatment of dementia: 2. Diagnosis. CMAJ. 2008;178(7):825–36.
85. Narayanan L, Murray AD. What can imaging tell us about cognitive impairment and dementia? World J Radiol. 2016;8(3):240–54.
86. Burrell JR, Piguet O. Lifting the veil: how to use clinical neuropsychology to assess dementia. J Neurol Neurosurg Psychiatry. 2015;86(11):1216–24.
87. Sancesario GM, Bernardini S. How many biomarkers to discriminate neurodegenerative dementia? Crit Rev. Clin Lab Sci. 2015;52(6):314–26.
88. Downing LJ, Caprio TV, Lyness JM. Geriatric psychiatry review: differential diagnosis and treatment of the 3 D's - delirium, dementia, and depression. Curr Psychiatry Rep. 2013;15(16):365.
89. Shatenstein B, Barberger-Gateau P, Mecocci P. Prevention of age-related cognitive decline: which strategies, when, and for whom? J Alzheimers Dis. 2015;48(1):35–53.
90. Cheng ST. Cognitive reserve and the prevention of dementia: the role of physical and cognitive activities. Curr Psychiatry Rep. 2016;18(9):85.
91. Norton S, Matthews FE, Barnes DE, et al. Potential for primary prevention of Alzheimer's disease: an analysis of population-based data. Lancet Neurol. 2014;13(8):788–94.
92. Barnes DE, Yaffe K. The projected effect of risk factor reduction on Alzheimer's disease prevalence. Lancet Neurol. 2011;10(9):819–28.
93. Anand R, Gill KD, Mahdi AA. Therapeutics of Alzheimer's disease: past, present and future. Neuropharmacology. 2014;76:27–50.

94. Tan CC, Yu JT, Wang HF, et al. Efficacy and safety of donepezil, galantamine, rivastigmine, and memantine for the treatment of Alzheimer's disease: a systematic review and meta-analysis. Alzheimer Dis. 2014;41(2):615–31.
95. Tsoi KK, Chan JY, Leung NW, et al. Combination therapy showed limited superiority over monotherapy for Alzheimer disease: a meta-analysis of 14 randomized trials. J Am Med Dir Assoc. 2016;17(9):863.e1–8.
96. Atri A, Hendrix SB, Pejović V, et al. Cumulative, additive benefits of memantine-donepezil combination over component monotherapies in moderate to severe Alzheimer's dementia: a pooled area under the curve analysis. Alzheimers Res Ther. 2015;7(1):28.
97. Kavirajan H, Schneider LS. Efficacy and adverse effects of cholinesterase inhibitors and memantine in vascular dementia: a meta-analysis of randomised controlled trials. Lancet Neurol. 2007;6(9):782–92.
98. Nardell M, Tampi RR. Pharmacological treatments for frontotemporal dementias: a systematic review of randomized controlled trials. Am J Alzheimers Dis Other Demen. 2014;29(2): 123–32.
99. Stinton C, McKeith I, Taylor JP, et al. Pharmacological Management of Lewy Body Dementia: a Systematic Review and Meta-Analysis. Am J Psychiatry. 2015;172(8):731–42.
100. Sarva H, Henchcliffe C. Evidence for the use of pimavanserin in the treatment of Parkinson's disease psychosis. Ther Adv Neurol Disord. 2016;9(6):462–73.
101. Bharucha AJ, Rosen J, Mulsant BH, et al. Assessment of behavioral and psychological symptoms of dementia. CNS Spectr. 2002;7(11): 797–802.
102. Lyketsos CG, Steinberg M, Tschanz JT, et al. Mental and behavioral disturbances in dementia: findings from the Cache County Study on Memory in Aging. Am J Psychiatry. 2000;157(5): 708–14.
103. Margallo-Lana M, Swann A, O'Brien J, et al. Prevalence and pharmacological management of behavioural and psychological symptoms amongst dementia sufferers living in care environments. Int J Geriatr Psychiatry. 2001;16(1):39–44.
104. Jost BC, Grossberg GT. The evolution of psychiatric symptoms in Alzheimer's disease: a natural history study. J Am Geriatr Soc. 1996;44(9):1078–81.
105. Lyketsos CG, Olin J. Depression in Alzheimer's disease: overview and treatment. Biol Psychiatry. 2002;52(3):243–52.
106. Burns A, Jacoby R, Levy R. Psychiatric phenomena in Alzheimer's disease. I: disorders of thought content. Br J Psychiatry. 1990;157:72–6, 92–4
107. Devanand DP, Jacobs DM, Tang MX, et al. The course of psychopathologic features in mild to moderate Alzheimer disease. Arch Gen Psychiatry. 1997;54:257–63.
108. Mega MS, Cummings JL, Fiorello T, et al. The spectrum of behavioral changes in Alzheimer's disease. Neurology. 1996;46:130–5.
109. Lee HB, Lyketsos CG. Depression in Alzheimer's disease: heterogeneity and related issues. Biol Psychiatry. 2003;54(3):353–62.
110. Olin JT, Katz IR, Meyers BS, et al. Provisional diagnostic criteria for depression of Alzheimer disease: rationale and background. Am J Geriatr Psychiatry. 2002;10(2):129–41.
111. Pearlson GD, Ross CA, Lohr WD, et al. Association between family history of affective disorder and the depressive syndrome of Alzheimer's disease. Am J Psychiatry. 1990;37:452–6.
112. Rose KM, Lorenz R. Sleep disturbances in dementia. J Gerontol Nurs. 2010;36(5):9.
113. White H, Pieper C, Schmader K. The association of weight change in Alzheimer's disease with severity of disease and mortality: a longitudinal analysis. J Am Geriatr Soc. 1998;46(10):1223–7.
114. Black B, Muralee S, Tampi RR. Inappropriate sexual behaviors in dementia. J Geriatr Psychiatry Neurol. 2005;18(3):155–62.
115. Zubenko GS, Moossy J, Martinez J, et al. Neuropathologic and neurochemical correlates of psychosis in primary dementia. Arch Neurol. 1991;48:619–24.
116. Victoroff J, Zarow C, Mack WJ, et al. Physical aggression is associated with preservation of substantia nigra pars compacta in Alzheimer's disease. Arch Neurol. 1996;53:428–34.
117. Farber NB, Rubin EH, Newcomer JW, et al. Increased neocortical neurofibrillary tangle density in subjects with Alzheimer disease and psychosis. Arch Gen Psychiatry. 2000;57(12):1165–73.
118. Tekin S, Mega MS, Masterman DM, et al. Orbitofrontal and anterior cingulate cortex neurofibrillary tangle burden is associated with agitation in Alzheimer disease. Ann Neurol. 2001;49(3):355–61.
119. Forstl H, Besthorn C, Burns A, et al. Delusional misidentification in Alzheimer's disease: a summary of clinical and biological aspects. Psychopathology. 1994;27(3–5):194–9.
120. Kotrla KJ, Chacko RC, Harper RG, et al. Clinical variables associated with psychosis in Alzheimer's disease. Am J Psychiatry. 1995;152(9):1377–9.

121. Starkstein SE, Vazquez S, Petracca G, et al. A SPECT study of delusions in Alzheimer's disease. Neurology. 1994;44(11):2055–9.
122. Mentis MJ, Weinstein EA, Horwitz B, et al. Abnormal brain glucose metabolism in the delusional misidentification syndromes: a positron emission tomography study in Alzheimer disease. Biol Psychiatry. 1995;38(7):438–49.
123. Sultzer DL, Mahler ME, Mandelkern MA, et al. The relationship between psychiatric symptoms and regional cortical metabolism in Alzheimer's disease. J Neuropsychiatry Clin Neurosci. 1995;7(4):476–84.
124. Hirono N, Mori E, Ishii K, et al. Alteration of regional cerebral glucose utilization with delusions in Alzheimer's disease. J Neuropsychiatry Clin Neurosci. 1998;10(4):433–9.
125. Cummings JL, Back C. The cholinergic hypothesis of neuropsychiatric symptoms in Alzheimer's disease. Am J Geriatr Psychiatry. 1998;6(2 Suppl 1):S64–78.
126. Strauss ME, Ogrocki PK. Confirmation of an association between family history of affective disorder and the depressive syndrome in Alzheimer's disease. Am J Psychiatry. 1996;153(10):1340–2.
127. Lyketsos CG, Tune LE, Pearlson G, et al. Major depression in Alzheimer's disease. An interaction between gender and family history. Psychosomatics. 1996;37(4):380–4.
128. Bacanu SA, Devlin B, Chowdari KV, et al. Heritability of psychosis in Alzheimer disease. Am J Geriatr Psychiatry. 2005;13(7):624–7.
129. Ballard C, Massey H, Lamb H, et al. Apolipoprotein E: non-cognitive symptoms and cognitive decline in late onset Alzheimer's disease. J Neurol Neurosurg Psychiatry. 1997;63(2):273–4.
130. Cacabelos R, Rodríguez B, Carrera C, et al. APOE-related frequency of cognitive and noncognitive symptoms in dementia. Methods Find Exp Clin Pharmacol. 1996;18(10):693–706.
131. Holmes C, Arranz MJ, Powell JF, et al. 5-HT2A and 5-HT2C receptor polymorphisms and psychopathology in late onset Alzheimer's disease. Hum Mol Genet. 1998;7(9):1507–9.
132. Sukonick DL, Pollock BG, Sweet RA, et al. The 5-HTTPR*S/*L polymorphism and aggressive behavior in Alzheimer disease. Arch Neurol. 2001;58(9):1425–8.
133. Sweet RA, Nimgaonkar VL, Kamboh MI, et al. Dopamine receptor genetic variation, psychosis, and aggression in Alzheimer disease. Arch Neurol. 1998;55(10):1335–40.
134. Holmes C, Smith H, Ganderton R, et al. Psychosis and aggression in Alzheimer's disease: the effect of dopamine receptor gene variation. J Neurol Neurosurg Psychiatry. 2001;71(6):777–9.
135. Meins W, Frey A, Thiesemann R. Premorbid personality traits in Alzheimer's disease: do they predispose to noncognitive behavioral symptoms? Int Psychogeriatr. 1998;10(4):369–78.
136. Chatterjee A, Strauss ME, Smyth KA, et al. Personality changes in Alzheimer's disease. Arch Neurol. 1992;49(5):486–91.
137. Lawlor B. Managing behavioural and psychological symptoms of dementia. Br J Psychiatry. 2002;181:463–5.
138. Coen RF, Swanwick GR, O'Boyle CA, et al. Behaviour disturbance and other predictors of carer burden in Alzheimer's disease. Int J Geriatr Psychiatry. 1997;12(3):331–6.
139. Kaufer DI, Cummings JL, Christine D, et al. Assessing the impact of neuropsychiatric symptoms in Alzheimer's disease: the Neuropsychiatric Inventory Caregiver Distress Scale. J Am Geriatr Soc. 1998;46(2):210–5.
140. O'Donnell BF, Drachman DA, Barnes HJ, et al. Incontinence and troublesome behaviors predict institutionalization in dementia. J Geriatr Psychiatry Neurol. 1992;5(1):45–52.
141. Steele C, Rovner B, Chase GA, et al. Psychiatric symptoms and nursing home placement of patients with Alzheimer's disease. Am J Psychiatry. 1990;147(8):1049–51.
142. Stern Y, Albert M, Brandt J, et al. Utility of extrapyramidal signs and psychosis as predictors of cognitive and functional decline, nursing home admission, and death in Alzheimer's disease: prospective analyses from the Predictors Study. Neurology. 1994;44:2300–7.
143. Stern Y, Mayeux R, Sano M, et al. Predictors of disease course in patients with probable Alzheimer's disease. Neurology. 1987;37:1649–53.
144. Beeri MS, Werner P, Davidson M, et al. The cost of behavioral and psychological symptoms of dementia (BPSD) in community dwelling Alzheimer's disease patients. Int J Geriatr Psychiatry. 2002;17(5):403–8.
145. Murman DL, Chen Q, Powell MC, et al. The incremental direct costs associated with behavioral symptoms in AD. Neurology. 2002;59(11):1721–9.
146. Robert PH, Verhey FR, Byrne EJ, et al. Grouping for behavioral and psychological symptoms in dementia: clinical and biological aspects. Consensus paper of the European Alzheimer disease consortium. Eur Psychiatry. 2005;20(7):490–6.
147. Jeon YH, Sansoni J, Low LF, et al. Recommended measures for the assessment of behavioral distur-

bances associated with dementia. Am J Geriatr Psychiatry. 2011;19(5):403–15.
148. Lanari A, Amenta F, Silvestrelli G, et al. Neurotransmitter deficits in behavioural and psychological symptoms of Alzheimer's disease. Mech Ageing Dev. 2006;127(2):158–65.
149. Livingston G, Johnston K, Katona C, et al. Old age task force of the world federation of biological psychiatry. Systematic review of psychological approaches to the management of neuropsychiatric symptoms of dementia. Am J Psychiatry. 2005;162(11):1996–2021.
150. Brodaty H, Arasaratnam C. Meta-analysis of nonpharmacological interventions for neuropsychiatric symptoms of dementia. Am J Psychiatry. 2012;169(9):946–53.
151. Seitz DP, Brisbin S, Herrmann N, et al. Efficacy and feasibility of nonpharmacological interventions for neuropsychiatric symptoms of dementia in long term care: a systematic review. J Am Med Dir Assoc. 2012;13(6):503–6.
152. Ballard CG, Waite J, Birks J. Atypical antipsychotics for aggression and psychosis in Alzheimer's disease. Cochrane Database Syst Rev. 2009;4:1–128.
153. Schneider LS, Dagerman K, Insel PS. Efficacy and adverse effects of atypical antipsychotics for dementia: meta-analysis of randomized, placebo-controlled trials. Am J Geriatr Psychiatry. 2006;14(3):191–210.
154. Schneider LS, Tariot PN, Dagerman KS, et al. Effectiveness and safety of atypical antipsychotic drugs in patients with Alzheimer's disease. N Engl J Med. 2006;355(15):1525–38.
155. Mittal V, Kurup L, Williamson D, et al. Review: risk of cerebrovascular adverse events and death in elderly patients with dementia when treated with antipsychotic medications: a literature review of evidence. Am J Alzheimers Dis Other Demen. 2011;26(1):10–28.
156. Herrmann N, Lanctot KL. Do atypical antipsychotics cause stroke? CNS Drugs. 2005;19(2):91–103.
157. Gill SS, Rochon PA, Herrmann N, et al. Atypical antipsychotic drugs and risk of ischaemic stroke: population based retrospective cohort study. BMJ. 2005;330(7489):445.
158. Liperoti R, Gambassi G, Lapane KL, et al. Cerebrovascular events among elderly nursing home patients treated with conventional or atypical antipsychotics. J Clin Psychiatry. 2005;66(9):1090–6.
159. Schneider LS, Dagerman KS, Insel P. Risk of death with atypical antipsychotic drug treatment for dementia: meta-analysis of randomized placebo-controlled trials. JAMA. 2005;294(15):1934–43.
160. Wang PS, Schneeweiss S, Avorn J, et al. Risk of death in elderly users of conventional vs. atypical antipsychotic medications. N Engl J Med. 2005;353(22):2335–41.
161. Reus V, Fochtmann L, Eyler A, et al. The American psychiatric association practice guideline on the use of Antipsychotics to treat agitation or Psychosis in patients with dementia. Am J Psychiatry. 2016;173(5):543–6.
162. Seitz DP, Adunuri N, Gill SS, et al. Antidepressants for agitation and psychosis in dementia. Cochrane Database Syst Rev. 2011;16(2):CD008191.
163. Henry G, Williamson D, Tampi RR. Efficacy and tolerability of antidepressants in the treatment of behavioral and psychological symptoms of dementia, a literature review of evidence. Am J Alzheimers Dis Other Demen. 2011;26(3):169–83.
164. Lonergan ET, Cameron M, Luxenberg J. Valproic acid for agitation in dementia. Cochrane Database Syst Rev. 2004;2:CD003945.
165. Konovalov S, Muralee S, Tampi RR. Anticonvulsants for the treatment of behavioral and psychological symptoms of dementia: a literature review. Int Psychogeriatr. 2008;20(2):293–308.
166. Trinh NH, Hoblyn J, Mohanty S, et al. Efficacy of cholinesterase inhibitors in the treatment of neuropsychiatric symptoms and functional impairment in Alzheimer disease: a meta-analysis. JAMA. 2003;289:210–6.
167. Maidment ID, Fox CG, Boustani M, et al. Efficacy of memantine on behavioral and psychological symptoms related to dementia: a systematic meta-analysis. Ann Pharmacother. 2008;42(1):32–8.
168. Tampi RR, Tampi DJ. Efficacy and tolerability of benzodiazepines for the treatment of behavioral and psychological symptoms of dementia: a systematic review of randomized controlled trials. Am J Alzheimers Dis Other Demen. 2014;29(7):565–74.
169. Jansen S, Forbes D, Duncan V, et al. Melatonin for cognitive impairment. Cochrane Database Syst Rev. 2006;25(1):CD003802.
170. Desk Reference to the Diagnostic Criteria from DSM-5. Washington DC: American Psychiatric Association. 2013. P. 292–8.
171. Saxena S, Lawley D. Delirium in the elderly: a clinical review. Postgrad Med J. 2009;85(1006):405–13.
172. Fong TG, Tulebaev SR, Inouye SK. Delirium in elderly adults: diagnosis, prevention and treatment. Nat. Rev Neurol. 2009;5(4):210–20.
173. Khan BA, Zawahiri M, Campbell NL, et al. Delirium in hospitalized patients: implications of

current evidence on clinical practice and future avenues for research-a systematic evidence review. J Hosp Med. 2012;7(7):580–9.
174. Miller MO. Evaluation and management of delirium in hospitalized older patients. Am Fam Physician. 2008;78(11):1265–70.
175. Inouye SK. Predisposing and precipitating factors for delirium in hospitalized older patients. Dement Geriatr Cogn Disord. 1999;10(5):393–400.
176. Inouye SK, Charpentier PA. Precipitating factors for delirium in hospitalized elderly persons. Predictive model and interrelationship with baseline vulnerability. JAMA. 1996;275(11): 852–7.
177. Laurila JV, Laakkonen ML, Tilvis RS, et al. Predisposing and precipitating factors for delirium in a frail geriatric population. J Psychosom Res. 2008;65(3):249–54.
178. Siddiqi N, House AO, Holmes JD. Occurrence and outcome of delirium in medical in-patients: a systematic literature review. Age Ageing. 2006;35(4):350–64.
179. Rockwood K, Cosway S, Carver D, et al. The risk of dementia and death after delirium. Age Ageing. 1999;28(6):551–6.
180. Leslie DL, Marcantonio ER, Zhang Y, et al. One-year health care costs associated with delirium in the elderly population. Arch Intern Med. 2008;168(1):27–32.
181. Young J, Inouye SK. Delirium in older people. BMJ. 2007;334(7598):842–6.
182. Wong CL, Holroyd-Leduc J, Simel DL, et al. Does this patients have delirium?: value of bedside instruments. JAMA. 2010;304(7):779–86.
183. Cole MG. Delirium in elderly patients. Am J Geriatr Psychiatry. 2004;12(1):7–21.
184. Luetz A, Heymann A, Radtke FM, et al. Different assessment tools for intensive care unit delirium: which score to use? Crit Care Med. 2010;38(2):409–18.
185. Adamis D, Sharma N, Whelan PJ, et al. Delirium scales: a review of current evidence. Aging Ment Health. 2010;14(5):543–55.
186. Zou Y, Cole MG, Primeau FJ, et al. Detection and diagnosis of delirium in the elderly: psychiatric diagnosis, confusion assessment method, or consensus diagnosis? Int Psychogeriatr. 1998;10(3):303–8.
187. Inouye SK, Bogardus ST Jr, Charpentier PA, Leo-Summers L, et al. A multicomponent intervention to prevent delirium in hospitalized older patients. N Engl J Med. 1999;340(9):669–76.
188. Rizzo JA, Bogardus ST, Leo-Summers L, et al. Multicomponent targeted intervention to prevent delirium in hospitalized older patients: what is the economic value? Med Care. 2001;39:740–52.
189. Leslie DL, Zhang Y, Bogardus ST, et al. Consequences of preventing delirium in hospitalized older adults on nursing home costs. J Am Geriatr Soc. 2005;53(3):405–9.
190. Marcantonio ER, Flacker JM, Wright RJ, et al. Reducing delirium after hip fracture: a randomized trial. J Am Geriatr Soc. 2001;49(5):516–22.
191. Caplan GA, Coconis J, Board N, et al. Does home treatment affect delirium? A randomised controlled trial of rehabilitation of elderly and care at home or usual treatment (The REACH-OUT trial). Age Ageing. 2006;35(1):53–60.
192. Milisen K, Lemiengre J, Braes T, et al. Multicomponent intervention strategies for managing delirium in hospitalized older people: systematic review. J Adv Nurs. 2005;52(1):79–90.
193. Clegg A, Siddiqi N, Heaven A, Young J, et al. Interventions for preventing delirium in older people in institutional long-term care. Cochrane Database Syst Rev. 2014;1:CD009537.
194. Martinez F, Tobar C, Hill N. Preventing delirium: should non-pharmacological, multicomponent interventions be used? A systematic review and meta-analysis of the literature. Age Ageing. 2015;44(2):196–204.
195. Teslyar P, Stock VM, Wilk CM, et al. Prophylaxis with antipsychotic medication reduces the risk of post-operative delirium in elderly patients: a meta-analysis. Psychosomatics. 2013;54(2):124–31.
196. Fok MC, Sepehry AA, Frisch L, et al. Do antipsychotics prevent postoperative delirium? A systematic review and meta-analysis. Int J Geriatr Psychiatry. 2015;30(4):333–44.
197. Cole MG, Fenton FR, Engelsmann F, et al. Effectiveness of geriatric psychiatry consultation in an acute care hospital: a randomized clinical trial. J Am Geriatr Soc. 1991;39(12):1183–8.
198. Cole MG, Primeau FJ, Bailey RF, et al. Systematic intervention for elderly inpatients with delirium: a randomized trial. CMAJ. 1994;151(7): 965–70.
199. Milisen K, Foreman MD, Abraham IL, et al. A nurse-led interdisciplinary intervention program for delirium in elderly hip-fracture patients. J Am Geriatr Soc. 2001;49(5):523–32.
200. Cole MG, McCusker J, Bellavance F, et al. Systematic detection and multidisciplinary care of delirium in older medical inpatients: a randomized trial. CMAJ. 2002;167(7):753–9.
201. Lonergan E, Britton AM, Luxenberg J, et al. Antipsychotics for delirium. Cochrane Database Syst Rev. 2007;2:CD005594.

202. Ozbolt LB, Paniagua MA, Kaiser RM. Atypical antipsychotics for the treatment of delirious elders. J Am Med Dir Assoc. 2008;9(1):18–28.
203. Liptzin B, Laki A, Garb JL, et al. Donepezil in the prevention and treatment of post-surgical delirium. Am J Geriatr Psychiatry. 2005;13(12):1100–6.
204. Sampson EL, Raven PR, Ndhlovu PN, et al. A randomized, double-blind, placebo-controlled trial of donepezil hydrochloride (Aricept) for reducing the incidence of postoperative delirium after elective total hip replacement. Int J Geriatr Psychiatry. 2007;22(4):343–9.
205. Gamberini M, Bolliger D, Lurati Buse GA, et al. Rivastigmine for the prevention of postoperative delirium in elderly patients undergoing elective cardiac surgery-a randomized controlled trial. Crit Care Med. 2009;37(5):1762–8.
206. Overshott R, Vernon M, Morris J, et al. Rivastigmine in the treatment of delirium in older people: a pilot study. Int Psychogeriatr. 2010;22(5):812–8.
207. Chakraborti D, Tampi DJ, Tampi RR. Melatonin and Melatonin Agonist for Delirium in the Elderly Patients. Am J Alzheimers Dis Other Demen. 2015;30(2):119–29.
208. Lonergan E, Luxenberg J, Areosa SA. Benzodiazepines for delirium. Cochrane Database Syst Rev. 2009;4:CD006379.
209. Treatment of Patients with Delirium. http://www.psychiatryonline.com/pracguidetopic_2.aspx. Accessed 5 Jun 2017.

17 Depressive Disorders and Bipolar and Related Disorders

Rajesh R. Tampi, Deena J. Tampi, M. Ingre Walters, Geetha Manikkara, Poorvanshi Alag, and Garima Garg

Depressive Disorders

Introduction

The *Diagnostic and Statistical Manual of Mental Disorders*, Fifth Edition (DSM-5), defines major depressive disorder (MDD) as a condition characterized by the presence of depressed mood or marked loss of interest or pleasure in activities [1]. Associated symptoms include changes in appetite or weight (5% of total body weight), sleep, energy, concentration, and psychomotor activity, as well as feelings of inappropriate guilt or worthlessness, and recurrent thoughts of death or suicide. In addition, these symptoms should cause clinically significant distress or impairments in social, occupational, or other areas of functioning. Furthermore, the episode of depression should not be attributable to the psychological effects of substances or to another medical condition. To meet the criteria for a MDD in addition to depressed mood or marked loss of interest or pleasure in activities, the individual should have four associated symptoms. These symptoms should have been present during the same 2-week period. Depression that occurs among individuals ≥65 years of age who have not had a previous history of depression is called late life depression (LLD) [2].

Epidemiology

The prevalence rates of depressive symptoms among older adults vary between 30 and 45% [3, 4]. However the rates of major depressive disorder (MDD) among community-dwelling older adults are low at about 2% [3, 5]. The prevalence of MDD increases to approximately 6–9% among individuals attending primary care clinics [6]. Among older adults who are admitted to acute care hospitals, the prevalence rate of MDD is 10–12%. Approximately 12–14% of older adults living in nursing homes meet the criteria for MDD [2]. Data indicates that almost half of older adults having MDD go undiagnosed [7]. One reason for this underdiagnosis is the fact that older adults are more likely to consult their primary physician for psychiatric symptoms than be evaluated by a psychiatrist when compared to the younger adults [8].

Presentation

MDD among older adults differs from MDD among younger individuals as older individuals with MDD are less likely to have a family history of depression, the symptoms of depression occur insidiously, and the individual is more likely to attribute the symptoms to the normal aging process [3, 9]. Older adults with depression are also more likely to present with more agitation, hypochondriasis, and general somatic as well as gastrointestinal symptoms, but with less guilt and loss of sexual interest when compared to younger adults with depression [10]. Older individuals with MDD also report higher rates of psychotic symptoms when compared to younger adults with

R. R. Tampi et al. (eds.), *Psychiatric Disorders Late in Life*, https://doi.org/10.1007/978-3-319-73078-3_17

MDD [11]. Available data indicates that psychotic symptoms occur among 16–23% of older adults [12]. Approximately 25–50% of admissions to the inpatient geriatric psychiatry units occur due to MDD with psychotic symptoms [13]. Older individuals with MDD may present with nihilistic, somatic, or poverty-based delusions, and these individuals have higher rates of insomnia, somatic symptoms, diurnal variation of mood, and poor insight into their illness [3, 13]. Hallucinations tend to occur infrequently among older individuals with MDD. Risk factors for the development of psychotic symptoms among older individuals with MDD include being single, widowed, or living alone [13]. The presence of psychotic symptoms among older individuals with MDD is a poor prognostic factor as individuals with these symptoms develop frequent recurrences of symptoms that require repeated hospitalizations [3]. Possible reasons for the greater rates of psychotic symptoms among older individuals with MDD include age-related deterioration of the cortical areas of the brain, neurochemical changes that are common with aging, comorbid medical conditions, social isolation, sensory deficits, cognitive decline, and polypharmacy [11].

Depression and dementia are two conditions among older adults that present similarly and share an important relationship [14, 15]. Depressive pseudodementia or depression-associated dementia refers to the presence of reversible cognitive deficits that are seen during an episode of depression and which tend to improve with the treatment of the depressive episode [2, 4]. Additionally, depression can be a presenting symptom of dementia. From the available data, it is unclear if an episode of depression is a prodrome for the onset of dementia, a risk factor for dementia, or an independent event [16]. The acute onset of symptoms, the presence of guilt or self-reproach, diurnal variations in mood, poor effort on cognitive testing, and impaired registration and recall occur primarily in depression-associated dementia when compared to a primary dementia. In addition, individuals with depression-associated dementia do not present with deficits in multiple cognitive domains. Furthermore, symptoms of depression-associated dementia improve with sleep deprivation, whereas symptoms of dementia worsen with sleep deprivation [17].

In Table 17-1 we have enumerated the essential diagnostic features for different types of depressive disorders according to the DSM-5. Readers who are interested in learning more about the various depressive disorders, the classification of their severity, and additional specifiers are

TABLE 17-1. Types of depressive disorders according to the DSM-5 [1]

Name	Essential diagnostic features
Disruptive mood dysregulation disorder	Verbal or physical temper outbursts that are severe and recurrent and out of proportion to the provocative situation. Mood is persistently irritable between outbursts. These outbursts occur ≥3 times/week. These symptoms have been present for ≥12 months. Symptoms occur before 10 years of age (≥6 years and ≤18 years)
Persistent depressive disorder (dysthymia)	Presence of depressed mood for most days for at least 2 years. Two or more of appetite change, sleep alteration, poor energy/fatigue, poor self-esteem, poor concentration, or feeling hopeless
Premenstrual dysphoric disorder	One or more of the following: affective lability, irritability or anger, depressed mood/hopeless, or anxiety
	One or more of the following: decreased interest in activities, poor concentration, poor energy/fatigue, sleep changes, feeling overwhelmed, breast tenderness/sweating/pain/bloating/weight gain
	Five or more of these symptoms should be present during the final week before menstruation with improvement after menses. Symptoms present for most menstrual cycles during the preceding year
Substance-/medication-induced depressive disorder	Depressed mood or decreased interest in activities that occurs during or soon after the exposure to substance (intoxication or withdrawal) or medication. These symptoms do not occur exclusively during a delirium episode
Depressive disorder due to another medical condition	Depressed mood or decreased interest in activities that occurs due to the direct pathophysiological consequences of a medical condition. These symptoms do not occur exclusively during a delirium episode

requested to kindly review the chapter on depressive disorder in the DSM-5 book.

Neurobiology

There are many biological, psychological, and sociological determinants for the development of depression among older adults [18]. The interaction between depression among older adults and medical disorders requires a special mention. Approximately 25% of older individuals who have a cerebrovascular accident develop MDD [19]. Similarly 40% of older individuals with Parkinson's disease develop MDD [19]. Among older adults who are status post myocardial ischemia, one-quarter develop MDD [20, 21].

Older adults with MDD are more likely to develop of cognitive impairment when compared to their age- and education-matched counterparts without depression [22–24]. Approximately 20–50% of older individuals with depression develop cognitive deficits including executive dysfunction [22–24]. Additional cognitive changes include deficits in information processing and visuospatial function [24]. Among older adults with depression and vascular disease of the brain, neuroimaging studies reveal the colocalization of atrophy and ischemic lesions especially in the frontostriatal, limbic, and subcortical regions [2, 3]. These individuals often present with psychomotor retardation, reduced interest in activities, and poor insight into their illness [2].

Older adults tend to use multiple medications that can result in or contribute to the development of depression. Antihypertensive medications like methyldopa, reserpine, clonidine, and hydralazine; antiparkinson drugs like levodopa; anticancer drugs like tamoxifen, vinblastine, and vincristine; and hormonal agents like estrogen and progesterone, benzodiazepines, corticosteroids, and cimetidine can cause or worsen symptoms of depression among older adults [2]. Controlled data indicates that beta-blockers do not cause alterations in mood [25].

Neuroticism, pessimistic thinking, and less open attitudes to new experiences are some of the psychological traits that have been found to predict the development of depression and suicidal ideation among older adults [26–28]. Isolation, bereavement, functional decline, and disability are social factors for the development of depression among older adults [3, 29]. The effect of these stressors on development of depression among older adults persists even after controlling for biological and physical health status variables. Additionally, the impact of these psychosocial risk factors on depression among older adults can be altered by personal or environmental factors [30]. An additional risk factor for development of depression among older adults is caregiving for someone. Depression tends to occur more commonly among older caregivers when caregiving is long-term, the person receiving the care has behavioral issues, and the caregiver has limited social supports [30].

The meta-analysis by Cole and Dendukuri concluded that bereavement, sleep disturbance, disability, prior depression, and female gender appear to be important risk factors for depression among older community-dwelling individuals [31].

Depression is a chronic and relapsing illness [32]. Almost one-quarter of older adults with depression will achieve full remission with or without any treatment. One-quarter of these individuals will never achieve any treatment response, and the remaining individuals will have a waxing-and-waning course [3]. The presence of physical disability, psychotic features, and comorbid medical illness and the lack of social supports are poor prognostic factors [3, 13]. A major risk factor for poor prognosis, poor treatment response, and poor antidepressant tolerability among older adults with depression is the presence of medical comorbidities [32].

Consequences

Rates of morbidity and mortality are higher among older adults with depression when compared to age-matched controls [33]. Older adults with depression have a 1.5–3 times greater morbidity when compared to those older adults without depression [1]. Older individuals with depression are more likely to have a comorbid anxiety disorder, substance use disorder, and chronic diseases such as arthritis and heart diseases when compared to older adults without depression [34]. Depression among older adults also appears to increase the risk for inflammatory activity, bone resorption, cancer, heart disease, and death from heart disease [33, 35, 36].

The relationship between medical comorbidity and depression appears to be bidirectional with depression being associated with poor outcomes with comorbid medical illness, and comorbid medical illness negatively affects the course of depression [37]. Depression is considered a risk factor for all-cause dementia including Alzheimer's disease and vascular dementia [38].

Older adults with depression are five times more likely to commit suicide than the general population [21]. Studies also indicate that older adults with depression have an approximately 15% greater lifetime risk for suicide when compared to those older adults without depression [1]. Additionally nearly 10% of these individuals die annually from completed suicides. Among the completers of suicide, approximately three-quarters of the individuals had depression and had visited their primary care physician within the preceding month [9]. Risk factors for suicide are comorbid medical disorders, psychiatric disorders, substance use disorders, certain personality traits, and severe social stressors [2, 3, 19, 39].

Depression among older adults is associated with reduced or lost workplace productivity and greater healthcare utilization [34, 40, 41]. It is estimated that yearly $26.1 billion is spent on the direct medical costs for depression and $51.5 billion is lost due to workplace costs including absenteeism [42]. Suicides due to depression costs the economy an additional $5.4 billion a year in mortality costs [42] (Table 17-2 describes consequences of depression among older adullts).

Assessment

Older adults with depression often present with somatic complaints, cognitive difficulties, and/or functional decline and not mood symptoms, and hence any older individual with these complaints should be screened for depression [37]. A thorough psychiatric evaluation of an older adult with depression includes a patient interview, interview of caregivers if any, a medical and psychosocial assessment, systematic assessment of suicide risk, cognitive screening, and a functional evaluation. The suicide risk assessment must weigh the individual's risk and protective factors and stratify the overall risk of suicide as low, moderate, or high [3, 43].

Standardized screening tools can assist in the diagnosis, suicide screening, identifying psychotic symptoms, grading of severity of depression, and assessing the response to treatments [44]. The Geriatric Depression Scale [GDS] is the most commonly used screening tool for evaluating depression among older adults in primary care clinics and day treatment programs. It is a reliable and valid instrument that is available in several languages. However it has limited validity in older individuals with cognitive impairment. Among older adults with depression and mild-to-moderate dementia, the Cornell Scale for Depression in Dementia [CSDD] is a more reliable screening tool for depression [44]. It's use is limited by the need for trained raters, caregiver input, and the longer time needed for its completion. Other standardized scales used in the assessment of older adults with depression including the Hamilton Rating Scale for Depression [HAM-D], Montgomery-Åsberg Depression Rating Scale [MADRS], and Zung Self-Rating Depression Scale [SDS] which are used in geriatric psychiatry clinics and research studies to evaluate patients with depression. When compared to the HAM-D, GDS was found to be a more sensitive instrument in eliciting depressive symptoms among older adults [44–46]. The use of MADRS is limited among older adults with depression by the lack of assessment of somatic symptoms. The sensitivity of SDS among older adults with depression is limited by the use of graded responses, lack of assessment of somatic symptoms, and high false-positive rates [44]. Among older individuals with depression and psychotic symptoms, the Brief Psychiatric Rating Scale [BPRS] is the most commonly used scale to detect and rate the severity of psychopathology [44].

Given the high rates of medical comorbidities among older adults with depression, a thorough

Table 17-2. Consequences of depression among older adults

Comorbidity with anxiety and substance use disorders
Comorbidity with chronic medical conditions like arthritis, cancer, and heart disease
Greater risk of cognitive decline and dementia
Decline in functional status
Worse quality of life
Higher rates of mortality including suicides
Greater use of services
Overall greater cost of care

physical examination is an essential part of the work-up in these individuals [37]. Routine laboratory studies should include a complete blood count to rule out anemia and infections and a complete metabolic panel including renal and liver function tests to rule out metabolic abnormalities. Thyroid function tests including TSH, T4, T3, and thyroid-binding globulin (TBG) can identify hypothyroidism, which may mimic symptoms of depression including psychomotor slowing, flat affect, and cognitive difficulties. Vitamin B12 and folate levels should be checked as low levels of vitamin B12 and folate contribute to anemia, depression, and cognitive decline. Syphilis screening tests including RPR or VDRL may identify the infection that can result in psychosis and cognitive decline. HIV testing is important among individuals with cognitive impairment as AIDS can lead to cognitive decline. A urine drug screen is essential in ruling out comorbid substance use disorder among individuals with depression. Structural and functional neuroimaging studies can identify cerebral abnormalities that can result in depression and cognitive impairment and contribute to the burden of illness and poorer prognosis among older adults with depression [47, 48] (Table 17-3 describes the assessment of depression among older adults).

TABLE 17-3. Assessment of depression among older adults

Obtain history	Course of illness, medical history, psychiatric history, current and past medications, premorbid personality, cognition, and functional status
Complete a standardized mental status examination and formal cognitive testing	
Complete standardized assessment scales	Neuropsychological testing if needed
Complete a focused physical examination	Rule out medical or neurological disorders
Order appropriate investigations	Blood and urine examination, vitamin B12 and folate levels, RPR/VDRL, HIV testing, urine drug screen, and neuroimaging studies
Treat medical, psychiatric, and neurological disorders	Remove offending drug(s)

Treatments

Current evidence indicates that when treatment for depression is offered in the primary care setting, older adults are more likely to accept the treatment [49]. The involvement of a skilled and empathic care manager has also been shown to improve the success of treatment of depression among older adults in primary care [50]. There is emerging data that a collaborative care approach can reduce symptoms of depression among older individuals [49, 51]. Data also indicates that prevention strategies implemented at skilled nursing facilities can reduce the incidence of depression among older adults living at these facilities [52].

The Improving Mood: Promoting Access to Collaborative Treatment [IMPACT] program found that collaborative care, which actively engages older adults in the treatment for depression, improves symptoms of depression, physical functioning, and the quality of life [53].

The Prevention of Suicide in Primary Care Elderly: Collaborative Trial [PROSPECT] found that when trained clinicians collaborate with the primary care physicians to implement a comprehensive depression management program, it improved outcomes for older adults with depression [54]. Additionally, the individuals in the intervention group had a greater degree and faster resolution of symptoms of depression and a faster rate of reduction in suicidal ideation when compared to individuals receiving usual care [55]. Furthermore, individuals in the intervention group had earlier remission of their depressive episode and the rates of remission were higher when compared to the group receiving usual care [56]. Individuals who were experiencing hopelessness and those individuals with low baseline anxiety were more likely to achieve remission.

The treatments that are currently available for older adults with depression include psychotherapy, pharmacotherapy, and/or electroconvulsive therapy [ECT] [57, 58]. Additionally, there is some data to support the use of aerobic and supervised group exercise regimens as nonmedical interventions to manage depressive symptoms among older individuals [59].

Psychotherapy

Available data indicates that cognitive behavioral therapy (CBT), reminiscence therapy (RT), brief dynamic therapy (BDT), problem-solving therapy (PST), and the combination of medication and interpersonal psychotherapy (IPT) are effective treatments for depression among older adults with moderate to large effect sizes [60–64]. Additionally there is no difference noted whether the therapy is delivered in the individual, group, or bibliotherapy format [61].

Pinquart et al. in their meta-analysis found that for CBT and RT, the effect sizes were large and for psychodynamic therapy, psychoeducation, physical exercise, and supportive interventions, the effect sizes were moderate [62]. The investigators found that in studies that used an active control group and in studies of physically ill or cognitively impaired individuals, the effect sizes were smaller. Higher dropout rates were noted among group interventions and studies involving longer interventions. Wilson et al. in their meta-analysis found that CBT was more effective than wait list controls for the treatment of depression among older adults and there was no evidence to suggest any significant treatment differences between CBT and psychodynamic therapy [63].

A meta-analysis by Cuijpers et al. that compared psychotherapies to control groups, other therapies, or pharmacotherapy for depression among older adults found that the effect size indicating the difference between psychotherapy and control groups was 0.64 with a number needed to treat of 3 [65]. These effects were maintained at 6 months or longer post randomization (effect size of 0.27). Psychotherapies that were found to be effective were CBT (effect size of 0.45), life review therapy (effect size of 0.59), and PST (effect size of 0.46). When treatments were compared to waiting list control groups, it resulted in larger effect sizes than when treatments were compared to care-as-usual and to other control groups ($p < 0.05$). The investigators found that studies with lower quality resulted in higher effect sizes than higher-quality studies ($p < 0.05$). CBT and PST were more effective than nondirective counseling and other psychotherapies. The systematic review and meta-analysis by Huang et al. also found that psychotherapy was effective for the treatment of LLD when compared to controls [66].

Data indicates that greater baseline anxiety and stress level, personality disorder, endogenous depression, and reduced self-rated health are associated with worse treatment outcomes for psychotherapy among older adults with depression [64].

Pharmacotherapy

Available data from a systematic review of placebo-controlled trials indicates that there are no significant differences in efficacy between different antidepressant classes (i.e., bupropion, mirtazapine, selective serotonin reuptake inhibitors [SSRIs], and tricyclic antidepressants [TCAs]) for the treatment of depression among older adults [6]. In this review, when the depression was measured using the HAM-D, the number needed to treat [NNT] for all antidepressants was eight, indicating that eight patients must be treated to have one additional patient achieve a 50% reduction in depressive symptom score [6]. A meta-analysis by Nelson et al. found that bupropion, mirtazapine, serotonin-norepinephrine reuptake inhibitors [SNRIs], and SSRIs have greater efficacy in treating symptoms of depression when compared to placebo among older adults, but the effects are modest [67]. The systematic review of literature by Mukai and Tampi found that dual-action antidepressants like SNRIs or TCAs have no superiority over single-action antidepressants like SSRIs in terms of efficacy or side effect profile for the treatment of depression among older adults [68].

As evidence indicates that the different antidepressant classes have equal efficacy for the treatment of depression among older adults, safety and tolerability often dictates the choice of the medication. The relatively benign adverse-effect profile of the SSRIs makes them first-line treatment for depression among older adults [19]. The most common side effects of SSRIs include nausea, diarrhea, anxiety, and sleep disturbance [69]. Venlafaxine and duloxetine [SNRIs] have been shown to be efficacious in the treatment of depression among older adults with fairly benign adverse effect profiles [70, 71]. In a trial of older adults with depression, mirtazapine was found to have equal efficacy when compared to paroxetine patients but with better tolerability profile [72]. The adverse-effect profile of mirtazapine including increased appetite and sedation is often beneficial to depressed older adults who have poor appetite and sleep [72].

Although efficacious, TCAs are not considered first-line treatment for depression among older adults [9, 23]. The use of TCAs is associated with multiple adverse effects due to their action on multiple neuroreceptors. Secondary amine TCAs [nortriptyline and desipramine] are thought to be safer for use among older adults when compared to the tertiary amine TCAs [imipramine and amitriptyline] [9, 23]. Tricyclic antidepressants are lethal in overdoses, which is particularly pertinent given the increased risk of suicide in the elderly population [23]. Common adverse effects of TCAs include sedation and weight gain due to their histamine receptor effects, orthostatic-hypotension due to their alpha-adrenergic receptor effects and tachycardia, dry mouth, visual problems, and dizziness due to their effects on the muscarinic receptors.

Augmentation and/or switching of medications are effective strategies for those younger adults who do not respond adequately to initial antidepressant treatment [73]. Evidence for the augmentation and/or switching of medications for the treatment of depression among older adults is limited, but available data indicates that augmentation of an antidepressant with lithium or another agent (antidepressant, buspirone, aripiprazole) or switching from one antidepressant class to another class produces similar rates and speed of response [74–80].

One systematic review of controlled studies for the treatment for psychotic depression among older adults found efficacy for nortriptyline, imipramine, mifepristone, fluoxetine, and olanzapine combination and electroconvulsive therapy in the treatment of these individuals [81]. Rothschild and Duval recommended that majority of individuals with psychotic depression do not require treatment with antipsychotic medications for more than 4 months [82].

Electroconvulsive Therapy

Available evidence indicates that electroconvulsive therapy [ECT] is an effective treatment for depression especially in cases that are resistant to psychotherapy and/or pharmacotherapy [83]. Current data indicates that ECT appears to work faster than medications for the treatment of severe depression among older individuals [84]. Unilateral and bilateral ECT appear to have similar efficacy in the treatment of depression among older adults, but unilateral ECT is preferred for short-term [≤5 weeks] and bilateral ECT for longer-term [≥3 weeks] treatments [83].

The Prolonging Remission in Depressed Elderly (PRIDE) study is a two-phase multisite study where phase 1 was an acute course of right unilateral ultra-brief pulse ECT augmented with venlafaxine and phase 2 compared two randomized treatment arms: a medication-only arm (venlafaxine plus lithium, over 24 weeks) and an ECT plus medication arm (four continuation ECT treatments over 1 month, plus additional ECT as needed, using the Symptom-Titrated, Algorithm-Based Longitudinal ECT [STABLE] algorithm while continuing venlafaxine plus lithium) [85]. In phase 1 of the study, the investigators found that overall, 61.7% of the participants met the remission criteria, 10.0% did not remit, 28.3% dropped out, and 70% met the response criteria. Among those who remitted, the average change from baseline scores for the depression scale scores was 79%, and the mean number of ECT treatments to remission was 7.3. In phase 2 of the study, the investigators found that at 24 weeks, the ECT plus medication group had statistically significantly lower depression scale scores than the medication-only group without any significant difference between the two groups on cognition [86]. The systematic review by Kumar et al. identified that the deleterious effects of ECT among older adults with depression were limited and transient, with better cognitive outcomes seen with unilateral ECT [87]. However, there is not enough evidence to fully characterize the long-term deleterious effects of ECT among older adults with depression. The use of brief-pulse stimulus, dose titration, and right unilateral and bitemporal lead placements has reduced the cognitive side effects of ECT among the elderly [88]. Cardiovascular side effects such as hypertension and tachycardia may occur more regularly among older adults, but they are mild and transient [83].

Repetitive Transcranial Magnetic Stimulation

Repetitive transcranial magnetic stimulation (rTMS) is FDA approved for the treatment of depression among adults who fail to respond to one medication trial [89]. It is a noninvasive neuromodulatory treatment where a potent but relatively focal electromagnetic field that is generated beneath a coil is positioned over the scalp to depolarize the neurons and modulate the cortical activity. The high frequency (10 Hz) over the left dorsolateral prefrontal cortex (DLPFC) with five sessions a week at 120% of the motor threshold for 3000 pulses per session for 4–6 weeks is the most commonly used stimulation parameter. The potential benefits of rTMS over ECT include the lack of need for anesthesia, the lack of seizure induction, and a lack of significant cognitive adverse effects [88]. rTMS is usually well tolerated, and the most common adverse effects are discomfort caused by scalp or facial muscle twitching and headaches [89]. The most serious but rare adverse effect is seizures. There is some concern that rTMS may be less effective among older individuals when compared to younger adults [90]. It is speculated that this lack of robust response among older adults is due to diminished brain volumes especially in the frontal lobes and the white matter cerebrovascular lesions that disrupt the connections between the DLPFC and mood-regulatory subcortical areas of the brain [89]. However in the review by Lisanby et al., the investigators did not find age (between ≤55 years and ≥55 years) to be a significant predictor of response to rTMS among individuals who are depressed [91]. They found that rTMS was more effective among individuals who failed to respond to one adequate trial of an antidepressant medication in the current episode. Other positive predictors of response were the absence of a comorbid anxiety disorder, a higher baseline depression severity, female gender, and a shorter duration of illness (<2 years).

Vagal Nerve Stimulation

Vagal nerve stimulation (VNS) was approved by the FDA as an adjunctive and long-term treatment for chronic or recurrent depression among adults ≥18 years of age who have a major depressive episode and did not have an adequate response to ≥4 adequate antidepressant trials [88]. In VNS, an electrode is attached to the left vagal nerve that is connected to a stimulator implanted in the chest wall. The electrical impulses are sent via the stimulator to different brain regions to exert its therapeutic effects.

In one study, the response rates for depression were 31% after 3 months, 44% after 1 year, and 42% after 2 years of adjunctive VNS [92]. The remission rates were 15% at 3 months, 27% at 1 year, and 22% at 2 years. At 2 years 81% of the individuals were still receiving VNS.

In our assessment of the literature, there are no controlled published studies that evaluated the efficacy of VNS among older adults with depression. In the only study we found on the use of VNS among older adults, VNS was used among individuals with Alzheimer's disease [AD] [93]. The investigators found that 41.2% of the individuals improved and 70.6% did not decline from baseline on the cognitive functioning. Seventy-one percent of the participants were rated as having no change or some improvement from baseline on a global score. The investigators did not identify any significant decline in mood, behavior, or quality of life during the 1 year of treatment. The VNS was well tolerated in this study. Additional studies are needed to assess the efficacy and safety of VNS before this treatment can be used regularly for the treatment of depression among the older individuals.

Expert Consensus Guideline for Treatment of Depression

A widely accepted expert consensus guideline for the treatment of depression among older adults indicates that for minor depressive episodes, an antidepressant combined with psychotherapy is the appropriate first-line treatment strategy, with either treatment alone being an acceptable alternative [19]. It is also recommended that a 4–7-week trial on the maximally tolerated dose of one antidepressant be completed before switching to another medication [23]. For more severe depressive episodes, an antidepressant combined with psychotherapy is the most widely accepted first-line treatment, with antidepressant alone being a suitable alternative first-line treatment [19]. The medications that are considered as first-line agents include the SSRIs [specifically citalopram and sertraline] and venlafaxine extended-release, with TCAs, bupropion, and mirtazapine being considered as second-line agents [19]. Electroconvulsive therapy is considered an appropriate alternate treatment for severe depressive episodes; when adequate trials of two or more antidepressants have failed, an acute suicide risk is present or the medical comorbidities make pharmacotherapy unviable [19]. This guideline did not recommend psychotherapy alone for more severe episodes of depression. The psychotherapies that are rated as being first-line include CBT, supportive psychotherapy, IPT, and PST [19].

Among older individuals with psychotic depression, the recommendation is to use a combination of an antidepressant and an antipsychotic medication as first-line agents, with an ECT trial if the individual did not respond adequately to pharmacotherapy [19]. The choice of antidepressants included SSRIs and venlafaxine as first-line treatment and TCAs being the alternative [23]. Atypical antipsychotics are to be preferred among these patients. The suggested duration of treatment for a first major depressive episode is 6 months, assuming that the individual tolerates the antidepressant and or psychotherapy well. More recent data among older adults indicates that longer-term treatment, i.e., ≥2 years, may prevent relapses especially among those individuals suffering from recurrent episodes of depression [94].

Conclusions

Available data indicates that depressive symptoms and depressive disorders are fairly common among older adults. Depression among older adults is associated with significant morbidity and mortality. Due to the lack of a standardized assessment protocol, limited standardized diagnostic criteria, and an ageist attitude toward older individuals, depression is often underdiagnosed among this population. In addition, the lack of prompt diagnosis and treatment results in worse outcomes among these individuals. Available data indicate efficacy for psychotherapy, pharmacotherapy, and neuromodulation treatments especially ECT for the treatment of depression among older adults.

Bipolar Disorder

Introduction

The *Diagnostic and Statistical Manual of Mental Disorders*, Fifth Edition (DSM-5), describes bipolar disorder (BD) as a condition characterized by recurrent and/or cyclical episodes of mania or hypomania and depression [95]. The DSM-5 describes two subtypes of BD including bipolar I disorder (BD-I) and bipolar II disorder (BD-II). Individuals with BD-I experience manic episodes with additional major depressive and/or hypomanic episodes. Individuals with BD-II report at least one hypomanic episode and at least one major depressive episode without any manic episodes.

Although the definition is still not clear, late-onset bipolar disorder usually refers to cases among individuals ≥50 years in age who exhibit symptoms of BD [96]. It has been reported that approximately 25% of all individuals with bipolar disorder are ≥60 years in age and >10% were ≥70 years in age [97].

Epidemiology

Current evidence indicates that the point prevalence of BD among older adults is between 0.1 and 0.5% and their lifetime prevalence is between 0.5 and 1.0% [98]. Approximately one-tenth to one-fourth of all older individuals with the diagnosis of a mood disorder has BD [99, 100]. Individuals with BD account for approximately 4–8% of the admissions to inpatient geriatric psychiatric units [100]. Among older individuals who come to the emergency room for a psychiatric evaluation, approximately 17% may have a diagnosis of BD [101]. Approximately 5–12% of older adults who are admitted to a hospital for psychiatric reasons have the diagnosis of mania [102]. It has been noted that the number of older adults who have been diagnosed with BD appears to be increasing [103, 104]. The relative frequency of diagnosis of BD among older adults appears to have increased from 1 to 11% between 1980 and 1998 [104].

Data indicates that 8–20% of individuals with new-onset BD are ≥60 years in age [103, 104].

Differences Between Late-Onset and Early-Onset Bipolar Disorder

Depression appears to be the usual presenting symptom rather than hypomania or mania among individuals with late-onset BD [105–107]. In addition, these individuals present with recurrent and more severe depressive symptoms [108]. Individuals with late-onset BD have longer latency period between the first and subsequent mood episodes when compared to individuals having early-onset BD [106].

Family history of a mood disorder is much less common among individuals with late-onset BD when compared to early-onset BD [105, 109]. Stressful life events (SLE) are common among individuals with late-onset BD when compared to age-matched controls [110].

Cerebrovascular disease and other neurological disorders are often seen in association with late-onset BD [98]. Manic symptoms are associated with vascular changes within the right cerebral hemisphere, whereas depressive symptoms are associated with vascular lesions within the left cerebral hemisphere [111, 112]. Individuals with late-onset BD also have greater number of medical comorbidities especially cardiovascular and metabolic disorders, and these comorbidities result in worse clinical outcomes including greater rates of suicide among these individuals [113–116]. Individuals with late-onset BD have a lifetime and 12-month prevalence rates of comorbid alcohol use disorder (38.1%, 38.1%), dysthymia (15.5%, 7.1%), generalized anxiety disorder (20.5%, 9.5%), and panic disorder (19.0%, 11.9%) which is significantly greater than among age-matched controls, but these rates are lower than among individuals with early-onset BD [117]. Older men with BD report a greater prevalence of alcoholism, whereas older women report a greater prevalence of panic disorder.

In a review of seven published studies that evaluated cognitive measures among older individuals with BD, all of the studies indicated that a majority of these individuals have some form of cognitive impairment [118]. The investigators found that these individuals had lower Mini-Mental State Examination (MMSE) scores ($P = 0.0007$) and the Mattis Dementia Rating Scale (DRS) scores ($P = 0.0003$) when compared to controls. The cognitive scores in these individuals did not correlate with the Young Mania Rating Scale scores. Individuals with late-onset bipolar disorder also have greater impairments in psychomotor performance and mental flexibility when compared to individuals with early-onset bipolar disorder [119]. Gildengers et al. found that approximately half of the older individuals with BD scored ≥1 standard deviation below the mean on the MMSE and the DRS total scores when compared to younger individuals with BD [120]. Among individuals with late-onset BD, a higher number of vascular risk factors and hospital admissions are associated with greater impairments in cognitive functioning [121]. In another study by Gildengers et al., the investigators found that the lifetime duration of BD had no significant relationship with overall cognitive function among older non-demented adults with BD [122]. However, greater vascular disease burden was associated with worse memory function. The investigators found no synergistic relationship between lifetime duration of BD and vascular disease burden on the overall cognition function.

Older adults with BD have higher total symptom severity, positive symptom scores, greater impaired community-living skills, and an earlier age at onset of illness than age-matched individuals with unipolar depression [123]. In addition, older individuals with BD tend to use mental health services four times more often and are four times more likely to have a psychiatric hospitalization over the previous 6 months when compared to age-matched controls.

Among individuals with BD, the life expectancy is reduced by approximately 9 years when compared to the general population [124]. The relative risk of all-cause mortality was reported to be 2.9 in the age group 65–75 years. The variables most strongly associated with natural deaths among individuals with BD were serum alanine aminotransferase levels (odds ratio [OR], 1.02–1.25) and leuko-

TABLE 17-4. Differences between late-onset and early-onset bipolar disorder

Features	*Late onset*	*Early onset*
Age of onset	≥50 years	≤50 years
Presenting symptom	Depression	Mania or hypomania
Mania	Less likely	More likely
Psychosis	Less likely	More likely
Latency between first and second episodes	Longer	Shorter
Family history	Less likely	More likely
Cerebrovascular disease	More likely	Less likely
Medical comorbidities	More likely	Less likely
Psychiatric comorbidities	Less likely	More likely
Cognitive dysfunction	More likely	Less likely
Healthcare service utilization	Greater use	Lesser use

cyte counts (OR, 1.01–2.50) [125]. The years of antipsychotic treatment prior to the last visit (OR, 0.77–0.98) and years of lithium treatment (OR, 0.74–0.97) were protective factors.

Individuals with BD are at greater risk for attempting suicides (BD-I = BD-II; women > men) [126]. Risks are highest with longer exposure, whereas the incidence rates decreased with longer time at risk, possibly due to "dilution" by longer exposure. In one study, the investigators found that when compared to other primary diagnosis suicides, those with BD were more likely to be female, to be more than 5 years post-diagnosis, to have a current/recent inpatient treatment, to have more than five inpatient admissions, and to have depressive symptoms [127]. Among individuals with BD who commit suicide, the most common comorbid diagnoses were personality disorder and alcohol dependence. Additionally, 40% of these individuals were not prescribed mood stabilizers at the time of death and more than 60% of individuals who committed suicide were in contact with services the week prior to suicide, but they were assessed as being of low suicide risk (Table 17-4 describes differences between late-onset and early-onset bipolar disorder).

Neurobiology

Individuals with late-onset life bipolar disorder are more likely to have comorbid medical and neurological illness but less family history of affective disorders when compared to younger-onset bipolar disorder individuals [128–130]. Common medical comorbidities seen among late-onset bipolar disorder individuals include cardiovascular disease, hypertension, hyperlipidemia, and obesity [114, 115].

Dysregulation of hypothalamic-pituitary-adrenal axis and abnormalities in the calcium signaling, glutamate toxicity, and glial cell changes are often seen among individuals with bipolar disorder [131]. Inflammatory processes including elevated cytokines, elevated neutrophils, and elevated products of oxidative stress are seen among individuals with bipolar disorder [132]. Abnormalities seen in the regulation of cellular plasticity that are responsible for the cell growth or atrophy and cell survival or death are being frequently noted among individuals with bipolar disorder [132].

Older adults with bipolar disorder have greater number of white matter hyperintensities in the brain [133–135]. These white matter hyperintensities are found in frontal, parietal, and putaminal areas in the brain [135]. There is no consistent evidence to indicate differences in grey matter, white matter, and total brain volumes among older adults with bipolar disorder when compared to younger individuals with bipolar disorder [136]. However, CT scan of the brain of certain older adults with mania was found to have greater cortical sulcal widening and lateral ventricle-brain ratio scores when compared to younger individuals [137]. When compared to individuals with early-onset bipolar disorder, individuals with late-onset bipolar disorder have greater morphological abnormalities on neuroimaging studies of the brain [112].

Diagnosis

A thorough history is essential in making a definitive diagnosis of bipolar disorder among older adults [98]. The sequelae of medical and/or neurological disorders and the effect of various drugs on the development of mood symptoms must be identified. A full physical examination that includes a neurological examination will help identify comorbid conditions that may cause mood instability [98]. Laboratory work-up including a complete blood count, a complete metabolic panel, and thyroid panel rules out common medical conditions that cause mood dysfunction including anemia, hypoglycemia, and hypo- or hyperthyroidism. Urine analysis, urine culture, and urine drug screen should be done to rule out urinary tract infection and illicit drug use. Neuroimaging studies like CT scans or MRI should only be obtained if there is concern for cerebrovascular disease or cognitive dysfunction [98].

Mood Disorder Questionnaire (MDQ) is a common screening tool used to identify individuals with bipolar disorder [138]. The MDQ screen has good sensitivity and specificity for detecting a lifetime history of mania or hypomania [138]. One known concern with the use of this instrument is the potential for overdiagnosis of bipolar disorder [139]. Other commonly used screening tools for BD are the Bipolar Spectrum Diagnostic Scale (BSDS), the Hypomanic Personality Scale (HPS), the Bipolar Depression Rating Scale (BDRS), and the Young Mania Rating Scale (YMRS) [140–143]. For the diagnosis of BD, the most widely used clinical assessment tool is the Structured Clinical Interview from the DSM-IV [140]. Although not specific to older adults, these scales can assist to quantify and qualify the symptoms of BD and help monitor their progress (Table 17-5 describes the assessment of BD among older adults).

TABLE 17-5. Assessment of BD among older adults

Obtain history	Course of illness, medical history, psychiatric history, current and past medications, premorbid personality, cognition, and functional status
Complete a standardized mental status examination and formal cognitive testing	
Complete standardized assessment scales	Neuropsychological testing if needed
Complete a focused physical examination	Rule out medical or neurological disorders
Order appropriate investigations	Blood and urine examination, vitamin B12 and folate levels, RPR/VDRL, HIV testing, urine drug screen, and neuroimaging studies
Treat medical, psychiatric, and neurological disorders	Remove offending drug(s)

Treatments

Psychosocial

Family-focused therapy, interpersonal social rhythm therapy, cognitive behavioral therapy (CBT), and individual or group psychoeducation are different forms of psychotherapies that have shown evidence in the treatment of individuals with BD [144, 145]. Evidence indicates that in combination with pharmacotherapy, these interventions can prolong time to relapse, reduce the symptom severity, and improve medication adherence.

Family-focused therapy aims to enhance communication skills among family members of individuals with BD, increase supportive behaviors, and improve problem-solving behaviors [144]. Interpersonal and social rhythm therapy (IPSRT) integrates interpersonal therapy with a behavioral component focusing on enhancing routines and structures of day-to-day events. CBT focuses on reducing and replacing cognitive distortions coupled with behavioral activation. Psychoeducation focuses on the development of self-management skills in coping with the illness via provision of education about the disorder and the importance of adherence, developing skills in identifying early warning signs and avoiding dangerous activities like using illicit drugs. Medication adherence skills training (MAST-BD) intervention for older individuals with BD has shown to improve medication adherence, medication management ability, depressive symptom, and selected health-related quality of life indices [146]. A manual-based medical care model (BCM) designed to improve medical outcomes in older individuals with bipolar disorder was shown to have high overall patient satisfaction with the intervention, high follow-through rates, and good tolerability with a dropout rate of <5% [147].

Pharmacotherapy

There is considerable dearth in the literature for evidence-based clinical practice guidelines and randomized controlled trials for the treatment of older adults with BD [148]. Available data indicates that the treatment for BD among older adults includes the use of lithium, anti-epileptics, antipsychotics, antidepressant, benzodiazepines, and ECT [148]. In a recent review of 34 national and international guidelines, Dols et al. found that among majority of the guidelines, there is no separate section for the treatment of older adults with bipolar disorder [149]. General principles recommended for treating older adults with bipolar disorder with medications are similar to those for younger adults but with special caution for side effects due to somatic comorbidities and concomitant use of other medications. The therapeutic lithium serum levels are suggested to be lower, but recommendations are very general and mostly are not informed by specific research evidence.

In the next section, we describe some of the medications/medication classes for BD among older adults.

Lithium

The prototypical drug for the treatment of BD among older adults is still lithium [148, 150]. Lithium appears to be most beneficial among individuals who present with manic symptoms and have limited number of neurological comorbidities [151]. Lithium also reduces the risk for suicide and may possibly decrease the risk of cognitive decline [152, 153]. It is suggested that older adults with BD require lower daily lithium dosage ranging from 25 to 50% of the adult daily dosage [154]. The targeted lithium levels for older adults with BD are between 0.4 and 0.7 mEq/L [148]. It is recommended that renal, thyroid, and cardiac functions be checked before starting treatment with lithium [155]. Older adults with bipolar disorder are more likely to experience adverse effects from lithium [148, 151]. Common adverse effects from lithium include sedation, weight gain, gait impairment, hypothyroidism, edema, renal dysfunction, and cognitive impairment [148, 151, 156]. When prescribing lithium to older adults, caution must be exercised as lithium interacts with several commonly used medications among older individuals including thiazide and loop diuretics, angiotensin-converting enzyme inhibitors, and NSAIDs [148, 154–156]. The risk for developing lithium toxicity due to reduced renal clearance, the presence of multiple medical comorbidities, and drug-drug interactions with commonly co-prescribed medications is greater among older adults with BD than among younger individuals with BD [144, 148, 151].

Anticonvulsants

Data on the use of antiepileptic medications as mood stabilizers among older adults with BD is limited [148]. Available evidence indicates that valproic acid (VPA) is being used more often for treating older adults with BD in lieu of lithium despite limited evidence for its superior efficacy and tolerability [148, 151, 157]. In addition, older adults require lower daily dosage of VPA to maintain a lower therapeutic level than those required among younger individuals [148, 157]. Furthermore, VPA may interact with other drugs including warfarin, phenytoin, phenobarbital, tricyclic antidepressants, and acetylsalicylic acid resulting in adverse effects [148]. Among older adults with bipolar disorder who are only partially responsive to lithium monotherapy or have a rapid cycling illness, a combination of VPA and lithium may be helpful [158, 159].

Available data indicates that there are no controlled clinical trials for the use of carbamazepine among older adults with BD [98, 148]. Trial data from mixed-age population indicates that lithium and VPA may be superior to carbamazepine for the treatment of acute mania and for the maintenance treatment of BD [160, 161]. However, among individuals who present with nonclassical or atypical features of BD, carbamazepine may be helpful [98]. But the side effect profile of carbamazepine and its potential for drug-drug interactions may result in the drug being less well tolerated among older adults [148].

Sajatovic et al. in a review of two maintenance studies of individuals $\geq$ 55 years of age found that lamotrigine significantly delayed time to intervention for any mood episode and for a depressive episode when compared to placebo [162]. Lithium also significantly delayed time to intervention for mania/hypomania/mixed episodes when compared to placebo. Lamotrigine was well tolerated in this study. Additionally, lamotrigine appears to have a favorable cognitive profile when compared to other anticonvulsant mood stabilizers [148].

Data on the efficacy and tolerability of other anticonvulsant mood stabilizers including gabapentin, oxcarbazepine, topiramate, and zonisamide among older adults with BD is limited, and their routine use among these individuals cannot be recommended at this time [148].

Antipsychotics

Aripiprazole, asenapine, olanzapine, quetiapine, quetiapine extended release (XR), risperidone, and ziprasidone are FDA approved for the treatment of BD [163]. Olanzapine-fluoxetine combination (OFC), quetiapine, and lurasidone are FDA approved for the acute treatment of bipolar depression [164]. Olanzapine-fluoxetine combination and quetiapine are approved as single-modality therapies, whereas lurasidone is approved as a monotherapy and as an adjunct to lithium or divalproex.

Risperidone was found to be effective for the treatment of older adults with BD in a small case series [165]. Clozapine was used to treat three older institutionalized male patients with BD disorder with mania and psychosis in an open trial [166]. These individuals were refractory or intolerant to treatment with lithium, valproate, benzodiazepines, and traditional antipsychotics as monotherapy or in combination treatment. There was sustained improvement in symptoms noted over an average of 11-month period, and there were no significant reductions in the granulocyte count.

Sajatovic et al. in a post hoc analysis of pooled data from two quetiapine monotherapy trials evaluated the efficacy and tolerability of quetiapine 400–800 mg a day among individuals ≥ 55 years in age with BD and mania [167]. The primary efficacy endpoint was the change from baseline in Young Mania Rating Scale (YMRS) total score at day 21. Individuals receiving quetiapine had significant improvements from baseline on the YMRS scores when compared with placebo-treated individuals. There was a sustained reduction in YMRS scores when compared to placebo that was apparent by day 4 of treatment. The most common adverse effects in the quetiapine group were dry mouth, somnolence, postural hypotension, insomnia, weight gain, and dizziness.

Sajatovic et al. conducted a 12-week prospective, open-label trial to assess the efficacy and tolerability of adjunct asenapine among non-demented older adults (≥ 60 years) with suboptimal previous response to BD treatments [168]. Asenapine was initiated at 5 mg a day and titrated as tolerated. Effects on global psychopathology were measured using the Clinical Global Impression-Bipolar Version (CGI-BP) and the Brief Psychiatric Rating Scale (BPRS). Mood polarity severity was measured using the Hamilton Depression Rating Scale (HDRS), Montgomery-Åsberg Depression Rating Scale (MADRS), and YMRS. Fifteen individuals with a mean age of 68.6 years were enrolled in the study. A total of 73% of the participants completed the study. The investigators noted significant improvements from baseline on the BPRS ($P < 0.05$), CGI-BP overall ($P < 0.01$), CGI-BP mania ($P < 0.05$), and depression ($P < 0.01$) subscales. The mean dose of asenapine was 11.2 mg a day. The most commonly reported side effects were gastrointestinal discomfort (33%), restlessness (13%), tremors (13%), cognitive difficulties (13%), and sluggishness (13%).

Sajatovic et al. conducted a post hoc analysis of two 6-week placebo-controlled, randomized, double-blind studies of lurasidone among individuals aged ≥55 years with bipolar depression [169]. The participants in these studies met the DSM-IV-TR criteria for bipolar I depression. The first study was a monotherapy study comparing fixed flexible-dose ranges of lurasidone 20–60 mg a day or 80–120 mg a day with placebo. The second study was an adjunctive therapy study comparing flexible doses of lurasidone 20–120 mg a day with placebo adjunctive to either lithium or valproate. The primary endpoint was mean change at week 6 in the Montgomery-Åsberg Depression Rating Scale (MADRS) total score. In the randomized sample, the proportion of individuals ≥55 years was 17.4% in the monotherapy study and 15.5% in the adjunctive therapy study. In this subgroup of individuals in the monotherapy study, the mean change at week 6 in the MADRS was significantly greater for lurasidone versus placebo ($P = 0.003$, effect size = 0.83), and in the adjunctive therapy study, the mean change for lurasidone was not significantly different from placebo ($P = 0.398$, effect size = 0.26). Discontinuation rates due to adverse events for lurasidone versus placebo were similar for the monotherapy (6.8 vs. 6.9%) and the adjunctive therapy (3.8 vs. 7.1%) studies. Lurasidone was found to have minimal effects on metabolic laboratory values.

Antipsychotic medications should be used with caution among older adults given the recent data on the metabolic changes and the risk of cerebrovascular events and deaths among those individuals with dementia and those individuals with cardiovascular and cerebrovascular diseases [170].

Antidepressants

In Gijsman et al.'s systematic review on the use of antidepressants among individuals ≤70 years of age with BD, the investigators concluded that antidepressants are effective in the short-term treatment of bipolar depression and that switching is not an early complication with the use of antidepressants in these patients [171]. Schaffer et al. in a population-based retrospective cohort study of individuals with BD aged ≥66 years found that antidepressants had significantly lower likelihood of admissions for manic/mixed (adjusted rate ratio [aRR], 0.5) but not depressive episodes (aRR, 0.7) when compared to patients not on antidepressants [172]. A recent meta-analysis of double-blind randomized controlled trials of individuals with BD found that individuals treated with antidepressants were not significantly more likely to achieve higher response and remission rates in the short-term or long-term treatment when compared to placebo and other medications [173]. In addition, antidepressants were not associated with an increased risk of discontinuation, relapse, or suicidality. When one antidepressant was compared with another, there were no significant difference noted for efficacy and tolerability.

Benzodiazepines

There are no controlled trials on the use of benzodiazepines among older adults with BD [148]. The available data is derived from studies of younger and mixed-age population with BD. Morishita and Aoki in a study of mixed-age population found that among individuals with unipolar depression or bipolar depression who were treated with clonazepam for 4 weeks, 84.2% of the individuals in unipolar depression group fulfilled the response criteria when compared to only 10.5% of the individuals in the bipolar depression group [174]. In a retrospective chart review of individuals with unipolar and bipolar disorder who had been treated with clonazepam either as monotherapy or as adjunctive therapy, Winkler et al. found that individuals with unipolar depression had significantly less depressive episodes ($P = 0.026$) after treatment with clonazepam, whereas individuals with bipolar disorder did not benefit from treatment with clonazepam [175]. Additionally, neither the frequency nor severity of manic/hypomanic or depressive episodes was reduced with the use of clonazepam.

Electroconvulsive Therapy

Among individuals with BD who need quick and robust clinical response, electroconvulsive therapy (ECT) remains the treatment of choice [98]. Additionally, ECT is effective among individuals with BD who are at immediate suicidal or homicidal risk or present in a catatonic, psychotic, agitated, or medically unstable state [98, 148]. The effectiveness of ECT for the treatment of BD is approximately 80% [148, 176]. There are no controlled studies of ECT among older individuals with BD [88, 148]. However, ECT is often used among older adults with BD where rapid treatment response is required and or where symptoms are refractory to pharmacotherapy [148]. Among older adults who are depressed, both right unilateral and bilateral ECT have been noted to have equal efficacy, although bilateral ECT is associated with greater time to postictal recovery and greater memory impairments [148, 177].

Additional Information Regarding Pharmacotherapy

For the treatment of bipolar disorder among older adults, there are no specialized algorithms [149]. However, available evidence indicates that the initial medication trial should last at least 3–4 weeks in duration [148]. If monotherapy is unsuccessful, then judicious combinations of medications that have some evidence of benefit for the treatment of BD should be considered [148]. Among individuals who respond appropriately to pharmacotherapy, medication(s) should be continued for at least the next 6–12 months

[148]. If the symptoms of BD are in remission for at least 12 months, then a slow taper and discontinuation of adjunctive medications may be attempted [178]. Despite significant advances in the treatment of BD, only 10% of older adults with BD experience a sustained clinical improvement with standardized treatment regimens [179].

Although monotherapy may be an ideal strategy for treating BD among older adults in order to maximize the efficacy of one drug, to minimize adverse effects, and to prevent unnecessary drug-drug interactions, that strategy may not be realistic in the real-world scenario. In a population-based cross-sectional study of individuals with BD who were aged ≥ 66 years and discharged from a psychiatric hospitalization, Rej et al. found that within 30 days post-discharge, a majority of these individuals (81.5%) were prescribed ≥2 psychotropic medications [180]. The most commonly prescribed medications were atypical antipsychotics (75.3%), benzodiazepines/zopiclone (42.3%), and antidepressants (38.5%). Less frequently prescribed medications were valproate (35.4%) and lithium (23.4%). Only 1.4% of the individuals were on lithium monotherapy, while 4.4 and 15.7% were on antidepressant or atypical antipsychotic monotherapy and 8.9% were using ≥2 atypical antipsychotics.

Available evidence indicates that poor adherence to prescribed medications, concomitant use of substances, and the presence of comorbid neurological illnesses reduce the response to treatment among older adults with BD [181]. Factors that affect functional outcomes among these individuals include premorbid levels of psychological, social, residential, and their occupational status (Table 17-6 provides a summary of treatments for bipolar disorder among older adults).

TABLE 17-6. Summary of treatments for bipolar disorder among older adults

Treatment	Details
Psychosocial therapies	Adjunctive treatment to medications
	As well tolerated among older adults as younger individuals
Lithium	More effective for manic and depressive symptoms
	Useful for maintenance treatment
	Decreases suicide risk and may be protective for cognition
	Less well tolerated than in younger patients
	Dosing: 25–50% of adult dosing
	Level: 0.4 –0.7 mEq/L
Anticonvulsant mood stabilizers	Effective for mixed episodes, in rapid cycling, individuals with medical and psychiatric comorbidities
	Lamotrigine is better for bipolar depression than mania
	Also useful for maintenance treatment
	Less well tolerated than among younger individuals
	Dosing: 25–50% of adult dosing
Atypical antipsychotics	Effective for manic episodes, for depressive episodes, and for maintenance treatment
	Less well tolerated than among younger patients
	Metabolic syndrome may develop with long-term use
	Risk of cerebrovascular events and death among individuals with dementia
	Dosing: 25–50% of adult dosing
Antidepressants	Limited evidence for the treatment of depressive episodes
	As well tolerated as among younger adults
	Risk of manic/hypomanic switch present but less than previously thought
	Dosing: Usual adult dosing
Benzodiazepines	Adjunctive treatment for manic or hypomanic episodes
	Less well tolerated than among younger adults
	High risk of cognitive and functional impairments
	Dosing: 25–50% of adult dosing
Electroconvulsive therapy	Similar efficacy for unilateral and bilateral treatments
	Effective for individuals with partial response or refractory to pharmacotherapy
	Effective for individuals with refractory, psychotic, or catatonic symptoms
	Effective for individuals with refractory suicidal or homicidal ideation
	Side effects are more than among younger adults

Conclusions

Bipolar disorder is not uncommon among older adults. BD among older adults is associated with greater morbidity, greater utilization of services, and worse outcomes when compared to the general population. Neurobiology of BD among older adults indicates greater burden of medical comorbidities especially neurovascular disease but less genetic preponderance. Assessment of older individuals with BD should include a thorough history, assessment of medical comorbidities, evaluation of medications, and assessment of illicit drug use. Standardized assessment tools help quantify and qualify symptoms associated with the disorder. Available evidence indicates efficacy for treatments that are used among younger adults with BD. Although there are no specific evidence-based guidelines for the treatment of BD among older adults, current evidence supports the use of pharmacotherapy as first-line treatment. Psychosocial therapies may be useful as adjunctive treatment and ECT is effective for refractory cases. Better understanding of phenomenology and pathophysiology of BD among older individuals will enable researchers to better assess and treat this disorder.

References

1. American Psychiatric Association. Desk reference to the diagnostic criteria from DSM-5, Depressive disorders. Washington DC: American Psychiatric Publishing; 2013. p. 93–114.
2. Alexopoulos GS. Depression in the elderly. Lancet. 2005;365(9475):1961–70.
3. Fountoulakis KN, O'Hara R, Iacovides A, et al. Unipolar late-onset depression: a comprehensive review. Ann Gen Hosp Psychiatry. 2003;2(1):11.
4. Alexopoulos GS. New concepts for prevention and treatment of late-life depression. Am J Psychiatry. 2001;158(6):835–8.
5. Harman JS, Schulberg HC, Mulsant BH, et al. The effect of patient and visit characteristics on diagnosis of depression in primary care. J Fam Pract. 2001;50(12):1068.
6. Taylor WD, Doraiswamy PMA. systematic review of antidepressant placebo-controlled trials for geriatric depression: limitations of current data and directions for the future. Neuropsychopharmacology. 2004;29(12):2285–99.
7. Mulsant BH, Ganguli M. Epidemiology and diagnosis of depression in late life. J Clin Psychiatry. 1999;60(Suppl 20):9–15.
8. Unutzer J, Katon W, Russo J, et al. Patterns of care for depressed older adults in a large-staff model HMO. Am J Geriatr Psychiatry. 1999;7(3):235–43.
9. Dunner DL. Treatment considerations for depression in the elderly. CNS Spectr. 2003;8(12 Suppl 3):14–9.
10. Hegeman JM, Kok RM, van der Mast RC, Giltay EJ. Phenomenology of depression in older compared with younger adults: meta-analysis. Br J Psychiatry. 2012;200(4):275–81.
11. Thorpe L. The treatment of psychotic disorders in late life. Can J Psychiatr. 1997;42(Suppl 1):19S–27S.
12. Myers JK, Weissman MM, Tischler GL, et al. Six-month prevalence of psychiatric disorders in three communities 1980 to 1982. Arch Gen Psychiatry. 1984;41(10):959–67.
13. Gournellis R, Lykouras L, Fortos A, et al. Psychotic (delusional) major depression in late life. Int J Geriatr Psychiatry. 2001;16(11):1085–91.
14. Raskind MA. The clinical interface of depression and dementia. J Clin Psychiatry. 1998;59(Suppl 10):9–12.
15. Wang S, Blazer DG. Depression and cognition in the elderly. Annu Rev. Clin Psychol. 2015;11:331–60.
16. Bennett S, Thomas AJ. Depression and dementia: cause, consequence or coincidence? Maturitas. 2014;79(2):184–90.
17. Reynolds CF 3rd, Smith GS, Dew MA, et al. Accelerating symptom-reduction in late-life depression: a double-blind, randomized, placebo-controlled trial of sleep deprivation. Am J Geriatr Psychiatry. 2005;13(5):353–8.
18. Weisenbach SL, Kumar A. Current understanding of the neurobiology and longitudinal course of geriatric depression. Curr Psychiatry Rep. 2014;16(9):463.
19. Alexopoulos GS, Katz IR, Reynolds CF, et al. Pharmacotherapy of depression in older patients: a summary of the expert consensus guidelines. J Psychiatr Pract. 2001;7(6):361–76.
20. Frasure-Smith N, Lesperance F, Talajic M. Depression following myocardial infarction. Impact on 6-month survival. JAMA. 1993;270(15):1819–25.
21. Carney RM, Freedland KE. Depression, mortality, and medical morbidity in patients with coronary heart disease. Biol Psychiatry. 2003;54(3):241–7.
22. Yaffe K, Blackwell T, Gore R, et al. Depressive symptoms and cognitive decline in nondemented

elderly women: a prospective study. Arch Gen Psychiatry. 1999;56(5):425–30.
23. Comijs HC, Jonker C, Beckman AT, Deeg DJ. The association between depressive symptoms and cognitive decline in community-dwelling elderly persons. Int J Geriatr Psychiatry. 2001;16(4):361–7.
24. Wilson RS, Barnes LL, Mendes de Leon CF, et al. Depressive symptoms, cognitive decline, and risk of AD in older persons. Neurology. 2002;59(3):364–70.
25. Ko DT, Hebert PR, Coffey CS, et al. Beta-blocker therapy and symptoms of depression, fatigue, and sexual dysfunction. JAMA. 2002;288(3):351–7.
26. Katon W, Lin E, von Korff M, et al. The predictors of persistence of depression in primary care. J Affect Disord. 1994;31(2):81–90.
27. Lynch TR, Johnson CS, Mendelson T, et al. New onset and remission of suicidal ideation among a depressed adult sample. J Affect Disord. 1999;56(1):49–54.
28. Duberstein PR. Openness to experience and completed suicide across the second half of life. Int Psychogeriatr. 1995;7(2):183–98.
29. Bruce ML. Psychosocial risk factors for depressive disorders in late life. Biol Psychiatry. 2002;52(3):175–84.
30. Clyburn LD, Stones MJ, Hadjistavropoulos T, Tuokko H, et al. Predicting caregiver burden and depression in Alzheimer's disease. J Gerontol B Psychol Sci Soc Sci. 2000;55(1):S2–S13.
31. Cole MG, Dendukuri N. Risk factors for depression among elderly community subjects: a systematic review and meta-analysis. Am J Psychiatry. 2003;160(6):1147–56.
32. Mitchell AJ, Subramaniam H. Prognosis of depression in old age compared to middle age: a systematic review of comparative studies. Am J Psychiatry. 2005;162(9):1588–601.
33. Hall CA, CF R-III. Late-life depression in the primary care setting: challenges, collaborative care, and prevention. Maturitas. 2014;79(2):147–52.
34. Goff VV. Depression: a decade of progress, more to do. NHPF Issue Brief. 2002;786:1–14.
35. Michelson D, Stratakis C, Hill L, et al. Bone mineral density in women with depression. N Engl J Med. 1996;335(16):1176–81.
36. Ferketich AK, Schwartzbaum JA, Frid DJ, et al. Depression as an antecedent to heart disease among women and men in the NHANES I study. National Health and Nutrition Examination Survey. Arch Intern Med. 2000;160(9):1261–8.
37. Glover J, Srinivasan S. Assessment of the person with late-life depression. Psychiatr Clin North Am. 2013;36(4):545–60.
38. Diniz BS, Butters MA, Albert SM, et al. Late-life depression and risk of vascular dementia and Alzheimer's disease: systematic review and meta-analysis of community-based cohort studies. Br J Psychiatry. 2013;202(5):329–35.
39. Turvey CL, Conwell Y, Jones MP, et al. Risk factors for late-life suicide: a prospective, community-based study. Am J Geriatr Psychiatry. 2002;10(4):398–406.
40. Johnson J, Weissman MM, Klerman GL. Service utilization and social morbidity associated with depressive symptoms in the community. JAMA. 1992;267(11):1478–83.
41. Croghan TW, Obenchain RL, Crown WE. What does treatment of depression really cost? Health Aff. 1998;17(4):198–208.
42. Greenberg PE, Kessler RC, Birnbaum HG, et al. The economic burden of depression in the United States: how did it change between 1990 and 2000? J Clin Psychiatry. 2003;64(12):1465–75.
43. http://www.psychiatryonline.com/content.aspx?aID=56046. Accessed 17 Feb 2017.
44. Mulkeen A, Zdanys K, Muralee S, et al. Screening tools for late-life depression: a review. Depression: Mind and Body. 2008;3(4):150–7.
45. Lichtenberg PA, Marcopulos BA, Steiner DA, et al. Comparison of the Hamilton Depression Rating Scale and the Geriatric Depression Scale: detection of depression in dementia patients. Psychol Rep. 1992;70:515–21.
46. Clayton AH, Holroyd S, Sheldon-Keller A. Geriatric depression scale vs Hamilton rating scale for depression in a sample of anxiety patients. Clin Gerontol. 1997;17:3–13.
47. Benjamin S, Steffens DC. Structural neuroimaging of geriatric depression. Psychiatr Clin North Am. 2011;34(2):423–35.
48. Gunning FM, Smith GS. Functional neuroimaging in geriatric depression. Psychiatr Clin North Am. 2011;34(2):403–22.
49. Bartels SJ, Coakley EH, Zubritsky C, et al. Improving access to geriatric mental health services: a randomized trial comparing treatment engagement with integrated versus enhanced referral care for depression, anxiety, and at-risk alcohol use. Am J Psychiatry. 2004;161(8):1455–62.
50. Hunkeler EM, Meresman JF, Hargreaves WA, et al. Efficacy of nurse telehealth care and peer support in augmenting treatment of depression in primary care. Arch Fam Med. 2000;9(8):700–8.
51. Sherbourne CD, Wells KB, Duan N, et al. Long-term effectiveness of disseminating quality improvement for depression in primary care. Arch Gen Psychiatry. 2001;58(7):696–703.

52. Cuijpers P, van Lammeren P. Secondary prevention of depressive symptoms in elderly inhabitants of residential homes. Int J Geriatr Psychiatry. 2001;16(7):702–8.
53. Hunkeler EM, Katon W, Tang L, et al. Long term outcomes from the IMPACT randomised trial for depressed elderly patients in primary care. BMJ. 2006;332(7536):259–63.
54. Mulsant BH, Alexopoulos GS, Reynolds CF, et al. Pharmacological treatment of depression in older primary care patients: the PROSPECT algorithm. Int J Geriatr Psychiatry. 2001;16(6):585–92.
55. Bruce ML, Ten Have TR, Reynolds CF, et al. Reducing suicidal ideation and depressive symptoms in depressed older primary care patients: a randomized controlled trial. JAMA. 2004;291(9):1081–91.
56. Alexopoulos GS, Katz IR, Bruce ML, et al. Remission in depressed geriatric primary care patients: a report from the PROSPECT study. Am J Psychiatry. 2005;162(4):718–24.
57. Mulsant BH, Blumberger DM, Ismail Z, et al. A systematic approach to pharmacotherapy for geriatric major depression. Clin Geriatr Med. 2014;30(3):517–34.
58. Knöchel C, Alves G, Friedrichs B, et al. Treatment-resistant late-life depression: challenges and perspectives. Curr Neuropharmacol. 2015;13(5):577–91.
59. Sjosten N, Kivela SL. The effects of physical exercise on depressive symptoms among the aged: a systematic review. Int J Geriatr Psychiatry. 2006;21(5):410–8.
60. Mackin RS, Areán PA. Evidence-based psychotherapeutic interventions for geriatric depression. Psychiatr Clin North Am. 2005;28(4):805–20, vii–viii
61. Cuijpers P, van Straten A, Smit F. Psychological treatment of late-life depression: a meta-analysis of randomized controlled trials. Int J Geriatr Psychiatry. 2006;21(12):1139–49.
62. Pinquart M, Duberstein PR, Lyness JM. Effects of psychotherapy and other behavioral interventions on clinically depressed older adults: a meta-analysis. Aging Ment Health. 2007;11(6):645–57.
63. Wilson KC, Mottram PG, Vassilas CA. Psychotherapeutic treatments for older depressed people. Cochrane Database Syst Rev. 2008;1:CD004853.
64. Kiosses DN, Leon AC, Areán PA. Psychosocial interventions for late-life major depression: evidence-based treatments, predictors of treatment outcomes, and moderators of treatment effects. Psychiatr Clin North Am. 2011;34(2):377–401, viii
65. Cuijpers P, Karyotaki E, Pot AM, et al. Managing depression in older age: psychological interventions. Maturitas. 2014;79(2):160–9.
66. Huang AX, Delucchi K, Dunn LB, Nelson JCA. systematic review and meta-analysis of psychotherapy for late-life depression. Am J Geriatr Psychiatry. 2015;23(3):261–73.
67. Nelson JC, Delucchi K, Schneider LS. Efficacy of second generation antidepressants in late-life depression: a meta-analysis of the evidence. Am J Geriatr Psychiatry. 2008;16(7):558–67.
68. Mukai Y, Tampi RR. Treatment of depression in the elderly: a review of the recent literature on the efficacy of single- versus dual-action antidepressants. Clin Ther. 2009;31(5):945–61.
69. Tollefson GD, Bosomworth JC, Heiligenstein JH, et al. A double-blind, placebo-controlled clinical trial of fluoxetine in geriatric patients with major depression. The Fluoxetine Collaborative Study Group. Int Psychogeriatr. 1995;7(1):89–104.
70. Allard P, Gram L, Timdahl K, et al. Efficacy and tolerability of venlafaxine in geriatric outpatients with major depression: a double-blind, randomised 6-month comparative trial with citalopram. Int J Geriatr Psychiatry. 2004;19(12):1123–30.
71. Nelson JC, Wohlreich MM, Mallinckrodt CH, et al. Duloxetine for the treatment of major depressive disorder in older patients. Am J Geriatr Psychiatry. 2005;13(3):227–35.
72. Schatzberg AF, Kremer C, Rodrigues HE, et al. Double-blind, randomized comparison of mirtazapine and paroxetine in elderly depressed patients. Am J Geriatr Psychiatry. 2002;10(5):541–50.
73. Posternak MA, Zimmerman M. Switching versus augmentation: a prospective, naturalistic comparison in depressed, treatment-resistant patients. J Clin Psychiatry. 2001;62(2):135–42.
74. Kamholz BA, Mellow AM. Management of treatment resistance in the depressed geriatric patient. Psychiatr Clin North Am. 1996;19(2):269–86.
75. Whyte EM, Basinski J, Farhi P, et al. Geriatric depression treatment in nonresponders to selective serotonin reuptake inhibitors. J Clin Psychiatry. 2004;65(12):1634–41.
76. Flint AJ, Rifat SL. The effect of sequential antidepressant treatment on geriatric depression. J Affect Disord. 1996;36(3–4):95–105.
77. Dew MA, Whyte EM, Lenze EJ, et al. Recovery from major depression in older adults receiving augmentation of antidepressant pharmacotherapy. Am J Psychiatry. 2007;164(6):892–9.

78. Karp JF, Whyte EM, Lenze EJ, et al. Rescue pharmacotherapy with duloxetine for selective serotonin reuptake inhibitor nonresponders in late-life depression: outcome and tolerability. J Clin Psychiatry. 2008;69(3):457–63.
79. Rutherford B, Sneed J, Miyazaki M, et al. An open trial of aripiprazole augmentation for SSRI non-remitters with late-life depression. Int J Geriatr Psychiatry. 2007;22(10):986–91.
80. Sheffrin M, Driscoll HC, Lenze EJ, et al. Pilot study of augmentation with aripiprazole for incomplete response in late-life depression: getting to remission. J Clin Psychiatry. 2009;70(2):208–13.
81. Shamsi A, Cichon D, Obey J, et al. Pharmacotherapy for late-life depression with psychotic features: a review of literature of randomized control trials. Curr Psychiatr Rev. 2010;6(3):219–22.
82. Rothschild AJ, Duval SE. How long should patients with psychotic depression stay on the antipsychotic medication? J Clin Psychiatry. 2003;64(4):390–6.
83. van der Wurff FB, Stek ML, et al. The efficacy and safety of ECT in depressed older adults: a literature review. Int J Geriatr Psychiatry. 2003;18(10):894–904.
84. Spaans HP, Sienaert P, Bouckaert F, et al. Speed of remission in elderly patients with depression: electroconvulsive therapy v. medication. Br J Psychiatry. 2015;206(1):67–71.
85. Kellner CH, Husain MM, Knapp RG, et al. Right unilateral Ultrabrief Pulse ECT in geriatric depression: phase 1 of the PRIDE Study. Am J Psychiatry. 2016;173(11):1101–9.
86. Kellner CH, Husain MM, Knapp RG, et al. A novel strategy for continuation ECT in geriatric depression: phase 2 of the PRIDE Study. Am J Psychiatry. 2016;173(11):1110–8.
87. Kumar S, Mulsant BH, Liu AY, et al. Systematic review of cognitive effects of electroconvulsive therapy in late-life depression. Am J Geriatr Psychiatry. 2016;24(7):547–65.
88. McDonald WM. Neuromodulation treatments for geriatric mood and cognitive disorders. Am J Geriatr Psychiatry. 2016;24(12):1130–41.
89. Riva-Posse P, Hermida AP, McDonald WM. The role of electroconvulsive and neuromodulation therapies in the treatment of geriatric depression. Psychiatr Clin North Am. 2013;36(4):607–30.
90. Figiel GS, Epstein C, McDonald WM, et al. The use of rapid-rate transcranial magnetic stimulation (rTMS) in refractory depressed patients. J Neuropsychiatry Clin Neurosci. 1998;10(1):20–5.
91. Lisanby SH, Husain MM, Rosenquist PB, et al. Daily left prefrontal repetitive transcranial magnetic stimulation in the acute treatment of major depression: clinical predictors of outcome in a multisite, randomized controlled clinical trial. Neuropsychopharmacology. 2009;34(2):522–34.
92. Nahas Z, Marangell LB, Husain MM, et al. Two-year outcome of vagus nerve stimulation (VNS) for treatment of major depressive episodes. J Clin Psychiatry. 2005;66(9):1097–104.
93. Merrill CA, Jonsson MA, Minthon L, et al. Vagus nerve stimulation in patients with Alzheimer's disease: additional follow-up results of a pilot study through 1 year. J Clin Psychiatry. 2006;67(8):1171–8.
94. Reynolds CF, Drew MA, Pollock BG, et al. Maintenance treatment of major depression in old age. N Engl J Med. 2006;354(11):1130–8.
95. American Psychiatric Association. Desk reference to the diagnostic criteria from DSM-5, Bipolar Disorders. Washington DC: American Psychiatric Publishing; 2013. p. 65–92.
96. Montes JM, Alegria A, Garcia-Lopez A, et al. Understanding bipolar disorder in late life. J Nerv Ment Dis. 2013;201(8):674–9.
97. Sajatovic M, Blow FC, Ignacio RV, Kales HC. Age-related modifiers of clinical presentation and health service use among veterans with bipolar disorder. Psychiatr Serv. 2004;55(9):1014–21.
98. Sajatovic M, Chen P. Geriatric bipolar disorder. Psychiatr Clin North Am. 2011;34(2):319–33.
99. Depp CA, Jin H, Mohamed S, et al. Bipolar disorder in middle-aged and elderly adults: is age of onset important? J Nerv Ment Dis. 2004;192(11):796–9.
100. Yassa R, Nair V, Nastase C, et al. Prevalence of bipolar disorder in a psychogeriatric population. J Affect Disord. 1988;14(3):197–201.
101. Depp CA, Lindamer LA, Folsom DP, et al. Differences in clinical features and mental health service use in bipolar disorder across the lifespan. Am J Geriatr Psychiatry. 2005;13(4):290–8.
102. Depp CA, Davis CE, Mittal D, et al. Health-relate quality of life and functioning of middle-aged and elderly adults with bipolar disorder. J Clin Psychiatry. 2006;67(2):215–21.
103. Räsänen P, Tiihonen J, Hakko H. The incidence and onset-age of hospitalized bipolar affective disorder in Finland. J Affect Disord. 1998;48(1):63–8.
104. Almeida OP, Fenner S. Bipolar disorder: similarities and differences between patients with illness onset before and after 65 years of age. Int Psychogeriatr. 2002;14(3):311–22.

105. Stone K. Mania in the elderly. Br J Psychiatry. 1989;155:220–4.
106. Shulman KI, Tohen M, Satlin A, et al. Mania compared with unipolar depression in old age. Am J Psychiatry. 1992;149(3):341–5.
107. Tohen M, Shulman KI, Satlin A. First-episode mania in late life. Am J Psychiatry. 1994;151(1):130–2.
108. García-López A, Ezquiaga E, De Dios C, Agud JL. Depressive symptoms in early- and late-onset older bipolar patients compared with younger ones. Int J Geriatr Psychiatry. 2017;32(2):201–7.
109. Hays JC, Krishnan KR, George LK, Blazer DG. Age of first onset of bipolar disorder: demographic, family history, and psychosocial correlates. Depress Anxiety. 1998;7(2):76–82.
110. Beyer JL, Kuchibhatla M, Cassidy F, Krishnan KR. Stressful life events in older bipolar patients. Int J Geriatr Psychiatry. 2008;23(12):1271–5.
111. Robinson RG, Starkstein SE. Current research in affective disorders following stroke. J Neuropsychiatry Clin Neurosci. 1990;2(1):1–14.
112. Steffens DC, Krishnan KR. Structural neuroimaging and mood disorders: recent findings, implications for classification, and future directions. Biol Psychiatry. 1998;43(10):705–12.
113. Gildengers AG, Whyte EM, Drayer RA, et al. Medical burden in late-life bipolar and major depressive disorders. Am J Geriatr Psychiatry. 2008;16(3):194–200.
114. Kilbourne AM, Post EP, Nossek A, et al. Improving medical and psychiatric outcomes among individuals with bipolar disorder: a randomized controlled trial. Psychiatr Serv. 2008;59(7):760–8.
115. McIntyre RS, Konarski JZ, Soczynska JK, et al. Medical comorbidity in bipolar disorder: implications for functional outcomes and health service utilization. Psychiatr Serv. 2006;57(8):1140–4.
116. Juurlink DN, Herrmann N, Szalai JP, et al. Medical illness and the risk of suicide in the elderly. Arch Intern Med. 2004;164(11):1179–84.
117. Goldstein BI, Herrmann N, Shulman KI. Comorbidity in bipolar disorder among the elderly: results from an epidemiological community sample. Am J Psychiatry. 2006;163(2):319–21.
118. Young RC, Murphy CF, Heo M, et al. Cognitive impairment in bipolar disorder in old age: literature review and findings in manic patients. J Affect Disord. 2006;92(1):125–31.
119. Schouws SN, Comijs HC, Dekker J, et al. Cognitive impairment in early and late bipolar disorder. Am J Geriatr Psychiatry. 2009;17(6):508–15.
120. Gildengers AG, Butters MA, Seligman K, et al. Cognitive functioning in late-life bipolar disorder. Am J Psychiatry. 2004;161(4):736–8.
121. Schouws SN, Stek ML, Comijs HC, et al. Risk factors for cognitive impairment in elderly bipolar patients. J Affect Disord. 2010;125(1–3):330–5.
122. Gildengers AG, Mulsant BH, Al Jurdi RK, et al. The relationship of bipolar disorder lifetime duration and vascular burden to cognition in older adults. Bipolar Disord. 2010;12(8):851–8.
123. Bartels SJ, Forester B, Miles KM, et al. Mental health service use by elderly patients with bipolar disorder and unipolar major depression. Am J Geriatr Psychiatry. 2000;8(2):160–6.
124. Kodesh A, Goldshtein I, Gelkopf M, et al. Epidemiology and comorbidity of severe mental illnesses in the community: findings from a computerized mental health registry in a large Israeli health organization. Soc Psychiatry Psychiatr Epidemiol. 2012;47(11):1775–82.
125. Tsai SY, Lee CH, Kuo CJ, Chen CCA. retrospective analysis of risk and protective factors for natural death in bipolar disorder. J Clin Psychiatry. 2005;66(12):1586–91.
126. Tondo L, Pompili M, Forte A, Baldessarini RJ. Suicide attempts in bipolar disorders: comprehensive review of 101 reports. Acta Psychiatr Scand. 2016;133(3):174–86.
127. Clements C, Morriss R, Jones S, Peters S, Roberts C, Kapur N. Suicide in bipolar disorder in a national English sample, 1996–2009: frequency, trends and characteristics. Psychol Med. 2013;43(12):2593–602.
128. Bartels SJ, Mueser KT, Miles KMA. comparative study of elderly patients with schizophrenia and bipolar disorder in nursing homes and the community. Schizophr Res. 1997;27(2–3):181–90.
129. Ahearn EP, Steffens DC, Cassidy F, et al. Familial leukoencephalopathy in bipolar disorder. Am J Psychiatry. 1998;155(11):1605–7.
130. Krishnan KR. Biological risk factors in late life depression. Biol Psychiatry. 2002;52(3):185–92.
131. Schloesser RJ, Huang J, Klein PS, et al. Cellular plasticity cascades in the pathophysiology and treatment of bipolar disorder. Neuropsychopharmacology. 2008;33(1):110–33.
132. Berk M. Neuroprogression: pathways to progressive brain changes in bipolar disorder. Int J Neuropsychopharmacol. 2009;12(4):441–5.
133. Subramaniam H, Dennis MS, Byrne EJ. The role of vascular risk factors in late onset bipolar disorder. Int J Geriatr Psychiatry. 2007;22(8):733–7.
134. Lloyd AJ, Moore PB, Cousins DA, et al. White matter lesions in euthymic patients

with bipolar disorder. Acta Psychiatr Scand. 2009;120(6):481–91.
135. Tamashiro JH, Zung S, Zanetti MV, et al. Increased rates of white matter hyperintensities in late-onset bipolar disorder. Bipolar Disord. 2008;10(7):765–75.
136. Sarnicola A, Kempton M, Germana C, et al. No differential effect of age on brain matter volume and cognition in bipolar patients and healthy individuals. Bipolar Disord. 2009;11(3):316–22.
137. Young RC, Nambudiri DE, Jain H, et al. Brain computed tomography in geriatric manic disorder. Biol Psychiatry. 1999;45:1063–5.
138. Hirschfeld RM, Williams JB, Spitzer RL, et al. Development and validation of a screening instrument for bipolar spectrum disorder: the Mood Disorder Questionnaire. Am J Psychiatry. 2000;157(11):1873–5.
139. Zimmerman M, Ruggero CJ, Galione JN, et al. Detecting differences in diagnostic assessment of bipolar disorder. J Nerv Ment Dis. 2010;198(5):339–42.
140. Baldassano CF. Assessment tools for screening and monitoring bipolar disorder. Bipolar Disord. 2005;7(Suppl 1):8–15.
141. Picardi A. Rating scales in bipolar disorder. Curr Opin Psychiatry. 2009;22(1):42–9.
142. Berk M, Malhi GS, Cahill C, et al. The Bipolar Depression Rating Scale (BDRS): its development, validation and utility. Bipolar Disord. 2007;9(6):571–9.
143. Young RC, Biggs JT, Ziegler VE, et al. A rating scale for mania: reliability, validity and sensitivity. Br J Psychiatry. 1978;133:429–35.
144. Miklowitz DJ. A review of evidence-based psychosocial interventions for bipolar disorder. J Clin Psychiatry. 2006;67(Suppl 11):28–33.
145. Lauder SD, Berk M, Castle DJ, et al. The role of psychotherapy in bipolar disorder. Med J Aust. 2010;193(4 Suppl):S31–5.
146. Depp CA, Lebowitz BD, Patterson TL, et al. Medication adherence skills training for middle-aged and elderly adults with bipolar disorder: development and pilot study. Bipolar Disord. 2007;9(6):636–45.
147. Kilbourne AM, Post EP, Nossek A, et al. Service delivery in older patients with bipolar disorder: a review and development of a medical care model. Bipolar Disord. 2008;10(6):672–83.
148. Aziz R, Lorberg B, Tampi RR. Treatment for late-life bipolar disorder. Am J Geriatr Pharmacother. 2006;4(4):347–64.
149. Dols A, Kessing LV, Strejilevich SA, et al. Do current national and international guidelines have specific recommendations for older adults with bipolar disorder? A brief report. Int J Geriatr Psychiatry. 2016;31(12):1295–300.
150. Sajatovic M, Madhusoodanan S, Coconcea N. Managing bipolar disorder in the elderly: defining the role of the newer agents. Drugs Aging. 2005;22(1):39–54.
151. Sajatovic M. Treatment of bipolar disorder in older adults. Int J Geriatr Psychiatry. 2002;17(9):865–73.
152. Kessing LV, Søndergård L, Kvist K, et al. Suicide risk in patients treated with lithium. Arch Gen Psychiatry. 2005;62(8):860–6.
153. Kessing LV, Forman JL, Andersen PK. Does lithium protect against dementia? Bipolar Disord. 2010;12(1):87–94.
154. Eastham JH, Jeste DV, Young RC. Assessment and treatment of bipolar disorder in the elderly. Drugs Aging. 1998;12(3):205–24.
155. American Psychiatric Association. Practice guideline for the treatment of patients with bipolar disorder (revision). Am J Psychiatry. 2002;159(Suppl 4):1–50.
156. Shulman KI, Rochon P, Sykora K, et al. Changing prescription patterns for lithium and valproic acid in old age: shifting practice without evidence. BMJ. 2003;326(7396):960–1.
157. Chen ST, Altshuler LL, Melnyk KA, et al. Efficacy of lithium vs. valproate in the treatment of mania in the elderly: a retrospective study. J Clin Psychiatry. 1999;60(3):181–6.
158. Schneider AL, Wilcox CS. Divalproate augmentation in lithium-resistant rapid cycling mania in four geriatric patients. J Affect Disord. 1998;47(1–3):201–5.
159. Goldberg JF, Sacks MH, Kocsis JH. Low-dose lithium augmentation of divalproex in geriatric mania. J Clin Psychiatry. 2000;61(4):304.
160. Greil W, Kleindienst N, Erazo N, et al. Differential response to lithium and carbamazepine in the prophylaxis of bipolar disorder. J Clin Psychopharmacol. 1998;18(6):455–60.
161. Vasudev K, Goswami U, Kohli K. Carbamazepine and valproate monotherapy: feasibility, relative safety and efficacy, and therapeutic drug monitoring in manic disorder. Psychopharmacology. 2000;150(1):15–23.
162. Sajatovic M, Gyulai L, Calabrese JR, et al. Maintenance treatment outcomes in older patients with bipolar I disorder. Am J Geriatr Psychiatry. 2005;13(4):305–11.
163. Atypical Antipsychotic Medications: Use in Adults.https://www.cms.gov/Medicare-Medicaid-Coordination/Fraud-Prevention/Medicaid-Integrity-

Education/Pharmacy-Education-Materials/Downloads/atyp-antipsych-adult-factsheet.pdf. Accessed 9 Feb 2017.
164. McIntyre RS, Cha DS, Kim RD, Mansur RB. A review of FDA-approved treatment options in bipolar depression. CNS Spectr. 2013;18(Suppl 1):4–20. quiz 21
165. Madhusoodanan S, Brenner R, Araujo L, et al. Efficacy of risperidone treatment for psychoses associated with schizophrenia, schizoaffective disorder, bipolar disorder, or senile dementia in 11 geriatric patients: a case series. J Clin Psychiatry. 1995;56(11):514–8.
166. Shulman RW, Singh A, Shulman KI. Treatment of elderly institutionalized bipolar patients with clozapine. Psychopharmacol Bull. 1997;33(1):113–8.
167. Sajatovic M, Calabrese JR, Mullen J. Quetiapine for the treatment of bipolar mania in older adults. Bipolar Disord. 2008;10(6):662–71.
168. Sajatovic M, Dines P, Fuentes-Casiano E, et al. Asenapine in the treatment of older adults with bipolar disorder. Int J Geriatr Psychiatry. 2015;30(7):710–9.
169. Sajatovic M, Forester BP, Tsai J, et al. Efficacy of lurasidone in adults aged 55 years and older with bipolar depression: post hoc analysis of 2 double-blind, placebo-controlled studies. J Clin Psychiatry. 2016;77(10):e1324–31.
170. Mittal V, Kurup L, Williamson D, et al. Risk of cerebrovascular adverse events and death in elderly patients with dementia when treated with antipsychotic medications: a literature review of evidence. Am J Alzheimers Dis Other Demen. 2011;26(1):10–28.
171. Gijsman HJ, Geddes JR, Rendell JM, et al. Antidepressants for bipolar depression: a systematic review of randomized, controlled trials. Am J Psychiatry. 2004;161(9):1537–47.
172. Schaffer A, Mamdani M, Levitt A, et al. Effect of antidepressant use on admissions to hospital among elderly bipolar patients. Int J Geriatr Psychiatry. 2006;21(3):275–80.
173. Zhang Y, Yang H, Yang S, et al. Antidepressants for bipolar disorder: a meta-analysis of randomized, double-blind, controlled trials. Neural Regen Res. 2013;8(31):2962–74.
174. Morishita S, Aoki S. Clonazepam augmentation of antidepressants: does it distinguish unipolar from bipolar depression? J Affect Disord. 2002;71(1–3):217–20.
175. Winkler D, Willeit M, Wolf R, et al. Clonazepam in the long-term treatment of patients with unipolar depression, bipolar and schizoaffective disorder. Eur Neuropsychopharmacol. 2003;13(2):129–34.
176. Mukherjee S, Sackeim HA, Schnur DB. Electroconvulsive therapy of acute manic episodes: a review of 50 years' experience. Am J Psychiatry. 1994;151(2):169–76.
177. Fraser RM, Glass IB. Unilateral and bilateral ECT in elderly patients. A comparative study. Acta Psychiatr Scand. 1980;62:13–31.
178. Young RC, Gyulai L, Mulsant BH, et al. Pharmacotherapy of bipolar disorder in old age: review and recommendations. Am J Geriatr Psychiatry. 2004;12(4):342–57.
179. Gildengers AG, Mulsant BH, Begley AE, et al. A pilot study of standardized treatment in geriatric bipolar disorder. Am J Geriatr Psychiatry. 2005;13(4):319–23.
180. Rej S, Herrmann N, Shulman K, et al. Current psychotropic medication prescribing patterns in late-life bipolar disorder. Int J Geriatr Psychiatry. 2016.
181. Sajatovic M, Strejilevich SA, Gildengers AG, et al. A report on older-age bipolar disorder from the International Society for Bipolar Disorders Task Force. Bipolar Disord. 2015;17(7):689–704.

18 Sleep Disorders

Nery A. Diaz

Introduction

This chapter will summarize important topics of sleep in older adults and will discuss sleep changes associated with aging, epidemiology, the clinical assessment, and treatment of sleep problems in the older adult.

The American Academy of Sleep Medicine (AASM) sets the clinical standards for the field of sleep medicine health care, education, and research [1]. A polysomnogram (PSG) is the gold standard for measuring sleep through the use of numerous electrodes and medical equipment each measuring physiological parameters of sleep including (1) the electrical activity of the brain with an encephalogram (EEG), (2) measurements of eye movement with an electrooculogram (EOG), and (3) the electrical activity of the muscles with an electromyogram (EMG) [2]. Respiratory data and heart electrophysiology data are also gathered. The sleep study is commonly gathered overnight in a controlled setting outside the patient's home, usually a sleep laboratory [2]. The objective data collected over the course of the night is aggregated to study the different stages of sleep and the accompanying physiological responses to aid in the evaluation, diagnosis, and treatment of sleep disorders [2].

Sleep is divided in two stages, NREM and REM sleep. NREM sleep is further divided into three stages of sleep, S1, S2, and S3 [3]. S1 and S2 stages are characterized by light sleep, and S3 is characterized by slow-wave sleep (SWS) or delta sleep [3]. Normal sleep cycles transition from NREM stages 1, 2, and 3 to REM every 90–120 min [3]. Slow-wave sleep is more abundant at the beginning of the night, and REM stage sleep tends to increase during the latter half of the night [3].

The suprachiasmatic nucleus (SCN), located in the anterior hypothalamus, controls circadian functions, such as the sleep-wake cycle, body temperature, and the secretion of endogenous melatonin [2]. Regulation of sleepiness and sleep onset is thought to occur through activation of melatonin, an endogenous hormone secreted by the pineal gland [3].

Sleep Changes Associated with Aging

Changes in sleep architecture are seen throughout the span of life [3, 4]. Most changes in adult sleep patterns occur between early adulthood and age 60, declining only minimally between the ages of 60 and 102 [3, 4]. Many studies support that, by itself, aging has minimal effects on sleep patterns [4, 5]. Instead, sleep problems in the elderly population are associated with illness, chronic diseases, and the medications used to treat those diseases [4–6]. Sleep difficulties are significantly associated with medical comorbidities such as heart disease, pulmonary disease, osteoarthritis, and depression [4]. Pain syndromes, stroke, and neurological disorders also adversely affect sleep in the older adult [3, 6]. The quality of sleep also

R. R. Tampi et al. (eds.), *Psychiatric Disorders Late in Life*, https://doi.org/10.1007/978-3-319-73078-3_18

decreases with increasing number of medical comorbidities [4, 6, 7].

The changes in sleep that are associated with aging are [3]:

- An incr ease in sleep fragmentation
- An increase in sleep latency
- An increase in nighttime awakenings
- Progressive increase in light sleep
- Decrease in S3, slow-wave sleep
- Decrease in sleep efficiency
- Decrease in REM sleep

Melatonin levels also appear to decline with age and are lower in elderly persons suffering from insomnia when compared with age-matched controls [4]. The circadian network also deteriorates with aging. The most common clinical consequence of these changes is an advance in the circadian rhythm resulting in sleep and wake times that are several hours earlier than societal norms [4]. Older adults feel sleepy in the early evening and awaken in the very early morning hours with women showing increased susceptibility to this pattern when compared with men [4].

There are other changes in sleep patterns that affect men and women differently [8]. For example, a progressive decrease of slow-wave sleep is seen in both men and women, but this decrease affects men more than women [3]. In a sleep study of 40 healthy seniors (19 men and 21 women, aged 58–82 years), men could not maintain sleep as well as women and experienced less S3 sleep [9]. The prevalence of obstructive sleep apnea (OSA) is higher in men than in women and increases with age and obesity [10]. Elderly men and woman also have differences in circadian temperature rhythms and the circadian timing system [11]. Sleep changes in aging women may also be associated with changes in estrogen levels that directly influence sleep, body temperature regulation, circadian rhythms, and stress reactivity [12].

Epidemiology

Age and gender are the most clearly identified demographic risk factors associated with insomnia, with an increased prevalence in women and older adults [13, 14]. The lifetime prevalence for insomnia in individuals aged 35 years and over is as high as 35% [7]. Insomnia affects 25–45% of adults over the age of 64 [15]. Other sleep disorders adversely affecting the older patient are sleep-related breathing disorders and periodic limb movement disorders [16]. Sleep apnea affects 24–42% of older adults, and periodic limb movement disorder affects 45% of older adults [17, 18].

Clinical Assessment

The management of sleep disorders begins with thoughtful attention to the patient's presenting complaint and inquiry into acute stressors that may be precipitating problems with sleep. A thorough sleep history is a priority. This history should include sleep symptoms, sleep schedule, leg discomfort, bedroom environment, exposure history, past medical history, past surgical history, pain syndromes, neurologic and psychiatric disorders, medications, family history, social history, physical examination, laboratory results, and imaging studies [19–22]. Each of those elements that are not self-explanatory will be discussed below.

Sleep Schedule

Understanding a patient's sleep schedule includes multiple variables:

- A thorough evaluation of sleep patterns, such as the normal bedtime and wake-up time.
- How many minutes are required for the patient to fall asleep ("sleep latency"), and how many times the patient wakes up during the night. It is important to understand the causes of multiple nighttime awakenings, including how many minutes it takes for the patient to return to sleep after waking up during the night ("wake time"). One study conducted in 2008 of the general American population reported that the prevalence of nightly awakenings significantly increases with age, reaching 34.6% in subjects aged 65 and older [23]. Previous studies have reported prevalence between 25% and 35% of people waking up at least three nights per week [7].

- Inquiries regarding life stressors that lead to excessive nighttime worry are important.
- Inquiries into whether the patient is feeling refreshed upon awakening in the morning.

Bedroom Environment

The bedroom should be dark, quiet, at a comfortable temperature, and used only for sleep or for sex. Watching television or using the computer or other electronic devices before going to sleep should be discouraged because the blue light in the screens promotes wakefulness [24–26]. The mattress should also be comfortable. The bed should feel secure. The habits of bedmates can also interrupt normal sleep patterns, and these should be investigated to determine how they affect the patient's sleep. Inquiring if the patient sleeps as well or worse in environments outside the home also yields important information.

Exposure History

Lifestyle patterns can also affect sleep. Inquiring about patterns of alcohol consumptions, illicit drug use, cigarette smoking, energy drinks, and caffeine use is important because these substances can adversely affect sleep [27, 28]. It is important to note the timing, dosing, and years of use. Caffeine consumption includes not only coffee but also decaffeinated coffee, sodas, and energy drinks.

Review of Medications

It is important to obtain a listing of all medications that the patient is using including prescribed, over-the-counter, and herbal medications. The review should encompass length of time used and the doses of medications. Medications and substances that may cause insomnia include alcohol, antidepressants, amphetamine, antihypertensives, diuretics, herbal remedies, laxatives, levodopa, phenytoin, pseudoephedrine, steroids, and theophylline [4, 10].

Sleep Symptoms, Including Snoring

Obtaining information on excessive daytime sleepiness is important in the diagnosis of sleep disorders. It is important to inquire how likely the patient is to doze off or fall asleep while sitting and reading, watching television, or sitting inactive in a public space, such as a movie theater or a business meeting. Inquiry should also be made into falling asleep in situations such as while a passenger in a car, sitting and talking to someone, sitting quietly after lunch, sitting in a chair, or while stopped in traffic. Documenting the severity of dosing off in these situations is also important. The Epworth Sleepiness Score is a tool that provides an efficient clinic assessment of the severity of daytime sleepiness [29]. A score of ten or greater indicates an increased need to investigate for a possible sleep disorder [10].

Gathering information about snoring is also important [10]. Specifically, does the patient snore and if so does the patient snore so loudly that it has bothered other people in the past? It is also important to know if the patient has been observed to stop breathing during sleep or wakes from sleep gasping for air or choking. If so, inquiry should be made regarding the frequency and severity of air choking. It is important to know if the patient awakens with a dry mouth or an acid taste in his mouth and whether he is experiencing daytime headaches. These symptoms are concerning for a sleep-related breathing disorder such as obstructive sleep apnea [10].

Leg Discomfort

Leg discomfort that disrupts sleep can be associated with restless legs syndrome (RLS) and periodic limb movement disorder (PLMD) [28, 30]. Both conditions are associated with medical comorbidities and mental disorders [30]. A diagnosis of RLS and PLMD is confirmed with an overnight polysomnography [31, 32].

Leg discomfort associated with an urge to move occurring in the evening and exacerbated by inactivity that is temporarily alleviated by movement can hint at restless legs syndrome ("RLS") [32]. Restless legs syndrome is common in the elderly, with an estimated prevalence of 10–35% in individuals over 65 years of age [32]. It is important to understand how many times per week the patient is experiencing, and the length of time the patient has experienced, these symptoms. Anemia can precipitate or worsen restless legs [32]. Evaluation with a complete blood count and, if warranted, treatment with iron supplementation may relieve symptoms [32].

RLS is associated with PLMD [30]. Unlike RLS, patients who experience PLMD are often unaware of the involuntary movement of the limbs [30]. Presenting complaints include daytime sleepiness and troubles with sleep onset and sleep maintenance. Symptoms can range from mild movements restricted to the lower extremities to vigorous movement of all four limbs [30]. PLMD is more common in the elderly female with up to 11% experiencing symptoms [30].

Pain

Sleep disturbances are common in patients suffering from chronic pain [33]. Chronic pain symptoms interfering with sleep may necessitate a referral to a multidisciplinary pain clinic for ongoing management of symptoms. Cancer of the pancreas and metastatic disease is also known to cause severe pain and lead to problems with sleep [34, 35]. A referral to the palliative care service for aggressive pain management would be appropriate in this case.

Common Sleep Disorders

In the elderly common sleep disorders are circadian rhythm sleep disorders, REM sleep behavior disorder, and sleep disorders due to neurodegenerative disorders [36, 37].

Circadian Rhythm Sleep Disorders

These disorders are categorized by a recurrent pattern of inappropriate bedtime and awake cycles that disrupts the normal rhythm of sleep. Circadian rhythms are regulated by melatonin. Melatonin synthesis in the human pineal gland is a culmination of chemical signals stimulated by darkness and inhibited by light entering the eye through the retina [2]. Melatonin is a hormone produced in the tryptophan/serotonin pathway [2]. During periods of darkness, melatonin is secreted from the pineal gland to induce chemical neural and endocrine effects that regulate circadian rhythms [2]. Light entering the retina inhibits the synthesis of melatonin via the retino-hypothalamic tract to the suprachiasmatic nucleus in the hypothalamus [2].

REM Sleep Behavior Disorder

REM sleep behavior disorder can also affect the quantity and quality of sleep not only for the patient but also for any bed partner. It is important to obtain information from reliable collateral informants about the patterns of sleep disturbance and the initiation and severity of the symptoms. These bizarre behaviors are associated with a loss of the muscle atonia that normally accompanies REM sleep [38]. As a consequence, the patient enacts their dreams, including punching, kicking, and crying often with severe consequences for the bed partner. The exact mechanism of the disease is unknown but may herald the onset of a synucleinopathy [39, 40]. Ongoing research studies are attempting to quantify the risk for conversion from idiopathic REM sleep behavior to a neurodegenerative alpha synucleinopathy such as Parkinson's disease, multiple systems atrophy, or dementias with Lewy bodies [38]. The sleep disorder episodes can be suppressed with the use of clonazepam 0.5–2.0 mg 30 min before bedtime [2, 3].

Neurodegenerative Disorders

The relationship between sleep disturbances and neurodegenerative disorders is well documented in the literature [41–44]. In patients with dementia, disruption in sleep patterns correlates with severity of disease [43]. Alzheimer's disease ("AD") and dementia with Lewy bodies are the two most prominent forms of dementia presenting with sleep disturbances [43, 45]. The type of sleep disturbance differs with sundowning and sleep apnea found most often in patients with AD, unlike Lewy body disease where motor movements and nocturnal disturbances in behavior predominate [43, 44].

A thorough discussion with the patient and caregiver about the risk and benefits of nonpharmacological and pharmacological interventions to target sleep disturbances is important. Attending to the concerns of the caregiver is a treatment priority with a goal of minimizing caregiver burnout and the risks factors for institutionalization [46, 47]. Referring the caregiver to a community support group and educating the caregiver on self-care and maintenance of healthy boundaries are also an important part of the treatment plan.

Alzheimer's Disease

The exact mechanisms for the sleep disturbances observed in AD are unknown [48]. The scope of the current research correlates dysfunction in the sleep-wake cycle to beta-amyloid deposition and tau aggregations in the pathogenesis and progression of AD [48].

The nature of sleep disturbances caused by AD is multifaceted and affects the quality of life of the patient and caregivers. Sleeping more than usual and early morning awakening were the most common sleep problems but the least disturbing for caregivers [49]. Nighttime awakening was less commonly reported by the patient but was more disturbing to the caregiver [49]. The factors most strongly associated with night awakening were male gender, greater memory problems, and decreased functional states [49]. Patients who awaken caregivers were characterized to have increased levels of fearfulness, fidgeting, and hallucinations [49]. There is little evidence of the effectiveness of sleep disorders treatment in this population, particularly for community-dwelling elderly individuals [50]. Sleep hygiene and bright light therapy are recommended due to low risk in comparison to psychopharmacological agents [51]. Using antidepressants, sedative hypnotics, antipsychotics, and nootropics is not supported by robust evidence and results in high risk for adverse events in the treatment of sleep disorders for patients with AD [52].

One prominent feature of AD is the phenomenon of "sundowning," which refers to the increased confusion, restlessness agitation, and insomnia that worsens in the late evening and leads to increased caregiver burden and institutionalization [46]. Sundowning may be precipitated by offending pharmacological agents, underlying medical illnesses, and delirium [45, 53]. Sundowning is correlated with degeneration of the acetylcholinergic nucleus basalis of Meynert in the basal forebrain and the innate circadian rhythm activity of the suprachiasmatic nucleus in the hypothalamus [54].

Dementia with Lewy Bodies

Typical signs and symptoms of this disease are prominent parkinsonian features, dementia, frequent episodes of nighttime delirium, and REM sleep behavior disorder [55–57]. In addition, states of anxiety with intermittent psychotic or delirious behavior also feature prominent in this neurodegenerative disease [2]. Response to treatment is variable as most patients are nonresponsive and/or sensitive to the side effects of L-dopa [2].

Treatment of Sleep Disorders

A conservative approach to the treatment of insomnia in late life is appropriate [3]. Eliminating the use of inappropriate medications, limiting the use of sedating medications, and emphasizing sleep hygiene are the most appropriate strategies when managing sleep complains in late life [50, 58, 59]. The efficacy and tolerability of sedating medications for sleep disorders among older adults are low, and the opportunities for adverse reactions are high [58, 59]. The management of sleep-related breathing disorders and REM sleep behavior disorder includes a referral to a sleep study center for a thorough evaluation that includes an overnight video polysomnogram [31].

Pharmacological Interventions

In the geriatric population, exploring non-pharmacological sleep therapies prior to initiating pharmacological interventions is the conservative approach to treatment [3]. Education on sleep hygiene is a first-line intervention followed by a thorough and thoughtful evaluation of all medications including prescription medications, OTC, and herbal supplements. The goal is to taper and gradually discontinue any medications that can lead to, or potentiate, problems with sleep.

Polypharmacy as defined as the use of five or more prescription drugs is on the rise among adults ≥65 and older with an increase from 24 to 39% in the years 2011–2012 [60]. Part of this increase includes drug classes such as antidepressants and muscle relaxants that are known to cause excessive sedation [60]. These rising trends persisted even when adjusting for the aging structure of the US population [60]. These studies suggest that polypharmacy may be an alarming and durable trend among all adult populations [60–63].

The most recent 2012 Beers list of prescription and OTC aids that should be avoided due to associated tolerance, confusion, and minimal efficacy includes benzodiazepines and non-benzodiazepine hypnotic medications [64].

Benzodiazepines

There is concern about the use of benzodiazepines in the elderly [62]. According to the 2012 American Geriatric Society Beers Criteria Update Expert Panel, good practice guidelines recommend limiting treatment with benzodiazepines to a few weeks [64, 65].

In addition, age-related pharmacokinetic and pharmacodynamics changes increase the potential for other side effects in the elderly, including excessive daytime sedation, cognitive slowing, impairment in driving skills, and increased risk for falls [3, 62, 65–67]. Among older patients, falls are associated with a high morbidity and mortality [68]. In a systemic review of the benefits of benzodiazepines in AD, no evidence was found for an improved quality of sleep when using a benzodiazepine [65]. Low-dose clonazepam is effective for managing the nighttime episodes associated with REM sleep behavior disorder [2, 3].

Non-benzodiazepine Hypnotics

These medications are listed on the Beers list of medications that should be avoided among older adults due to adverse side effect profile similar to those reported by benzodiazepines [64]. The more common side effects of non-benzodiazepine hypnotics are somnolence, headache, dizziness, nausea, diarrhea, confused behaviors, somnambulism, hallucinations, and memory impairment [69]. Eszopiclone is known to cause an unpleasant metallic taste [70].

Melatonin

Melatonin when prescribed to older adults decreases sleep latency, decreases sleep fragmentation, increases sleep efficiency (the ratio of total time lying in bed sleeping divided by total time lying in bed), and increases total sleep duration [71, 72]. No objective benefit has been found for the use of melatonin to treat sleep disturbances in elderly patients with AD [73]. A large multicenter, randomized, placebo-controlled clinical trial of oral melatonin coordinated by the National Institute of Aging found no statistically significant difference in objective measures of sleep time when compared with placebo among older adults with sleep disturbances due to AD, although caregivers' subjective measures reported improvement in the quality of sleep [74].

Ramelteon

Several clinical trials using sleep diary data and polysomnographic data support the efficacy of ramelteon when prescribed to older adults by showing a statistically significant decrease in sleep latency and increase in total sleep time [75, 76]. One study, examining a subset of elderly individuals presenting with severe sleep initiation difficulties of greater than or equal to 60 min at baseline, demonstrated a statistically significant improvement from baseline in the ramelteon group when compared with placebo at weeks 1 and 5 [77]. That study also reported statistically significant decreases in sleep latency at week 1 (7.5 min for placebo control group and 23.2 min for the ramelteon group) and week 5 (17.1 min for the placebo-controlled group and 37.4 min for the ramelteon group) [77]. When compared to placebo, ramelteon is not associated with abuse, sedation or impairment in alertness, ability to concentrate, or memory recall [75, 78].

Trazodone

Trazodone is prescribed off-label at a sub-therapeutic antidepressant dose for the treatment of insomnia [79–81]. Trazodone is on the Beers list and is known to cause side effects that include daytime sedation, constipations, nausea, vomiting, headache, blurred vision, dry mouth hypotension, anxiety, and fatigue [64, 81]. Priapism is an uncommon side effect of trazodone that is more commonly reported among young and middle-aged men [82].

Mirtazapine

Mirtazapine is an antidepressant that is prescribed in low doses for the treatment of insomnia [81]. Although the exact mechanism of action is unknown, it postulated that at low doses the medication works on the histaminergic receptors thereby promoting sedation. Side effects include excessive daytime sedation weight gain, urinary retention, and agranulocytosis [83–85]. Due to potential for increase in weight, mirtazapine should be used with caution in patients who are obese or diabetic [86, 87]. Several case reports of mirtazapine-induced hyponatremia and SIADH are reported in the literature [88, 89].

Amitriptyline

Amitriptyline is a tricyclic antidepressant commonly prescribed in low doses to treat insomnia. Common side effects include dry mouth, blurry vision, constipation, urinary retention, and cardiac conduction abnormalities [85, 90]. Amitriptyline is on the Beers list as a medication to avoid in the geriatric population due to its highly anticholinergic properties [64, 90]. Overdoses with tricyclic antidepressants can be lethal due to their anticholinergic and cardiotoxic effects [91].

Complementary and Alternative Medicines

Treatment of insomnia with complementary and alternative medicines is becoming more popular among individuals who are concerned about taking traditional prescription medications [92, 93]. Some of the more commonly used complementary and alternative medicines for insomnia include herbs such as valerian, chamomile, lavender, hops, cannabis, L-arginine L-aspartate, S-adenosyl-L-homocysteine, passion flower, and delta sleep-inducing peptide (DSIP). Alternative medications are not FDA-approved and may contain harmful fillers, be processed with contaminants such as herbicides, and adversely interact with other prescribed and OTC medications [92]. The paucity of research that is available offers limited evidence of the efficacy of treatment of insomnia with these agents [93]. More research trials are needed to evaluate the efficacy of OTC and herbal supplements for the treatments of insomnia. It is important to engage in frank discussions with patients about these potential risk factors when discussing complementary and alternative medicines for insomnia [94].

Traditional Chinese Medicine

In traditional Chinese medicine, harmonizing the liver and spleen is the main principle in the treatment of insomnia [95]. According to classic Chinese medicine theory, Chaihuguizhiganjiang decoctions are beneficial for eliminating liver-heat syndrome, while suanzaoren decoctions aid in replenishing the spleen [95]. It is believed that together, these two classical compounds, Chaihuguizhiganjiang-suanzaoren granule (CSG), act synergistically to nourish the spleen and clear liver heat. A study published in the Clinical Journal of Chinese medicine in 2014 reported that Chaihuguizhiganjiang decoctions plus acupuncture had remarkable effects on improving sleep quality [95]. Although a few studies are available to support the efficacy and safety of these traditional Chinese medications, some trials are underway. A major limitation of many of these studies is the absence of polysomnographic sleep parameters with results relying on patient's subjective sleep outcomes [95]. With the DSM-5 shift to more data-driven diagnostic criteria for sleep disorders, the absence of objective parameters calls into question the reliability of the data [95].

Non-pharmacological Interventions

Sleep Education

Educating geriatric patients on the facts regarding sleep and aging is important. A report from a panel of experts assembled by the American Academy of Sleep Medicine recommends that between 7 and 9 h of sleep may be appropriate for adults ages 26–64 [96]. For those individuals who are 65 and older, 7 to 8 h is the daily amount of sleep that is recommended with less than 5 h of sleep deemed to be inappropriate and greater than 9 h of sleep not recommended [96].

Sleep Hygiene

The usual clinical recommendations for good sleep hygiene include the following guidelines:

1. Going to bed and rising at the same time each day including weekends [97].
2. The bed should be comfortable, and the bedroom should only be used for sleep [97].
3. The bedroom should also be quiet, dark, relaxing, and at a comfortable temperature that is neither too hot nor cold [97].
4. Avoiding reading, watching TV, listening to music, or the use of electronic devices in the bedroom. These behaviors can promote a state of arousal and negatively associate the bedroom with activities other than sleep [97, 98].
5. Avoiding both going to bed hungry and consuming large meals before bedtime [97].
6. Avoiding diuretics and excessive liquids in the evening to minimize nighttime awakenings to void [97].
7. Avoiding activities that are mentally activating and physically vigorous too close to bedtime, including exercise and emotionally disturbing conversations [97].
8. Daytime naps are helpful in situations of sleep loss when sufficient amount of sleep is not possible, such as work involving extended duty hours [97].
9. Avoiding nicotine and caffeine can have a positive impact on the quality of sleep. Nicotine has deleterious effects on overall health and well-being [99]. The negative consequences of the use of nicotine and caffeine on the quality of sleep may be partially explained by withdrawal phenomenon during the night as the result of their half-lives of 1–2 and 3–7 h, respectively [100].
10. Avoiding alcohol use, which has a series of negative consequences on sleep physiology. Alcohol has a modest increase in sleep promotion in the first half of the night and severe disruptions of sleep during the second half of the night [101]. Withdrawal from alcohol is also associated with severe rebound insomnia [101]. Alcoholism and older age have an additive effect in decreasing total sleep time [101].
11. Avoiding cannabis, which also negatively impacts sleep, especially in the setting of chronic use [102]. Subjective reports of strange dreams, insomnia, and poor sleep quality have been objectively corroborated with PSG studies [102]. PSG studies of cannabis withdrawal have also demonstrated increases in sleep latency and wakefulness, together with reductions in total sleep time, sleep efficiency, and slow-wave sleep [102]. Changes in objective PSG measures can start the first night of abstinence with more noticeable changes among heavy users [102]. Disturbances may progress over the first 2 weeks of abstinence and persist for more than 45 days into a marijuana abstinence period [102].

Sleep Restriction

The goal of sleep restriction is to increase the amount of time spent in bed sleeping ("sleep efficiency") by decreasing the time needed to get to sleep ("sleep latency") and decreasing the time needed to fall back to sleep if person wakes during sleep ("wake time") [103]. This treatment establishes a fixed time to arise and decreases time spent in bed by prescribing a progressively later bedtime [103]. Initially, this strategy will lead to a reduction in total sleep time; however, over the course of several days, this therapy results in decreased sleep latency and decreased wake time after sleep onset [96], leading to increased sleep efficiency [103]. Throughout the therapy, patients may be asked to "roll back" their bedtime in 15-min increments until efficient sleep is achieved [103]. Efficient sleep is defined as 90% or more of the total sleep time calculated as total sleep time divided by the time in bed and multiplied by 100 [104]. Sleep restriction is contraindicated in patients with history of mania, seizure disorder, and parasomnias because it may aggravate these conditions [104].

Stimulus Control

The goal of stimulus control therapy is to teach patients suffering from insomnia to decrease sleep latency and increase the efficiency of sleep [98]. The goal of treatment is to strengthen the bedroom as a cue for sleep by eliminating activities other than sleep in the bedroom and eliminating sleep in places other than the bedroom [98]. Stimulus control is contraindicated in geriatric patients with mobility problems or who are at risk for slips and falls [105]. This practice is also limited by small or shared sleep environments [105].

Cognitive Behavioral Therapy-Insomnia (CBT-I)

Cognitive Behavioral Therapy-Insomnia ("CBT-I") is a behavioral therapy focusing on sleep hygiene, including sleep restrictions and stimulus control [106–109]. Formal cognitive therapy is not part of the intervention, and therefore non-pharmacological interventions with CBT-I can be helpful even in patients with dementia [110]. Although more research is needed to test the adaptation of CBT-I to other psychiatric and medical conditions, CBT-I is a good treatment for patients with medical and psychiatric comorbidities [108, 111].

CBT-I Session Summary [109]

- **Session 1, clinical evaluation and 2-week baseline:** During this session, the patient's sleep complaints are reviewed, and the patient is instructed to keep a sleep diary for a baseline period of 2 weeks [109]. The sleep diary data is reviewed at all subsequent sessions [109]. Session 2 is scheduled 2 weeks after session 1 [109]. All other sessions are scheduled at 1-week intervals [109].
- **Session 2, sleep restriction and stimulus control therapy:** In this session, the clinician explains in detail the rationale and procedures for sleep restriction and stimulus control components [34, 103]. The information obtained from the patient and the data noted on the sleep diary are used to identify the parameters for sleep restriction and stimulus control components of the therapy [109]. Also, the clinician emphasizes the focus of treatment with the goal of debunking "the positive correlation fallacy, the belief that the more time spent lying in bed the more sleep the patient will get" [109].
- **Session 3, sleep hygiene and sleep restriction therapy adjustments:** After discussing and charting the sleep diary data, the sleep hygiene instructions are reviewed [97, 109].
- **Sessions 4 to 7, adjustments to sleep restriction:** After discussing and charting the sleep diary data, any patient nonadherence to treatment guidelines are addressed [109].
- **Session 8, relapse prevention:** This final session is predominantly educational with a review of the triggers of insomnia and a review of strategies to minimize the risk for extended episodes of insomnia [109].

Adjunctive Therapies

Relaxation training, including progressive muscle relaxation, diaphragmatic breathing, biofeedback, hypnosis, mindfulness, and aromatherapy are all adjunctive therapies for insomnia that can assist the patient with entering a state of calmful rest [109].

Conclusion

Sleep disorders are not a normal part of aging, although complaints of difficulty with sleep are not uncommon in late life. The cause of sleep disorders in the elderly is usually multifactorial and often associated with declining health. A thorough evaluation with appropriate treatment is an important part of the geriatric psychiatric evaluation. More research studies are needed that examine objective sleep measures in old age with the goal of designing novel treatment strategies aimed at reducing the burden of sleep disorders for the patient, caregivers, and families.

References

1. AASM: The American Academy of Sleep Medicine - Association for Seep Clinicians and Researchers. http://www.aasmnet.org.
2. Ropper AH, Adams RD, Victor M, Samuels MA. Adams and Victor's principles of neurology. 9th ed. New York: McGraw-Hill Medical; 2009.
3. Fetveit A. Late-life insomnia: a review. Geriatr Gerontol Int. 2009;9(3):220–34.
4. Ancoli-Israel S. Sleep and its disorders in aging populations. Sleep Med. 2009;10(Suppl 1): S7–11.

5. Vitiello MV, Moe KE, Prinz PN. Sleep complaints cosegregate with illness in older adults: clinical research informed by and informing epidemiological studies of sleep. J Psychosom Res. 2002;53(1):555–9.
6. Foley D, Ancoli-Israel S, Britz P, Walsh J. Sleep disturbances and chronic disease in older adults: results of the 2003 National Sleep Foundation Sleep in America Survey. J Psychosom Res. 2004;56(5):497–502.
7. Ohayon MM. Epidemiology of insomnia: what we know and what we still need to learn. Sleep Med Rev. 2002;6(2):97–111.
8. Zdanys KF, Steffens DC. Sleep disturbances in the elderly. Psychiatr Clin North Am. 2015;38(4):723–41.
9. Reynolds CF, Kupfer DJ, Taska LS, Hoch CC, Sewitch DE, Spiker DG. Sleep of healthy seniors: a revisit. Sleep. 1985;8(1):20–9.
10. Franklin KA, Lindberg E. Obstructive sleep apnea is a common disorder in the population-a review on the epidemiology of sleep apnea. J Thorac Dis. 2015;7(8):1311–22.
11. Moe KE, Prinz PN, Vitiello MV, Marks AL, Larsen LH. Healthy elderly women and men have different entrained circadian temperature rhythms. J Am Geriatr Soc. 1991;39(4):383–7.
12. Moe KE. Reproductive hormones, aging, and sleep. Semin Reprod Endocrinol. 1999;17(4):339–48.
13. Roth T. Insomnia: definition, prevalence, etiology, and consequences. J Clin Sleep Med. 2007;3(5 Suppl):S7–10.
14. NIH State-of-the-Science Conference Statement on manifestations and management of chronic insomnia in adults. NIH Consens State Sci Statements. 2005;22(2):1-30.
15. Mellinger GD, Balter MB, Uhlenhuth EH. Insomnia and its treatment. Prevalence and correlates. Arch Gen Psychiatry. 1985;42(3):225–32.
16. Young T, Shahar E, Nieto FJ, et al. Predictors of sleep-disordered breathing in community-dwelling adults: the Sleep Heart Health Study. Arch Intern Med. 2002;162(8):893–900.
17. Ancoli-Israel S, Kripke DF, Klauber MR, Mason WJ, Fell R, Kaplan O. Sleep-disordered breathing in community-dwelling elderly. Sleep. 1991;14(6):486–95.
18. Ancoli-Israel S, Kripke DF. Prevalent sleep problems in the aged. Biofeedback Self Regul. 1991;16(4):349–59.
19. Woodward M. Insomnia in the elderly. Aust Fam Physician. 1999;28(7):653–8.
20. Rajput V, Bromley SM. Chronic insomnia: a practical review. Am Fam Physician. 1999;60(5):1431–8. discussion 1441-1432
21. Woodward M. Hypnosedatives in the elderly. CNS Drugs. 1999;11(4):263–79.
22. Vgontzas AN, Kales A. Sleep and its disorders. Annu Rev Med. 1999;50:387–400.
23. Ohayon MM. Nocturnal awakenings and comorbid disorders in the American general population. J Psychiatr Res. 2008;43(1):48–54.
24. Rahman SA, Flynn-Evans EE, Aeschbach D, Brainard GC, Czeisler CA, Lockley SW. Diurnal spectral sensitivity of the acute alerting effects of light. Sleep. 2014;37(2):271–81.
25. Hattar S, Liao HW, Takao M, Berson DM, Yau KW. Melanopsin-containing retinal ganglion cells: architecture, projections, and intrinsic photosensitivity. Science. 2002;295(5557):1065–70.
26. Hubbard J, Ruppert E, Gropp CM, Bourgin P. Non-circadian direct effects of light on sleep and alertness: lessons from transgenic mouse models. Sleep Med Rev. 2013;17(6):445–52.
27. Patterson TL, Jeste DV. The potential impact of the baby-boom generation on substance abuse among elderly persons. Psychiatr Serv. 1999;50(9):1184–8.
28. Neubauer DN. Sleep problems in the elderly. Am Fam Physician. 1999;59(9):2551–8, 2559-2560
29. Johns MW. A new method for measuring daytime sleepiness: the Epworth sleepiness scale. Sleep. 1991;14(6):540–5.
30. Ohayon MM, Roth T. Prevalence of restless legs syndrome and periodic limb movement disorder in the general population. J Psychosom Res. 2002;53(1):547–54.
31. Kushida CA, Littner MR, Morgenthaler T, et al. Practice parameters for the indications for polysomnography and related procedures: an update for 2005. Sleep. 2005;28(4):499–521.
32. Milligan SA, Chesson AL. Restless legs syndrome in the older adult: diagnosis and management. Drugs Aging. 2002;19(10):741–51.
33. Pilowsky I, Crettenden I, Townley M. Sleep disturbance in pain clinic patients. Pain. 1985;23(1):27–33.
34. Wyse JM, Chen YI, Sahai AV. Celiac plexus neurolysis in the management of unresectable pancreatic cancer: when and how? World J Gastroenterol. 2014;20(9):2186–92.
35. Habermehl D, Brecht IC, Debus J, Combs SE. Palliative radiation therapy in patients with metastasized pancreatic cancer - description of a rare patient group. Eur J Med Res. 2014; 19:24.
36. Cooke JR, Ancoli-Israel S. Normal and abnormal sleep in the elderly. Handb Clin Neurol. 2011;98:653–65.

37. Stepnowsky CJ, Ancoli-Israel S. Sleep and its disorders in seniors. Sleep Med Clin. 2008;3(2):281–93.
38. Postuma RB, Gagnon JF, Vendette M, Fantini ML, Massicotte-Marquez J, Montplaisir J. Quantifying the risk of neurodegenerative disease in idiopathic REM sleep behavior disorder. Neurology. 2009;72(15):1296–300.
39. Postuma RB, Gagnon JF, Montplaisir J. Rapid eye movement sleep behavior disorder as a biomarker for neurodegeneration: the past 10 years. Sleep Med. 2013;14(8):763–7.
40. Iranzo A, Molinuevo JL, Santamaría J, et al. Rapid-eye-movement sleep behaviour disorder as an early marker for a neurodegenerative disorder: a descriptive study. Lancet Neurol. 2006;5(7):572–7.
41. Drogos LL, Gill SJ, Tyndall AV, et al. Evidence of association between sleep quality and APOE ε4 in healthy older adults: a pilot study. Neurology. 2016;87(17):1836–42.
42. Gottlieb DJ, DeStefano AL, Foley DJ, et al. APOE epsilon4 is associated with obstructive sleep apnea/hypopnea: the Sleep Heart Health Study. Neurology. 2004;63(4):664–8.
43. Grace JB, Walker MP, McKeith IG. A comparison of sleep profiles in patients with dementia with lewy bodies and Alzheimer's disease. Int J Geriatr Psychiatry. 2000;15(11):1028–33.
44. Bliwise DL, Mercaldo ND, Avidan AY, Boeve BF, Greer SA, Kukull WA. Sleep disturbance in dementia with Lewy bodies and Alzheimer's disease: a multicenter analysis. Dement Geriatr Cogn Disord. 2011;31(3):239–46.
45. Weldemichael DA, Grossberg GT. Circadian rhythm disturbances in patients with Alzheimer's disease: a review. Int J Alzheimers Dis. 2010;2010.
46. Pollak CP, Perlick D. Sleep problems and institutionalization of the elderly. J Geriatr Psychiatry Neurol. 1991;4(4):204–10.
47. Gibson RH, Gander PH, Jones LM. Understanding the sleep problems of people with dementia and their family caregivers. Dementia. 2014;13(3):350–65.
48. Lim MM, Gerstner JR, Holtzman DM. The sleep-wake cycle and Alzheimer's disease: what do we know? Neurodegener Dis Manag. 2014;4(5): 351–62.
49. McCurry SM, Logsdon RG, Teri L, et al. Characteristics of sleep disturbance in community-dwelling Alzheimer's disease patients. J Geriatr Psychiatry Neurol. 1999;12(2):53–9.
50. Bloom HG, Ahmed I, Alessi CA, et al. Evidence-based recommendations for the assessment and management of sleep disorders in older persons. J Am Geriatr Soc. 2009;57(5):761–89.
51. Dauvilliers Y. Insomnia in patients with neurodegenerative conditions. Sleep Med. 2007;8(Suppl 4):S27–34.
52. Deschenes CL, McCurry SM. Current treatments for sleep disturbances in individuals with dementia. Curr Psychiatry Rep. 2009;11(1):20–6.
53. Khachiyants N, Trinkle D, Son SJ, Kim KY. Sundown syndrome in persons with dementia: an update. Psychiatry Investig. 2011;8(4):275–87.
54. Bedrosian TA, Nelson RJ. Sundowning syndrome in aging and dementia: research in mouse models. Exp Neurol. 2013;243:67–73.
55. Schneider JA, Arvanitakis Z, Yu L, Boyle PA, Leurgans SE, Bennett DA. Cognitive impairment, decline and fluctuations in older community-dwelling subjects with Lewy bodies. Brain. 2012;135(Pt 10):3005–14.
56. Donaghy PC, McKeith IG. The clinical characteristics of dementia with Lewy bodies and a consideration of prodromal diagnosis. Alzheimers Res Ther. 2014;6(4):46.
57. Zupancic M, Mahajan A, Handa K. Dementia with lewy bodies: diagnosis and management for primary care providers. Prim Care Companion CNS Disord 2011;13(5).
58. Gooneratne NS, Vitiello MV. Sleep in older adults: normative changes, sleep disorders, and treatment options. Clin Geriatr Med. 2014;30(3):591–627.
59. Sack RL, Auckley D, Auger RR, et al. Circadian rhythm sleep disorders: part II, advanced sleep phase disorder, delayed sleep phase disorder, free-running disorder, and irregular sleep-wake rhythm. An American Academy of Sleep Medicine review. Sleep. 2007;30(11):1484–501.
60. Kantor ED, Rehm CD, Haas JS, Chan AT, Giovannucci EL. Trends in prescription drug use among adults in the United States from 1999-2012. JAMA. 2015;314(17):1818–31.
61. Tannenbaum C. Inappropriate benzodiazepine use in elderly patients and its reduction. J Psychiatry Neurosci. 2015;40(3):E27–8.
62. Madhusoodanan S, Bogunovic OJ. Safety of benzodiazepines in the geriatric population. Expert Opin Drug Saf. 2004;3(5):485–93.
63. Mojtabai R, Olfson M. National trends in psychotropic medication polypharmacy in office-based psychiatry. Arch Gen Psychiatry. 2010;67(1):26–36.
64. Panel AGSBCUE. American Geriatrics Society updated Beers Criteria for potentially inappropriate medication use in older adults. J Am Geriatr Soc. 2012;60(4):616–31.

65. Defrancesco M, Marksteiner J, Fleischhacker WW, Blasko I. Use of benzodiazepines in Alzheimer's disease: a systematic review of literature. Int J Neuropsychopharmacol. 2015;18(10):pyv055.
66. Bakken MS, Engeland A, Engesæter LB, Ranhoff AH, Hunskaar S, Ruths S. Risk of hip fracture among older people using anxiolytic and hypnotic drugs: a nationwide prospective cohort study. Eur J Clin Pharmacol. 2014;70(7):873–80.
67. de Jong MR, Van der Elst M, Hartholt KA. Drug-related falls in older patients: implicated drugs, consequences, and possible prevention strategies. Ther Adv Drug Saf. 2013;4(4):147–54.
68. Tinetti ME. Clinical practice. Preventing falls in elderly persons. N Engl J Med. 2003;348(1):42–9.
69. Wagner J, Wagner ML. Non-benzodiazepines for the treatment of insomnia. Sleep Med Rev. 2000;4(6):551–81.
70. Doty RL, Treem J, Tourbier I, Mirza N. A double-blind study of the influences of eszopiclone on dysgeusia and taste function. Pharmacol Biochem Behav. 2009;94(2):312–8.
71. Brzezinski A, Vangel MG, Wurtman RJ, et al. Effects of exogenous melatonin on sleep: a meta-analysis. Sleep Med Rev. 2005;9(1):41–50.
72. Wurtman RJ, Zhdanova I. Improvement of sleep quality by melatonin. Lancet. 1995;346(8988):1491.
73. Serfaty M, Kennell-Webb S, Warner J, Blizard R, Raven P. Double blind randomised placebo controlled trial of low dose melatonin for sleep disorders in dementia. Int J Geriatr Psychiatry. 2002;17(12):1120–7.
74. Singer C, Tractenberg RE, Kaye J, et al. A multicenter, placebo-controlled trial of melatonin for sleep disturbance in Alzheimer's disease. Sleep. 2003;26(7):893–901.
75. Roth T, Seiden D, Wang-Weigand S, Zhang J. A 2-night, 3-period, crossover study of ramelteon's efficacy and safety in older adults with chronic insomnia. Curr Med Res Opin. 2007;23(5):1005–14.
76. Roth T, Seiden D, Sainati S, Wang-Weigand S, Zhang J, Zee P. Effects of ramelteon on patient-reported sleep latency in older adults with chronic insomnia. Sleep Med. 2006;7(4):312–8.
77. Mini LJ, Wang-Weigand S, Zhang J. Self-reported efficacy and tolerability of ramelteon 8 mg in older adults experiencing severe sleep-onset difficulty. Am J Geriatr Pharmacother. 2007;5(3):177–84.
78. Johnson MW, Suess PE, Griffiths RR. Ramelteon: a novel hypnotic lacking abuse liability and sedative adverse effects. Arch Gen Psychiatry. 2006;63(10):1149–57.
79. Mendelson WB. A review of the evidence for the efficacy and safety of trazodone in insomnia. J Clin Psychiatry. 2005;66(4):469–76.
80. Bayer AJ, Pathy MS, Ankier SI. Pharmacokinetic and pharmacodynamic characteristics of trazodone in the elderly. Br J Clin Pharmacol. 1983;16(4):371–6.
81. Thase ME. Antidepressant treatment of the depressed patient with insomnia. J Clin Psychiatry. 1999;60(Suppl 17):28–31. discussion 46-28
82. Raskin DE. Trazodone and priapism. Am J Psychiatry. 1985;142(1):142–3.
83. Thase ME, Nierenberg AA, Keller MB, Panagides J, Group RPS. Efficacy of mirtazapine for prevention of depressive relapse: a placebo-controlled double-blind trial of recently remitted high-risk patients. J Clin Psychiatry. 2001;62(10):782–8.
84. de Boer T. The pharmacologic profile of mirtazapine. J Clin Psychiatry. 1996;57(Suppl 4):19–25.
85. Verhamme KM, Sturkenboom MC, Stricker BH, Bosch R. Drug-induced urinary retention: incidence, management and prevention. Drug Saf. 2008;31(5):373–88.
86. Laimer M, Kramer-Reinstadler K, Rauchenzauner M, et al. Effect of mirtazapine treatment on body composition and metabolism. J Clin Psychiatry. 2006;67(3):421–4.
87. Fava M. Weight gain and antidepressants. J Clin Psychiatry. 2000;61(Suppl 11):37–41.
88. Viramontes TS, Truong H, Linnebur SA. Antidepressant-induced hyponatremia in older adults. Consult Pharm. 2016;31(3):139–50.
89. Tripathi P, Tomar LR, Goyal P, Singh P. An unusual presentation of dose dependent SIADH secondary to mirtazapine therapy. Aust N Z J Psychiatry. 2015;49(11):1070–1.
90. Remick RA. Anticholinergic side effects of tricyclic antidepressants and their management. Prog Neuro-Psychopharmacol Biol Psychiatry. 1988;12(2-3):225–31.
91. Mandour RA. Antidepressants medications and the relative risk of suicide attempt. Toxicol Int. 2012;19(1):42–6.
92. Pearson NJ, Johnson LL, Nahin RL. Insomnia, trouble sleeping, and complementary and alternative medicine: analysis of the 2002 national health interview survey data. Arch Intern Med. 2006;166(16):1775–82.
93. Meolie AL, Rosen C, Kristo D, et al. Oral nonprescription treatment for insomnia: an evaluation of products with limited evidence. J Clin Sleep Med. 2005;1(2):173–87.
94. Tariq SH. Herbal therapies. Clin Geriatr Med. 2004;20(2):237–57.

95. Liu QQ, Zhang J, Guo RJ, et al. Efficacy and safety of the Chaihuguizhiganjiang-suanzaoren granule on primary insomnia: study protocol for a randomised controlled trial. BMJ Open. 2016;6(2):e008459.
96. Watson NF, Badr MS, Belenky G, et al. Joint consensus statement of the American Academy of Sleep Medicine and Sleep Research Society on the recommended amount of sleep for a healthy adult: methodology and discussion. J Clin Sleep Med. 2015;11(8):931–52.
97. Stepanski EJ, Wyatt JK. Use of sleep hygiene in the treatment of insomnia. Sleep Med Rev. 2003;7(3):215–25.
98. Bootzin RR, Epstein D, Wood JM. Stimulus control instructions. In: Hauri P, editor. Case studies in insomnia. New York: Plenum Medical; 1991. p. 19–23.
99. Alberg AJ, Shopland DR, Cummings KM. The 2014 Surgeon General's report: commemorating the 50th Anniversary of the 1964 Report of the Advisory Committee to the US Surgeon General and updating the evidence on the health consequences of cigarette smoking. Am J Epidemiol. 2014;179(4):403–12.
100. Ogeil RP, Phillips JG. Commonly used stimulants: sleep problems, dependence and psychological distress. Drug Alcohol Depend. 2015;153:145–51.
101. Brower KJ, Hall JM. Effects of age and alcoholism on sleep: a controlled study. J Stud Alcohol. 2001;62(3):335–43.
102. Angarita GA, Emadi N, Hodges S, Morgan PT. Sleep abnormalities associated with alcohol, cannabis, cocaine, and opiate use: a comprehensive review. Addict Sci Clin Pract. 2016;11(1):9.
103. Spielman AJ, Saskin P, Thorpy MJ. Treatment of chronic insomnia by restriction of time in bed. Sleep. 1987;10(1):45–56.
104. Harsora P, Kessmann J. Nonpharmacologic management of chronic insomnia. Am Fam Physician. 2009;79(2):125–30.
105. Smith MT, Perlis ML. Who is a candidate for cognitive-behavioral therapy for insomnia? Health Psychol. 2006;25(1):15–9.
106. Edinger JD, Olsen MK, Stechuchak KM, et al. Cognitive behavioral therapy for patients with primary insomnia or insomnia associated predominantly with mixed psychiatric disorders: a randomized clinical trial. Sleep. 2009;32(4):499–510.
107. Jacobs GD, Pace-Schott EF, Stickgold R, Otto MW. Cognitive behavior therapy and pharmacotherapy for insomnia: a randomized controlled trial and direct comparison. Arch Intern Med. 2004;164(17):1888–96.
108. Smith MT, Huang MI, Manber R. Cognitive behavior therapy for chronic insomnia occurring within the context of medical and psychiatric disorders. Clin Psychol Rev. 2005;25(5):559–92.
109. Perlis ML. Cognitive behavioral treatment of insomnia: a session-by-session guide. New York, NY: Springer; 2005.
110. Shub D, Darvishi R, Kunik ME. Nonpharmacologic treatment of insomnia in persons with dementia. Geriatrics. 2009;64(2):22–6.
111. JQ W, Appleman ER, Salazar RD, Ong JC. Cognitive behavioral therapy for insomnia comorbid with psychiatric and medical conditions: a meta-analysis. JAMA Intern Med. 2015;175(9):1461–72.

19 Schizophrenia Spectrum and Other Psychotic Disorders

Michael Reinhardt, Dina Ghoneim, Bronwyn Huggins, Anup Mani, Tessa Murante, and Carl Cohen

Introduction

The term psychosis can be traced in origin to two individuals, Karl Friedrich Canstatt (1841) and Ernst von Feuchtersleben (1845) as an amalgam of the Greek words for "psyche" (life, soul, mind) and "osis" (an abnormal condition thereof) [1]. The DSM-5 defines psychosis as a condition characterized by abnormalities in one or more of the following five domains: delusions, hallucinations, disorganized thinking (speech), grossly disorganized or abnormal motor behavior (including catatonia), and negative symptoms [2].

Psychosis among older adults is a highly prevalent and heterogeneous condition which presents in approximately 5–62% of older adults depending on the population that is sampled [3, 4]. Late-life psychosis has assumed more prominence recently as its prevalence has increased in tandem with the rapid worldwide growth in the aging population. Late-life psychosis remains a diagnostic conundrum in many cases due to a multitude of potential etiologies. This chapter will focus on late-life primary psychotic disorders, including schizophrenia, schizoaffective disorder, and delusional disorder.

Epidemiology

Psychosis

The risk of developing psychotic symptoms in late life has been estimated to be up to 23%—primarily due to incident dementia [3, 4]. The prevalence of psychotic symptoms in the general population of noncognitively impaired, community-dwelling older adults has been estimated in various population samples to range between 0 and 4%, with the prevalence increasing correspondingly with age [5]. In clinical populations, the prevalence of psychosis in late life is more dramatic: 5–15% of geriatric psychiatry inpatients and up to 62% of nursing home patients [3, 4].

It is important epidemiologically and clinically to distinguish between "primary" (not attributable to other medical conditions) and "secondary" (contributable to other medical conditions) forms of psychosis [6]. Primary psychotic disorders include schizophrenia spectrum illnesses and affective spectrum illnesses. These disorders comprise approximately 40% of cases in older adults.

R. R. Tampi et al. (eds.), *Psychiatric Disorders Late in Life*, https://doi.org/10.1007/978-3-319-73078-3_19

TABLE 19-1. The etiologies and relative prevalence of primary and secondary psychoses [2, 3, 7]

Etiology	Primary/secondary psychosis	Relative prevalence (%)
Dementia (all types)	Secondary	40
Disease, drugs, alcohol, toxins	Secondary	11
Delirium	Secondary	7
Affective spectrum illness	Primary	38
Schizophrenia spectrum illness	Primary	3

Secondary psychotic disorders include those attributable to major neurocognitive disorders (dementia), delirium, substance use, and other medical conditions. These disorders comprise the majority of cases in late life (60%) [2, 3, 7]. Table 19-1 outlines the etiologies and relative prevalence of primary and secondary psychoses in late life.

Schizophrenia Spectrum Illness

While the lifetime prevalence of schizophrenia has been estimated at 1%, the prevalence in older adults is estimated between 0.1 and 0.5% [8, 9]. This relative decrease in prevalence is likely due to historically lower life expectancies in persons with schizophrenia owing to increased mortality from various causes (e.g., other medical conditions, suicide) [10, 11]. The prevalence is expected to rise in the coming decades as increasing numbers of persons with schizophrenia survive into later life, with roughly one quarter of persons in developed countries being 55 or older by 2025 [12].

Although the DSM-5 and ICD10 do not classify schizophrenia by age of onset, the International Late-Onset Schizophrenia Group proposed subdividing schizophrenia into three groups based on age of onset: early-onset schizophrenia (EOS, before age 40), late-onset schizophrenia (LOS, ages 40–60), and very late-onset schizophrenia-like psychosis (VLOS, after age 60) [13]. Early-onset schizophrenia comprises the majority of late-life cases, or approximately 75–80%, with late-onset schizophrenia comprising the remaining 20–25% [14].

Older adults with early-onset schizophrenia have been described as experiencing an enhanced "paradox of aging" compared to the general population. This is characterized by:

(a) An early and magnified physical comorbidity and mortality accompanied by accelerated physiologic aging.
(b) An initial incidence of neurocognitive disorder at illness onset that is followed by a rate of cognitive decline similar to their healthy age peers; this results in cognitive deficits comparable to mild dementia for roughly half of older adults with schizophrenia.
(c) In contrast, psychosocial function tends to improve, psychosis decreases, relapse/hospitalization declines, and there are improvements in well-being and self-management [15].

Schizophrenia in later life, like its counterpart in younger adults, is associated with increased rates of depression (32–75%) and resultant suicide although suicide rates are lower in the older group.

Late-Onset Schizophrenia (LOS)

Compared to early onset, persons with LOS are more likely to be female, have lower burden of positive symptoms, require lower doses of antipsychotics, have increased organization of their delusions and increased persecutory-type delusions, but have equal family history and childhood history of maladjustment [16, 17]. Deficits in hearing and vision may be risk factors for late-onset schizophrenia [18].

There are conflicting data with respect to cognitive deficits in older patients with early-onset schizophrenia and late-onset schizophrenia, with some finding higher, lower, or no differences in cognition. Notably, Rajji and Mulsant's literature review found that "all the cross-sectional and most of the longitudinal studies were unable to distinguish patients with early-onset schizophrenia from those with late onset in terms of their cognitive profiles" (p. 138) [19]. In a large comparative study, Vahia and colleagues found that when the duration of illness was considered, the only differences between early- and late-onset schizophrenia were in the processing speed and perceptual organization, which were more impaired in the former [17]. Socio-occupationally, individuals with late-onset schizophrenia have higher rates of occupational and marital success.

Very Late-Onset Schizophrenia-Like Psychosis (VLOS)

Compared to EOS and LOS, very late-onset schizophrenia-like psychosis (VLOS) has higher rates of brain abnormalities and a greater burden of neuropsychological deficit—suggestive of a neurodegenerative condition. Clinically, VLOS is differentiated by lower genetic load; much larger female preponderance; increased partition and persecutory delusions; higher incidence of visual, tactile, and olfactory hallucinations; and typically an absence of negative symptoms and thought disorders [13].

Schizoaffective Disorder

While there is a paucity of studies available on schizoaffective disorder in older adults, the available data are consistent in finding schizoaffective disorder more like schizophrenia than bipolar disorder, both epidemiologically and clinically.

In their 2012 study, Meesters et al. estimated the 12-month prevalence of schizoaffective disorder in adults over the age of 60 at 0.14% [20]. Clinically, the features of schizoaffective disorder in older adults include increased treatment resistance, risk of suicide, and severity of illness [21]. Increased mortality rates, negative symptom burden, clinical global impression of impairment, lower likelihood of marriage, and independent living have been found to be similar to schizophrenia [22]. In comparison to depressive and bipolar types of schizoaffective disorder, patients with depressive type appear to be at higher risk for suicide [23].

Delusional Disorder

Delusional disorder in older adults, which is characterized by non-bizarre delusions without prominent hallucinations, has been inadequately studied [24]. The lifetime prevalence of delusional disorder is estimated at 0.18%, with the preponderance of cases occurring after the age of 45 years [25]. Within the subpopulation of older adults, the prevalence of delusional disorder in the elderly is estimated at 0.03%, with a slight preponderance of women affected by the condition [26]. The disorder typically first appears in middle to late adulthood, with an average age at onset of 40–49 years for men and 60–69 years for women. In general, when delusional disorder occurs in later life, social functioning is impaired, but cognitive functioning, personality, and vocational functioning are minimally impaired or unimpaired [10].

Secondary Psychoses

Approximately 60% of psychoses in older adults are due to another medical condition. The relative prevalence of these secondary psychotic disorders are noted in Table 19-1.

Risk Factors and Neurobiology of Psychosis in Late Life

Schizophrenia spectrum and other psychotic disorders have an etiology and pathophysiology that remain to be fully elucidated. With advances in science, it is becoming clear that schizophrenia—along with many other mental illnesses—represents the manifestation of complex interactions between genetic, neurodevelopmental, environmental, and social factors.

Social and Clinical Risk Factors

A number of age-related factors have been associated with a risk for psychosis in older adults, including hearing and vision deficits, isolation, decline in cognition, physical and mental disorder comorbidity, polypharmacy, pharmacokinetic changes, pharmacodynamic changes, changes in cerebral structures, and neurochemical changes [27].

With respect to late-onset schizophrenia and early-onset schizophrenia, the greater prevalence of female gender in the former is the only well-established risk factor [28]. Both types have several shared risk factors: a family history of schizophrenia (10–15%), minor physical anomalies, and a history of childhood maladjustment [28, 29]. By contrast, VLOS has a very large predominance of females, a low family history for schizophrenia, lower risk of childhood maladjustment, possibly higher risk in immigrant populations, and greater abnormalities in brain structures [13].

With respect to delusional disorder, Manglione and coauthors' (2015) literature review identified several risk factors including a family history of schizophrenia or avoidant personality and paranoid or schizoid personality disorder, possible hearing loss, immigrant status, and lower socioeconomic status [10].

Genetics

To date, there have been no published genome-wide association studies of late-onset schizophrenia to allow comparison to the growing body of literature on early-onset schizophrenia. Schizophrenia carries a well-documented heritability risk, ranging from 60 to 85% [30, 31]. A multitude of candidate genes, loci, and noncoding RNAs have been identified over the past decade, with more recent genome-wide association studies (GWAS) increasingly replicating and augmenting these findings. The 2014 study by the Schizophrenia Working Group of the Psychiatric Genomics Consortium, with a sample size of 36,989 subjects and 113,075 controls, demonstrated 108 genomic loci significantly associated with schizophrenia [32]. Importantly, many of the loci identified in this study corroborate currently held pathophysiologic models of schizophrenia and are highly expressed in brain tissue. This study amplified the hypothesis that schizophrenia is a disorder of polygenic risk—with risk spread across genes associated with neurodevelopment, synaptic plasticity and function, immunity, neuronal calcium signaling, neurotransmission (dopamine, glutamate), neuronal ion channels, and suppression of neuronal transcription [21]. Furthermore, this polygenic risk appears to be further enriched by the presence of a family history [33].

To date there is very limited data to provide guidance on the genetic risk determinants of LOS and VLOS. One recent study by Voisey and coauthors pointed to a polymorphism of the DDR2 gene, rs2734839, that may be predictive of late-onset illness [34]. There has been some evidence of more rapid cognitive decline in older adults with schizophrenia after age 65, especially among institutionalized persons. However, there is little evidence that such persons are genetically similar to persons with Alzheimer's disease. For example, Liebers and colleagues, who followed middle-aged and older adults for an average of over 10 years, found evidence of varying degrees of association regarding cognitive function and decline between genetic risk for Alzheimer's disease and polygenic risk for schizophrenia [35]. There is/are little data on the genetic determinants of schizoaffective disorder and delusional disorder in late life.

Neurodevelopment and Neurocircuitry

Schizophrenia

A prevailing theory of the pathogenesis of schizophrenia is one of aberrant neurodevelopment. This has been corroborated by recent genetic findings and further validated by postmortem neurohistological studies showing synaptic changes such as decreased density of dendritic spines in prefrontal neurons and abnormal connectivity in hippocampal neurons [36, 37]. Decreases in brain volume with corresponding increase in size of the ventricles have been reproducibly reported. Functional neuroimaging studies have examined the function and circuitry of the brain in schizophrenia. PET imaging studies have implicated a "hypofrontal" state in schizophrenia, with decreased cerebral metabolism in the frontal cortex and corresponding increases in activity in temporal and occipital cortices [38].

Structural and microstructural changes in LOS and VLOS remain active areas of study. Comparatively, persons with late-onset schizophrenia tend to have increased structural abnormalities and larger thalamic volumes on MRI and may also show changes in white matter integrity

[39–41]. Reduced cerebral blood flow differences have also been noted between EOS and LOS on 99mTc-EDC SPECT, with EOS exhibiting reduced blood flow in the precentral gyrus and inferior frontal gyrus and LOS exhibiting reduced blood flow in the postcentral gyrus bilaterally [42]. A recent study has suggested that age of onset is an important modulating factor in gray matter volume changes, with LOS experiencing relatively less volume loss as compared to EOS [43]. The latter corroborates clinical reports associating earlier age of onset with increased severity of illness. Nevertheless despite these findings, definitive biological markers of schizophrenia with a later onset have been elusive, and no specific neuropathological substrate has been identified [17]. Hahn et al.'s review of neuroimaging studies that compared early-onset and late-onset schizophrenia reported differences in eight of ten studies, but these were not consistent across studies [44].

Delusional Disorder

Two smaller neuroimaging studies of delusional disorder are available, only one of which focuses on older adults. A 1994 study by Howard and colleagues indicates increased lateral ventricle volumes in older adults with delusional disorder which is greater than that of schizophrenics and twice that of controls [45].

Pathophysiology

Schizophrenia spectrum and other psychotic disorders likely represent the manifestation of complex interactions between genetic, neurodevelopmental, environmental, and social stressors.

Schizophrenia and Schizoaffective Disorder

Most of the pathophysiological studies have been conducted on mixed cohorts of individuals with schizophrenia and schizoaffective disorders. There is a confluence of evidence indicating the roles of dopamine, glutamate, serotonin, and GABA in the pathophysiology of schizophrenia [46, 47]; and like many aspects of aging human physiology, there are well-established changes in neurotransmitter concentrations and receptor densities. Age-related declines have been found in dopamine and glutamate concentration, serotonin receptors (5-HT2) and transporter (5-HTT), decreased dopamine- and serotonin-binding capacities, and D1, D2, and D3 receptor densities [48–56]. Notably, D2 receptor density has been shown to decline an additional 5–10% with each decade [57, 58]. Age-related declines in dopamine function are thought to be responsible for frequent neurological complaints in older adults including rigidity, decreased arm swing, and diminished cognitive flexibility [59].

These declines are also likely responsible for increased adverse effect rates in older adults treated with antipsychotic medications which include increased falls, extrapyramidal symptoms (EPS), and mortality [60, 61]. Decreased dosage requirements are also likely explicable through these changes in aging physiology. Increased EPS rates are noted in older adults at lower D2 receptor occupancy rates (34–79%) than expected of younger adults where EPS is rare at occupancy less than 80%. Graff-Guerrero and colleagues proposed aiming for a D2/D3R occupancy of 50–60% to minimize adverse effects and improve disease-specific measures [62]. Moreover, Rajii et al. indicated that antipsychotic dose reduction has the benefit of enhancing overall cognition in addition to EPS reduction [63].

There is a paucity of pathophysiological study of older adults with schizoaffective disorder or delusional disorder.

Diagnosis

Psychotic disorders in the elderly can be a diagnostic dilemma as there can be a multitude of causes. Primary psychotic illnesses are those that are caused by a psychiatric illness, while secondary psychoses are caused by medical or neurological illness.

The differential diagnosis is broad and necessitates obtaining a good clinical history: delirium (onset, days to weeks), psychotic disorder due to another medical condition (onset, days to months), substance-/medication-induced psychotic disorders (onset, days to months), neurocognitive disorders (onset, months to years), affective spectrum disorders with psychotic features (onset, weeks to months), and schizophrenia spectrum disorders (onset, months to decades. Importantly, clinicians should also consider the possibility of elder abuse and neglect in their diagnostic process, as some cases of paranoia or suspiciousness may be justified [64].

When attempting to diagnose the etiology of late-life psychosis, it is important to keep two principles in mind:

1. Roughly 60% of late-life psychotic disorders are secondary psychoses. Thus, one should operate under the assumption that new onset psychotic disorders in the elderly are secondary until proven otherwise.
2. There are no signs/symptoms that are pathognomonic for any type of psychotic illness.

That said, characteristics that may help differentiate secondary psychoses from primary psychotic disorders include acute onset (days to weeks), atypical age of onset, visual hallucinations in the absence of auditory hallucinations, absent family and past psychiatric histories, symptoms that are worse than expected or resistant to treatment, symptoms that occur after a change in personality, symptoms that occur in conjunction with a medical disorder known to cause psychotic symptoms, cognitive abnormalities, and medication/substance abuse [65].

A careful history, including collateral information from family members and caregivers, physical exam, cognitive testing, and collateral history are essential in diagnosis of late-life psychoses. Typical diagnostic testing includes complete blood count (CBC), comprehensive metabolic panel (CMP), thyroid stimulating hormone (TSH), vitamin B12, folate, rapid plasma regain (RPR) and erythrocyte sedimentation rate (ESR), and urine toxicology. A brain MRI or CT scan is often obtained to rule out structural intracranial pathology. Additional tests such as autoimmune panels, HIV, toxicology, and EEG may be ordered on a case-by-case basis [6].

Schizophrenia spectrum disorders should be considered only after other causes are excluded. Following this exclusion, the diagnosis of a primary mental illness should be established for older adults according to DSM-5 diagnostic criteria.

Diagnostic Criteria

- Delusional disorder: Diagnosis requires the presence of at least one delusion for 1 month or greater. Psychosocial functioning is minimally impaired surrounding only the delusional belief. Diagnostic criteria for schizophrenia cannot be simultaneously met, and affective symptoms of limited co-occurrence cannot be better explained by substance use, another medical condition, or another mental disorder [2].
- Brief psychotic disorder, schizophreniform disorder, and schizophrenia: Brief psychotic disorder and schizophreniform disorder are diagnosed in the same way as schizophrenia with only a difference of duration: brief psychotic disorder (1 day to 1 month), schizophreniform disorder (1 month to 6 months), and schizophrenia (greater than 6 months). Psychosocial dysfunction is not necessary for the diagnosis of schizophreniform disorder. A diagnosis of schizophrenia is established when at least two core symptoms of psychosis are present actively for 1 month with signs of illness for greater than 6 months. Psychosocial dysfunction must be present and symptoms cannot be better explained by substance use, another medical condition, or another mental disorder [2].
- Schizoaffective disorder: The diagnosis is established by the concomitant presence of a major mood episode with two core symptoms of psychosis (as in schizophrenia). Delusions or hallucinations must be present for at least 2 weeks without the presence of an affective episode, while an episode of depression or mania must be present for the majority of the person's illness. Psychosocial dysfunction must be present, and symptoms cannot be bet-

ter explained by substance use, another medical condition, or another mental disorder [2].

- Substance-/medication-induced psychotic disorder: The diagnosis requires the presence of delusions or hallucinations that are directly attributable to the neurobiological activity of a substance or medication, and symptoms cannot be better explained by substance use, another medical condition, or another mental disorder [2].
- Psychotic disorder due to another medical condition: This requires the presence of marked delusions or hallucinations with plausible evidence of direct causation by another medical condition, and symptoms cannot be better explained by substance use, another medical condition, or another mental disorder [2].
- Catatonia associated with another mental disorder/medical condition: This is a diagnostic specifier used when at least 3 of the 12 clinical features of catatonia are present during the course of another mental disorder or are directly contributable to another medical condition. These criteria include stupor, catalepsy, waxy flexibility, mutism, negativism, posturing, mannerism, stereotypy, agitation, grimacing, echolalia, and echopraxia [2].

Table 19-2 outlines the clinical differentiation of schizophrenia and schizophrenia spectrum illnesses in late life.

TABLE 19-2. Outlines the clinical differentiation of schizophrenia and schizophrenia spectrum illnesses in late life

	Early-onset schizophrenia	Late-onset schizophrenia	Very late-onset schizophrenia-like psychosis	Schizoaffective disorder	Delusional disorder
Prevalence [8, 9, 14, 16, 20, 25, 66–69]	Lifetime* Ages 45–64, 1% Ages >65, 0.3% 1-year prevalence* Ages 45–64, 0.6% Ages >65, 0.1–0.5%	14–36% of cases 1-year prevalence, 0.14%	1-year prevalence, 0.05%	Lifetime All ages, 0.32% 1-year prevalence Ages <40, 0.09 Ages >40, 0.04	Lifetime All ages, 0.18% 1-year prevalence Ages >60, 0.03%
Age of onset [13, 25]	<40	40–60	>60	<40 (late-onset cases have been reported)	45 (mean)
Gender [68]	Female = male	Female > male	Female >> male	Female > male	Female
Family history [68]	+	+	−	+	+
Early childhood maladjustment [68]	++	+	−	+	Limited available data
Neuroimaging findings [68]	Variable	Variable	>> Incidence of brain abnormality compared to EOS and LOS	Limited available data	Limited available data
Neuropsychological deficits [10, 68]	Deficits [68] + Mild to moderate + Generalized + Heterogeneous + Spared: retention, verbal knowledge	Deficits [68] + Mild to moderate + Generalized + Heterogeneous ++ Spared: retention, verbal knowledge	Variable	Limited available data	Minimal
Cognitive decline/ neurodegeneration [10, 68–70]	Community dwelling: initial decline, then stable compared to healthy, age-matched peers Institutionalized: progressive dementia reported	Initial decline, then stable compared to healthy, age-matched peers	Initial and progressive decline; variable	Limited available data	Minimal

(continued)

TABLE 19-2. (continued)

	Early-onset schizophrenia	Late-onset schizophrenia	Very late-onset schizophrenia-like psychosis	Schizoaffective disorder	Delusional disorder
Minor physical abnormalities [68]	+	+	–	Limited available data	Limited available data
Delusions [2, 13]	+ Persecutory, partition	++ Persecutory, partition	+++ Persecutory, partition	+	+ (Non-bizarre)
Hallucinations [2, 13]	+ Auditory > others	+ Visual, olfactory, tactile more common than in EOS	+ Visual, olfactory, tactile more common than in EOS	+	–
Negative symptoms [2, 13]	++	+	–	+	–
Thought disorder [2, 13, 28]	++	+	–	+/++	–
Affective symptoms [2, 11, 22, 23]	+ Depression common (32 to 75%) [11] + Increased suicide risk	+ Depression + Increased suicide risk	Limited available data	+ Depressed type > bipolar type + Increased suicide risk	–
Dosage requirements [17, 62, 63, 71, 72]	+ Decreased	++ Decreased	++ Decreased	+ Decreased	Limited available data
Tardive dyskinesia risk [73]	+	+	++	+	+
Increased mortality risk [74, 75]	+ Male > female	+ Male > female	++ Male > female	Limited available data	Limited available data

*, likely underestimates; +, associated; ++, strongly associated; +++, very strongly associated; –, not associated

Treatment

The major goals of the treatment for older adults with psychotic symptoms are improving the quality of life, maintaining tenure in the least restrictive setting possible, and limiting admission to acute and long-term care settings. Certain general guidelines should be followed regarding the use of all drugs in older psychotic adults. A pretreatment medical evaluation is essential to all older adults who present with psychotic symptoms. As an individual ages, the ratio of lean body mass decreases, while body fat increases causing changes in distribution and the duration of action for lipophilic psychotropic medications. Thus, the adage "start low, go slow" should be followed closely, using the lowest possible dosage to achieve the desired therapeutic response. Additionally, liquid preparations are readily available for many medications (or can be prepared by compounding pharmacies) and are useful for patients who cannot swallow tablets [76]. In general, the treatment of psychosis in late life is based on the etiology of the illness.

Currently available evidence to guide the pharmacological treatment of older adults with schizophrenia is limited, with available evidence supporting the short-term use of antipsychotic treatment and little guidance available for long-term treatment. Older adults are more likely to suffer from the adverse effects of antipsychotic medications, and treatment should be initiated and maintained cautiously. Typical antipsychotic medications have more favorable metabolic profiles but carry a substantially increased risk of newly incident tardive dyskinesia [77]. Atypical antipsychotics have diminished risk of tardive dyskinesia but are metabolically problematic. Careful consideration of each person's physical state and comorbidities should be undertaken prior to treatment. Initial antipsychotic dosing should be approximately half the normal adult starting dose and increased gradually to the minimum effective dose [78].

The data on the evidence-based pharmacological treatment of late-life LOS and VLOS patients is limited. The most recent Cochrane review on the topic found a dearth of studies meeting their quality criteria to allow for a critical review [79]. Available data for the treatment of EOS in late life indicates possible benefit for the use of risperidone and olanzapine, with limited evidence supporting the use of clozapine in treatment-resistant elderly [80]. Paliperidone has shown efficacy over placebo in the treatment of older adults with schizophrenia [81].

Expert consensus is available regarding recommended dosing: risperidone 1.25–3.5 mg/day (first line), quetiapine 100–300 mg/day, olanzapine 7.5–15 mg/day, and aripiprazole 15–30 mg/day [82]. Extrapyramidal symptoms resulting from treatment are managed similarly to younger adults with emphasis on dose reduction or change of medication to minimize symptoms. Anticholinergic agents should be avoided or used only sparingly—a general rule for all older adults.

There is limited data to suggest tapering and discontinuing antipsychotic medications in older persons with chronic schizophrenia [83]. Potential targets for such a strategy would include one-fourth of older adults who are in long-standing clinical remission or persons whose symptoms have not responded to any anti-antipsychotic medication. Combining the tapering of medication with cognitive behavioral approaches to psychotic symptoms might optimize outcomes. Although it may be impossible to completely eliminate medications in some individuals, dosage reductions may be the option available for these individuals.

Finally, genetic tests are now readily available that can personalize treatment so as to avoid medications that are poorly metabolized and likely to cause more side effects or to identify rapid metabolizers in whom higher doses of medications are required to attain clinical effects.

The greatest benefits for treatment are likely to be found in the combination of pharmacotherapy and psychosocial modalities. While further study is needed, promising work has shown benefit from functional adaptation skills training (FAST), cognitive behavioral social skills training (CBSST), the HOPES intervention (social skills training combined with a preventive healthcare program), and supported employment [84–89].

Conclusion

Schizophrenia spectrum and other psychotic disorders in late life represent a varied group of conditions. Given the aging of the global population, increasing incidence, prevalence, and the associated morbidity and mortality of these psychotic disorders can be expected. These illnesses are best evaluated cautiously and thoroughly recognizing that most psychotic disorders in late life are secondary to other medical conditions. Treatment must be carefully targeted, utilizing minimum effective dosing and making full consideration of each individual's unique history, comorbidity, and pharmacological profiles. Furthermore, attempts to reduce or discontinue antipsychotic treatment must be made at regular intervals to limit associated morbidity and mortality.

References

1. Bürgy M. The concept of psychosis: historical and phenomenological aspects. Schizophr Bull. 2008;34(6):1200–10.
2. Association, A.P. Diagnostic and statistical manual of mental disorders (DSM-5®). Virginia: American Psychiatric Pub; 2013.
3. Holroyd S, Laurie S. Correlates of psychotic symptoms among elderly outpatients. Int J Geriatr Psychiatry. 1999;14(5):379–84.
4. Webster R, Holroyd S. Prevalence of psychotic symptoms in delirium. Psychosomatics. 2000;41(6):519–22.
5. Östling S, et al. Paranoid symptoms and hallucinations among the older people in Western Europe. Int J Geriatr Psychiatry. 2013;28(6):573–9.
6. Reinhardt MM, Cohen CI. Late-life psychosis: diagnosis and treatment. Curr Psychiatry Rep. 2015;17(2):1.
7. Manepalli JN, et al. Differential diagnosis of the older patient with psychotic symptoms. Pri Psychiatry. 2007;14(8):55–62.
8. Castle DJ, Murray RM. The epidemiology of late-onset schizophrenia. Schizophr Bull. 1993;19(4):691–700.

9. Copeland JRM, et al. Schizophrenia and delusional disorder in older age: community prevalence, incidence, comorbidity, and outcome. Schizophr Bull. 1998;24(1):153–61.
10. Maglione JE, Vahia IV, Jeste DV. Schizophrenia spectrum and other psychotic disorders. In: The American Psychiatric publishing textbook of geriatric psychiatry. 5th ed.; 2015.
11. Diwan S, et al. Depression in older adults with schizophrenia spectrum disorders: prevalence and associated factors. Am J Geriatr Psychiatry. 2007;15(12):991–8.
12. Cohen CI, et al. Schizophrenia in later life: clinical symptoms and social well-being. Psychiatr Serv. 2008;59(3):232–4.
13. Howard R, et al. Late-onset schizophrenia and very-late-onset schizophrenia-like psychosis: an international consensus. Am J Psychiatr. 2000;157(2):172–8.
14. Harris MJ, Jeste DV. Late-onset schizophrenia: an overview. Schizophr Bull. 1988;14(1):39.
15. Jeste DV, Wolkowitz OM, Palmer BW. Divergent trajectories of physical, cognitive, and psychosocial aging in schizophrenia. Schizophr Bull. 2011;37(3):451–5.
16. Palmer BW, McClure FS, Jeste DV. Schizophrenia in late life: findings challenge traditional concepts. Harv Rev Psychiatry. 2001;9(2):51–8.
17. Vahia IV, et al. Is late-onset schizophrenia a subtype of schizophrenia? Acta Psychiatr Scand. 2010;122(5):414–26.
18. Howard R, Almeida O, Levy R. Phenomenology, demography and diagnosis in late paraphrenia. Psychol Med. 1994;24(02):397–410.
19. Rajji TK, Mulsant BH. Nature and course of cognitive function in late-life schizophrenia: a systematic review. Schizophr Res. 2008;102(1):122–40.
20. Meesters PD, et al. Schizophrenia spectrum disorders in later life: prevalence and distribution of age at onset and sex in a dutch catchment area. Am J Geriatr Psychiatr. 2012;20(1):18–28.
21. Post F. Schizo-affective symptomatology in late life. Br J Psychiatry. 1971;118(545):437–45.
22. Gupta S, et al. Comparison of older patients with bipolar disorder and schizophrenia/schizoaffective disorder. Am J Geriatr Psychiatry. 2007;15(7):627–33.
23. Baran XY, Young RC. Bipolar and depressive types of schizoaffective disorder in old age. Am J Geriatr Psychiatr. 2006;14(4):382–3.
24. Kendler KS. Demography of paranoid psychosis (delusional disorder): a review and comparison with schizophrenia and affective illness. Arch Gen Psychiatry. 1982;39(8):890–902.
25. Perälä J, et al. Lifetime prevalence of psychotic and bipolar I disorders in a general population. Arch Gen Psychiatry. 2007;64(1):19–28.
26. Maher B. Delusional thinking and cognitive disorder. Integr Physiol Behav Sci. 2005;40(3):136–46.
27. Brunelle S, Cole MG, Elie M. Risk factors for the late-onset psychoses: a systematic review of cohort studies. Int J Geriatr Psychiatry. 2012;27(3):240–52.
28. Jeste DV, et al. Nondementia nonpraecox dementia praecox?: late-onset schizophrenia. Am J Geriatr Psychiatry. 1997;5(4):302–17.
29. Lohr JB, et al. Minor physical anomalies in older patients with late-onset schizophrenia, early-onset schizophrenia, depression, and Alzheimer's disease. Am J Geriatr Psychiatry. 1997;5(4):318–23.
30. MacDonald AW, Schulz SC. What we know: findings that every theory of schizophrenia should explain. Schizophr Bull. 2009;35(3):493–508.
31. Bienvenu O, Davydow D, Kendler K. Psychiatric 'diseases' versus behavioral disorders and degree of genetic influence. Psychol Med. 2011;41(01):33–40.
32. Ripke S, et al. Biological insights from 108 schizophrenia-associated genetic loci. Nature. 2014;511(7510):421.
33. Bigdeli TB, et al. Genome-wide association study reveals greater polygenic loading for schizophrenia in cases with a family history of illness. Am J Med Genet B Neuropsychiatr Genet. 2016;171(2):276–89.
34. Voisey J, et al. A novel DRD2 single-nucleotide polymorphism associated with schizophrenia predicts age of onset: HapMap tag-single-nucleotide polymorphism analysis. Genet Test Mol Biomarkers. 2012;16(2):77–81.
35. Liebers DT, et al. Polygenic risk of schizophrenia and cognition in a population-based survey of older adults. Schizophr Bull. 2016;42(4):984–91.
36. LEWIS DA, et al. Altered cortical glutamate neurotransmission in schizophrenia. Ann N Y Acad Sci. 2003;1003(1):102–12.
37. Harrison PJ. The hippocampus in schizophrenia: a review of the neuropathological evidence and its pathophysiological implications. Psychopharmacology. 2004;174(1):151–62.
38. Ingvar D, Franzén G. Distribution of cerebral activity in chronic schizophrenia. Lancet. 1974;304(7895):1484–6.
39. Sachdev P, et al. Schizophrenia with onset after age 50 years. 2: neurological, neuropsychological and MRI investigation. Br J Psychiatry. 1999;175(5):416–21.

40. Corey-Bloom J, et al. Quantitative magnetic resonance imaging of the brain in late-life schizophrenia. Am J Psychiatr. 1995;152(3):447–9.
41. Chen L, et al. White matter microstructural abnormalities in patients with late-onset schizophrenia identified by a voxel-based diffusion tensor imaging. Psychiatry Res Neuroimaging. 2013;212(3):201–7.
42. Wake R, et al. Regional cerebral blood flow in late-onset schizophrenia: a SPECT study using 99mTc-ECD. Eur Arch Psychiatry Clin Neurosci. 2016;266(1):3–12.
43. Tordesillas-Gutierrez D, et al. Grey matter volume differences in non-affective psychosis and the effects of age of onset on grey matter volumes: a voxelwise study. Schizophr Res. 2015;164(1):74–82.
44. Hahn C, Lim HK, Lee CU. Neuroimaging findings in late-onset schizophrenia and bipolar disorder. J Geriatr Psychiatry Neurol. 2014;27(1):56–62.
45. Howard RJ, et al. Quantitative magnetic resonance imaging volumetry distinguishes delusional disorder from late-onset schizophrenia. Br J Psychiatry. 1994;165(4):474–80.
46. Grace AA. Dysregulation of the dopamine system in the pathophysiology of schizophrenia and depression. Nat Rev Neurosci. 2016;17(8):524–32.
47. Selvaraj S, et al. Alterations in the serotonin system in schizophrenia: a systematic review and meta-analysis of postmortem and molecular imaging studies. Neurosci Biobehav Rev. 2014;45:233–45.
48. Wang Y, et al. Age-dependent decline of dopamine D1 receptors in human brain: a PET study. Synapse. 1998;30(1):56–61.
49. Kaasinen V, et al. Age-related dopamine D2/D3 receptor loss in extrastriatal regions of the human brain. Neurobiol Aging. 2000;21(5):683–8.
50. Chang L, Jiang CS, Ernst T. Effects of age and sex on brain glutamate and other metabolites. Magn Reson Imaging. 2009;27(1):142–5.
51. Iyo M, Yamasaki T. The detection of age-related decrease of dopamine D1, D2 and serotonin 5-HT2 receptors in living human brain. Prog Neuro-Psychopharmacol Biol Psychiatry. 1993;17(3):415–21.
52. Wong DF, et al. Effects of age on dopamine and serotonin receptors measured by positron tomography in the living human brain. Science. 1984;226(4681):1393–6.
53. Rinne JO, Lönnberg P, Marjamäki P. Age-dependent decline in human brain dopamine D1 and D2 receptors. Brain Res. 1990;508(2):349–52.
54. Hof PR, Mobbs CV. Handbook of the neuroscience of aging. Burlington, MA: Academic Press; 2009.
55. Sailasuta N, Ernst T, Chang L. Regional variations and the effects of age and gender on glutamate concentrations in the human brain. Magn Reson Imaging. 2008;26(5):667–75.
56. Yamamoto M, et al. Age-related decline of serotonin transporters in living human brain of healthy males. Life Sci. 2002;71(7):751–7.
57. Wong DF, et al. Quantification of neuroreceptors in the living human brain: IV. Effect of aging and elevations of D2-like receptors in schizophrenia and bipolar illness. J Cereb Blood Flow Metab. 1997;17(3):331–42.
58. Wong DF, et al. Quantification of neuroreceptors in the living human brain: III. D2-like dopamine receptors: theory, validation, and changes during normal aging. J Cereb Blood Flow Metab. 1997;17(3):316–30.
59. Wang E, Snyder DS. Handbok of the aging brain. San Diego: Academic Press; 1998.
60. Finkelstein E, Prabhu M, Chen H. Increased prevalence of falls among elderly individuals with mental health and substance abuse conditions. Am J Geriatr Psychiatry. 2007;15(7):611–9.
61. Ayd FJ. A survey of drug-induced extrapyramidal reactions. JAMA. 1961;175(12):1054–60.
62. Graff-Guerrero A, et al. Evaluation of antipsychotic dose reduction in late-life schizophrenia: a prospective dopamine D2/3 receptor occupancy study. JAMA Psychiat. 2015;72(9):927–34.
63. Rajji TK, et al. Cognition and dopamine D 2 receptor availability in the striatum in older patients with schizophrenia. Am J Geriatr Psychiatry. 2017;25(1):1–10.
64. Vahia IV, Lanouette NM, Jeste DV. Schizophrenia and paranoid disorders. In: Clinical manual of geriatric psychiatry. Virginia: American Psychiatric Publishing; 2013.
65. Marsh L, et al. Psychiatric comorbidities in patients with Parkinson disease and psychosis. Neurology. 2004;63(2):293–300.
66. Robins LN, Regier DA. Psychiatric disorders in America: the epidemiologic catchment area study. New York: Free Press; 1991.
67. Copeland JRM, et al. Alzheimers-disease, other dementias, depression and pseudodementia - prevalence, incidence and 3-year outcome in liverpool. Br J Psychiatry. 1992;161:230–9.
68. Iglewicz A, Meeks TW, Jeste DV. New wine in old bottle: late-life psychosis. Psychiatr Clin N Am. 2011;34(2):295–318.
69. Harvey PD, et al. Cognitive decline in late-life schizophrenia: a longitudinal study of geriatric chronically hospitalized patients. Biol Psychiatry. 1999;45(1):32–40.

70. Davidson M, et al. Severity of symptoms in chronically institutionalized geriatric schizophrenic patients. Am J Psychiatry. 1995;152(2):197–207.
71. Uchida H, et al. Sensitivity of older patients to antipsychotic motor side effects: a PET study examining potential mechanisms. Am J Geriatr Psychiatry. 2009;17(3):255–63.
72. Uchida H, et al. Therapeutic window for striatal dopamine D 2/3 receptor occupancy in older patients with schizophrenia: a pilot PET study. Am J Geriatr Psychiatry. 2014;22(10):1007–16.
73. Jeste DV. Tardive dyskinesia in older patients. J Clin Psychiatry. 2000;61(Suppl 4):27–32.
74. Meesters PD, et al. Mortality and its determinants in late-life schizophrenia: a 5-year prospective study in a Dutch catchment area. Am J Geriatr Psychiatry. 2016;24(4):272–7.
75. Talaslahti T, et al. Patients with very-late-onset schizoprhenia-like psychosis have higher mortality rates than elderly patients with earlier onset schizophrenia. Int J Geriatr Psychiatry. 2015;30(5):453–9.
76. Sadock BJ, Ruiz P, Sadock VA. In: Sadock BJ, Ruiz P, Sadock VA, editors. Kaplan & Sadock's synopsis of psychiatry: behavioral sciences/ clinical psychiatry. 11th ed. Philadelphia, PA: Lippincott Williams & Wilkins; 2015.
77. Jeste D, et al. Conventional vs. newer antipsychotics in elderly patients. Am J Geriatr Psychiatry. 1999;7(1):70.
78. Lehman AF, et al. Practice guideline for the treatment of partients with schizophrenia. Am J Psychiatr. 2004;161(2 Suppl):1–56.
79. Essali A, Ali G. Antipsychotic drug treatment for elderly people with late-onset schizophrenia. Cochrane Database Syst Rev. 2012;2:CD004162.
80. Rothenberg KG, et al. Clozapine in geriatric population-clinical indication and safety monitoring. Am J Geriatr Psychiatry. 22(3):S73–S74.
81. Tzimos A, et al. Safety and tolerability of oral paliperidone extended-release tablets in elderly patients with schizophrenia: a double-blind, placebo-controlled study with six-month open-label extension. Am J Geriatr Psychiatry. 2008;16(1):31–43.
82. Alexopoulos GS, Streim JE, Carpenter D. Commentary: expert consensus guidelines for using antipsychotic agents in older patients. J Clin Psychiatry. 2004;65(suppl 2):100–2.
83. Takeuchi H, et al. Effects of risperidone and olanzapine dose reduction on cognitive function in stable patients with schizophrenia: an open-label, randomized, controlled, pilot study. Schizophr Bull. 2013;39(5):993–8.
84. Granholm E, et al. A randomized, controlled trial of cognitive behavioral social skills training for middle-aged and older outpatients with chronic schizophrenia. Am J Psychiatry. 2005;162(3):520–9.
85. Granholm E, et al. Randomized controlled trial of cognitive behavioral social skills training for older people with schizophrenia: 12-month follow-up. J Clin Psychiatry. 2007;68(5):730–7.
86. Patterson TL, et al. Functional Adaptation Skills Training (FAST): a randomized trial of a psychosocial intervention for middle-aged and older patients with chronic psychotic disorders. Schizophr Res. 2006;86(1–3):291–9.
87. Bartels SJ, et al. Long-term outcomes of a randomized trial of integrated skills training and preventive healthcare for older adults with serious mental illness. Am J Geriatr Psychiatry. 2014;22(11):1251–61.
88. Mueser KT, et al. Randomized trial of social rehabilitation and integrated health care for older people with severe mental illness. J Consult Clin Psychol. 2010;78(4):561–73.
89. Cohen-Mansfield J, Libin A, Marx MS. Nonpharmacological treatment of agitation: a controlled trial of systematic individualized intervention. J Gerontol A Biol Sci Med Sci. 2007;62(8):908–16.

20 Substance-Related and Addictive Disorders

Rachel D. Maree and Craig A. Riccelli

Introduction

Substance use is a widely recognized medical and public health problem affecting patients across the lifespan [1]. The US Census Bureau has estimated that the population aged 65 years and older will be 72.1 million in 2030, almost double its estimated population of 40.3 million in 2010. This significant increase is due to the aging of the baby boomer cohort, as they began turning 65 years old in 2011 [2]. It has been established that substance use disorders both exist and persist among older adults [3]. As the baby boomers, who have had higher rates of substance use than those previously 65+ continue to age, it is estimated that older adults will have increasing rates of substance use, likely due to cohort effects. In fact, it is estimated that at least 5.7 million Americans aged 50 years and older (50+) will need substance misuse treatment in the year 2020 [4, 5]. Majority of substance use literature to date as it relates to older adults has been published on alcohol. There is limited published research on national prevalence rates of other specific substance use disorders among older adults and even fewer investigations into specialized treatments and interventions targeted toward this age group. As the baby boomer generation continues to age, older adults will increasingly present for first time substance use treatment [6]. The aging of the baby boomer cohort and the noted increase in substance use among those 65+ are areas of concern that require special thought for practitioners and providers.

Epidemiology

Alcohol

Previous National Survey on Drug Use and Health (NSDUH) results have shown significant levels of current, binge and heavy alcohol use for persons age 50+ [7]. The 2013 NSDUH results showed that 41.7% of adults aged 65+ used alcohol within the past month and considered 9.1% of those users to engage in binge drinking (5+ drinks on same occasion on at least 1 day in the past 30 days) and 2.1% to engage in heavy alcohol use (5+ drinks on same occasion on 5+ days in the past 30 days) [8]. Of note, estimates of alcohol problems are higher among health-care seeking populations as drinkers are more likely to seek medical care [9]. Older adults with medical, social, and emotional problems are also at higher risk for alcohol and other substance use, and this substance use can aggravate other medical comorbidities [10]. In a 2010 study of 3308 drinkers aged 60+ in primary care clinics, 21.5% of participants were identified as at risk of harm due to combined use of alcohol in the context of comorbidities, 21.2% were noted to be at risk of harm due to combined use of alcohol and medications, and 22.3% were found to be at risk based on alcohol use alone. Over half of the participants (56.1%) fell into more than one risk category [11].

Cannabis

Data from the 1999 to 2001 NSDUH estimated that 719,000 older adults aged 50+ used marijuana

R. R. Tampi et al. (eds.), *Psychiatric Disorders Late in Life*, https://doi.org/10.1007/978-3-319-73078-3_20

in the past year (1.1% of older adults). This was estimated to increase to 3.3 million in 2020 (355% increase), reflecting the increase in population and a 190% increase in rate of marijuana use, from 1.0 to 2.9% [12]. Based on data from the NSDUH from 2005 to 2006, 2.6% of respondents reported marijuana use in the last year. The use of marijuana was more prevalent in the 50–64 age groups (4%), rather than 65+ group (0.7%). This data also found that major depression was associated with higher prevalence of marijuana use (6.54%). Other subsets of the population associated with higher prevalence of marijuana use were sex (male 3.96% vs. female 1.39%), race/ethnicity (highest being American Indian or Alaskan Native 5.29% followed by African-American 3.78%), and marital status (never married, 5.23%) [13]. In 2012, 4.6 million adults aged 50+ reported past-year marijuana use [14]. These numbers reflect a rapid increase in the number of older adult marijuana users than previously projected. Nearly half of the United States and Washington D.C. have legalized marijuana use in some capacity. The increasing number of states legalizing the use of medicinal marijuana and decriminalizing recreational use will likely contribute to the rapidly growing number of older adult marijuana users [15].

Tobacco

Estimates have shown that among adults aged 65+, 14% reported tobacco use in the last 12 months. Another study estimates that nearly seven million adults aged 60+ are smokers [16]. Older adult smokers also tend to be long-term, heavy smokers. Tobacco use is independently associated with greater mortality, including increased risks of coronary events, cardiac deaths, smoking-related cancers, chronic obstructive lung disease, decline in pulmonary function, development of osteoporosis, risk of hip fractures, and poorer physical functioning. Rates of cardiovascular disease among adults 50+ are higher among individuals with comorbid drug use and cigarette smoking as compared to individuals with drug use alone (74 vs. 44%, respectively). Similarly, rates of pulmonary disease are higher in the comorbid smoking and drug use group as well (38 vs. 13%, respectively) [14, 17]. These stark differences highlight the potentially adverse physiologic effects of tobacco use.

Prescription Drug Use

The number of older adults age 50+ misusing prescription substances, defined as using pain relievers, stimulants, tranquilizers, and sedatives without a prescription or taking them for the feeling or experience they caused) is projected to increase approximately 190%, from 911,000 based on 1999 to 2001 data to 2.7 million in 2020. This reflects a doubling in the rate of use from 1.2 to 2.4%. Men accounted for 44% of prescription drug misuse in 1999–2001 and are expected to account for 52% in 2020. The age distribution in 1999–2001 showed 62% in their 50s and 19% in their 60s; in 2020, the age distribution of projected users is expected to show 48% in their 50s and 37% in their 60s, reflecting a significant increase in an almost 20-year time span [4]. In 2007, 4.62% of Medicare Part D recipients received greater than 90 days of prescriptions for combined schedule II/III opioids, and this percentage was noted to be 7.35% in 2012 [18]. Factors associated with prescription drug abuse in older adults include female sex, social isolation, history of a substance use or mental health disorder, and medical exposure to prescription drugs with abuse potential [19].

In 2007, an analysis of the Treatment Episode Data Set (TEDS) that assesses national admissions to substance abuse treatment services found that methamphetamine/ amphetamine was the primary substance for 7.87% (142,832 admissions) of all admissions, of which 3.75% were 50+. Other stimulants were the primary substances for 896 admissions, of which 8.4% were age 50+ [20, 21]. Data from 2013 showed that amphetamines and other stimulants were the primary substances used for 8.2% of admissions with the following age distributions: 51–55, 7.5%, 56–60, 2.9%, 61–65, 0.8%, and 66+ 0.1% [22]. These data do not show dramatic changes in the percentages for this demographic but do show that stimulant use among older adults has been consistent and should not be overlooked.

Illicit Substance Use

Based upon the 1999–2001 data, the overall number of illicit drug users, characterized in this study as marijuana, cocaine, inhalants, hallucinogens, heroin, and prescription type psychotherapeutic drugs, is projected to increase from 1.6 to 3.5 million in 2020. The sex distribution of users is expected to remain stable at 48% women and 52% men. Distribution by race/ethnicity will not change radically, but the proportion in their 50s will decline from 74 to 51%, whereas representation of persons in their 60s is expected to increase from 14 to 37% [4].

Neurobiology Including Risk Factors

Many neurotransmitters are involved in the effects of various types of drugs of abuse (Table 20-1). However, dopamine has been shown to have significant effects on reinforcing use. Research has shown that drugs of abuse promote faster and longer extracellular dopamine release than other natural factors that reinforce drug use. This increase in dopamine can occur by inhibiting dopamine reuptake from the synaptic cleft or by promoting the release of dopamine into the cytoplasm [23].

Urine drug screens are useful for screening and as confirmation of verbal reports of substance use. Depending on the type of drug and frequency of use, it can be detected in the urine up to periods ranging from 12 h to several weeks.

TABLE 20-1. Neurotransmitter targets of commonly misused substances [24]

Drug	Neurotransmitter
Cocaine, amphetamines	Dopamine, serotonin, norepinephrine
Opioids	Endogenous opiates
Nicotine	Acetylcholine
Alcohol	GABA, glutamate
Marijuana	Endogenous cannabinoids
PCP, ketamine	Glutamate
LSD and other hallucinogens	Serotonin

GABA, γ-aminobutyric acid; *PCP*, Phencyclidine; *LSD*, lysergic acid diethylamide

Additional biomarkers have been studied for alcohol use. Liver function tests, including alanine transaminase (ALT), aspartate transaminase (AST), and gamma-glutamyl transpeptidase (GGT), can be tested in the blood and are sometimes used as indicators of chronic or more acute alcohol use. It should be noted that elevations in these biomarkers are not specific to alcohol use. Other markers of chronic alcohol use include percent carbohydrate-deficient transferrin (% CDT), mean corpuscular volume (MCV), and high-density lipoproteins (HDL), each of which would be elevated in the setting of chronic alcohol use [25].

Adverse events associated with substance use in older adults are in part related to altered hepatic metabolism and changing proportions of body fat and water which may impact effective dosing of various substances. Drug interactions also increase with age due to the likelihood of a higher number of pharmacologic agents being prescribed and because of changes in metabolism associated with age [26, 27].

Diagnosis

The general diagnostic criteria from the *Diagnostic and Statistical Manual of Mental Disorders* Fifth Edition (DSM-5) can be found in Table 20-2. These criteria can be applied to all

TABLE 20-2. DSM-5 substance use criteria and considerations for older adults [28, 29]

DSM-5 substance use disorder criteria At least two of the following over a 12-month period	Considerations for DSM criteria in older adults
Substance is taken in larger amounts or over a longer period than was intended	Substance use can exacerbate cognitive impairment and ability to self-monitor
Persistent desire or unsuccessful efforts to cut down or control substance use	
A great deal of time is spent in activities necessary to obtain, use, or recover from effects of substance	

(continued)

TABLE 20-2. (continued)

DSM-5 substance use disorder criteria At least two of the following over a 12-month period	Considerations for DSM criteria in older adults
Craving or a strong desire or urge to use substance	Older adults may have chronic habits related to substance use that they do not identify as cravings
Recurrent use resulting in a failure to fulfill major role obligations at work, school, or home	Role obligations for older adults can be significantly different given life transitions (i.e., retirement)
Continued use despite persistent or recurrent social or interpersonal problems caused or exacerbated by the effects of the substance	Older adults may have limited insight regarding substance use as a cause of their problems
Important social, occupational, or recreational activities are given up or reduced because of use	Older adults may not have a reduction in these activities despite substance use
Recurrent use in situations in which it is physically hazardous Use is continued despite knowledge of having a persistent or recurrent physical or psychological problem that is likely to have been caused or exacerbated by the substance	Older adults may have limited insight regarding substance use as a cause of their problems
Tolerance—need for markedly increased amounts OR markedly diminished effect with continued use of the same amount	Older adults can have increased sensitivity due to physiological changes with metabolism
Withdrawal—the characteristic withdrawal syndrome OR substance is taken to relieve or avoid withdrawal symptoms	May not develop physiologic dependence depending on the onset and type of substance used

classes of substances with the exception of caffeine. Severity of substance use disorders as per the DSM can be defined as mild (2–3 symptoms), moderate (4–5 symptoms), and severe (6 or more symptoms).

Complicating the identification of substance misuse problems in late life is the fact that substance use or intoxication may present similarly to depression, delirium, or dementia [30, 31]. Hence, practitioners should make every effort to screen and assess for these comorbidities that may present similarly or in addition to comorbid substance use. Data from the 2009 NSDUH found that some of the DSM-5 criteria, as listed in Table 20-2, need special consideration in older adults due to the physiology of aging and unique social circumstances older adults may face. With this in mind, strictly using the DSM-5 may result in under diagnosis of older adults with SUDs [14].

Another approach in diagnosing older adults with SUDs is a two-tier categorical classification: at risk and problem use. The first tier is defined by use of a substance more than the recommended amount. Problem use emphasizes the potential negative impact associated with use instead of the quantity and frequency of use [14]. When considering prescribed substances, there is also the potential for misuse of substances. Misuse can include adjusting doses without direction from a prescriber, unintentionally taking larger doses than prescribed or taking medication for indications other than the intended use [32]. Assessment for misuse may help patients adhere to medications as prescribed and reduce the potential for adverse effects associated with some prescription medications.

Most of the screening and diagnostic research in older adults has been done with alcohol. The National Institute on Alcohol Abuse and Alcoholism (NIAAA) and the American Geriatrics Society (AGS) recommend no more than three drinks per day or seven drinks per week for adults over age 65 who are healthy and do not take medications [33]. There are several tools that can be used to screen and assess for alcohol use in older adults.

The CAGE questionnaire is a brief measure that asks four lifetime questions regarding cutting down use, being annoyed by others, feeling guilty about use, and needing an eye-opener in the morning. More than two responses indicate substance use disorder. A major limitation of the CAGE is that it does not distinguish between current and lifetime use. This is an especially difficult issue among those who are aging and have a history of problematic use without having a current problem. Because of the brief nature of the CAGE, it can be a useful screening tool, but it should not be a substitute for a more thorough assessment. It also does poorly in detecting heavy or binge drinkers. In a study assessing potentially hazardous alcohol use among 5065 patients aged 60+ in primary care settings, the CAGE had 35% sensitivity and 96% specificity in detecting binge drinkers [34]. The CAGE-AID, with the AID meaning adapted to include drugs, is a modified version of the CAGE that assesses for alcohol and other drug use as well. It has not been validated in older adults.

The Michigan Alcohol Screening Test comes in a geriatric form (MAST-G) and a short, geriatric form (S-MAST-G) (Table 20-3). Both are used to identify those at risk for negative outcomes related to alcohol use. The MAST-G focuses more on potential stressors and behaviors relevant to alcohol use in late life, as opposed to questions toward family, vocational, and legal consequences of use. The short version has ten questions with two or more positive responses indicating a positive test. Although useful as an indicator of lifetime problem use, it lacks information about frequency, quantity, and current problems important for intervention [14, 35].

The AUDIT was developed and validated in older adults to identify formal alcohol disorders and hazardous drinkers. In a sample of almost 200 adults aged 65+ in primary care centers, the AUDIT was found to have a sensitivity of 66.7% and specificity of 95.3%. The AUDIT-C, which is a shorter version of the AUDIT, had a sensitivity of 100% and specificity of 80.7%. The cutoff threshold to indicate alcohol use disorder among a general population is eight. The AUDIT uses amount of drinking to define hazardous drinking, which may be useful in younger populations, but in older adults, the consideration of any amount of drinking must be weighed with other medical comorbidities and social and environmental problems [36, 37].

TABLE 20-3. Short Michigan alcohol screening test-geriatric (S-MAST-G) [14, 35]

1. When talking with others, do you ever underestimate how much you drink?
2. After a few drinks, have you sometimes not eaten or been able to skip a meal because you didn't feel hungry?
3. Does having a few drinks help decrease your shakiness or tremors?
4. Does alcohol sometimes make it hard for you to remember parts of the day or night?
5. Do you usually take a drink to relax or calm your nerves?
6. Do you drink to take your mind off your problems?
7. Have you ever increased your drinking after experiencing a loss in your life?
8. Has your doctor or nurse ever said they were worried or concerned about your drinking?
9. Have you ever made rules to manage your drinking?
10. When you feel lonely, does having a drink help?

To date, there have not been any validated screening measures developed to assess for misuse of other substances in older adults. However, smaller studies have provided some ideas for screening and monitoring. There are screening tools available for benzodiazepine misuse, such as the benzodiazepine dependence self-report questionnaire and the severity of dependence scale [38, 39]. Asking about tolerance and attempts to stop have the greatest evidence as screening measures for older adults with benzodiazepine misuse [40]. Additionally, as substance use in older adults continues to be researched and understood, it will be important for practitioners to familiarize themselves with the most recent legal and medical regulations when evaluating older adults for cannabis use disorder [14].

Treatments

The proportion of older adults seeking substance abuse treatment for the first time is growing at a rate faster than that of younger adults, making the focus on the specific needs of this population crucial [41]. Many of the well-studied interventions for older adults with substance use disorders have been conducted with alcohol. Nonetheless, evidence thus far shows that older adults do engage in substance use treatment, are able to complete treatment, and tend to respond well to age-appropriate interventions [42–45]. While there remains much to be discovered in order to tailor non-pharmacologic interventions toward this population, research thus far is promising.

Non-pharmacologic

Alcohol

Non-pharmacologic treatments for alcohol use disorders in the geriatric population have been studied in various settings. Older adults may benefit from community options, including twelve-step groups such as "Alcoholics Anonymous" and other self-help groups; however, it is important to consider mobility and travel when making these recommendations [46]. Non-pharmacologic interventions have also been studied in inpatient and outpatient settings as well.

The Florida Brief Intervention and Treatment for Elders (BRITE) project, a 3-year pilot program of screening and brief intervention for older adult substance misusers, demonstrated improvements by using a series of brief interventions that included completion of a workbook and cognitive behavioral therapy (CBT) sessions [45, 47]. Additional studies have shown the benefits of addressing alcohol misuse in the primary care setting and utilizing other modes and combinations of treatment including one randomized controlled trial where there were reductions in the amount of drinking at 12 months with multifaceted treatment approach that included a personalized report, booklet about alcohol and aging, a drinking diary, brief advice from a care provider, and telephone counseling [48]. Other modes of treatment can include motivational interviewing (MI), contracting with a physician, CBT, and using care coordination services to maintain long-term sobriety. Positive effects have been noted from these modes of treatment in reducing alcohol use among older adults [45, 49].

Cannabis

Overall, there is a dearth of literature for non-pharmacologic treatment of cannabis use disorder in older adults. However, available evidence indicates efficiency for motivational enhancement therapy (MET), CBT, and contingency management. According to the literature, combining all three modalities had the best results, specifically in reducing frequency and quantity of use [50].

Tobacco

In a study that evaluated treatments specifically tailored for individuals aged 50–74 years, the investigators found that this population prefers clear evidence of the negative consequences of smoking [16]. In addition, they found that potential medical problems associated with smoking are a motivating factor for cessation of tobacco use. Furthermore, this study found that self-help was preferred to group programs for smoking cessation. The smoking cessation guide for smokers aged 50–74 years, "Clear Horizons," was developed based on the findings from this study. After 12 months, the self-reported quit rate of standard versus tailored treatment was 15 and 20%, respectively. Motivational interviewing has been shown to be effective for smoking cessation in older adults [51]. In a study examining MI-enhanced care in older adults, there was a statistically significant increase in attempts to stop smoking and decrease in number of cigarettes smoked that was demonstrated for as long as 12 months post intervention.

Prescription Drugs

Available evidence indicates that sending an intervention letter advising patients to gradually taper their benzodiazepine use, assessing benzodiazepine craving in a treatment intervention aimed at long-term benzodiazepine users, conducting brief interventions, and providing self-help booklets from primary care physicians are methods that can be utilized in the outpatient setting to target prescription drug misuse among older adults [3–5, 31, 47, 52, 53]. Other community and self-help groups like "Narcotics Anonymous," adapted from Alcoholics Anonymous are available for individuals with prescription drug to utilize to reduce their substance use.

Pharmacological

Alcohol

Older adults are at higher risk for medical complications during alcohol withdrawal including myocardial ischemia, delirium tremens, and convulsions when compared to the younger adults [54]. Short-acting benzodiazepines, specifically lorazepam and oxazepam, are recommended for management of acute withdrawal among these individuals. Given the potential physiological changes associated with aging, the effective dosages of these medications are less than those required among the general adult population. Additionally, lorazepam and oxazepam are not hepatically metabolized and can be safely taken by individuals with liver dysfunction [55].

One randomized controlled trial demonstrated that older adults with alcohol use disorder who were given naltrexone were significantly less likely to relapse when exposed to alcohol when compared to the control group of older adults who did not receive naltrexone [14]. The long-acting, injectable formulation of naltrexone may be particularly helpful in older adults with cognitive disorders [54].

Acamprosate has been shown to be effective for alcohol use disorder among older adults with treatment outcomes similar to the general adult population; however, there are no controlled studies assessing the efficacy of this medication specifically for older adults [14]. Studies that have looked at outcomes when combining naltrexone and acamprosate have found limited efficacy for the combined treatment among individuals with alcohol use disorders [54].

Disulfiram has demonstrated some benefit in adults 50+ with alcohol use disorder, but given the significant adverse effects including increased cardiovascular strain associated with its use, it is generally not recommended for use among older adults [14, 54] (Table 20-4).

Although not FDA approved for alcohol use disorder, topiramate and gabapentin are being researched as potential treatments for this disorder. The adverse side effect profile of topiramate, including effects on cognition and increased risk of falls, should be taken into account when considering this medication as a possible treatment for alcohol use disorders among older adults [58]. It should also be taken into account that gabapentin has the potential for misuse and should be prescribed with caution among the older adult population [59].

Cannabis

Based on the most recent review of the available literature, no specific pharmacological agents have demonstrated clear efficacy for treatment of cannabis use disorder in the general adult population or for the older adult population. One study did find a significant decrease in cannabis use among adults with comorbid depression when treated with fluoxetine. Medications such as nefazodone, extended-release bupropion, dronabinol, divalproex, and buspirone have been researched in the general population with non-specific results. As the number of older adults with cannabis use disorder continues to rise, this area proves to be imperative for future research [50].

TABLE 20-4. FDA-approved medications for alcohol dependence [56, 57]

Medication	Naltrexone	Acamprosate	Disulfiram
Dosage	Oral: 50 mg/day OR 100 mg on Monday and Wednesday and 150 mg on Friday Injectable: 380 mg every 4 weeks	666 mg three times daily	250–500 mg/day; do not take until 12 h after drinking
Mechanism of action	Opioid receptor antagonist	Reduces excitatory glutamate transmission; blocks certain glutamate receptors; increases inhibitory GABA transmission	Aldehyde dehydrogenase inhibitor
General physiologic considerations	Cannot be used in patients using opioid therapy	Can be used in patients prescribed opioids for pain control	Tachycardia, diaphoresis, nausea, and vomiting can be experienced if alcohol is used with this medication
Adverse side effects	Dizziness, headache, GI distress	Diarrhea, nausea	Dermatitis, drowsiness, metallic taste
Special considerations	Use with caution in those with decreased liver function	Can be used in patients with severe liver disease; cautious use in patients with renal insufficiency/ chronic renal failure	Avoid in patients with cognitive impairment, cardiac disease, severe liver disease, or alcohol intoxication

Tobacco

Nicotine replacement therapy (NRT), bupropion, and varenicline are all effective and safe pharmacologic agents for tobacco cessation in the general adult population; however, these have been understudied in the geriatric population [60]. There are a variety of NRT products available in the United States, both prescription and over the counter (OTC). The OTC products include the patch, lozenge, and gum, while the prescription products include nasal spray and an oral inhaler each of which has special considerations in older adults (Table 20-5). Of note, a nicotine mouth spray and sublingual tablet are available in other countries but not in the United States [61].

It has been shown that older adults metabolize nicotine slower than young adults; however, it has not been empirically demonstrated that this impacts efficacy of NRT. There is a theoretical risk of increased cardiovascular events with NRT; however, the risk is less than that associated with active tobacco use. Although studies have not demonstrated an increased risk, special consideration should be used with NRT in older adults immediately following a cardiovascular event [60]. Combination NRT (patch plus gum or lozenge) has been shown to be more efficacious in the general population without clear evidence if this is consistent with older adults [61].

Bupropion has been shown to be effective in smoking cessation in adults; however, there is a dearth of information regarding its efficacy among older adults. Blood pressure should be monitored before and during treatment with bupropion. This medication is known to lower the seizure threshold and is contraindicated in those with seizure disorders or certain conditions with high seizure risk [56]. The two most common adverse effects among individuals taking bupropion for smoking cessation are insomnia and dry mouth with discontinuation rates around 10%. The most recent review did not detect a significant difference between bupropion and NRT [60]. The recommended dosing of varenicline is no different in the geriatric population when compared to the general population. Special consideration should be given when using this medication in older adults with comorbid psychiatric conditions as there is limited data for this specific patient population [56]. The most recent review for older adults is limited but suggests that it is more efficacious than bupropion and NRT [60].

Illicit and Prescription Drug Use

There are no widespread, validated measures of treatment for substance use disorders, namely, opioid and sedative/hypnotic/anxiolytic use disorders in older adults. However, previous studies have shown that engaging older adults in a slow, stepwise taper (reduction of 25% of dose every 2 weeks) for benzodiazepines has been effective with reduced risk of complex side effects [63]. Older adults are and will also be engaged in various treatment modalities for drugs including methadone, buprenorphine, buprenorphine/naloxone, and naltrexone, but there are limited studies assessing differences in treatment need and special considerations for this population. Medical comorbidities should be considered when starting or continuing these treatments in older adults. Recent research on pharmacological interventions for cocaine use disorder includes

TABLE 20-5. Nicotine replacement therapy (NRT) and special considerations for older adults [62]

Type of NRT	Available dosage	Side effects	Considerations in older adults
Patch	7 mg, 14 mg and 21 mg	Local skin irritation	Daily dosing, which may be particularly beneficial in those with cognitive
Gum	2 mg and 4 mg	Buccal mucous irritation, sore jaw and nicotine related as listed below	Requires specific dosing for maximal results; should not be use in those with poor dentition, temporomandibular joint disorders, or dental appliances
Lozenge	2 mg and 4 mg	Abdominal pain, nausea, vomiting, diarrhea, headache, and palpitations	Easier to use than gum

clinical trials assessing medications impacting the dopamine neurotransmitter pathways, a cocaine vaccine, and plant-based therapy. None of these interventions have been specifically studied in older adults [64]. Studies assessing the efficacy of gabapentin for cocaine use disorder have shown this approach to be inappropriate. Gabapentin has also been shown to be ineffective in treating methamphetamine and opioid use disorders [59].

Conclusion

Substance use among older adults provides a unique challenge with regard to both diagnosis and treatment. This chapter highlights the most up-to-date review of the available literature including specialized diagnostic approach and treatment modalities. Most of the evidence basis is for alcohol use; however, epidemiologic studies show the high prevalence of other substance use including cannabis, prescription medications, and illicit substances. The use of these substances is projected to significantly increase as the aging baby boomer generation ages. Given this projected demand for treatment of substance use among older adults, it is imperative that there be continued research for additional epidemiological data in addition to further studies that target specific treatments and interventions for older adults.

References

1. Schulden J, Lopez M, Compton W. Clinical implications of drug abuse epidemiology. Psychiatr Clin North Am. 2012;35(2):411–23. https://doi.org/10.1016/j.psc.2012.03.007.Clinical.
2. Ortman J, Velkoff V, Hogan H. An aging nation: the older population in the United States. Current population reports. http://www.census.gov/library/publications/2014/demo/p25-1140.html. Published 2014. Accessed 5 April 2016.
3. Reynolds K, Pietrzak RH, El-Gabalawy R, Mackenzie CS, Sareen J. Prevalence of psychiatric disorders in U. S. older adults: findings from a nationally representative survey. World Psychiatry. 2015;14(1):74–81. https://doi.org/10.1002/wps.20193.
4. Han B, Gfroerer J, Colliver J, Penne M. Substance use disorder among older adults in the United States in 2020. Addiction. 2009;104(1):88–96.
5. Gfroerer J, Penne M, Pemberton M, Folsom R. Substance abuse treatment need among older adults in 2020: the impact of the aging baby-boom cohort. Drug Alcohol Depend. 2003;69(2):127–35.
6. Centers for Disease Control and Prevention. Vital signs: overdoses of prescription opioid pain relievers -- United States, 1999-2008. Morb Mortal Wkly Rep. 2011;60(43):1487–92.
7. Blazer DG, Wu L-T. The epidemiology of at-risk and binge drinking among middle-aged and elderly community adults national survey on drug use and health. Psychiatry Interpers Biol Process. 2011;166(10):1162–9. https://doi.org/10.1176/appi.ajp.2009.09010016.
8. U.S. Department of Health and Human Services Substance Abuse and Mental Health Services Administration (SAMSHA). Results from the 2013 national survey on drug use and health: summary of national findings. Rockville, MD; 2013.
9. Oslin D. Late-life alcoholism: issues relevant to the geriatric psychiatrist. Am J Geriatr Psychiatry. 2004;12(6):571–83.
10. Lynskey M, Day C, Hall W. Alcohol and other drug use disorders among older-aged people. Drug Alcohol Rev. 2003;22(2):125–33.
11. Barnes AJ, Moore AA, Xu H, et al. Prevalence and correlates of at-risk drinking among older adults: the project SHARE study. J Gen Intern Med. 2010;25(8):840–6. https://doi.org/10.1007/s11606-010-1341-x.
12. Dinitto DM, Choi NG. Marijuana use among older adults in the U.S.A.: user characteristics, patterns of use, and implications for intervention. Int Psychogeriatr. 2011;23(5):732–41. https://doi.org/10.1017/S1041610210002176.
13. Blazer DG, Wu L-T. The epidemiology of substance use and disorders among middle aged and elderly community adults: national survey on drug use and health (NSDUH). Am J Geriatr Psychiatry. 2009;17(3):237–45. https://doi.org/10.1097/JGP.0b013e318190b8ef.
14. Kuerbis A, Sacco P, Blazer DG, Moore AA. Substance abuse among older adults. Clin Geriatr Med. 2014;30(3):629–54. https://doi.org/10.1016/j.cger.2014.04.008.
15. ProCon.org. 24 legal medical marijuana states and DC. Medical marijuana home. http://medicalmarijuana.procon.org/view.resource.php?resourceID=000881. Published 2004. Accessed 1 Jan 2016.
16. Rimer BK, Orleans CT. Tailoring smoking cessation for older adults. Cancer. 1994;74(7 Suppl):2051–4.

17. Li-Tzy W, Blazer DG. Illicit and nonmedical drug use among older adults: a review. J Aging Health. 2011;23(3):481–504. https://doi.org/10.1177/0898264310386224.Illicit.
18. Kuo YF, Raji MA, Chen NW, Hasan H, Goodwin JS. Trends in opioid prescriptions among part D medicare recipients from 2007 to 2012. Am J Med. 2015;129(221):21–30. https://doi.org/10.1016/j.amjmed.2015.10.002.
19. Simoni-Wastila L, Yang H. Psychoactive drug abuse in older adults. Am J Geriatr Pharmacother. 2006;4(4):380–94.
20. Kalapatapu RK, Sullivan MA. Prescription use disorders in older adults. Am J Addict. 2010;19(6):515–22. https://doi.org/10.1111/j.1521-0391.2010.00080.x.
21. Becker W, Tobin D, Feillin D. Nonmedical use of opioid analgesics obtained directly from physicians: prevalence and correlates. Arch Intern Med. 2011;171(11):1034–5.
22. Center for Behavioral Health Statistics and Quality Substance Abuse and Mental Health Services Administration. Treatment episode data set (TEDS). April 2016. http://wwwdasis.samhsa.gov/webt/quicklink/US13.htm. Published 2013. Accessed 1 April 2016.
23. Volkow N, Warren K. Drug addiction: the neurobiology of behavior gone awry. In: Ries RK, Fiellin DA, Miller SC, Saitz R, editors. The ASAM principles of addiction medicine. Fifth ed. Beijing: Wolters Kluwer; 2014. p. 4–5.
24. Moeller FG. Drug abuse and dependence. In: Nabel E, Federman D, editors. Scientific American medicine. Hamilton, ON: Decker Intellectual Properties; 2016. p. 1–16. https://doi.org/10.2310/7900.1191.
25. Mavandadi S, Oslin D. Substance-related and addictive disorders. In: Steffens D, Blazer D, Thakur M, editors. The American psychiatric publishing textbook of geriatric psychiatry. 5th ed. Arlington, VA: American Psychiatric Publishing; 2015.
26. Ries RK, Fiellin DA, Miller SC, Saitz R. American Society for addiction medicine principles of addiction medicine. 5th ed. Philadelphia, PA: Lippincott, Williams and Wilkins; 2014.
27. Mulsant BH, Pollock BG. Psychopharmacology. In: Thakur ME, Blazer DG, Steffens DC, editors. Clinical manual of geriatric psychiatry. 1st ed. Washington, D.C.: American Psychiatric Publishing; 2014. p. 17–82.
28. American Psychiatric Association. American Psychiatric Association: diagnostic and statistical manual of mental disorders. 5th ed. (American Psychiatric Association, ed.). Arlington, VA: American Psychiatric Publishing; 2013.
29. Angelica MD, Fong Y. Substance abuse among older adults. 2008;141(4):520–529. https://doi.org/10.1016/j.surg.2006.10.010.Use.
30. Koechl B, Unger A, Fischer G. Age-related aspects of addiction. Gerontology. 2012;58(6):540–4. https://doi.org/10.1159/000339095.Age-related.
31. Mcinnes E, Powell J. Drug and alcohol referrals : are elderly substance abuse diagnoses and referrals being missed ? Br Med J. 1994;308(6926):444–6.
32. Gilson AM, Kreis PG. The burden of the nonmedical use of prescription opioid analgesics. Pain Med. 2009;10(S2):S89–S100. https://doi.org/10.1111/j.1526-4637.2009.00668.x.
33. NIAAA. Alcohol and your health. National Institute on Alcohol Abuse and Alcoholism. https://www.niaaa.nih.gov/alcohol-health/special-populations-co-occurring-disorders/older-adults. Published 2014. Accessed 1 April 2016.
34. Adams W, Barry K, Flemin M. Screening for problem drinking in older primary care patients. J Am Med Assoc. 1996;276(24):1964–7.
35. O'Connell H, Chin A, Hamilton F, et al. A systematic review of the utility of self-report alcohol screening instruments in the elderly. Int J Geriatr Psychiatry. 2004;19(11):1074–86.
36. Gómez A, Conde A, Santana JM, Jorrín A, Serrano IM, Medina R. The diagnostic usefulness of AUDIT and AUDIT-C for detecting hazardous drinkers in the elderly. Aging Ment Health. 2006;10(5):558–61. https://doi.org/10.1080/13607860600637729.
37. Piccinelli M, Tessari E, Bortolomasi M, et al. Efficacy of the alcohol use disorders identification test as a screening tool for hazardous alcohol intake and related disorders in primary care: a validity study. BMJ. 1997;314(7078):420–4.
38. Kan CC, Breteler MH, van der Ven AH, Zitman FG. Cross-validation of the benzodiazepine dependence self-report questionnaire in outpatient benzodiazepine users. Compr Psychiatry. 2001;42(5):433–9. https://doi.org/10.1053/comp.2001.26275.
39. de las Cuevas C, Sanz EJ, de La Fuente JA, Padilla J, Berenguer JC. The Severity of Dependence Scale (SDS) as screening test for benzodiazepine dependence: SDS validation study. Addiction. 2000;95(2000):245–50.
40. Voyer P, Roussel ME, Berbiche D, Préville M. Effectively detect dependence on benzodiazepines among community-dwelling seniors by asking only two questions. J Psychiatr Ment Health Nurs. 2010;17(4):328–34. https://doi.org/10.1111/j.1365-2850.2009.01529.x.
41. Arndt S, Clayton R, Schultz S. Trends in substance abuse treatment 1998-2008: increasing older adult

first time admissions for illicit drugs. Am J Geriatr Psychiatry. 2011;19(8):704–11.
42. Oslin D, Pettinati H, Volpicelli J. Alcoholism treatment adherence: older age predicts better adherence and drinking outcomes. Am J Geriatr Psychiatry. 2002;10(6):740–7.
43. Oslin D, Slaymaker V, Blow F, Owen P, Colleran C. Treatment outcomes for alcohol dependence among middle-aged and older adults. Addict Behav. 2005;30(7):1431–6.
44. Jonas D, Garbutt J, Amick H, et al. Behavioral counseling after screening for alcohol misuse in primary care: a systematic review and meta-analysis for the U.S. Preventive Services Task Force. Ann Intern Med. 2012;157(9):645–54.
45. Kuerbis A, Sacco P. A review of existing treatments for substance abuse among the elderly and recommendations for future directions. Subst Abuse. 2013;7:13–37.
46. Alcoholics Anonymous, edoitors. Twelve steps and twelve traditions. New York: Alcoholics Anonymous; 2004.
47. Schonfeld L, King-Kallimanis BL, Duchene DM, et al. Screening and brief intervention for substance misuse among older adults: the Florida BRITE project. Am J Public Health. 2010;100(1):108–14. https://doi.org/10.2105/AJPH.2008.149534.
48. Ayalon L, Jin C, Mcculloch CE, et al. Integrated specialty mental health care among older minorities improves access but not outcomes: results of the PRISMe study. Int J Geriatr Psychiatry. 2008;23(August):1086–92. https://doi.org/10.1002/gps.
49. Barry K, Blow F. Drinking over the lifespan. Alcohol Res. 2016;38(1):115–20.
50. Ramesh D, Haney M. Treatment of cannabis use disorders. In: Textbook of addiction treatment: international perspectives; 2015. P. 367–380. https://doi.org/10.1007/978-88-470-5322-9_14.
51. Ryrie I. Motivational interviewing. In: Norman I, Ryrie I, editors. The art and science of mental health nursing: principles and practice; 2013. P. 356–366.
52. Petrovic M, Vandierendonck A, Mariman A, Van Maele G, Afschrift M, Pevernagie D. Personality traits and socio-epidemiological status of hospitalised elderly benzodiazepine users. Int J Geriatr Psychiatry. 2002;17(8):733–8.
53. Tannenbaum C, Martin P, Tamblyn R, Benedetti A, Ahmed S. Reduction of inappropriate benzodiazepine prescriptions among older adults through direct patient education: the EMPOWER cluster randomized trial. JAMA Intern Med. 2014;174(6):890–8. https://doi.org/10.1001/jamainternmed.2014.949.
54. Caputo F, Vignoli T, Leggio L, Addolorato G, Zoli G, Bernardi M. Alcohol use disorders in the elderly: a brief overview from epidemiology to treatment options. Exp Gerontol. 2012;47(6):411–6. https://doi.org/10.1016/j.exger.2012.03.019.
55. Letizia M, Reinbolz M. Identifying and managing acute alcohol withdrawal in the elderly. Geriatr Nurs. 2005;26:176–83.
56. Stahl S. Stahl's essential psychopharmacology - prescriber's guide. 5th ed. New York: Cambridge University Press; 2014.
57. Substance Abuse and Mental Health Services Administration. Incorporating alcohol pharmacotherapies into medical practice treatment improvement protocol (TIP) series, no. 49. Rockville, MD; 2009.
58. Litten R, Wilford B, Falk D, Ryan M, Fertig J. Potential medications for the treatment of alcohol use disorder: an evaluation of clinical efficacy and safety. Subst Abus. 2016;37(2):286–98.
59. Berlin R, Butler P, Perloff M. Gabapentin therapy in psychiatric disorders: a systematic review. Prim Care Companion CNS Disord. 2015;17(5). https://doi.org/10.4088/PCC.15r01821.
60. Cawkwell PB, Blaum C, Sherman SE. Pharmacological smoking cessation. Drugs Aging. 2015;32(6):443–51.
61. Hartmann-Boyce J, Aveyard P. Drug for smoking cessation. Br Med J. 2016;352(571):1–5.
62. Siu AL. Behavioral and pharmacotherapy interventions for tobacco smoking cessation in adults, including pregnant women: U.S. preventive services task force recommendation statement. Ann Intern Med. 2015;163(8):622–34. https://doi.org/10.7326/M15-2023.
63. Tannenbaum MD, MSc C. Inappropriate benzodiazepine use in elderly patients and its reduction. J Psychiatry Neurosci. 2015;40(3):E27–8. https://doi.org/10.1503/jpn.140355.
64. Shorter D, Kosten TR. Novel pharmacotherapeutic treatments for cocaine addiction. BMC Med. 2011;9(1):119. https://doi.org/10.1186/1741-7015-9-119.

21 Anxiety Disorders

Rajesh R. Tampi, Deena J. Tampi, Suneela Cherlopalle, and Silpa Balachandran

Introduction

Available data indicates that the population of individuals ≥65 years of age in the United States will rise from 46.2 million or 14.5% of the total population to approximately 21.7% of the US population by the year 2040 [1]. It is also estimated that approximately one among five older adults has a diagnosable psychiatric disorder in the United States [2]. A recent study by Reynold et al. found that the proportion of older adults in the United States who experienced any past-year anxiety and mood disorders was 11.4 and 6.8%, respectively [3]. The investigators also found that a total of 3.8% of older adults met the criteria for any past-year substance use disorder and 14.5% had one or more personality disorders. Additionally, they found that men had higher rates of substance use disorders and any personality disorder, whereas women experienced greater rates of mood and anxiety disorders. Emerging data indicates that among older adults, anxiety disorders are more prevalent than previously identified [4, 5]. In this chapter, we review the most up-to-date information on anxiety disorders among older adults and their treatments.

Epidemiology

Data indicates that across the life span, anxiety symptoms are much more prevalent than diagnosable anxiety disorders among all the age groups [6]. Among older adults, the rates of anxiety symptoms range between 15 and 20% among the community- dwelling and primary care samples [5]. However, their prevalence increases to over 40% among individuals with disability or chronic medical conditions [5]. Clinically significant anxiety symptoms were noted to occur in approximately 17.1% of older men and 21.5% of older women in one study [7]. Another study found that among older adults, the prevalence of phobias was between 3.1 and 10%, the prevalence of panic disorder was between 0.1 and 1.0%, and the prevalence of obsessive compulsive disorder (OCD) was approximately 0.6–0.8% [4].

The Longitudinal Aging Study Amsterdam (LASA) found that the overall prevalence of anxiety disorders was approximately 10.2% among older adults. Among the anxiety disorders, generalized anxiety disorder (GAD) was the most common with a prevalence of 7.3% followed by phobic disorders with a prevalence rate of 3.1%. The prevalence of panic disorder was 1.0% and that of OCD was 0.6% [8]. The prevalence of post-traumatic stress disorder (PTSD) among Holocaust survivors and prisoners of war in World War II was found to be approximately 70% and among these individuals the symptoms were found to be chronic [4]. In a population-based study of older adults, the 6-month prevalence of subthreshold PTSD and PTSD were 13.1 and 0.9%, respectively [9].

R. R. Tampi et al. (eds.), *Psychiatric Disorders Late in Life*, https://doi.org/10.1007/978-3-319-73078-3_21

The National Comorbidity Survey Replication (NCS-R) study found that among older adults, the prevalence of any anxiety disorder was approximately 15.3% [10]. Among the anxiety disorders, specific phobia was found to have the highest prevalent rate of 7.5% followed by social phobia (6.6%), GAD (3.6%), PTSD (2.5%), panic disorder (2%), agoraphobia without panic (1%), and OCD at 0.7%. The ESA (Enquête sur la Santé des Aînés) study found that among community-dwelling older adults, the 12-month prevalence rate for any anxiety disorder that was diagnosed using the DSM-IV criteria was approximately 5.6% [11]. In this study, specific phobia was the most common anxiety disorder with a prevalence rate of 2% followed by OCD (1.5%), GAD (1.2%), social phobia (0.7%), panic disorder (0.6%), and agoraphobia (0.3%). However, the prevalence of anxiety disorders rose to approximately 26.2% when the total prevalence of cases was calculated using the subthreshold and the threshold DSM-IV criteria. Using this calculation, the highest prevalence was noted for specific phobia with prevalence rate of 9.8% followed by agoraphobia (4.5%), GAD (4.1%), panic (3.2%), OCD (3.0%), and social phobia (1.4%).

Neurobiology and Risk Factors

Current evidence indicates that anxiety disorders are heritable, and the genes influence the development of one's temperament and personality through altering their brain functions [12–15]. Personality traits that are related to anxiety, i.e., neuroticism, introversion, and harm avoidance, have been found to be heritable [12, 13]. Twin studies indicate that the comorbidity of PTSD with anxiety disorders, depressive disorders, and substance use disorders appears to be partly attributable to common additive genetic and non-shared environmental influences [12, 14]. It has been noted that adult children of Holocaust survivors with PTSD had a greater risk of developing PTSD following trauma when compared to adult children of Holocaust survivors without PTSD [14]. This suggests that genetic factors may influence the exposure to potentially traumatic events and a possible gene-environment correlation where the selection of environment and the subsequent potential for exposure to trauma is partly determined by genetic factors [12, 14].

Functional imaging studies indicate that proneness to anxiety and vulnerability to anxiety disorders are associated with the activation of limbic brain circuits especially the reactivity of amygdala in response to emotional stimuli [15]. The increased limbic reactivity is also associated with the functional variability in genes involved in serotonergic neurotransmission, including tryptophan hydroxylase 2, serotonin transporter and receptors, and catechol-o-methyltransferase (COMT) [12, 15]. Functional imaging studies also indicate that adults with anxiety disorders show greater activity in their amygdala and the insula to negative emotional responses than the matched comparators [15]. Smaller hippocampal volumes have been found among the PTSD and trauma-exposed groups without PTSD when compared to the trauma-unexposed group [16]. In the PTSD group, the right hippocampus was noted to be smaller when compared to the trauma-exposed group without PTSD. The right hippocampal volume was found to be larger than the left among the PTSD and trauma-unexposed groups but not in the trauma-exposed group without PTSD [16]. Reduced sizes of amygdala and hippocampus have been noted among individuals with social phobia when compared to controls, and the smaller right-sided hippocampal volumes are correlated with the disorder severity [17]. It has also been noted that subjects with hoarding behaviors have brain lesions in the anterior ventromedial prefrontal and cingulate cortex [18, 19]. Additionally, lower glucose metabolism has been noted in the bilateral dorsal and ventral anterior cingulate cortex among these individuals when compared to controls.

Hyperactivity of the HPA (hypothalamic-pituitary-adrenal) axis has been linked to the development of generalized anxiety disorder (GAD) among older adults [20]. In addition, the pharmacological treatment of GAD has been shown to reduce salivary cortisol levels and an improvement in anxiety levels among older individuals.

Based on the available evidence, the risk factors for the development of anxiety among older adults can be divided into two types: internal and external [8]. The internal factors (vulnerability factors) included personality traits of neuroticism and low self-efficacy. The external factors (stress factors) included chronic medical illnesses, disability, and major illness in the spouse.

Consequences

Although anxiety has been developed as a natural evolutionary response to stressful stimuli, pathologic anxiety is often debilitating and harmful to the individual [21, 22]. Anxiety symptoms among older adults are associated with reduced physical activity, reduced functional status, poorer self-perceptions of health, decreased life satisfaction, and increased loneliness [23–25]. Additionally, anxiety among older adults is associated with poorer quality of life, greater service use, and the overall higher cost of care [26, 27].

Available data indicates that anxiety and depressive disorders are highly comorbid conditions [28–30]. Anxiety disorders among older adults often progress to either a depressive disorder or depressive disorder with a comorbid anxiety disorder [30]. The remission rates at follow-up are worse among individuals who have comorbid anxiety and depressive disorders when compared to individuals who just have an anxiety or depressive disorder. Among older adults, majority of individuals with an anxiety disorder also have a comorbid alcohol use disorder [31]. One recent study found that among older adults with GAD, approximately 55% of the individuals endorsed alcohol use in the past month [34]. Approximately 42% of the participants drank moderately (average of ≤7 drinks per week), 9% of the participants reported at-risk drinking (an average of 8–14 drinks per week), and 5% indicated heavy drinking (average of >14 drinks per week). The use of alcohol in this study was higher than what has been reported in a previous study of older veterans [35]. Data indicates that one-quarter of the older adults with comorbid anxiety and alcohol use disorders also have a personality disorder [31]. Furthermore, many of these individuals have chronic health problems and poorer health-related quality of life.

Emerging data indicates that higher levels of anxiety are associated with greater risk of developing Alzheimer's disease (AD) and a more rapid decline in global cognition among older adults [32, 33].

Anxiety disorders among older adults are associated with chronically painful conditions like arthritis, back pain, and migraines and other commonly occurring diseases including allergies, cataracts, and gastrointestinal, lung, and heart diseases [36]. The comorbidity of anxiety disorders with allergies, cataracts, arthritis, and lung disease among older adults results in worse self-rated physical and/or mental health.

Data from a longitudinal study indicates that among older men, a baseline diagnosis of an anxiety disorder was associated with an adjusted mortality risk of 1.78 [37]. However, this increased risk of mortality was not seen among older women. Another study found that among older individuals with GAD and mixed anxiety-depression, there was no increase in the risk of mortality [38]. Table 21-1 summarizes the consequences of anxiety disorders among older adults.

Assessment

Anxiety disorders among older adults are very often under-recognized and poorly treated [5]. One study found that primary care physicians correctly made the diagnosis of GAD in only 1.5% of the older adults with anxiety disorders, whereas the diagnosis of any anxiety disorder

TABLE 21-1. Consequences of anxiety disorders among older adults

Reduced physical activity
Reduced functional status
Poorer self-perceptions of health
Decreased life satisfaction
Increased loneliness
Worse quality of life
Increased service use
Overall greater cost of care
Comorbidity with depression, alcohol abuse, and personality disorder
Greater risk of cognitive decline and dementia
Comorbidity with arthritis, back pain, migraine, cataract, lung disease, and heart disease
Greater rate of mortality

was made in approximately 9% of the individuals [39]. This is in contrast to the data from another study where the primary care physicians made the correct diagnosis of GAD in 34.4% of younger individuals [40]. The current diagnostic criteria for anxiety disorders were developed for use among younger individuals leading to poor sensitivity in detecting these disorders among older adults [41]. In addition, anxiety disorders among older adults are often comorbid with depression, substance use disorders, and cognitive disorders resulting in greater complexity in making an appropriate diagnosis [41]. Furthermore, physical symptoms associated with anxiety including poor sleep, easy fatigability, restlessness, and poor concentration tend to overlap with medical disorders that occur commonly among older adults resulting in the underdiagnosis of anxiety disorders [39].

A comprehensive history aids in making a diagnosis of an anxiety disorder among older adults [41]. Collateral information from well-informed caregivers and or family members should be obtained for older adults with cognitive disorders [42]. A thorough mental status examination and formal cognitive testing assist in differentiating various psychiatric disorders including comorbid cognitive illness. A focused physical examination and appropriate laboratory testing rule out medical disorders and drug effects that may mimic symptoms of anxiety disorders.

Standardized assessment scales assist in qualifying and quantifying the symptoms of anxiety disorders [43]. These scales can be divided into self-reported and clinician-rated scales. The common self-reported scales used among older adults with anxiety disorders include the Worry Scale (WS), the State-Trait Anxiety Inventory (STAI), the Penn State Worry Questionnaire (PSWQ), Padua Inventory (PI), and the Beck Anxiety Inventory (BAI) [43–45]. The clinician-rated scales include the Structured Clinical Interview for the DSM (SCID), the Diagnostic Interview Schedule (DIS), the Anxiety Disorders Interview Schedule (ADIS-R), and the Hamilton Anxiety Rating Scale (HARS) [43, 44]. Neuropsychological assessment is useful among cases where the diagnosis of anxiety disorders is complicated by the presence of comorbid personality disorder and/or cognitive disorders. Table 21-2 summarizes the assessment of anxiety disorders among older adults.

TABLE 21-2. Assessment of anxiety disorders among older adults

Obtain history	Course of illness, medical history, psychiatric history, current and past medications, premorbid personality, cognition and functional status
Complete a standardized mental status examination and formal cognitive testing	
Complete a focused physical examination	Rule out medical or neurological disorders
Order appropriate investigations	Blood and urine examination, vitamin B 12 and folate levels, VDRL, urine drug screen, and neuroimaging
Treat medical, psychiatric, and neurological disorders	Remove offending drug(s)
Complete standardized assessment scales	Neuropsychological testing if needed

Prevention

In a randomized controlled trial (RCT) of older adults with subthreshold symptom levels of anxiety or depression who did not meet the full diagnostic criteria for these disorders, the participants were randomly assigned to receive either a preventive stepped-care program or usual care [46]. In the stepped-care program, the participants sequentially received a watchful waiting approach, cognitive behavior therapy-based bibliotherapy, cognitive behavior therapy-based problem-solving treatment, and a referral to a primary care clinician for medications if required. The investigators found that among the stepped-care group, the 12-month incidence of anxiety and depressive disorders was one-half that of the incidence among the usual care group: 12 vs. 24%, relative risk (RR) = 0.49. The stepped-care program also reduced the cost of care significantly for these individuals indicating that it was good value for the money spent [47]. In a follow-up to the trial by van't Veer-Tazelaar et al., the investigators found that the cumulative incidence rate of *Diagnostic and Statistical Manual of Mental Disorders*, Fourth

Edition (DSM IV), anxiety or major depressive disorders over a 24-month period was one-half in the intervention group when compared to the usual care group (19.8 vs. 39.3%, OR = 0.38, $P = 0.006$) and the number needed to treat (NNT) in this study was five [48].

Treatments

Evidence indicates that both non-pharmacological and pharmacological treatments benefit older adults with anxiety disorders [5, 43, 49]. In this section, we will review the data on the treatment of anxiety disorders in older adults from RCTs and meta-analyses.

Non-pharmacological

Randomized Controlled Trials

In the study by Barrowclough et al., individuals with a mean age of 72 years and a diagnosis of anxiety disorder were randomized to receive either 8–12 sessions of individual and home-delivered cognitive behavioral therapy (CBT) or supportive counseling (SC) [50]. All individuals had been stabilized on medications at least 3 months prior to study enrollment. At the end of treatment and at 12 months, CBT was found to be superior to SC on BAI. However, on the HAMA and STAI-T, CBT was equal to SC at the end of treatment but better than SC at the 12-month follow-up period.

In the study by Wetherell et al., individuals with a mean age of 67.1 years and a diagnosis of GAD were randomly assigned to be part of a CBT group, a discussion group (DG) organized around worry-provoking topics, or a waiting period group (WPG) [51]. When compared to participants in the waiting list group, participants in both active treatment groups improved significantly. Individuals in the CBT group improved on more measures than the DG group participants immediately after treatment, but there were no differences between the two groups noted at the 6-month follow-up period. The CBT group showed a large effect size, whereas the DG group showed only a medium effect size.

In the study by Stanley et al., individuals ≥60 years of age with a diagnosis of GAD were randomized to either 15 sessions of CBT group or to the minimal contact control (MCC) group [52]. The investigators found that posttreatment, there were significant improvements in worry, anxiety, depression, and quality of life among the CBT group when compared to the MCC group. Forty-five percent of individuals in the CBT group were classified as being responders when compared to only 8% of the individuals in the MCC group. The treatment gains noted among individuals in the CBT group were maintained at the 12-month follow-up period. However, the posttreatment scores for individuals in the CBT group did not reach normative functioning.

In the study by Gorenstein et al., individuals with anxiety disorders who were ≥60 years of age were randomized to receive either 13 sessions of CBT plus medical management (MM) for medication taper (CBT-MM) or MM only [53]. The investigators found that the CBT-MM was superior to MM in reducing scores on several of the Hopkins Symptom Checklist-90 subscales. However, both groups were similar in reducing the use of anxiolytic medications. Additionally, both groups were similar on scales for worry, state, or trait anxiety and depression. The investigators also found that despite monthly booster sessions, there was loss of treatment gains at the 6 month follow-up period in both groups. Posttreatment response rates on the CGI were better in CBT-MM group when compared to the MM group.

Schuurmans et al. conducted a randomized, controlled trial of individuals ≥60 years of age with a diagnosis of GAD, panic disorder, agoraphobia, or social phobia. The participants were randomized to the 15 sessions of CBT group, sertraline (maximum dosage 150 mg a day) group, or a waitlist control group (WLC) [54]. The investigators found that both the CBT and sertraline groups had significant improvements in anxiety, worry, and depressive symptoms both at posttreatment and at the 3-month follow-up period. However, the sertraline group showed superior results on the worry symptoms. The effect size for CBT was in the small-to-medium range at posttreatment and at 3-month follow-up compared to the large effect size for sertraline group. The waitlist group did not show any improvement in symptoms.

In a study by Stanley et al., the investigators randomized individuals with a mean age of 66.9 years who were receiving treatment for GAD to receive either CBT or enhanced usual care (EUC) for 3 months [55]. They found that individuals receiving CBT had less worry, less depressive symptoms, and better general mental health when compared to the group receiving EUC. There was no difference in GAD severity in patients receiving CBT vs. those receiving EUC. However, in the intention-to-treat analyses, response rates defined according to worry severity were higher in the CBT group when compared to the EUC group.

In a pilot study by Wetherell et al., 31 individuals who were ≥60 years of age with a diagnosis of GAD or anxiety disorder not otherwise specified were randomized to receive either modular form of psychotherapy (MP) or enhanced community treatment (EnCT) [56]. Both treatment groups showed substantial improvements in anxiety symptoms, worry, depressive symptoms, and mental health-related quality of life. In the enhanced community treatment group, most individuals also reported receiving medications or some other form of professional treatment for their anxiety. Smaller treatment gains were reported in individuals who had major life events or stressors and among those who used involvement in activities as a coping strategy than those who did not use these interventions. Table 21-3 summarizes the important psychotherapy trials for anxiety disorders among older adults.

Meta-Analyses

In the meta-analysis by Nordhus and Pallesen, the investigators evaluated the efficacy of non-pharmacological interventions for late-life anxiety disorders [57]. They included a total of 15 outcome studies in their analysis. These studies included a total of 495 participants with a mean age of 69.5 years and provided 20 separate treatment interventions. The investigators found that psychological interventions were definitely more effective than no treatment on self-rated and clinician-rated measures of anxiety with an effect size of 0.55. However, the data regarding maintenance of treatment gains for a minimum of 6 months follow-up was insufficiently reported preventing a reliable estimation of overall long-term efficacy.

In a meta-analysis by Thorp et al., the investigators evaluated the efficacy of cognitive behavior therapy [CBT] alone, CBT with relaxation training [RT], and RT alone for late-life anxiety from 19 studies [58]. They compared the post-treatment and pretreatment scores and effects relative to control conditions for anxiety. When the treatment samples were compared to active control conditions on anxiety measures, the mean controlled effect sizes were 0.90 for RT, 0.33 for CBT, and 0.00 for CBT without RT. These effect sizes are comparable to the mean controlled effect size of 0.71 for CBT for GAD in the general population and 0.83 for pharmacotherapy for anxiety among older adults.

TABLE 21-3. Psychotherapy trials for anxiety disorders among older adults

Name of study	Diagnosis	Age of participants	Number of participants	Comparators	Outcomes
Barrowclough et al. [50]	Anxiety disorders	Mean age of 72 years	55	CBT vs. SC	CBT > SC on BAI All other scales CBT = SC
Wetherell et al. [51]	GAD	Mean age of 67.1 years	75	CBT vs. DG vs. WPG	CBT = DG > WPG
Stanley et al. [52]	GAD	≥60 years of age	85	CBT vs. MCC	CBT > MCC
Gorenstein et al. [53]	Anxiety disorders	≥60 years of age	42	CBT-MM vs. MM	CBT-MM > MM
Schuurmans et al. [54]	Anxiety disorders	≥60 years of age	84	CBT vs. sertraline vs. WLC	CBT < sertraline CBT and sertraline > WLC
Stanley et al. [55]	GAD	Mean age of 66.9 years	70	CBT vs. EUC	CBT > EUC
Wetherell et al. [56]	GAD or other anxiety disorders	≥60 years of age	31	MP vs. EnCT	MP = EnCT

In a recent meta-analysis by Hall et al., the investigators evaluated the efficacy of CBT for GAD among older adults [59]. The investigators included data from 14 RCTs in this review. They found that the end of treatment population effect size estimate for CBT when compared with any control favored CBT with a medium effect size (0.66). The population effect size estimate for CBT when compared with waitlist controls favored CBT and was large (1.10). For CBT when compared with TAU, the population effect size was medium (0.67). The number of patients that needed to be treated for one additional beneficial outcome (NNTB) was three for CBT when compared with treatment as usual (TAU) at the end of treatment. When CBT was compared with active controls, the population effect size estimate was small (0.42) and nonsignificant indicating that CBT was not significantly superior to active treatments. The corresponding NNTB was four. The population effect size estimate for CBT when compared with any control group at 6-month follow-up favored CBT but was in the small-to-medium range (0.46). The follow-up population effect size estimate for CBT when compared with passive controls favored CBT and was large (0.83). The population effect size estimate for CBT when compared with active controls at follow-up was near zero (0.06) and nonsignificant indicating that there was no significant advantage for either CBT or active controls at follow-up.

Pharmacotherapy

Antidepressants

There is a dearth of RCTs of antidepressants for the treatment of anxiety disorders among older adults. There are only four such studies in the published literature.

In the earliest of the four studies, Sheikh and Swales randomized 25 individuals 55–73 years of age with a DSM-III-R diagnosis of panic disorder to receive alprazolam, imipramine, or placebo for 8 weeks [60]. The main outcomes were global change ratings—Hamilton Anxiety and Depression Scales (HAM-A & HAM-D), the Physicians Global Impression ratings, and panic diaries. Both alprazolam and imipramine reduced the number of panic attacks per week and resulted in an improvement on the HAM-A and HAM-D scores at the end of the study when compared to baseline. There were no dropouts in the alprazolam group, whereas 10% of the individuals in the imipramine group dropped out, and 86% of the individuals in the placebo group dropped out. The daily doses of the drugs were about half the normal adult doses.

Katz et al. in their pooled secondary analysis of five Phase-III RCTs included 184 individuals ≥60 years of age with a DSM-IV diagnosis of GAD and total scores of ≥18 on the HAM-A [61]. All five trials were 8 weeks in duration with three trials having extension phases. The participants received fixed or flexible doses of venlafaxine ER with a dose range of 37.5–225 mg a day or matched placebo. The primary efficacy variables were the HAM-A total score and the psychic anxiety factor, the anxiety subscale of the Hospital Anxiety and Depression (HAD) Scale, and the Clinical Global Impression of Improvement (CGI-I). On the CGI, 66% of the individuals in the venlafaxine ER group responded when compared with only 41% in the placebo group ($P < 0.01$). There were no main effects noted for age and no age-by-treatment interactions for any of the primary or secondary efficacy outcome measures. Higher levels of depression were associated with decreased responses of anxiety symptoms. Twenty-three percent of older adults in the venlafaxine ER group discontinued the treatment prematurely when compared to 31% of the individuals in the placebo group. Discontinuation rates due to adverse events were 15% in the venlafaxine ER group when compared to 14% among the placebo group.

In a RCT by Lenze et al., 34 individuals ≥60 years of age with a DSM-IV diagnosis of anxiety disorder (mainly GAD) and a HAM-A score of ≥17 were assigned to receive either citalopram or placebo for a period of 8 weeks [62]. Response was defined as a score of 1 (very much improved) or 2 (much improved) on the Clinical Global Improvement (CGI) scale or a 50% reduction in the HAM-A scores. Eleven (65%) of the 17 citalopram-treated participants responded by 8 weeks when compared to only 4 (24%) of the 17 placebo-treated participants. Among individuals with GAD, the response rates in the citalopram group was 10 of 15 participants (67%) when compared to 4 of 15 participants (27%) in the placebo group ($P < 0.03$). The most common and problematic adverse effect in the citalopram group was sedation. Twelve of the 17 citalopram-treated participants complained of at least 1 side effect when compared to 9 of the 17 placebo-treated participants. The most common adverse effects in both groups were dry mouth, nausea, and fatigue. The investigators found that adverse effects decrease over time in the citalopram group when compared to no change over time in the placebo group.

In the study by Alaka et al., individuals with GAD who were ≥65 years of age were randomly assigned to receive either duloxetine or placebo [63]. The primary efficacy measure was the HAM-A total score at week 10. Global functioning was assessed by using the Sheehan Disability Scale (SDS). At week 10, duloxetine was found to be superior to placebo on mean changes from baseline in HAM-A total scores ($P < 0.001$) and in the SDS global scores ($P < 0.001$). Treatment-emergent adverse events occurred in ≥5% of duloxetine-treated individuals which was twice the rate in the placebo group including constipation ($P = 0.06$), dry mouth ($P = 0.02$), and somnolence ($P = 0.14$). Table 21-4 summarizes the important antidepressant trials for anxiety disorders among older adults.

Benzodiazepines

A literature review indicates that there are only four published RCTs of benzodiazepines for anxiety disorders among older adults.

In the first of these trials, Koepke et al. randomized 220 individuals with a mean age of 67.5 years and a primary diagnosis of anxiety disorder to receive oxazepam or placebo over a 4-week period [64]. The investigators found that oxazepam reduced symptoms of anxiety more than placebo on the HAM-A ($P = 0.01$), Physician's Target Symptom Scale ($P = 0.001$), Hopkins 35-Item Symptom Checklist ($P = 0.002$), and Physician's and the Patient's Global Improvement Scale ($P < 0.001$). The drug was well tolerated in this study with minimal adverse effects.

In a double-blind trial, Bresolin et al. randomized 63 older adults with GAD to receive either 15 mg a day of ketazolam or placebo for 15 days [65]. If at the end of this trial period the total scores on the HAM-A had decreased by at least 25%, then the treatment was continued unchanged for another 15 days. For those individuals who did not respond to treatment, the dose of ketazolam was increased to 30 mg a day. During the initial 15-day period, 83% of the ketazolam-treated individuals responded to treatment compared to 43% of the placebo-treated individuals ($P < 0.01$). During the second 15-day period, the anxiety scores in the ketazolam-treated individuals continued to decline, whereas the individuals in the placebo group showed no improvements.

In the RCT by Frattola et al., 40 individuals between the ages of 65 and 80 years with a diagnosis of anxiety disorder were randomized to receive either alpidem or placebo after a 7-day placebo run-in period for 3 weeks [66]. The investigators found that alpidem reduced symptoms of anxiety on all the rating scales when compared to placebo with the anxiolytic effect of the drug being evident from day 7 of the study. There were no significant adverse effects observed in either group.

In the study by Small and Bystritsky, the investigators randomized 182 individuals with a mean age of 68.3 years to receive high-dose abecarnil, low-dose abecarnil, or placebo for 6 weeks for the treatment of anxiety disorders after a 7-day placebo

TABLE 21-4. Antidepressant trials for anxiety disorders among older adults

Name of study	Diagnosis	Age of participants	Number of participants	Comparators	Outcomes
Sheikh and Swales [60]	Panic disorder	55–73 years	25	Alprazolam, imipramine, or placebo	Alprazolam = imipramine > placebo
Katz et al. [61]	GAD	≥60 years	184	Venlafaxine XR or placebo	Venlafaxine XR > placebo
Lenze et al. [62]	Anxiety disorder (mainly GAD)	≥60 years	34	Citalopram or placebo	Citalopram > placebo
Alaka et al. [63]	GAD	≥65 years	291	Duloxetine or placebo	Duloxetine > placebo

lead-in period [67]. This was followed by an abrupt discontinuation of drug and a 2-week follow-up period. The low-dosage abecarnil was found to be superior to placebo in reducing symptoms of anxiety at weeks 2, 3, 4, and 6 and was superior to high-dosage abecarnil at weeks 4, 5, and 6. More than half of the individuals in the placebo group also showed at least moderate global improvement at weeks 3 and 6. One week after the discontinuation of abecarnil, the placebo-treated group had less anxiety than did both active drug groups. The discontinuation rate from adverse events during the treatment period was greater for the high-dosage abecarnil group (44%) when compared to low-dosage abecarnil (14%) or placebo (12%) groups. The most commonly reported adverse effects were drowsiness and insomnia and the most common withdrawal effects were headache and insomnia.

Three of the four benzodiazepines used in these studies are not currently available in the United States (abecarnil, alpidem, ketazolam). These drugs appear to reduce anxiety and were fairly well tolerated. But, these studies were of short duration as they only lasted between 3 and 6 weeks. Additionally, the American Geriatrics Society (AGS) Beers Criteria include benzodiazepines in the potentially inappropriate medications class to be used among older adults and recommend that there is strong evidence for avoiding their use in this population [68]. Furthermore, benzodiazepines are included in the potentially inappropriate medications and classes that are to be avoided in older adults with certain diseases and syndromes that these drugs can exacerbate including cognitive impairment and dementia. Table 21-5 summarizes the important benzodiazepine trials for anxiety disorders among older adults.

Sequenced Treatments

In a study by Wethrell et al., the investigators provided a sequenced treatment that combined pharmacotherapy and cognitive behavioral therapy (CBT) for GAD to 73 individuals ≥60 years of age [69]. The participants initially received 12 weeks of open-label escitalopram (10–20 mg a day) [69]. At the end of 12 weeks, participants who exhibited at least a 20% improvement in HAM-A symptoms were randomly assigned to one of four groups: 16 weeks of treatment with escitalopram (10–20 mg a day) plus modular CBT, followed by 28 weeks of maintenance escitalopram; escitalopram alone, followed by maintenance escitalopram; escitalopram plus CBT, followed by pill placebo; and escitalopram alone, followed by placebo. The investigators found that escitalopram augmented with CBT increased response rates on the PSWQ ($P = 0.01$) but not on the HAM-A ($P = 0.15$) when compared to escitalopram alone. For response, according to the PSWQ, after controlling for score at the start of augmentation, participants who received CBT were approximately three times more likely to respond by the end of augmentation than those who did not receive CBT ($P < 0.05$). Both escitalopram ($P < 0.001$) and CBT ($p = 0.009$) prevented relapse when compared to placebo.

Controlled data indicates that psychotherapy and pharmacotherapy have shown benefit in the treatment for anxiety disorders among older adults [70]. Current data indicates that there is no superiority noted for any particular psychotherapy modality for the treatment of anxiety disorders among older adults. Among the pharmacotherapeutic agents, antidepressants have shown superior efficacy to placebo in the treatment of anxiety

TABLE 21-5. Benzodiazepine trials for anxiety disorders among older adults

Name of study	Diagnosis	Age of participants	Number of participants	Comparators	Outcomes
Koepke et al. [64]	Anxiety disorders	Mean age of 67.5 years	220	Oxazepam or placebo	Oxazepam > placebo
Bresolin et al. [65]	GAD	Unclear	63	Ketazolam or placebo	Ketazolam > placebo
Frattola et al. [66]	Anxiety disorders	65–80 years	40	Alpidem or placebo	Alpidem > placebo
Small and Bystritsky [67]	Anxiety disorders	Mean age 68.3 years	182	Abecarnil or placebo	Abecarnil > placebo

disorders among older adults with a good tolerability profile. Benzodiazepines appear to have short-term efficacy in the treatment of anxiety disorders among older adults, but their use must be balanced with their significant adverse effect profile. Sequenced treatment from one study indicates that a combination of escitalopram and CBT was beneficial in treating GAD in older adults.

Conclusions

Older adults often present with anxiety disorders. Phobias and GAD are the most common anxiety disorders noted among the older adults. These disorders among older adults are associated with significant comorbidity. Available data indicates that these anxiety disorders among older adults are often underdiagnosed or misdiagnosed. Despite a dearth of evidence, current evidence indicates efficacy for both psychotherapy and pharmacotherapy for the treatment of anxiety disorders among older adults. The development of standard diagnostic criteria for anxiety disorders among older adults, the education of clinicians regarding the diagnosis of these disorders, and the critical appraisal of treatment modalities available for these disorders will improve the diagnosis and treatment of these disorders.

References

1. Aging Statistics. https://aoa.acl.gov/Aging_Statistics/index.aspx. Accessed 19 Dec 2016.
2. Mental health and older adults. http://www.who.int/mediacentre/factsheets/fs381/en/. Accessed 19 Dec 2016.
3. Reynold K, Pietrzak RH, El-Gabalawy R, Mackenzie CS, Sareen J. Prevalence of psychiatric disorders in U.S. older adults: findings from a nationally representative survey. World Psychiatry. 2015; 14(1):74–81.
4. Flint AJ. Epidemiology and comorbidity of anxiety disorders in the elderly. Am J Psychiatry. 1994;151(5):640–9.
5. Wetherell JL, Lenze EJ, Stanley MA. Evidence-based treatment of geriatric anxiety disorders. Psychiatr Clin North Am. 2005;28(4):871–96.
6. Olfson M, Broadhead EW, Weissman MM, et al. Subthreshold psychiatric symptoms in a primary care group practice. Arch Gen Psychiatry. 1996;53:880–6.
7. Himmelfarb S, Murrell SA. The prevalence and correlates of anxiety symptoms in older adults. J Psychol. 1984;116(2d Half):159–67.
8. Beekman AT, Bremmer MA, Deeg DJ, et al. Anxiety disorders in later life: a report from the longitudinal aging study Amsterdam. Int J Geriatr Psychiatry. 1998;13(10):717–26.
9. van Zelst WH, de Beurs E, Beekman AT, et al. Prevalence and risk factors of posttraumatic stress disorder in older adults. Psychother Psychosom. 2003;72(6):333–42.
10. Kessler RC, Berglund P, Demler O, et al. Lifetime prevalence and age-of-onset distributions of DSM-IV disorders in the National Comorbidity Survey Replication. Arch Gen Psychiatry. 2005; 62(6):593–602.
11. Grenier S, Préville M, Boyer R, et al. The impact of DSM-IV symptom and clinical significance criteria on the prevalence estimates of subthreshold and threshold anxiety in the older adult population. Am J Geriatr Psychiatry. 2011;19(4):316–26.
12. Hettema JM, Neale MC, Kendler KS. A review and meta-analysis of the genetic epidemiology of anxiety disorders. Am J Psychiatry. 2001; 158(10):1568–78.
13. Bienvenu OJ, Hettema JM, Neale MC, et al. Low extraversion and high neuroticism as indices of genetic and environmental risk for social phobia, agoraphobia, and animal phobia. Am J Psychiatry. 2007;164(11):1714–21.
14. Afifi TO, Asmundson GJ, Taylor S, Jang KL. The role of genes and environment on trauma exposure and posttraumatic stress disorder symptoms: a review of twin studies. Clin Psychol Rev. 2010; 30(1):101–12.
15. Etkin A, Wager TD. Functional neuroimaging of anxiety: a meta-analysis of emotional processing in PTSD, social anxiety disorder, and specific phobia. Am J Psychiatry. 2007;164(10):1476–88.
16. Woon FL, Sood S, Hedges DW. Hippocampal volume deficits associated with exposure to psychological trauma and posttraumatic stress disorder in adults: a meta-analysis. Prog Neuro-Psychopharmacol Biol Psychiatry. 2010;34(7):1181–8.
17. Irle E, Ruhleder M, Lange C, et al. Reduced amygdalar and hippocampal size in adults with generalized social phobia. J Psychiatry Neurosci. 2010;35(2):126–31.
18. Pertusa A, Frost RO, Fullana MA, et al. Refining the diagnostic boundaries of compulsive hoarding: a critical review. Clin Psychol Rev. 2010; 30(4):371–8618.
19. Saxena S. Neurobiology and treatment of compulsive hoarding. CNS Spectr. 2008;13(9 Suppl 14): 29–36.

20. Lenze EJ, Mantella RC, Shi P, et al. Elevated cortisol in older adults with generalized anxiety disorder is reduced by treatment: a placebo-controlled evaluation of escitalopram. Am J Geriatr Psychiatry. 2011; 19(5):482–90.
21. Marks IM, Nesse RM. Fear and fitness: an evolutionary analysis of anxiety disorders. Ethol Sociobiol. 1994;15:247–61.
22. Lydiard RB. The role of GABA in anxiety disorders. J Clin Psychiatry. 2003;64(suppl 3):21–7.
23. Tinetti ME, Inouye SK, Gill TM, et al. Shared risk factors for falls, incontinence, and functional dependence. Unifying the approach to geriatric syndromes. JAMA. 1995;273(17):1381–3.
24. Dew MA, Karp JF, et al. The burden of late-life generalized anxiety disorder: effects on disability, health-related quality of life, and healthcare utilization. Am J Geriatr Psychiatry. 2009;17(6): 473–82.
25. de Beurs E, Beekman AT, van Balkom AJ, et al. Consequences of anxiety in older persons: its effect on disability, well-being and use of health services. Psychol Med. 1999;29(3):583–93.
26. Porensky EK, Dew MA, Karp JF, et al. The burden of late-life generalized anxiety disorder: effects on disability, health-related quality of life, and healthcare utilization. Am J Geriatr Psychiatry. 2009;17(6):473–82.
27. Vasiliadis HM, Dionne PA, Préville M, et al. The excess healthcare costs associated with depression and anxiety. Am J Geriatr Psychiatry. 2013; 21(6):536–48.
28. Beekman AT, de Beurs E, van Balkom AJ, et al. Anxiety and depression in later life: co-occurrence and communality of risk factors. Am J Psychiatry. 2000;157(1):89–95.
29. van Balkom AJ, Beekman AT, de Beurs E, et al. Comorbidity of the anxiety disorders in a community-based older population in The Netherlands. Acta Psychiatr Scand. 2000;101(1):37–45.
30. Schoevers RA, Deeg DJ, van Tilburg W, et al. Depression and generalized anxiety disorder: co-occurrence and longitudinal patterns in elderly patients. Am J Geriatr Psychiatry. 2005;13(1): 31–9.
31. Mackenzie CS, Reynolds K, Chou KL, et al. Prevalence and correlates of generalized anxiety disorder in a national sample of older adults. Am J Geriatr Psychiatry. 2011;19(4):305–15.
32. Wilson RS, Begeny CT, Boyle PA, et al. Vulnerability to stress, anxiety, and development of dementia in old age. Am J Geriatr Psychiatry. 2011;19(4):327–34.
33. Potvin O, Forget H, Grenier S, et al. Anxiety, depression, and 1-year incident cognitive impairment in community-dwelling older adults. J Am Geriatr Soc. 2011;59(8):1421–8.
34. Ivan MC, Amspoker AB, Nadorff MR, et al. Alcohol use, anxiety, and insomnia in older adults with generalized anxiety disorder. Am J Geriatr Psychiatry. 2014;22(9):875–83.
35. Kirchner JE, Zubritsky C, Cody M, et al. Alcohol consumption among older adults in primary care. J Gen Intern Med. 2007;22(1):92–7.
36. El-Gabalawy R, Mackenzie CS, Shooshtari S, Sareen J. Comorbid physical health conditions and anxiety disorders: a population-based exploration of prevalence and health outcomes among older adults. Gen Hosp Psychiatry. 2011;33(6):556–64.
37. van Hout HP, Beekman AT, de Beurs E, et al. Anxiety and the risk of death in older men and women. Br J Psychiatry. 2004;185:399–404.
38. Holwerda TJ, Schoevers RA, Dekker J, et al. The relationship between generalized anxiety disorder, depression and mortality in old age. Int J Geriatr Psychiatry. 2007;22(3):241–9.
39. Calleo J, Stanley MA, Greisinger A, et al. Generalized anxiety disorder in older medical patients: diagnostic recognition, mental health management and service utilization. J Clin Psychol Med Settings. 2009;16(2):178–85.
40. Wittchen HU, Kessler RC, Beesdo K, Krause P, Höfler M, Hoyer J. Generalized anxiety and depression in primary care: prevalence, recognition, and management. J Clin Psychiatry. 2002; 63(Suppl 8):24–34.
41. Kogan JN, Edelstein BA, McKee DR. Assessment of anxiety in older adults: current status. J Anxiety Disord. 2000;14(2):109–32.
42. Seignourel PJ, Kunik ME, Snow L, et al. Anxiety in dementia: a critical review. Clin Psychol Rev. 2008;28(7):1071–82.
43. Stanley MA, Beck JG. Anxiety disorders. Clin Psychol Rev. 2000;20(6):731–54.
44. Beck JG, Stanley MA, Zebb BJ. Characteristics of generalized anxiety disorder in older adults: a descriptive study. Behav Res Ther. 1996;34(3): 225–34.
45. Stanley MA, Beck JG, Zebb BJ. Psychometric properties of four anxiety measures in older adults. Behav Res Ther. 1996;34(10):827–38.
46. van't Veer-Tazelaar PJ, van Marwijk HW, van Oppen P, et al. Stepped-care prevention of anxiety and depression in late life: a randomized controlled trial. Arch Gen Psychiatry. 2009;66(3):297–304.
47. van't Veer-Tazelaar P, Smit F, van Hout H, et al. Cost-effectiveness of a stepped care intervention to prevent depression and anxiety in late life: randomised trial. Br J Psychiatry. 2010;196(4): 319–25.

48. van't Veer-Tazelaar PJ, van Marwijk HW, van Oppen P, et al. Prevention of late-life anxiety and depression has sustained effects over 24 months: a pragmatic randomized trial. Am J Geriatr Psychiatry. 2011;19(3):230–9.
49. Blay SL, Marinho V. Anxiety disorders in old age. Curr Opin Psychiatry. 2012;25(6):462–7.
50. Barrowclough C, King P, Colville J, et al. A randomized trial of the effectiveness of cognitive-behavioral therapy and supportive counseling for anxiety symptoms in older adults. J Consult Clin Psychol. 2001;69(5):756–62.
51. Wetherell JL, Gatz M, Craske MG. Treatment of generalized anxiety disorder in older adults. J Consult Clin Psychol. 2003;71(1):31–40.
52. Stanley MA, Beck JG, Novy DM, et al. Cognitive-behavioral treatment of late-life generalized anxiety disorder. J Consult Clin Psychol. 2003;71(2):309–19.
53. Gorenstein EE, Kleber MS, Mohlman J, et al. Cognitive-behavioral therapy for management of anxiety and medication taper in older adults. Am J Geriatr Psychiatry. 2005;13(10):901–9.
54. Schuurmans J, Comijs H, Emmelkamp PM, et al. A randomized, controlled trial of the effectiveness of cognitive-behavioral therapy and sertraline versus a waitlist control group for anxiety disorders in older adults. Am J Geriatr Psychiatry. 2006;14(3):255–63.
55. Stanley MA, Wilson NL, Novy DM, et al. Cognitive behavior therapy for generalized anxiety disorder among older adults in primary care: a randomized clinical trial. JAMA. 2009;301(14):1460–7.
56. Wetherell JL, Ayers CR, Sorrell JT, et al. Modular psychotherapy for anxiety in older primary care patients. Am J Geriatr Psychiatry. 2009;17(6):483–92.
57. Nordhus IH, Pallesen S. Psychological treatment of late-life anxiety: an empirical review. J Consult Clin Psychol. 2003;71(4):643–51.
58. Thorp SR, Ayers CR, Nuevo R, et al. Meta-analysis comparing different behavioral treatments for late-life anxiety. Am J Geriatr Psychiatry. 2009; 17(2):105–15.
59. Hall J, Kellett S, Berrios R, et al. Efficacy of cognitive behavioral therapy for generalized anxiety disorder in older adults: systematic review, meta-analysis, and meta-regression. Am J Geriatr Psychiatry. 2016;24(11):1063–73.
60. Sheikh JI, Swales PJ. Treatment of panic disorder in older adults: a pilot study comparison of alprazolam, imipramine, and placebo. Int J Psychiatry Med. 1999;29(1):107–17.
61. Katz IR, Reynolds CF 3rd, Alexopoulos GS, Hackett D. Venlafaxine ER as a treatment for generalized anxiety disorder in older adults: pooled analysis of five randomized placebo-controlled clinical trials. J Am Geriatr Soc. 2002;50(1): 18–25.
62. Lenze EJ, Mulsant BH, Shear MK, et al. Efficacy and tolerability of citalopram in the treatment of late-life anxiety disorders: results from an 8-week randomized, placebo-controlled trial. Am J Psychiatry. 2005;162(1):146–50.
63. Alaka KJ, Noble W, Montejo A, et al. Efficacy and safety of duloxetine in the treatment of older adult patients with generalized anxiety disorder: a randomized, double-blind, placebo-controlled trial. Int J Geriatr Psychiatry. 2014;29(9):978–86.
64. Koepke HH, Gold RL, Linden ME, Lion JR, Rickels K. Multicenter controlled study of oxazepam in anxious elderly outpatients. Psychosomatics. 1982;23(6):641–5.
65. Bresolin N, Monza G, Scarpini E, et al. Treatment of anxiety with ketazolam in elderly patients. Clin Ther. 1988;10(5):536–42.
66. Frattola L, Piolti R, Bassi S, et al. Effects of alpidem in anxious elderly outpatients: a double-blind, placebo-controlled trial. Clin Neuropharmacol. 1992;15(6):477–87.
67. Small GW, Bystritsky A. Double-blind, placebo-controlled trial of two doses of abecarnil for geriatric anxiety. J Clin Psychiatry. 1997;58(Suppl 11):24–9.
68. By the American Geriatrics Society 2015 Beers Criteria Update Expert Panel. American Geriatrics Society 2015 updated beers criteria for potentially inappropriate medication use in older adults. J Am Geriatr Soc. 2015;63(11):2227–46.
69. Wetherell JL, Petkus AJ, White KS, et al. Antidepressant medication augmented with cognitive-behavioral therapy for generalized anxiety disorder in older adults. Am J Psychiatry. 2013;170(7): 782–9.
70. Bower ES, Wetherell JL, Mon T, Lenze EJ. Treating anxiety disorders in older adults: current treatments and future directions. Harv Rev Psychiatry. 2015;23(5):329–42.

22 Sexual Dysfunctions, Gender Dysphoria, and Paraphilic Disorders

Raman Marwaha, Poorvanshi Alag, and Amit Thour

Sexual Dysfunctions

Introduction

Sexual health is defined as "a state of physical, emotional, mental, social well being in relation to sexuality. It is not merely the absence of disease, dysfunction or infirmity. It requires a positive and respectful approach to sexuality and sexual relationships, as well as possibility of having pleasurable and safe sex experiences, free of coercion, discrimination and violence" [1]. Therefore, healthy sexual functioning is a part of good health.

Sexual dysfunctions are disorders that interfere with a full sexual response cycle. This makes it difficult for a person to enjoy or to have sexual intercourse. It not only affects physical health but also takes a heavy toll on a person's psychological health, bringing on depression and debilitating feelings of inadequacy. It is, therefore, essential to understand the effect of aging on sexual functioning. And, thus, sexual disorders are important to be assessed and treated by geriatric psychiatrists.

The Sexual Response Cycle

Researchers have developed a four-stage model of normal sexual response. This cycle takes place in the body during sexual activity. The four stages are excitement/arousal, plateau, orgasm, and resolution. Later a fifth stage was added, desire, to account for psychological and physiological component of sexuality [2] (Figure 22-1).

Sexual Dysfunction Diagnostic Criteria

The Diagnostic and Statistical Manual of Mental Disorder, Fourth Edition, Text Revision (DSM-IV-TR) defined sexual dysfunction as sexual pain or disturbance in one or more phases of the sexual response cycle [3]. The diagnostic criteria for DSM-IV-TR were criticized, firstly due to imprecise duration and secondly there was no clear differentiation between normal sexual function and sexual disorder that may merit medical intervention. Now, according to *Diagnostic and Statistical Manual of Mental Disorders*, Fifth Edition (DSM-5) [4], duration of at least 6 months is required for diagnosis of sexual dysfunction that should be present in at least 75% of the occasions to meet threshold of diagnosis. One of the exceptions that do not have to follow duration criterion is substance- or medication-induced sexual dysfunction. As per DSM-5, sexual dysfunction has been classified in the following categories (Table 22-1):

Epidemiology

Majority of studies have shown that most older adults continue to engage in sexual activities. The most significant predictors of sexual interest and activity are relationship status, physical health, and previous level of activity [5, 6]. Physical health is the most influencing factor for older men versus the quality of relationship in older women.

R. R. Tampi et al. (eds.), *Psychiatric Disorders Late in Life*, https://doi.org/10.1007/978-3-319-73078-3_22

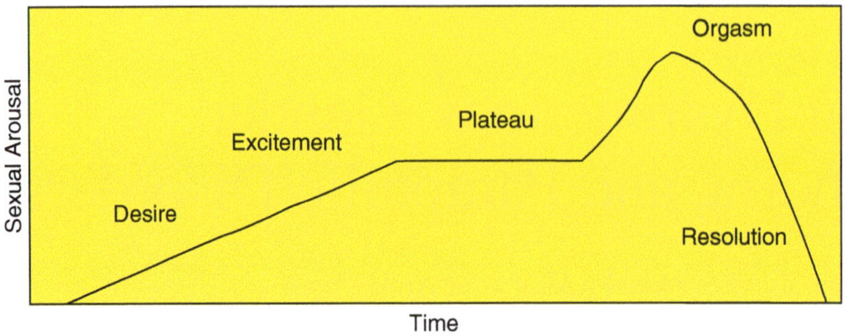

FIGURE. 22-1. Sexual response cycle

TABLE 22-1. Categories of sexual dysfunction as per DSM-5 [4]

Female sexual interest/arousal disorder: absence or significantly reduced sexual interest/arousal for at least 6 months (with at least three of the following symptoms)
• Absent/reduced interest in sexual activity
• Absent/reduced sexual/erotic thoughts or fantasies
• No/reduced initiation of sexual activity, unresponsive to partner's attempt to initiate sexual activity
• Absent/reduced sexual excitement/pleasure during sexual activity in at least 75% of encounters
• Absent/reduced sexual interest/arousal in response to any internal or external cues (e.g., written, verbal, visual)
• Absent/reduced genital or non-genital sensations during sexual activity in at least 75% of sexual encounters
Male hypoactive sexual desire disorder: diagnosis made by persistently deficient or absent sexual/erotic thoughts of fantasies and desire for sexual activity for 6 months
Erectile disorder: at least one of the three following symptoms must be experienced on almost all or all (75–100%) occasions of sexual activity for minimum of 6 months, causing significant distress and not better explained by nonsexual mental disorder, consequence of relationship distress, and is not attributed to substance or another medical condition
• Marked difficulty in obtaining an erection during sexual activity
• Marked difficulty in maintaining an erection until the completion of sexual activity
• Marked decrease in erectile rigidity
Delayed ejaculation: either of the following symptoms must be experienced on almost all or all (75–100%) occasions of sexual activity for a minimum of 6 months, causing clinically significant distress and not better explained by nonsexual mental disorder, consequence of relationship distress, and is not attributed to substance or another medical condition
• Marked delay in ejaculation
• Marked infrequency or absence of ejaculation
Female orgasmic disorder: either of the following symptoms must be experienced on almost all or all (75–100%) occasions of sexual activity for minimum of 6 months, causing clinically significant distress and not better explained by nonsexual mental disorder, consequence of relationship distress, and is not attributed to substance or another medical condition
• Marked delay in, marked infrequency of, or absence of orgasm
• Markedly reduced intensity of orgasmic sensations
Premature (early) ejaculation: diagnosed by a persistent pattern of ejaculation occurring during partnered sexual activity within approximately 1 min following vaginal penetration and before the individual wishes it for 6 months
Substance-/medication-induced sexual dysfunction: significant disturbance in sexual function during substance intoxication or withdrawal or after exposure to a medication
Genito-pelvic pain/penetration disorder: diagnosis made when there are persistent difficulties with one or more of the following for 6 months
• Vaginal penetration during intercourse
• Marked vulvovaginal or pelvic pain during vaginal intercourse
• Marked fear or anxiety about vulvovaginal pain in anticipation of, during, or a result of penetration
• Marked tensing or tightening of pelvic floor muscles during attempted vaginal penetration

Epidemiological studies for sexual dysfunction are limited due to lack of consistent definitions. However, in 2007, prevalence of sexual activity, behavior, and problems in 3005 adults aged 57–85 years in the United States was studied, and the association of these variables with age and health status was described [7]. Sexual activity was found in 73 % of individuals aged between 57 and 64 years, while it declined to 53% for ages between 65 and 74 years. The percentage went down to 26% for individuals 75 years of age and older. The rate of having sex two or three times per month went down from 65.4% for both men and women in middle cohort to 54.2% of men and 54.1% of women in oldest cohort.

Available data indicates that the prevalence of sexual dysfunction increases with age [8]. About 40–45% of adult women and 20–30% of adult men have at least one manifestation of sexual dysfunction [7]. Among all the sexual disorders, erectile disorder is the most common sexual dysfunction in older men, affecting 20–40% of men in their 60s and 50–70% of men in their 70s and 80s [8, 9]. In females, the most common type is hypoactive sexual desire, followed by female orgasmic disorder and dyspareunia as per DSM-IV-TR [5].

Neurobiology

Various factors are associated with development of sexual dysfunctions in late life. These include normal age-related changes, medical and psychiatric conditions, and medication-induced sexual dysfunction [10–22]. Additionally, an important association to be considered is the interaction between psychological factors and sexual dysfunction in late life. The psychological factors include stress, performance anxiety, relationship problems, psychological fear of trauma or abuse, anxiety, and depression (Table 22-2).

Diagnosis

The evaluation of sexual dysfunction in late life involves a detailed history including medical, sexual and psychiatric histories, and the use of medications. The interviewer should also evaluate the patient for age-related physical and psychological issues [23, 24]. An important aspect for a good assessment of sexual dysfunction in late life is the patient-doctor relationship, where on the one hand, the patient along with his/her partner feels comfortable and secure enough to disclose adequate history, while on the other hand, the physician can ask relevant questions and perform an appropriate evaluation.

The medical workup for sexual dysfunction also involves a physical examination, with the focus being the assessment of genital and urological anatomy and functions. In addition the neurological and vascular systems should be thoroughly assessed. Laboratory testing typically involves blood count, serum electrolytes, blood glucose, testosterone and prolactin levels, lipid profile, thyroid function, and the PSA levels (in men). Specialized diagnostic tests include nocturnal penile tumescence and rigidity testing and penile duplex ultrasonography (Figure. 22-2).

Treatments

It is important to preserve and enhance sexual activity in older adults. This essentially requires recognition of the fact that many of these individuals, despite having changes in physical and sexual functioning, intend to continue having sex. An integration of medical and psychological treatment has been thought to be most helpful in the treatment of sexual dysfunction among older adults. A first step in the treatment of sexual dysfunction among older adults is the education of both partners regarding normal and dysfunctional sexuality [25]. This not only helps in building trust between patient and the doctor but also reduces that patient and partners' anxiety regarding the problem.

Many older adults suffer from chronic medical conditions that limit them from engaging in normal sexual activity due to fatigue, loss of muscle strength, and pain [22, 24]. The use of analgesics for pain and physical therapy for joint and muscle weakness will improve sexual functioning by alleviating the physical problems. If the patient has an underlying psychiatric illness, then appropriate treatment of the condition should improve sexual functioning.

Pharmacotherapy

Several options can be considered when sexual functions get impaired due to medication side

TABLE 22-2. Factors are associated with the development of sexual dysfunctions among older adults

Normal age-related changes	**Women** • Decreased testosterone levels • Vaginal atrophy • Reduced blood supply to pelvic region • During orgasm, strength and amount of vaginal contractions are decreased • During arousal, vaginal lubrication is decreased **Men** • Due to decrease in blood flow and smooth muscle relaxation, penile rigidity decreases • Production of testosterone is reduced, yet it does not have uniform effect on sexual function • Amount of functional sperms decreases despite no change in sperm count • Erections take longer to achieve and are more difficult to sustain • Refractory period decreases from hours to days • No change in sexual desire
Psychological	• Stress • Anxiety and depression • Anger • Guilt • Relationship problems • Psychological trauma and abuse
Hormonal	• Hypothyroidism • Pituitary dysfunction
Vascular	• High blood pressure and atherosclerosis • Diabetes • Cardiovascular diseases • Hyperlipidemia
Neurological	• Spinal cord injury • Diabetes • Parkinson's disease • Multiple sclerosis • Pelvic fracture • Obstructive sleep apnea
Musculoskeletal	• Arthritis and other degenerative joint diseases
Genitourinary	• Lower urinary tract infection • Chronic renal failure • Prostate disease and surgery • Genital and urological cancers
Psychiatric	• Anxiety disorder (generalized anxiety disorders, panic disorder) • Obsessive-compulsive disorder • Major depressive disorder and other mood disorders • Schizophrenia and other psychotic disorders • Substance abuse
Medications	• Alpha adrenergic blockers (prazosin, phentolamine) • Antidepressants (monoamine oxidase inhibitors, tricyclic antidepressants, selective serotonin reuptake inhibitors, venlafaxine) • Antihistamines • Antihypertensives (thiazides, diuretics, beta blockers, ACE inhibitors, clonidine, spironolactone, calcium channel blockers, reserpine) • Benzodiazepines • Antipsychotics (conventional and atypical)

effects [11–16]. One of the options is to continue administering the medication and wait for tolerance to develop. If no change is seen, then a reduction in dose should be considered. If still no improvements are noted, then changing the medication would be next appropriate step in the treatment plan.

It has been studied that elderly men benefit more from medical treatment [26]. For certain medications like antidepressants, the clinician can consider replacing the medication with other medications that have less potential for sexual side effects such as mirtazapine or bupropion [27, 28]. With respect to

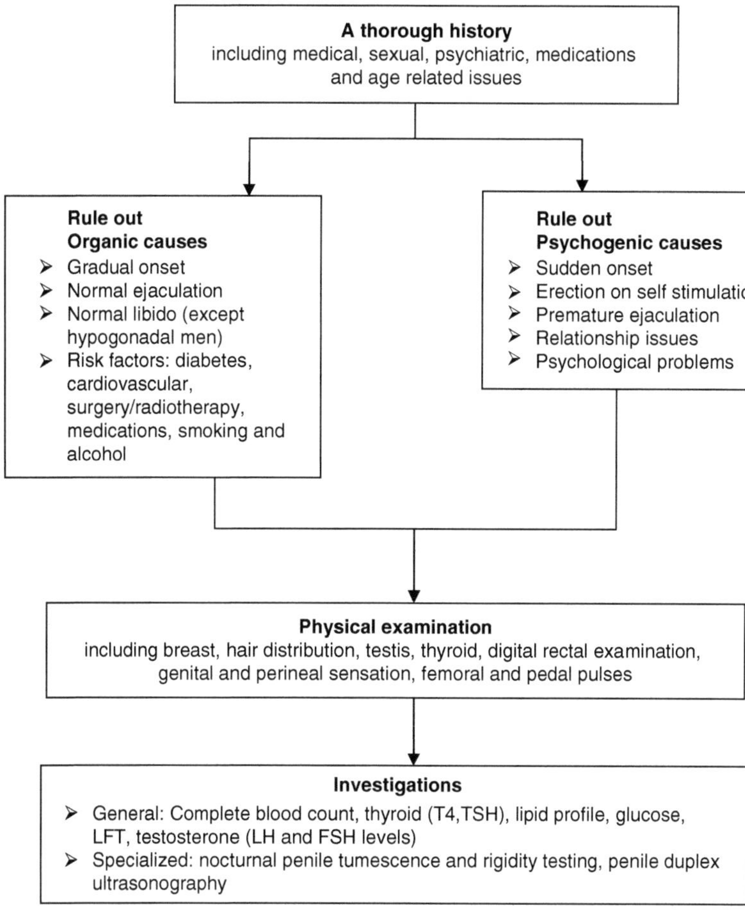

FIGURE. 22-2. Assessment of sexual dysfunction among older adults

antipsychotics, more potent agents with less anticholinergic side effects may cause less sexual dysfunction [29, 30]. Some antidotes have been reported in a Cochrane review that can reverse sexual side effects of medications which include yohimbine, amantadine, bethanechol, methylphenidate, buspirone, bromocriptine (for antipsychotic-induced sexual dysfunction), bupropion, nefazodone, mirtazapine, and trazodone [31]. The drugs used for the treatment of erectile dysfunction are phosphodiesterase (PDE-5) inhibitors—sildenafil, tadalafil, and vardenafil—that have shown success rates of 70–80% among affected men [32–34]. These medications have also shown to reverse antidepressant-induced erectile dysfunction [31, 35, 36].

Sex Therapy

Sex therapy is most beneficial when both partners participate together toward finding a solution for the sexual problems. Cognitive behavioral technique is the current treatment of model used in sex therapy [36]. During sex therapy, the therapist works with the couple over their problem and helps them in overcoming resistance that inevitably arises during treatment. Regardless of age, most couples feel that during sex therapy not only does the sexual interest and pleasure reemerge but also the enjoyment and happiness in their relationship get reestablished (Table 22-3).

Gender Dysphoria

Introduction

Gender dysphoria is the condition of a person feeling that their gender identity is opposite to their biological sex. Gender dysphoria has been introduced as a new diagnostic class in DSM-5,

Table 22-3. Specific treatments for sexual dysfunctions

Female sexual interest/arousal disorder	Sex education and counseling to counter psychological barriers Estrogen replacement therapy may help improve sexual arousal and comfort
Erectile disorder	Educating and counseling both patient and partner Lifestyle change and risk factor modification Phosphodiesterase (PDE-5) inhibitors—sildenafil, tadalafil, and vardenafil Increased nitric oxide (NO) which relaxes smooth muscles in the penis and increases blood flow. Side effects—headache, low BP, flushing, dyspepsia Intraurethral alprostadil Vacuum pump devices
Female orgasmic disorder	Sex therapy involving relaxation techniques and guided masturbation Testosterone and sildenafil have also proven to be beneficial
Premature (early) ejaculation	Behavior technique "squeeze method" Topical anesthetic agent like lidocaine Selective serotonin reuptake inhibitors (cause delayed ejaculation)

while previously in DSM-IV-TR, it was covered in sexual and gender identity disorders. DSM-5 considers gender dysphoria to be multicategory and diminishes the use of gender variance. Gender nonconformity in itself is not a disorder, but if it is associated with clinically significant distress, then it is a disorder and is called gender dysphoria. It is a unique condition as mental health providers make the diagnosis although the treatments are mainly endocrinological and/or surgical.

Gender dysphoria has been further classified as gender dysphoria in children and gender dysphoria in adolescents and adults. Among adults, the DSM-5 mentions a subtype that is present with a disorder of sex development (e.g., congenital adrenal hyperplasia) and a specifier of posttransition.

The DSM-5 diagnostic criteria for gender dysphoria in adults are as follows:

1. There is a marked incongruence between one's experienced/expressed gender and assigned gender which is of at least 6 months duration and is manifested by two or more of the following:
   (a) A marked incongruence between one's experienced/expressed gender and primary and/or secondary sex characteristics
   (b) A strong desire to be rid of one's primary and/or secondary sex characteristics because of a marked incongruence with one's experienced/expressed gender
   (c) A strong desire for the primary and/or secondary sex characteristics of the other gender
   (d) A strong desire to be of the other gender (or some alternative gender different from one's assigned gender)
   (e) A strong desire to be treated as the other gender (or some alternative gender different from one's assigned gender)
   (f) A strong conviction that one has the typical feelings and reactions of the other gender (or some alternative gender different from one's assigned gender)
2. The gender dysphoria leads to clinically significant distress and/or social, occupational, and other functioning impairments. Additionally, there may be an increased risk of suffering, distress, or disability.

Epidemiology

It is difficult to estimate the incidence and prevalence of gender dysphoria in geriatric population due to lack of epidemiological studies. While DSM-5 does not give any specific prevalence rates in geriatric age group, the estimated prevalence in adults is 0.005–0.014% for males and 0.002–0.003% for females. Cohen-Kettenis noted that 0.009% male and 0.003% female seek treatment for gender dysphoria at specialized clinics [37].

Twenty-five percent of men who have gender dysphoria are attracted toward women, while majority of these individuals identify themselves as being attracted toward men. Among females who have gender dysphoria, there are conflicting reports about whether they are sexually attracted toward women or men. Chivers and Bailey indicated that female to male transsexuals are not a homogeneous group and vary in ways that may be useful in understanding the relation between sexual orientation and gender identity [38].

Male to female and female to male are used to identify the direction of transition and the gender identity the person has chosen.

Substance use disorders are commonly found in men and women with gender dysphoria with studies showing that 28% of these individuals have reported problems with substance use [39]. Lifetime prevalence of suicidal ideation was reported as 76.1% in male to female and 71.9% in female to male patients [40]. Anxiety, depression, and personality disorders are also common comorbidities. One study by Madeddu in 2009 found that personality disorder was comorbid in 52% of cases, and the most common was Cluster B personality disorders [41].

Etiology

It is unclear what causes gender dysphoria, and there is a lot of controversy surrounding its etiology. The etiology in geriatric population is considered to be the same as in children and adults. Zucker has postulated a biopsychosocial model of development in children [42].

Coolidge et al. described a significant genetic component in gender dysphoria accounting for 62% of the variance and a non-shared environmental component accounting for the remaining 38% of the variance, which showed the significant role played by biology [43]. Sexual differentiation of the human brain can get affected during the intrauterine period depending on exposure to testosterone or its absence, and it has been postulated that gender dysphoria can possibly be explained by abnormal exposure to hormones [44].

Gender dysphoria can be present in congenital adrenal hyperplasia or partial androgen insensitivity syndrome, and DSM-5 recognizes this as a specifier.

Cohen-Kettenis and Gooren report that certain parental factors seem to be associated with cross-gender identification including parents being less emotionally warm, more rejecting, and/or more (over)controlling [37].

Diagnosis

The DSM-5 criteria help in differentiating "transsexual" behaviors with gender dysphoria as the latter should lead to clinically significant distress and/or social, occupational, and other functioning impairments. Geriatric population will either present with a past history of gender dysphoria or rarely as a new diagnosis. Diagnosis of gender dysphoria should be made carefully and warrant an extensive evaluation including detailed history and examination. A multidisciplinary team consisting of a psychiatrist, psychologist, endocrinologist, surgeon, and geriatrician may help in evaluating the patient. It is important to make sure that gender dysphoria is consistent, persistent, and insistent. Differential diagnosis including medical problems and psychiatric disorders such as psychotic disorders and personality disorders should be considered.

Treatments

Management of gender dysphoria includes working in a multidisciplinary team. Some patients may only need counseling, while others may want hormonal therapy or surgery.

Hormonal treatments include giving estrogens to male to female patients with gender dysphoria and testosterone to female to male patients. Hormonal therapy can provide certain desired results but can also cause adverse effects, and patients should be educated about the risks and benefits.

Physical interventions include electrolysis, chest/breast surgery, other cosmetic surgery, or genital surgery. Plastic surgeons can conduct gender-confirming surgeries like top surgery (mastectomy or breast augmentation) and bottom surgery (vaginoplasty or phalloplasty). Aydin et al. did a 20-year follow-up study on transgender surgery in Denmark and reported that 126 gender-confirming surgeries were performed from 1994 to 2015 [45]. They also noted that median age at the time of surgery decreased from 40 to 27 years during the 20-year period.

The World Professional Association for Transgender Health (WPATH) has published the Standards of Care (SOC), to provide clinical guidelines for health care of transsexual, transgender, and gender-nonconforming persons in order to maximize health and well-being of patients with gender dysphoria [46]. All treatment options should be offered, and depending on an individual's goals and expectations, the most appropriate surgical technique should be performed. The Standards of Care outlined by WPATH recommend against physical interventions before the age of 16 years. They recommend that surgery only be performed after the age of 18 and after the individual has lived in their desired gender role for at least 2 years. In order for people to undergo physical (hormonal or surgical) interventions to make their body more in line with their gender identity, they must be assessed by a mental health professional that has special competence in this area, and often recommendations are required from two such mental health professionals.

Murad et al. looked at prognosis in patients with gender dysphoria and suggested that sex reassignment that includes hormonal interventions improves gender dysphoria, psychological functioning and comorbidities, sexual function, and overall quality of life [47].

Paraphilic Disorder

Introduction

Paraphilia is defined as a type of sexual disorder, where sexual function is intact but sexual excitement depends on a particular stimulus or an activity that is unusual or even bizarre [48]. These remain at the center of controversy and political decisions.

In DSM-5, paraphilic disorder is a paraphilia that is currently causing distress or impairment or that has entailed harm or risk of harm to others [49]. Previously in the DSM-IV-TR, the above criterion had been necessary but not sufficient for having a paraphilic disorder [50]. The definition of paraphilia, according to DSM-IV-TR (which was not redefined in DSM-5), is recurrent, intense sexually arousing fantasies, sexual urges, or behavior generally involving:

1. Nonhuman objects
2. The suffering or humiliation of oneself or one's partner
3. Children or other non-consenting person that occurs over a period of at least 6 months (Table 22-4)

Epidemiology

Due to cultural differences and constant changes in criteria over time, it has also been difficult to obtain accurate prevalence rates of paraphilic disorders among adults [52]. In late life, paraphilic disorders are thought to be seen more in men than women. In a surveyed sample of 1915 men, aged 40–79 years, it was found that 62.4% had at least one paraphilia-associated sexual arousal pattern, and it caused distress in only 1.7% of cases [53].

When a nonclinical sample of men and women was examined for the prevalence of paraphilic interest, a correlation between the sex drive and paraphilic interests was noted. There are various comorbidities that are associated with different paraphilic interests including mood and anxiety disorders. In men paraphilic interests often represent long-standing behaviors or occur due to brain damage, mostly involving the frontotemporal region [54, 55]. In a recent systematic review of paraphilias and paraphilic disorders in Parkinson's disease, patients revealed that both could emerge as a rare iatrogenic consequence in Parkinson's disease treatment [56].

TABLE 22-4. DSM-5 classification of paraphilic disorders [51]

Voyeuristic disorder	Sexual arousal by watching an unsuspecting person naked/in sexual activity/disrobing
Exhibitionistic disorder	Exposure of genitals to strangers in public
Frotteuristic disorder	Sexual arousal by touching or rubbing non-consenting person
Sexual masochism disorder	Sexual pleasure from physical or mental abuse or humiliation
Sexual sadism disorder	Sexual arousal from causing mental or physical suffering to another person
Pedophilic disorder	Sexual fantasies, urges, or activity with prepubescent child. Must be at least 16 years old and be 5 years older than the child
Fetishistic disorder	Sexual arousal with nonliving objects
Transvestic disorder	Sexual disorder from cross-dressing

Neurobiology

Paraphilias usually emerge during adolescence [57]. These can occur due to a connection with an event or relationships in early childhood which include childhood emotional abuse and family dysfunction, childhood behavior problems, and childhood sexual abuse. Once established, paraphilias tend to be chronic, although research has shown that these behaviors reduce as the individual ages [58]. Although biological factors contribute to the development of paraphilias, psychological factors seem to play a central role in their development.

Diagnosis

It is essential to differentiate between paraphilic disorders and normal variation of sexual behavior. Inappropriate sexual behavior is not always a paraphilic disorder, for example, a psychotic patient may cross-dress due to his delusional belief or a patient with dementia may behave in a sexually inappropriate behavior due to cognitive impairment, but those are not considered as paraphilias. It is therefore important to evaluate and assess every patient carefully before diagnosing them with a paraphilic disorder.

A detailed history including psychiatric and psychosexual history should be obtained. It is often difficult to interview people with paraphilic disorders due to their feelings of guilt and reluctance to be forthcoming with the information. It is therefore required to establish a good patient-doctor relationship, so as to allow the individual to voice their concerns freely. In addition to history, a complete mental status examination and physical and neurological examinations are required to assist with the evaluation and rule out any other disease process. Investigations that may be considered in the assessment of patients with paraphilic disorder include complete blood count, thyroid function tests, phallometric testing, and EEG if indicated.

Treatments

There is very limited data regarding the treatment of paraphilia among the elderly. Treatments largely depend on the nature of the paraphilia [59]. In some cases of paraphilia, events that occurred during childhood may have led to the developmental of a paraphilia (by associating sexual pleasure with that event or object). Thus psychotherapy is required to explore the sexual experiences and fantasies that caused and maintained the paraphilia. It has been reported that cognitive behavioral therapy, couple therapy, and psychodynamic therapy have all shown good benefits with low rates of relapse [60, 61].

Currently the most common treatment for paraphilic disorders is cognitive behavioral therapy (CBT) and includes all of the following:

1. Covert conditioning which typically causes undesirable behavior to become less desirable [62]. This type of intervention can be used for any type of paraphilic disorder.
2. Aversive therapy which involves pairing arousal to the deviant fantasy with either mild electric shock or unpleasant smell [63].
3. Orgasmic conditioning aims at redirecting the arousal pattern by looking at "appropriate" objects and providing themselves with positive reinforcement. This type of treatment is helpful for individuals who have a fetish [61].
4. Group therapy is also beneficial in treating paraphilic disorders [62]. This therapy focuses on building social skills, establishing family support, and cognitive reconstruction.

Medication treatments are reserved for more severe cases of paraphilia, especially for individuals who are at high risk to reoffend and who do not respond to other interventions [59]. Medications include antiandrogens, gonadotropin-releasing hormone agonist, and selective serotonin reuptake inhibitors (SSRI). Antiandrogens are reported to cause a reduction in sexual behaviors but are associated with significant side effects including hot flushes, leg cramps, hair loss, bone mineral loss, and cardiac issues. Gonadotropin-releasing hormone agonists desensitize gonadotropin-releasing hormone receptors, which results in a reduction of luteinizing hormones (luteinizing hormone stimulus releases testosterone from testes). SSRI are also used to treat various forms of paraphilias including voyeurism, exhibitionism, and pedophilia [64–66]. It is important to understand that these medications do not cure paraphilic disorders and should not generally be used as the sole form of treatment. It is generally recommended to combine medications with some form of CBT to maximize benefits of the treatment for paraphilic disorders.

Conclusions

Although majority of older adults continue to engage in sexual activity, there is a decline in the rate and frequency of sexual activity with increasing age. Currently there is limited research on the epidemiology, etiology, assessment, and management of sexual dysfunctions, gender dysphoria, and paraphilic disorders among the geriatric population. However, available evidence indicates efficacy for non-pharmacological and pharmacological treatments for these disorders. The availability of data from controlled studies of sexual dysfunctions, gender dysphoria, and paraphilic disorders specifically among older adults will enable clinicians to diagnose and treat these disorders appropriately. Appropriate diagnosis and treatment of these disorders will help reduce the morbidity due to these disorders and reduce the suffering of the individuals and their families.

References

1. Glasier A, Gülmezoglu A, Schmid GP, et al. Sexual and reproductive health: a matter of life and death. Lancet. 2006;368(9547):1595–607.
2. Archer J, Lloyd B. Sex and gender. Cambridge. Retrieved 2002: Cambridge University Press; 2012. p. 85–8.
3. Balon R. The DSM criteria of sexual dysfunction: need for a change. J Sex Martial Ther. 2008;34(3):186–97.
4. Hoeksema SN. Abnormal psychology. New York, NY: McGraw-Hill; 2014. p. 366–7.
5. Lindua ST, Schumm LP, Laumann EO, et al. A study of sexuality and health among older adults in the United States. N Engl J Med. 2007;357(8): 762–74.
6. Schick V, Herbenick D, Reece M, et al. Sexual behaviors, condom use and sexual health of Americans over 50; implications for sexual health promotion for older adults. J Sex Med. 2010;7(5):315–29.
7. Lewis RW, Fugl-Meyer KS, Bosch R, et al. Epidemiology/risk factors of sexual dysfunction. J Sex Med. 2004;1:35–9.
8. Laumann EO, Waite LJ. Sexual dysfunction among older adults: prevalence and risk factors from a nationally representative U.S. probability sample of men and women 57-85 years of age. J Sex Med. 2008;5(10):2300–11.
9. Feldman HA, Goldstein I, Hatzichristou DG, et al. Impotence and its medical and psychosocial correlates: results of the Massachusetts male ageing study. J Urol. 1994;151:54–61.
10. Abdallah RT, Simon JA. Testosterone therapy in women: its role in the management of hypoactive sexual desire disorder.
11. Ludwig W, Phillips M. Organic causes of erectile dysfunction in men under 40. Urol Int. 2003;92(3):553–62.
12. Thomas DR. Medications and sexual function. Clin Geriatr Med. 2003;19(3):535–62.
13. Liu L, Zhao S, Zhang T, et al. Sexual dysfunction in patients with obstructive sleep apnea: a systematic review and meta-analysis. J Sex Med. 2015;12:1992–2003.
14. Nicolai MPJ, Liem SS, Both S, et al. A review of positive and negative effects of cardiovascular drugs on sexual function: a proposed table for use in clinical practice. Neth Heart J. 2014;22(1):11–9.
15. Segraves RT, Balon R. Antidepressant induced sexual dysfunction in men. Pharmacol Biochem Behav. 2014;121:132–7.
16. Zajecka J. Stratergies for the treatment of antidepressant related sexual dysfunction via avoidance, switching antidepressants, antidotes and adaptation. J Clin Psychiatry. 2003;64(Suppl 10):11–9.
17. McVary K. Lower urinary tract symptoms and sexual dysfunction: epidemiology and pathophysiology. BJU Int. 2006;97(Suppl 2):23–8.
18. Hansen BL. Lower urinary tract symptoms (LUTS) and sexual function in both sexes. Eur Urol. 2004;46: 229–34.
19. Currey HLF. Osteoarthritis of hip joint and sexual activity. Ann Rheum Dis. 1970;29:488–93.
20. Nikoobakht M, Nasseh H, Pourkasmaee M. The relationship between lipid profile and erectile dysfunction. Int J Impot Res. 2005;17:523–36.
21. Billups KL, et al. Erectile dysfunction is a marker of cardiovascular disease: results of the minority health institute expert advisory panel. J Sex Med. 2005;2:40–52.
22. Morley JE, Tariq SH. Sexuality & disease. Clin Geriatr Med. 2003;19:563–73.

23. Agronin ME. Sexuality and ageing. In: Binik YM, Hall KSK, editors. Principles and practice of sex therapy. 5th ed. New York: Guilford; 2014. p. 529–39.
24. Dunn KM, Croft PR, Hackett GI. Association of sexual problems with social, psychological, and physical problems in men and women: a cross sectional population survey. J Epidemiol Community Health. 1999;53:144–8.
25. Bitzer J, Platano G, Tschudin S, et al. Sexaul counseling in elderly couples. J Sex Med. 2008; 5(9):2027–43.
26. Segraves RT, Lee J, Stevenson R. Tadalafil for treatment of erectile dysfunction in men on antidepressant. J Clin Psychopharmacol. 2007;27(1):62–6.
27. Clayton AH, Croft HA, Handiwala L. Antidepressants and sexual dysfunction: mechanisms & clinical implications. Postgrad Med. 2014;126(2):91–9.
28. Reichenpfader U, Gartlehner G, Morgon LC, et al. Sexual dysfunction associated with second generation antidepressants in patients with major depressive disorder: results from systematic review with network metaanalysis. Drug Saf. 2014;37(1):19–31.
29. Baggaley M. Sexual dysfunction in schizophrenia: focus on recent evidence. Hum Psychopharmacol. 2008;23(3):201–9.
30. Serretti A, Chiesa A. A meta analysis of sexual dysfunction in psychiatric patients taking antipsychotics. Int Clin Psychopharmacol. 2011;26(3): 30–140.
31. Taylor MJ, Rudkin L, Bullemor-Day P, et al. Strategies for managing sexual dysfunction induced by antidepressant medications. *Cochrane Database Syst Rev*. 2013;5:CD003382.
32. Boolell M, Gepi AS, Gingell JC, et al. Sildenafil a novel effective oral therapy for male erectile dysfunction. Br J Urol. 1996;78(2):257–61.
33. Porst H, Young JM, Schmidt AC, et al. Efficacy and tolerability of vardenafil for treatment of erectile dysfunction in pt subgroups. Urology. 2003;62(3):519–23.
34. Porst H, Montorsi F, Rosen RC, et al. The premature ejaculations prevalence and attitudes survey: prevalence comorbidites and professional help seeking. Eur Urol. 2006;51(3):816–23.
35. Berigan T. Antidepressant induced sexual dysfunction treated with vardenafil. Can J Psychiatr. 2004; 49(9):643.
36. Brotto L, Luria M. Sexual interest/arousal disorder in women, principles and practice of sex therapy. 5th ed. New York: Guilford; 2014. p. 17–41.
37. Cohen-Kettenis PT, Gooren LJ. Transsexualism: a review of etiology, diagnosis and treatment. J Psychosom Res. 1999;46(4):315–33.
38. Chivers ML, Bailey JM. Sexual orientation of female-to-male transsexuals: a comparison of homosexual and nonhomosexual types. Arch Sex Behav. 2000;29(3):259–78.
39. Collier CM, O'Boyle M, Emory LE, et al. Co-morbidity of gender dysphoria and other major psychiatric diagnoses. Arch Sex Behav. 1997;26(1): 13–26.
40. Hoshiai M, Matsumoto Y, Sato T, et al. Psychiatric co-morbidity among patients with gender identity disorder. Psychiatry Clin Neurosci. 2010;64(5): 514–9.
41. Madeddu F, Prunas A, Hartmann D, et al. Prevalence of Axis II disorders in a sample of clients undertaking psychiatric evaluation for sex reassignment surgery. Psychiatr Q. 2009;80(4):261–7.
42. Zucker KJ, Wood H, Singh D, et al. A developmental, biopsychosocial model for the treatment of children with gender identity disorder. J Homosex. 2012;59(3):369–97.
43. Coolidge FL, Thede LL, Young SE. The heritability of gender identity disorder in a child and adolescent twin sample. Behav Genet. 2002;32(4): 251–7.
44. Bao AM, Swaab DF. Sexual differentiation of the human brain: relation to gender identity, sexual orientation and neuropsychiatric disorders. Front Neuroendocrinol. 2011;32(2):214–26.
45. Aydin D, Buk LJ, Partoft S, et al. Transgender surgery in Denmark from 1994 to 2015: 20-year follow-up study. J Sex Med. 2016;13(4):720–5.
46. Selvaggi G, Dhejne C, Landen M, et al. The 2011 WPATH standards of care and penile reconstruction in female-to-male transsexual individuals. Adv Urol. 2012;2012:581712.
47. Murad MH, Elamin MB, Garcia MZ, et al. Hormonal therapy and sex reassignment: a systematic review and meta-analysis of quality of life and psychosocial outcomes. Clin Endocrinol. 2010;72(2):214–31.
48. Balon R. Politics of diagnostic criteria: specifies of pedophilic disorders in DSM-5. Arch Sex Behav. 2014;43:1235–6.
49. American Psychiatric Association. "Paraphilic Disorders". Diagnostic and statistical manual of mental disorders. 5th ed. Virginia: American Psychiatric Publishing; 2013. p. 685–6.
50. Konrad N, Welke J, Opitz- Welke A. Paraphilias. Curr Opin Psychiatry. 2015;28(6):440–4.

51. Campbell MM, Artz L, Stein DJ. Sexual disorders in DSM-5 and ICD-11: a conceptual framework. Curr Opin Psychiatry. 2015;28(6):435–9.
52. Bhugra D, Popelyuk D, McMullen I. Paraphilias across cultures: contexts and controversies. J Sex Res. 2010;4:242–56.
53. Ahlers CJ, Schaefer GA, Mundt IA. How unusual are the contents of paraphilia- associated sexual arousal patterns in a community based sample of men. J Sex Med. 2011;8:1362–70.
54. Leo RJ, Kim RY. Clomipramine treatment of paraphilias on elderly demented patients. J Geriatr Psychiatry Neurol. 1995;8:123–4.
55. Philpot CD. Paraphilia and aging. Clin Geriatr Med. 2003;19(3):629–36.
56. Sollo P, Bortolato M, Cannas A, et al. Paraphilias and paraphilic disorders in parkinson's disease: a systematic review of the literature. Mov Disord. 2015;30:604–13.
57. Lee JKP, Jackson H, Pattison P. Developmental risk factors for sexual offending. Child Abuse Negl. 2002;26(1):73–92.
58. Barbaree HE, Langton CM, Blanchard R, et al. Predicting recidivism in sex offenders using SUR-20: the contribution of age at release. Int J Forensic Ment Health. 2008;7:47–64.
59. Thibaut F, De La Barra F, Gordon H, et al. The world federation of societies of biological psychiatry guidelines for the biological treatment of paraphilias. World J Biol Psychiatry. 2010;11: 604–55.
60. Sorrentino RM. Paraphilias in Kaplan & Sadock's comprehensive textbook of psychiatry. 9th ed. Philadelphia, PA: Lippincott Williams & Wilkins; 2009. p. 2090–8.
61. Beech AR, Harkins L. DSM-IV paraphilias: description, demographics and treatment intervention. Aggress Violent Behav. 2012;17:527–39.
62. Morin JW, Levenson JS. Exhibitionism: assessment & treatment. In: Laws DL, O'Donohue WT, editors. Sexual deviance: theory, assessment, and treatment. 2nd ed.; 2008. p. 76–107.
63. Plaud JJ. Sexual disorders. In: Sturmey P. editors. Functional analysis of clinical treatment; 2007. p. 357–378.
64. Kraus C, Strohm K, Hill A, et al. Selective serotonin reuptake inhibitor in the treatment of paraphilia. Fortschr Neurol Psych. 2007;75(6): 351–6.
65. Emmanuel NP, Lydiard RB, Ballenger JC. Fluoxetine treatment of voyeurism. Am J Psychiatry. 1991;148(7):950.
66. Bourgeois JA, Klein M. Risperidone and fluoxetine in treatment of pedophilia with comorbid dysthymia. J Clin Psychopharmacol. 1996;16: 257–8.

23 Intellectual Disability in the Elderly

Joanna C. Lim, Laurel J. Bessey, Pallavi Joshi, and Lisa L. Boyle

Introduction

Formerly classified as mental retardation, intellectual disability (ID) is defined in the *Diagnostic and Statistical Manual of Mental Disorders, Fifth Edition* (DSM-5) as a disorder with onset in the developmental period that is characterized by deficits in general mental abilities that result in impairments of adaptive functioning. Persons with ID have deficits in functions such as reasoning, problem-solving, abstract thinking, academic learning, communication, social participation, and independent living [1].

People with ID are a heterogeneous group. They consist of individuals who have syndrome-specific illnesses and individuals who have had central nervous system injury during the developmental period that caused ID. Advances in medical treatment and social care over the last century have resulted in increased longevity in this population. The mean life expectancy of a person with ID increased from 19 years in the 1930s to 66 years in the 1990s [2–4]. With the increase in life expectancy, middle and old age become important for this population, and many face similar age-associated health problems as older adults without ID [5, 6]. Among older adults with ID, the most studied are individuals with Down syndrome due to the relatively high rates of Alzheimer's disease (AD) among these individuals [7]. Limited data exist on the typical aging process of adults with other syndrome-specific disorders.

In this subchapter, we will review and discuss what is currently known about the epidemiology, neurobiology, diagnosis, and available treatments of older adults with ID.

Epidemiology

The global prevalence of ID is approximately 1%, with higher rates observed in males in both child and adult populations. The prevalence is almost two times higher in lower and middle income countries [8]. Although life expectancy of individuals with ID has increased, individuals with ID continue to have a lower life expectancy when compared to the general population [9], with the exception of individuals with mild ID, who have a life expectancy close to the general population [10].

Fragile X syndrome (FXS) is the most common identifiable inherited cause of ID with a prevalence of one in 4000 males and one in 8000 females [11–13]. The average age of death based on a mortality study among 348 males and 433 females is approximately 12 years lower than the general population. The most common causes of death in this group are comparable with those in the general population [14].

Down syndrome (DS) is another common identifiable cause of ID with an incidence of 1 in every 700 live births in the United States [15]. The mean age of death increased from 9 years in the 1920s to 56 years in 1999 [2–4, 16], likely from better

R. R. Tampi et al. (eds.), *Psychiatric Disorders Late in Life*, https://doi.org/10.1007/978-3-319-73078-3_23

treatments of congenital heart disease and respiratory infections in early life [16, 17]. Middle-aged adults with DS are at risk for premature aging: development of early menopause in women, early onset of visual and hearing impairment, epilepsy, hypothyroidism, obesity, early decline in functioning, and increased risk of developing AD [18–25]. Age, presence of dementia, and restrictions in mobility are important predictors of mortality in a population-based cohort of individuals with DS who are 45 years and older. Individuals with a physical handicap and severe to profound level of ID and those living in institutions are more likely to die [26]. In some studies, life expectancy is influenced by gender with males on average outliving females by more than 3 years [3]. Dementia is the most important cause of morbidity and mortality among adults with DS. Better understanding of the underlying neurochemical, biochemical, and neuropathological processes of AD in DS may improve life expectancy and quality of life in this population [23, 26].

Dementia in non-DS ID individuals is less studied. Reported prevalence rates vary from 18.3 to 21.6% of adults with non-DS ID aged over 65 years, which are higher when compared to a younger group of individuals with ID and the general population over age 65 [26–29].

Overall, individuals with ID have poorer health status when compared to the general population due to genetic predispositions to health conditions, poor access to health-care services, social environment, and residential situations that promote inactivity [5]. Older adults with ID are more likely to live in psychiatric hospitals, nursing homes, and other large institutions [30].

Low physical activity and consumption of a high-calorie diet increase the prevalence of obesity, cardiovascular disease, Type 2 diabetes, constipation, osteoporosis, incontinence, and arthritis in older adults with ID [64]. The prevalence of epilepsy is also greater in people with ID than in the general population [31]. A negative association exists between survival and severity of ID [2, 26, 32].

Psychiatric disorders are more common in older adults with ID, which effect caregiver burden and cost of care [17, 33]. Depression becomes more prevalent with increasing age. Risk of psychiatric disorders appears to increase with the severity of ID, especially when mild ID is excluded from the analysis [34]. The most predominant psychiatric disorder in adults with ID is affective disorders, followed by anxiety disorders, psychosis, and autism spectrum disorders [35]. Substance abuse is observed in only 0.8% and attention-deficit hyperactivity disorder in 0.5% of adults with ID [36]. Problem behavior (aggression toward others and oneself) can occur in approximately 61% of adults with ID according to a study from a mixed-age community sample in the UK [37].

Individuals with ID experience higher rates of physical, sexual, verbal, and psychological abuse, neglect, and financial exploitation compared to adults without ID [38, 39]. Due to the physical and mental handicap prevalent in this population, individuals with ID may have difficulty verbalizing the abuse or advocating for themselves. Thus, the presence of abuse may be diagnosed only via physical or behavioral symptoms such as inappropriate sexual behavior, alterations in bowel- or bladder-emptying patterns, changes in sleep, sexually transmitted infections, or pregnancy. It is therefore important for practitioners to screen all individuals with ID for physical and sexual abuse [38, 40].

Neurobiology

Individuals with ID comprise of a diverse group of individuals with unique biological and psychological impairments. To describe the neurobiological characteristics of this group, it is best to look at the most common genetic syndromes that present with ID. In general, individuals with ID have reduced brain reserve, smaller brain size, and fewer neurons or synapse count [29].

Fragile X Syndrome (FXS)

FXS is caused by an expansion of a trinucleotide CGG repeat (>200) on the promoter region of the fragile X mental retardation 1 gene (FMR1). Individuals with a full mutation (>200 repeats), premutation (50–200 repeats), and intermediate allele carriers (40–55 repeats) experience a range of psychological and physical effects of FXS [41].

Expansion in full mutation individuals results in hypermethylation of the CGG that leads to silencing of the FMR1 gene and loss of the encoded gene product, fragile X mental retardation protein (FMRP) [42]. FMRP is commonly expressed in neurons and plays a vital role in synaptogenesis and synaptic plasticity, which is why learning and memory are affected in this syndrome. FXS in males presents with mild to moderate ID that is consistent with an IQ of 35–70 [43]. Hypermethylation in FXS also leads to the behavioral and physical abnormalities of FXS which includes hyperactivity, anxiety, attention problems, hand flapping, hand biting, gaze avoidance, loose connective tissue, prominent ears, and flat feet [44]. Reduced FMRP has been shown to increase levels of APP (beta-amyloid peptides) that can predispose an individual with FXS to dementia in later life [7, 45, 46]. Global atrophy, Purkinje cell loss, heterotopias, deterioration of the corticospinal tract, and dendritic spine abnormalities have also been observed in brains of individuals with FXS [7].

Individuals who are carriers of premutations in the *FMR1* gene, 40–75% of males and 16–20% of females, develop a fragile X-associated tremor/ataxia (FXTAS) that presents on average at >60 years of age with a median survival of 21 years [47]. FXTAS is characterized by cerebellar gait ataxia, intention tremor, and cognitive decline with characteristic white matter changes on MRI [48–52]. The contribution of FXTAS to morbidity and mortality of older adults with ID requires further study.

Autism is a common problem in individuals with FXS and is most commonly seen in males [53]. Females with the full mutation are less likely affected due to X-inactivation with a diluting effect of the second, normal X chromosome. A third of females have mild intellectual impairment with associated autistic behaviors such as poor eye contact and shyness [54].

Down Syndrome (DS)

DS is caused by a trisomy of chromosome 21, except in rare instances of translocation (4–5%) or mosaicism (2–4%) [55]. The genetic defect leads to the overexpression of over 300 HSA21 genes that result in aberrant genetic and molecular processes altering neural structure and function, which result in cognitive deficits [56]. Reduced brain volumes are primarily seen in the cerebellum, frontal lobe, and temporal lobe based on MRI studies and postmortem observations [57]. Age-related increase in the volume of cerebrospinal fluid has also been observed [58]. Premature aging is thought to result from overexpression of genes on chromosome 21 and genes related to oxidative stress including superoxide dismutase (SOD1), Ets-2 transcription factors, and S100 [59]. This accelerated aging can lead to premature age-related cognitive decline and AD in individuals with DS.

Increasing age is the strongest predictor of AD in individuals with DS. Although the physiological processes leading to Aβ deposition is similar in the general population, the deposition in individuals with DS occurs 20–30 years earlier. The triplication of the APP gene on chromosome 21 leads to the overexpression of this gene and is believed to cause the increase of Aβ deposition in the brain. This predisposes individuals with DS to AD at an earlier age [59].

Studies on sex difference in AD in DS are limited. One study in a population aged 35–79 years found that women with DS had a greater incidence of AD when compared to men, as is seen in the general population [60]. This is likely due to estrogen deficiency that occurs with menopause onset [18]. Further studies are required to prove this association.

Diagnosis

The criteria for the diagnosis of intellectual disability (ID) are outlined in the DSM-5. Notable updates from DSM-IV TR include changes to terminology (from mental retardation) and the severity of impairment being based on adaptive functioning rather than IQ test scores alone [1]. Although diagnosis of ID is made at any age, ID, by definition, has onset during the developmental period. Therefore, diagnosis of ID is often made prior to reaching the geriatric age.

Clinical assessment, standardized measures, and speaking with knowledgeable informants in addition to the patient can establish ID diagnosis based on three criteria:

1. Deficits in intellectual functions (i.e., reasoning, problem-solving, abstract thinking, judgment, academic learning, and learning from experience) must be present and confirmed by clinical assessment and standardized intelligence testing.
2. Deficits in adaptive functions (i.e., communication skills, social participation, personal hygiene) that result in failure to meet societal standards for independence must be present.
3. Onset of the above deficits must occur during the developmental period [1].

Severity of ID is categorized into mild, moderate, severe, and profound based on adaptive functioning deficits in three domains outlined in Table 23-1. More specific diagnosis of a syndrome, such as Down's or Rett's, is made based on genetics.

Given that IQ and other standardized test scores may be affected by an individual's sociocultural background and comorbid disorders, they are no longer included in the criteria for severity or diagnosis of ID. However, IQ scores and other standardized tests can still be helpful in approximating an individual's intellectual functioning. ID is still considered two standard deviations or more below the population average for the test (IQ score of 70 or below) though clinical correlation to patient functioning should be done when interpreting IQ or other test scores [1].

Distinguishing ID from other categories of cognitive deficits that arise in the elderly is important to provide appropriate treatment. ID is a neurodevelopmental disorder where first deficits occur during childhood. In some cases, ID can be acquired from illness such as encephalitis or head trauma. Cognitive deficits of neurocognitive disorders (dementia), however, are acquired after the developmental period.

Both neurodevelopmental and neurocognitive causes of deficits can be comorbid in the elderly, which pose diagnostic challenges. Large variability in baseline cognitive and functional abilities in populations with ID throughout the lifetime further complicates assessment [6].

Although no consensus guideline exists for evaluating comorbid neurocognitive disorders in the intellectually disabled [6], an approach to diagnosis by using a battery of recommended tests has been proposed [61]. Since "normal" functioning in an individual with ID varies greatly from the general population, individual data from standardized cognitive and memory testing during adulthood is the most useful. One group proposed testing individuals with DS prior to age 40 and all other individuals with ID prior to age 50 to establish a baseline. This group also recommended gathering descriptive information from caregivers who know the patient's functional status and behavior in different settings at the time the baseline testing is done. Later in life, if a decline in function is suspected, standardized testing can be re-administered and new descriptive data can be compared to baseline, which can help clinicians diagnose dementia [61]. However, this approach may not work for individuals with profound ID because memory and cognition may be so impaired that repeat standardized testing would not detect a decline. In these cases, descriptive data of the patient's functioning and behavior from caregivers at baseline and when a decline is suspected are more useful [62]. In the future, standards for diagnosing dementia in the intellectually disabled will be needed to ensure older adults with ID are able to benefit from dementia treatments [6].

TABLE 23-1. Domains used to assess functioning deficits among individuals with ID [1]

Domain	Conceptual	Social	Practical
Associated functions	• Academic competence • Memory • Language • Math	• Awareness of other's experiences • Empathy • Social judgment • Interpersonal communication	• Money management • Job responsibilities • Personal care

Treatments

Available treatments for older adults with ID include both non-pharmacological and pharmacological interventions. Below is a summary of the currently recommended treatments based on available research data.

Non-pharmacological

A report prepared by the Aging Special Interest Research Group of the International Association for the Scientific Study of Intellectual Disabilities (IASSID) in collaboration with other organizations examined the health status of adults with ID and provided recommendations to support healthy aging and improve quality of life in this population [63]. The report emphasized the importance of improving lifestyle and environment conditions, health promotion, disease prevention, access to support services, public attitudes on individuals with ID, and education among health-care providers about recognizing special needs of older adults with ID.

Educating older adults with ID and their caregivers about nutrition, exercise, oral hygiene, and safety is important to discourage older adults with ID from engaging in risky behaviors such as substance abuse, unprotected or multiple partner sexual activity, and following a sedentary lifestyle [63]. In one review, physical activity interventions and multicomponent interventions (physical activity plus health education) led to improvement of physical and health behavior and psychosocial outcomes in older adults with ID. Incorporating health-screening interventions during health-care visits also increased overall screening adherence and decreased challenging behavior. Other interventions such as volunteering and civic engagement also improved self-rated health, neurocognitive plasticity and reduced depression [64].

Health-care providers are encouraged to perform careful assessments as medical conditions can present atypically in this population due to the high prevalence of sensory impairment and cognitive and language deficits. This includes regularly screening for visual and hearing impairments, evaluating for functional decline and assessing for undiagnosed conditions. Functional decline, in particular, should not be attributed solely to behavior issues or dementia as more thorough evaluations have yielded high rates of treatable conditions such as delirium, depression, and sensory impairments in older adults with ID [65–67]. Screening for possible infectious diseases such as tuberculosis, hepatitis B, and *Helicobacter pylori* is also encouraged, especially if the individual resides or has previously lived in a large institution, which could put them at risk for exposure to these illnesses.

Improved training for caregivers of older adults with ID is equally important to ensure that basic health status and needs of the impaired adult are accurately reported to health-care providers [68]. Case management can also assist in optimizing the utilization of health-care services and improving access to care in cases that require multidisciplinary expertise [69].

Behavioral and psychiatric symptoms associated with aging in older adults with ID are challenging to treat. In one study, older adults in the UK with dementia and behavior symptoms resulted in increased caregiver burden and cost of care, with the existence of a mental health disorder being an important predictor of costs [70]. Although pharmacological treatment is widely used to treat behavior and psychiatric symptoms in adults with ID, non-pharmacological interventions are equally important. However, research supporting non-pharmacological interventions in older adults with ID and behavior problems is limited. Assessing for pain and other modifiable conditions and ensuring access to assistive devices such as walkers, dentures, eyeglasses, and hearing aids are examples of non-pharmacological interventions that can help alleviate behavior issues in an older adult with ID. Additionally, educating health-care providers about possible confusion, fear, and frustration that older adults with ID may have during a health-care visit can be helpful [63].

One study attempted to examine the role of cognitive rehabilitation of dementia in adults with DS; however, few or limited studies were found [71]. Additionally, studies of other interventions, such as memory training, behavior modification, and psychoeducation for caregivers, to treat behavior issues in comorbid dementia and DS, are lacking, and available studies are limited by study design (low power, lack of generalizability, lack of follow-up period) [71].

Pharmacological

Adults with ID often suffer from psychiatric disorders, display challenging behavior, and are at higher risk for certain medical illnesses. Thus, they are often on multiple medications. The efficacy and safety of the use of multiple medications in this population, however, is not well studied [72]. Additionally, some studies have shown that individuals with ID and comorbid mental disorders are undertreated compared to the general population, resulting in poorer outcomes. The use of psychotropic drugs for older adults with ID and behavior problems remains controversial, especially in those with dementia [73].

One review looked at several studies that treated adults with ID with more than one psychoactive drug to address behavior and psychiatric issues. They found that adults and especially older adults with ID are more susceptible to side effects from polypharmacy [72]. Therefore, monotherapies are encouraged as initial treatment to address behavior and should be exhausted before adding a second agent. Furthermore, adults with ID show amplified side effects at low doses, and the rule of "start low, go slow" should be applied when initiating medication in this population [72].

Treatment of mental health disorders in individuals with ID is important, as these disorders are often treatable. However, guidance on medication selection and prescribing practice is lacking as people with ID have been underrepresented or excluded in many randomized medication trials [72].

With respect to mood disorder, one review of older adults with ID found that depression is positively correlated with age and is associated with chronic diseases such as heart failure, stroke, chronic obstructive pulmonary disease, coronary artery disease, and diabetes mellitus [73]. Although no specific treatment guidelines exist for treatment of depression in older adults with ID, use of antidepressants such as SSRIs in the ID population has increased since the mid-1990s in the United States and has not been known to cause significant side effects [74]. It is therefore assumed that general population guidelines for depression treatment can be applied to this population.

With respect to antipsychotic medication use, a large survey in the UK found that psychotic illness, anxiety, and behavior issues such as aggression, threatening behavior, and self-harm were the most common reasons for prescribing antipsychotics to individuals (all ages) with ID [75]. Guidelines exist on the use of newer antipsychotic drugs and clozapine in adults with ID and recommend caution in this population, particularly with comorbid dementia and medical conditions [76, 77]. The use of newer antipsychotic drugs in individuals with ID and dementia or cerebrovascular disease has led to an increased risk for stroke [73]. Additionally, the use of quetiapine and olanzapine, in combination with other antimuscarinic agents, could significantly impact the cognition of older adults with ID or lead to decreased gastrointestinal motility, urinary retention, and narrow-angle glaucoma [77].

Some evidence exists to support the use of medication for behavior problems in adults with ID, particularly those with autism [78]. Risperidone has the best evidence for efficacy [79]. Careful prescribing and monitoring practices are encouraged. Regular follow-up visits should be arranged, and dose reduction or discontinuation of medication should be considered during the course of treatment [72].

Dementia in older adults with ID can be separated into those with DS and those without DS. For older adults with ID and dementia without DS, no specific treatment guidelines are available. Clinicians can use anti-dementia medications available to the general population, though efficacy and safety for this group is unknown. Studies are available to support the use of donepezil in older adults with ID and dementia with DS. However, efficacy measures are lacking as the controlled trials used to support the use of donepezil had small sample size and lacked an adequate length of follow-up [80–82]. Similarly, more research is needed to assess the long-term efficacy of rivastigmine in this population [83].

In one study, transdermal rivastigmine showed better patient compliance versus oral formulation because of its once a day dosing and minimal side effect profile [84]. Additionally, current literature does not support the use of NMDA antagonists in individuals with DS and dementia [85].

Conclusion

The population of older adults with ID represents a heterogeneous group. Adults with ID are living longer due to improvements in medical and social care; however, older adults with ID tend to have more medical and psychiatric comorbidities and overall poorer health outcomes compared with the general population. Providers need to consider comorbid medical, psychiatric, and neurocognitive comorbidities when evaluating and managing the mental health of their aging patients with ID. More research is needed to better understand the growing and unique needs of older adults living with ID and how to best optimize identification and management of comorbid psychiatric and neurocognitive disorders.

References

1. American Psychiatric Association D-TF. Intellectual disabilities. In: Diagnostic and statistical manual of mental disorders. 5th Ed. DSM-5. Arlington, VA: American Psychiatric Association; 2013. P. 33–41.
2. Bittles AH, Petterson BA, Sullivan SG, Hussain R, Glasson EJ, Montgomery PD. The influence of intellectual disability on life expectancy. J Gerontol A Biol Sci Med Sci. 2002;57(7):M470–2.
3. Glasson EJ, Sullivan SG, Hussain R, Petterson BA, Montgomery PD, Bittles AH. Comparative survival advantage of males with Down syndrome. Am J Hum Biol. 2003;15(2):192–5.
4. Bigby J, Perez-Stable E. The challenges of understanding and eliminating racial and ethnic disparities in health. J Gen Intern Med. 2004;19(2):201–3.
5. Fisher K, Kettl P. Aging with mental retardation: increasing population of older adults with MR require health interventions and prevention strategies. Geriatrics. 2005;60(4):26–9.
6. Krinsky-McHale SJ, Silverman W. Dementia and mild cognitive impairment in adults with intellectual disability: issues of diagnosis. Dev Disabil Res Rev. 2013;18(1):31–42.
7. Dykens EM. Aging in rare intellectual disability syndromes. Dev Disabil Res Rev. 2013;18(1):75–83.
8. Maulik PK, Mascarenhas MN, Mathers CD, Dua T, Saxena S. Prevalence of intellectual disability: a meta-analysis of population-based studies. Res Dev Disabil. 2011;32(2):419–36.
9. Coppus AM, Schuur M, Vergeer J, et al. Plasma beta amyloid and the risk of Alzheimer's disease in Down syndrome. Neurobiol Aging. 2012;33(9):1988–94.
10. Patja K, Iivanainen M, Vesala H, Oksanen H, Ruoppila I. Life expectancy of people with intellectual disability: a 35-year follow-up study. J Intellect Disabil Res. 2000;44(Pt 5):591–9.
11. Crawford DC, Acuna JM, Sherman SL. FMR1 and the fragile X syndrome: human genome epidemiology review. Genet Med. 2001;3(5):359–71.
12. Turner G, Webb T, Wake S, Robinson H. Prevalence of fragile X syndrome. Am J Med Genet. 1996;64(1):196–7.
13. Coffee B, Keith K, Albizua I, et al. Incidence of fragile X syndrome by newborn screening for methylated FMR1 DNA. Am J Hum Genet. 2009;85(4):503–14.
14. Partington MW, Robinson H, Laing S, Turner G. Mortality in the fragile X syndrome: preliminary data. Am J Med Genet. 1992;43(1–2):120–3.
15. Centers for Disease Control and Prevention. Down syndrome: data and statistics. Updated October 21, 2014; http://www.cdc.gov/ncbddd/birthdefects/downsyndrome/data.html. Accessed 28 Oct 2016.
16. Janicki MP, Dalton AJ, Henderson CM, Davidson PW. Mortality and morbidity among older adults with intellectual disability: health services considerations. Disabil Rehabil. 1999;21(5–6):284–94.
17. Day K. Male mentally handicapped sex offenders. Br J Psychiatry. 1994;165(5):630–9.
18. Schupf N, Pang D, Patel BN, et al. Onset of dementia is associated with age at menopause in women with Down's syndrome. Ann Neurol. 2003;54(4):433–8.
19. Seltzer GB, Schupf N, Wu HSA. prospective study of menopause in women with Down's syndrome. J Intellect Disabil Res. 2001;45(Pt 1):1–7.
20. Coppus AM, Evenhuis HM, Verberne GJ, et al. Early age at menopause is associated with increased risk of dementia and mortality in women with Down syndrome. J Alzheimers Dis. 2010;19(2):545–50.
21. Evenhuis HM, Theunissen M, Denkers I, Verschuure H, Kemme H. Prevalence of visual and hearing impairment in a Dutch institutionalized

population with intellectual disability. J Intellect Disabil Res. 2001;45(Pt 5):457–64.
22. Prasher VP. Down syndrome and thyroid disorders: a review. Downs Syndr Res Pract. 1999;6(1):25–42.
23. Janicki MP, Davidson PW, Henderson CM, et al. Health characteristics and health services utilization in older adults with intellectual disability living in community residences. J Intellect Disabil Res. 2002;46(Pt 4):287–98.
24. Oliver C, Crayton L, Holland A, Hall S, Bradbury J. A four year prospective study of age-related cognitive change in adults with Down's syndrome. Psychol Med. 1998;28(6):1365–77.
25. van Schrojenstein Lantman-de Valk HM, Haveman MJ, Maaskant MA, Kessels AG, Urlings HF, Sturmans F. The need for assessment of sensory functioning in ageing people with mental handicap. J Intellect Disabil Res. 1994;38(Pt 3):289–98.
26. Coppus AM, Evenhuis HM, Verberne GJ, et al. Survival in elderly persons with Down syndrome. J Am Geriatr Soc. 2008;56(12):2311–6.
27. Cooper SA. Epidemiology of psychiatric disorders in elderly compared with younger adults with learning disabilities. Br J Psychiatry. 1997;170:375–80.
28. Cooper SA. High prevalence of dementia among people with learning disabilities not attributable to Down's syndrome. Psychol Med. 1997;27(3):609–16.
29. Strydom A, Hassiotis A, King M, Livingston G. The relationship of dementia prevalence in older adults with intellectual disability (ID) to age and severity of ID. Psychol Med. 2009;39(1):13–21.
30. Haveman M, Perry J, Salvador-Carulla L, et al. Ageing and health status in adults with intellectual disabilities: results of the European POMONA II study. J Intellect Develop Disabil. 2011;36(1):49–60.
31. Matthews T, Weston N, Baxter H, Felce D, Kerr M. A general practice-based prevalence study of epilepsy among adults with intellectual disabilities and of its association with psychiatric disorder, behaviour disturbance and carer stress. J Intellect Disabil Res. 2008;52(Pt 2):163–73.
32. Blair E, Watson L, Badawi N, Stanley FJ. Life expectancy among people with cerebral palsy in Western Australia. Dev Med Child Neurol. 2001;43(8):508–15.
33. Nottestad JA, Linaker OM. Psychiatric health needs and services before and after complete deinstitutionalization of people with intellectual disability. J Intellect Disabil Res. 1999;43(Pt 6):523–30.
34. Cooper SA, van der Speck R. Epidemiology of mental ill health in adults with intellectual disabilities. Curr Opin Psychiatry. 2009;22(5):431–6.
35. Cooper SA, Smiley E, Morrison J, Williamson A, Allan L. Mental ill-health in adults with intellectual disabilities: prevalence and associated factors. Br J Psychiatry. 2007;190:27–35.
36. Kessler RC, Demler O, Frank RG, et al. Prevalence and treatment of mental disorders, 1990 to 2003. N Engl J Med. 2005;352(24):2515–23.
37. Deb S, Thomas M, Bright C. Mental disorder in adults with intellectual disability. 2: the rate of behaviour disorders among a community-based population aged between 16 and 64 years. J Intellect Disabil Res. 2001;45(Pt 6):506–14.
38. Horner-Johnson W, Drum CE. Prevalence of maltreatment of people with intellectual disabilities: a review of recently published research. Ment Retard Dev Disabil Res Rev. 2006;12(1):57–69.
39. Evans E, Bhardwaj A, Brodaty H, Sachdev P, Draper B, Trollor JN. Dementia in people with intellectual disability: insights and challenges in epidemiological research with an at-risk population. Int Rev Psychiatry. 2013;25(6):755–63.
40. Ross WT, Olsen M. Care of the adult patient with Down syndrome. South Med J. 2014;107(11):715–21.
41. Turk J, Fragile X. syndrome: lifespan developmental implications for those without as well as with intellectual disability. Curr Opin Psychiatry. 2011;24(5):387–97.
42. Utari A, Adams E, Berry-Kravis E, et al. Aging in fragile X syndrome. J Neurodev Disord. 2010;2(2):70–6.
43. Backes M, Genc B, Schreck J, Doerfler W, Lehmkuhl G, von Gontard A. Cognitive and behavioral profile of fragile X boys: correlations to molecular data. Am J Med Genet. 2000;95(2):150–6.
44. Hagerman RJ, Hagerman PJ. The fragile X premutation: into the phenotypic fold. Curr Opin Genet Dev. 2002;12(3):278–83.
45. Kamenetz F, Tomita T, Hsieh H, et al. APP processing and synaptic function. Neuron. 2003;37(6):925–37.
46. Westmark CJ, Malter JS. FMRP mediates mGluR5-dependent translation of amyloid precursor protein. PLoS Biol. 2007;5(3):e52.
47. Hagerman RJ, Hagerman P. Fragile X-associated tremor/ataxia syndrome—features, mechanisms and management. Nat Rev Neurol. 2016;12(7):403–12.
48. Jacquemont S, Hagerman RJ, Hagerman PJ, Leehey MA. Fragile-X syndrome and fragile X-associated tremor/ataxia syndrome: two faces of FMR1. Lancet Neurol. 2007;6(1):45–55.

49. Hagerman PJ, Greco CM, Hagerman RJ. A cerebellar tremor/ataxia syndrome among fragile X premutation carriers. Cytogenet Genome Res. 2003;100(1–4):206–12.
50. Leehey MA. Fragile X-associated tremor/ataxia syndrome: clinical phenotype, diagnosis, and treatment. J Investig Med. 2009;57(8):830–6.
51. Berry-Kravis E, Abrams L, Coffey SM, et al. Fragile X-associated tremor/ataxia syndrome: clinical features, genetics, and testing guidelines. Mov Disord. 2007;22(14):2018–30. quiz 2140
52. Jacquemont S, Hagerman RJ, Leehey M, et al. Fragile X premutation tremor/ataxia syndrome: molecular, clinical, and neuroimaging correlates. Am J Hum Genet. 2003;72(4):869–78.
53. Budimirovic DB, Kaufmann WE. What can we learn about autism from studying fragile X syndrome? Dev Neurosci. 2011;33(5):379–94.
54. Terracciano A, Chiurazzi P, Neri G. Fragile X syndrome. Am J Med Genet C Semin Med Genet. 2005;137c(1):32–7.
55. Coppus AM. People with intellectual disability: what do we know about adulthood and life expectancy? Dev Disabil Res Rev. 2013;18(1):6–16.
56. Sturgeon X, Gardiner KJ. Transcript catalogs of human chromosome 21 and orthologous chimpanzee and mouse regions. Mamm Genome. 2011;22(5–6):261–71.
57. Ruparelia A, Pearn ML, Mobley WC. Aging and intellectual disability: insights from mouse models of Down syndrome. Dev Disabil Res Rev. 2013;18(1):43–50.
58. Beacher F, Daly E, Simmons A, et al. Brain anatomy and ageing in non-demented adults with Down's syndrome: an in vivo MRI study. Psychol Med. 2010;40(4):611–9.
59. Zigman WB. Atypical aging in Down syndrome. Dev Disabil Res Rev. 2013;18(1):51–67.
60. Lai F, Kammann E, Rebeck GW, Anderson A, Chen Y, Nixon RA. APOE genotype and gender effects on Alzheimer disease in 100 adults with Down syndrome. Neurology. 1999;53(2):331–6.
61. Burt DB, Aylward EH. Test battery for the diagnosis of dementia in individuals with intellectual disability. Working Group for the Establishment of Criteria for the Diagnosis of Dementia in Individuals with Intellectual Disability. J Intellect Disabil Res. 2000;44(Pt 2):175–80.
62. Aylward EH, Burt DB, Thorpe LU, Lai F, Dalton A. Diagnosis of dementia in individuals with intellectual disability. J Intellect Disabil Res. 1997;41(Pt 2):152–64.
63. Evenhuis H, Henderson M, Beange H, Lennox N, Chicoine B. Healthy ageing—adults with intellectual disabilities: physical health issues. J Appl Res Intellect Disabil. 2001;14:175–94.
64. Heller T, Fisher D, Marks B, Hsieh K. Interventions to promote health: crossing networks of intellectual and developmental disabilities and aging. Disabil Health J. 2014;7(1 Suppl):S24–32.
65. Evenhuis HM. Medical aspects of ageing in a population with intellectual disability: III. Mobility, internal conditions and cancer. J Intellect Disabil Res. 1997;41(Pt 1):8–18.
66. Thorpe L. Psychiatric disorders. Print Book: English ed. Philadelphia, PA: Brunner/Mazel; 1999.
67. Chicoine B, McGuire D, Rubin S. Specialty clinic perspectives. Print Book: English ed. Castletown, NY: Hamilton Printing; 1999.
68. Bromley J, Emerson E, Caine A. The development of a self-report measure to assess the location and intensity of pain in people with intellectual disabilities. J Intellect Disabil Res. 1998;42(Pt 1):72–80.
69. Walsh KK, Kastner T, Criscione T. Characteristics of hospitalizations for people with developmental disabilities: utilization, costs, and impact of care coordination. Am J Ment Retard. 1997;101(5):505–20.
70. Strydom A, Shooshtari S, Lee L, et al. Dementia in older adults with intellectual disabilities—epidemiology, presentation, and diagnosis. J Policy Pract Intellect Disabil. 2010;7(2):96–110.
71. Fonseca LM, Navatta AC, Bottino CM, Miotto EC. Cognitive rehabilitation of dementia in adults with Down syndrome: a review of non-pharmacological interventions. Dement Geriatr Cogn Dis Extra. 2015;5(3):330–40.
72. Häβler F, Thome J, Reis O. Polypharmacy in the treatment of subjects with intellectual disability. J Neural Transm. 2015;122(Supplement 1):93–100.
73. Eady N, Courtenay K, Strydom A. Pharmacological management of behavioral and psychiatric symptoms in older adults with intellectual disability. Drugs Aging. 2015;32(2):95–102.
74. Tsiouris JA, Kim SY, Brown WT, Pettinger J, Cohen IL. Prevalence of psychotropic drug use in adults with intellectual disability: positive and negative findings from a large scale study. J Autism Dev Disord. 2013;43(3):719–31.
75. Paton C, Flynn A, Shingleton-Smith A, et al. Nature and quality of antipsychotic prescribing practice in UK psychiatry of intellectual disability services. J Intellect Disabil Res. 2011;55:665–74.
76. de Leon J, Greenlee B, Barber J, Sabaawi M, Singh NN. Practical guidelines for the use of new generation antipsychotic drugs (except clozapine) in adult individuals with intellectual disabilities. Res Dev Disabil. 2009;30(4):613–69.

77. Sabaawi M, Singh NN, de Leon J. Guidelines for the use of clozapine in individuals with developmental disabilities. Res Dev Disabil. 2006;27(3):309–36.
78. Sawyer A, Lake J, Lunsky Y, Liu S-K, Desarkar P. Psychopharmacological treatment of challenging behaviours in adults with autism and intellectual disabilities: A systematic review. Res Autism Spectr Disord. July 2014;8(7):803–13.
79. Cohen D, Raffin M, Canitano R, et al. Risperidone or aripiprazole in children and adolescents with autism and/or intellectual disability: a Bayesian meta-analysis of efficacy and secondary effects. Res Autism Spectr Disord. 2013;7(1):167–75.
80. Lott IT, Osann K, Doran E, Nelson L. Down syndrome and Alzheimer disease: response to donepezil. Arch Neurol. 2002;59(7):1133–6.
81. Prasher VP, Huxley A, Haque MS. Group DsAS. A 24-week, double-blind, placebo-controlled trial of donepezil in patients with Down syndrome and Alzheimer's disease—pilot study. Int J Geriatr Psychiatry. 2002;17(3):270–8.
82. Prasher VP, Adams C, Holder R, Group DSR. Long term safety and efficacy of donepezil in the treatment of dementia in Alzheimer's disease in adults with Down syndrome: open label study. Int J Geriatr Psychiatry. 2003;18(6):549–51.
83. Prasher VP, Fung N, Adams C. Rivastigmine in the treatment of dementia in Alzheimer's disease in adults with Down syndrome. Int J Geriatr Psychiatry. 2005;20(5):496–7.
84. Prasher VP, Sachdeva N, Adams C, Haque MS. Rivastigmine transdermal patches in the treatment of dementia in Alzheimer's disease in adults with Down syndrome-pilot study. Int J Geriatr Psychiatry. 2013;28(2):219–20.
85. Hanney M, Prasher V, Williams N, et al. Memantine for dementia in adults older than 40 years with Down's syndrome (MEADOWS): a randomised, double-blind, placebo-controlled trial. Lancet. 2012;379(9815):528–36.

24 Personality Disorders

Karin Kerfoot

Introduction

The Diagnostic and Statistical Manual of Mental Disorders, Fifth Edition (DSM-5) defines personality disorder (PD) as an enduring pattern of inner experiences and behaviors that deviates markedly from the individual's culture. The enduring pattern must be inflexible and pervasive, lead to clinically significant distress or functional impairments, and be of long duration with onset in adolescence or early adulthood. Finally, it cannot be better explained as a manifestation or consequence of another mental disorder or attributable to the physiological effects of substances or another medical condition [1]. During the development process of the DSM-5, several proposed revisions were drafted within the category of personality disorders which would have resulted in substantial changes to the definition and diagnosis of personality disorders. However, it was ultimately decided to retain the DSM-IV categorical approach with the same ten personality disorders. These ten personality disorders have been grouped into three clusters based on descriptive similarities. Cluster A includes the paranoid, schizoid, and schizotypal personality disorders: individuals who often appear odd or eccentric. Cluster B includes antisocial, borderline, histrionic, and narcissistic personality disorders: individuals who often appear dramatic, emotional, or erratic. Cluster C includes the avoidant, dependent, and obsessive-compulsive personality disorders: individuals who often appear anxious or fearful. In contrast to the multiaxial system of DSM-IV, DSM-5 has shifted to a single-axis system. Therefore, personality disorders are no longer delegated to "Axis II," as the first three axes present in past editions of the DSM have been combined into one, encompassing all mental and other medical diagnoses.

Despite available evidence that personality disorders complicate the course and treatment of other psychiatric disorders and adversely impact the quality of life among older adults, personality disorders in late life have received relatively little attention in the medical literature [2, 3]. These disorders often present with significant issues including a plethora of psychiatric symptoms, vague physical complaints and medical issues, significant interpersonal conflicts, and variable cognitive difficulties. As there are significant medical comorbidities among older adults and cognitive disorders often present with personality changes, the accurate identification and diagnosis of personality disorders among older adults can be difficult. Additionally, treatments are often time-intensive and challenging. However, the outcomes for the treatment of personality disorders among older adults appear to hold promise.

Epidemiology

Prevalence estimates for the personality disorders vary widely across studies and samples, but they are generally thought to be less common among older adults than in younger individuals. Available data indicates that the prevalence rates

R. R. Tampi et al. (eds.), *Psychiatric Disorders Late in Life*, https://doi.org/10.1007/978-3-319-73078-3_24

for personality disorders among older adults living in the community are approximately 10% [4]. The prevalence rate for personality disorders are comparable to or higher than the community-based prevalence rates for many other disorders among older adults including major depressive disorder, substance use disorders, and dementia [5]. The prevalence rates for personality disorders in clinical samples are higher (13–63%) than those among community-dwelling elders although these estimates vary depending on the samples evaluated and the method of assessment [4].

Inconsistencies in the diagnostic process result in the underdiagnosis of personality disorders among older adults [6]. Reasons for this underdiagnosis include the unavailability/unreliability of longitudinal histories and the lack of age-adjusted diagnostic instruments. In addition, the current diagnostic criteria often fail to appropriately account for age-related issues including the changes in social and cognitive functioning and the effects of comorbid medical or psychiatric illnesses.

Available evidence indicates that older individuals with personality disorders are more likely to be living alone (single, separated, or divorced), exhibit more marital problems, and/or have multiple marriages but few numbers of children [5]. These individuals also tend to have lower educational and occupational attainments.

Personality disorders and depressive disorders are highly comorbid among older adults. In addition, older adults with depression and personality disorders are more likely to have earlier onset and recurrent depressive episodes, a history of suicide attempts, and a current anxiety disorder diagnosis than those depressed older adults without personality disorders [7]. Symptoms of personality disorders also worsen the long-term prognosis for depressive disorders among older individuals [3].

Among older adults, personality changes may be heralded by or co-occur with various common medical or neurological conditions [5]. Evidence indicates that personality changes frequently precede the onset and diagnosis of Alzheimer's disease [8]. Early in the course of neurocognitive disorders, the cognitive difficulties can be masked by personality or behavioral changes such as egocentricity, rigidity, apathy, or emotional instability [5]. Additionally, personality changes may occur among older adults as a direct pathophysiological consequence of another medical condition. These individuals should then be classified as having a personality change due to another medical condition as per the DSM-5 diagnostic criteria [1].

Neurobiology

The development of personality disorders is associated with different biological, psychological, and social factors. The existing assumption is that the origins of personality disorders are ingrained in early childhood [9, 10]. Abnormal attachment with primary caregivers at an early age may result in patterns of maladaptive relationships in adulthood [11]. Evidence also indicates that stress and trauma during critical developmental periods in life may result in abnormalities in brain structure and/or functions, contributing to the development of personality disorders [10, 12].

Experiences of neglect and physical or sexual abuse during childhood years have been identified as potentially important risk factors for the development of personality disorders with early abuse experiences resulting in maladaptive changes in personality [10]. A low family socioeconomic status, being on family welfare support, being raised by a single parent, parental conflicts, paternal and maternal sociopathy, parental illness and/or death, lack of parental figures, parental overcontrol, and being the result of an unwanted pregnancy are other known early risk factors for the subsequent development of personality disorders [13]. The exposure to intrauterine influenza, prenatal stress, birth complications, and early malnutrition are factors associated with the development of schizotypal features [12].

Long-term predictors across the three personality disorder clusters include the presence of early disruptive behavior and depressive disorders [10]. Additionally, abnormalities in early temperament may precede the development of personality disorders in adulthood [9]. The presence of low intelligence quotient [IQ], social isolation, poor health in childhood, and academic difficulties are also risk factors for the development of personality disorders [13].

Although there is substantial stability over time for major personality traits, such as those described by Costa and McCrae's five-factor model, a recent meta-analysis found that changes in personality traits across the life course are possible [14, 15]. Evidence suggests that individuals with cluster B personality disorders may experience favorable changes with age due to various biopsychosocial factors [5].

Diagnosis

There are many challenges when making a diagnosis of personality disorders among older adults. In the DSM-5, personality disorders are noted to be enduring with onset in adolescence or early adulthood [1]. Hence by definition personality disorders cannot arise for the first time among elderly individuals, except when they are temporally related to medical or neurological conditions that occur among the elderly. It is usually an arduous task to gather reliable information regarding the individual's personality across their life span. In addition there is often significant doubt about the stability of personality traits through an individual's life to make a confident diagnosis of a personality disorder [16].

Available data does not clarify the extent to which the natural process of aging, life events, and previous treatments alter an individual's personality. While there is some evidence to suggest that specific features of certain personality disorders like schizoid personality disorder may increase in frequency with age, other personality disorders like antisocial and borderline personality disorder appear to be less frequent with age [17]. It is also hypothesized that certain personality disorders may relapse in old age following a period of relative dormancy in middle adulthood.

The current classification systems contain measurement bias across the age groups [18]. Criteria like involvement in solitary activities and the lack of interest in having sexual experiences with another person that are often seen among individuals with cluster A personality disorders may occur among older adults due to lack of social supports, losses of loved ones, or physical illnesses, and not due to a personality pathology [16]. In addition, many cluster B traits including physical fights, sexual impulsivity, reckless driving, and sexual seductiveness may not occur among older adults [16]. Furthermore, symptoms like impairments in occupational activities and loss of productivity at work that are associated with cluster C personality disorders among younger individuals are not necessarily relevant to older adults.

Personality disorders among older adults may be underdiagnosed for various reasons [19]. The elderly may underreport personality traits that are considered to be socially undesirable. In addition, ageist attitudes toward the elderly including stereotypes that portray the older adults as being rigid, withdrawn, or cognitively impaired may also result in the underdiagnosis of personality disorders in late life [19]. Furthermore, clinicians may preferentially overlook personality issues in favor of other major psychiatric disorders during the assessment of older adults [20]. Finally, the presence of cognitive disorders among the elderly may also veil the diagnosis of personality disorders among older adults.

There has been recent dialogue on changing the diagnostic system to accommodate for personality disorders among older adults [2, 6]. A proposal to create a geriatric subclassification for personality disorders that will be more reliable and valid has been proposed [6]. In addition, the development of age-neutral measurement systems that take into consideration dimensions and not categories may allow for a more consistent assessment of personality disorders across the life span [10].

Outcomes

There are numerous consequences to having certain personality traits including their effects on health, life span, and social and personal relationships and the adjustment to life events [17]. Personality disorders have a negative impact on the outcomes for primary psychiatric disorders like depression where there is a decline in global functioning, interpersonal relationships, and quality of life among those older adults with depression and comorbid personality disorders when compared to those individuals with only depression [3, 5, 20, 21]. Additionally, the presence of certain personality traits can increase the risk of death by suicide among older adults including narcissism, obsessiveness, and anxiety acting as predictors for late-life suicides [22, 23].

Treatment

Available data indicates that the combination of psychotherapy and pharmacotherapy is beneficial among older adults with personality disorders [19]. The main aim of treatment among these individuals is to maximize coping strategies while minimizing the maladaptive behaviors [19].

Non-pharmacological

The applicability of therapies like dialectical behavior therapy (DBT), interpersonal therapy (IPT), cognitive behavioral therapy (CBT), and problem-solving therapy (PST) to older adults with personality disorders has not been specifically evaluated [2]. However, emerging data indicates that these therapies may benefit older individuals with personality disorders, especially individuals with borderline personality disorder [9]. Focusing on achieving small gains in the present (rehabilitation), rather than cure, may offer practicality and consistency for both the individual and the treating clinician.

There is limited evidence for the use of open-ended psychotherapies based on psychoanalysis for the treatment of personality disorders among older adults [24]. Intermittent psychotherapy with periods of breaks during treatment may be useful given the remission and relapses seen during the natural life history of personality disorders. Additionally, this form of psychotherapy where individuals take breaks in treatment with return to therapy when new issues arise is consistent with a life span perspective and is ideologically different from other methods of therapy.

Pharmacological

Available evidence indicates that personality pathology is often associated with neurochemical abnormalities [25]. The pharmacological treatments for personality disorders are geared to target individual symptoms rather than the whole personality disorder [2]. Medications that are often prescribed include antidepressants for low mood and anxiety symptoms, mood stabilizers for affective instability, and antipsychotics for psychotic-like symptoms. Although there is emerging evidence for the pharmacotherapy of personality disorders among younger adults, the literature that specifically examines pharmacological treatment of personality disorders among older adults is still lacking [19].

Evidence indicates that older adults with psychiatric disorders and comorbid personality disorders have worse outcomes and poorer response to treatments when compared to age-matched individuals who have psychiatric disorders without comorbid personality disorders [19, 26]. But the presence of a comorbid personality disorder should not be an exclusion criteria for treating psychiatric disorders among older adults, and specific symptoms may respond to psychotropic medications [7]. In cases where older individuals with comorbid psychiatric and personality disorders have residual symptoms, additional treatments may be required [20].

Conclusion

Available evidence indicates that personality disorders are not uncommon among older adults. Many older adults continue to experience personality dysfunction in their later years with poor clinical outcomes, although there is still controversy regarding the natural history of personality disorders over the life span. There is emerging evidence that personality disorders among older adults represent a very important diagnostic consideration and are critical in the assessment of the risk of self-harm [26]. Although personality disorders among older adults are often underdiagnosed and undertreated, emerging data indicates efficacy for psychotherapy, pharmacotherapy, and combination treatments for these disorders.

References

1. Association AP. Diagnostic and statistical manual of mental disorders. 5th ed. Washington, DC: American Psychiatric Association; 2013.
2. Abrams RC, Bromberg CE. Personality disorders in the elderly: a flagging field of inquiry. Int J Geriatr Psychiatry. 2006;21(11):1013–7.

3. Abrams RC, Alexopoulos GS, Spielman LA, et al. Personality disorder symptoms predict declines in global functioning and quality of life in elderly depressed patients. Am J Geriatr Psychiatry. 2001;9(1):67–71.
4. Widiger TA, Seidlitz L. Personality, psychopathology, and aging. J Res Pers. 2002;36:335–62.
5. Zweig RA. Personality disorder in older adults: assessment challenges and strategies. Prof Psychol Res Pr. 2008;39(3):298–305.
6. Agronin ME, Maletta G. Personality disorders in late life. Understanding and overcoming the gap in research. Am J Geriatr Psychiatry. 2000;8(1):4–18.
7. Kunik ME, Mulsant BH, Rifai AH, et al. Personality disorders in elderly inpatients with major depression. Am J Geriatr Psychiatry. 1993;1(1):38–45.
8. Balsis S, Carpenter BD, Storandt M. Personality change precedes clinical diagnosis of dementia of the Alzheimer type. J Gerontol B Psychol Sci Soc Sci. 2005;60(2):P98–P101.
9. Paris J. Personality disorders over time: precursors, course and outcome. J Personal Disord. 2003;17(6):479–88.
10. Tackett JL, Balsis S, Oltmanns TF, Krueger RF. A unifying perspective on personality pathology across the life span: developmental considerations for the fifth edition of the diagnostic and statistical manual of mental disorders. Dev Psychopathol. 2009;21(3):687–713.
11. Sroufe LA, Carlson EA, Levy AK, Egeland B. Implications of attachment theory for developmental psychopathology. Dev Psychopathol. 1999;11(1):1–13.
12. Raine A. Schizotypal personality: neurodevelopmental and psychosocial trajectories. Annu Rev Clin Psychol. 2006;2:291–326.
13. Cohen P, Crawford TN, Johnson JG, et al. The children in the community study of developmental course of personality disorder. J Personal Disord. 2005;19(5):466–86.
14. Costa PT, McCrae RR. Personality in adulthood: a six-year longitudinal study of self-reports and spouse ratings on the NEO Personality Inventory. J Pers Soc Psychol. 1988;54(5):853–63.
15. Roberts BW, Walton KE, Viechtbauer W. Patterns of mean-level change in personality traits across the life course: a meta-analysis of longitudinal studies. Psychol Bull. 2006;132(1):1–25.
16. Van Alphen SPJ, Engelen GJJA, Kuin Y, et al. The relevance of a geriatric sub-classification of personality disorders in the DSM-V. Int J Geriatr Psychiatry. 2006;21(3):205–9.
17. Oltmanns TF, Balsis S. Studying personality disorders in later life: questions about the measurement, course, and impact of disorders. Annu Rev Clin Psychol. 2011;7:321–49.
18. Balsis S, Woods CM, Gleason MEJ, Oltmanns TF. Overdiagnosis and underdiagnosis of personality disorders in older adults. Am J Geriatr Psychiatry. 2007;15(9):742–53.
19. Morse JQ, Lynch TR. Personality disorders in late life. Curr Psychiatry Rep. 2000;2(1):24–31.
20. Abrams RC, Spielman LA, Alexopoulos GS, et al. Personality disorder symptoms and functioning in elderly depressed patients. Am J Geriatr Psychiatry. 1998;6(1):24–30.
21. Morse JQ, Pilkonis PA, Houck PR, et al. Impact of cluster C personality disorders on outcomes of acute and maintenance treatment in late-life depression. Am J Geriatr Psychiatry. 2005;13(9):808–14.
22. Heisel MJ, Links PS, Conn D, et al. Narcissistic personality and vulnerability to late-life suicidality. Am J Geriatr Psychiatry. 2007;15(9):734–41.
23. Harwood D, Hawton K, Hope T, et al. Psychiatric disorder and personality factors associated with suicide in older people: a descriptive and case-control study. Int J Geriatr Psychiatry. 2001;16(2):155–65.
24. Paris J. Intermittent psychotherapy: an alternative to continuous long-term treatment for patients with personality disorders. J Psychiatr Pract. 2007;13(3):153–8.
25. Markovitz PJ. Recent trends in the pharmacotherapy of personality disorders. J Personal Disord. 2004;18(1):90–101.
26. Mattar S, Khan F. Personality disorders in older adults: diagnosis and management. Prog Neurol Psychiatry. 2017;21(2):22–7.

Part V
Treatments

25 Pharmacology and Psychopharmacology

Rajesh R. Tampi, Deena J. Tampi, and Mallika Lavakumar

Introduction

The World Health Organization reports that between 2015 and 2050, the proportion of the world's older adults (≥60 years) will double from about 12% to almost 22% of the total population [1]. This means that the population of older adults will increase from 900 million to approximately 2 billion. Data indicates that there will be a similar growth of the population of individuals 65 years and older in the United States from 46.2 million or 14.5% of the total population to roughly 21.7% of the US population by 2040 [2].

It is estimated that over 20% of older adults have a diagnosable psychiatric disorder [1]. A recent study found that the proportion of older adults in the United States who experienced any past-year anxiety disorder and mood disorders was 11.4% and 6.8%, respectively [3]. A total of 3.8% of older adults also met criteria for any past-year substance use disorder, and 14.5% had one or more personality disorder. Men had higher rates of substance use disorders and any personality disorder, whereas women experienced higher rates of mood and anxiety disorders.

Available data indicates that approximately 20% of the community-dwelling older adults have been prescribed with psychotropic medications [4]. It is also estimated that among community-dwelling older adults, about 10% take antidepressants, 7.5% take anxiolytics, and approximately 5% take sedative/hypnotic medications. In nursing homes approximately 85% of the residents are prescribed with psychotropic medication within 3 months of admission, and 19% of the residents are on four or more psychoactive medications [5]. Benzodiazepines and antipsychotics are among the potentially inappropriately used psychotropic drugs in nursing homes [6]. One nursing home study found that antipsychotics, antidepressants, and sedatives/hypnotics were the most common medications that were associated with preventable adverse drug events [7]. Among these adverse drug events, neuropsychiatric events were the most common types of events that were preventable. Data also indicates that treatment with psychotropic medications can result in significant functional decline, cognitive decline, cerebrovascular adverse events, and also death among older adults [8–11].

The 2015 American Geriatrics Society (AGS) Beers Criteria include medications/medication classes that are divided into five different categories: the potentially inappropriate medication class to be avoided in older adults, the potentially inappropriate medication class to be avoided in older adults with certain diseases and syndromes as the drugs can exacerbate the disease or syndrome, the medication class that is to be used with caution among older adults, the medication class for which dose adjustment is required based on kidney function, and the medication class that can result in drug–drug interactions [12]. The AGS Beers Criteria include antipsychotics and benzodiazepines among the potentially inappropriate medication class and

R. R. Tampi et al. (eds.), *Psychiatric Disorders Late in Life*, https://doi.org/10.1007/978-3-319-73078-3_25

recommend that there is strong evidence for avoiding their use in older adults especially for the treatment of insomnia, agitation, or delirium. Antipsychotics, antidepressants, and carbamazepine are included among the potentially inappropriate medications to be used with caution among older adults. Antipsychotics, antidepressants, and benzodiazepines are also included in the potentially inappropriate medication class to avoid in older adults with certain diseases and syndromes as the drugs listed can exacerbate syncope, seizures, delirium, cognitive impairment/dementia, and also falls.

Available data from psychopharmacological trials that are specific to older adults to guide evidence-based treatments for psychiatric disorders in late life are limited [13]. Additionally, the treatment responses among older adults who are prescribed with psychoactive medications are variable due to individual differences in the pharmacokinetics, pharmacodynamics, and central nervous system functioning of these individuals. The judicious use of pharmacoepidemiology, population-based pharmacokinetic modeling, and pharmacogenetics has resulted in an improvement in drug safety and personalization of drug and dose selections for the treatment of psychiatric disorders among older adults [13]. In this chapter we review important psychopharmacological treatment principles that will help guide the treatment of psychiatric disorders among older adults.

Pharmacokinetics and Pharmacodynamics

Pharmacokinetics is the study of the effects of the human body on the drug that is administrated [14]. Pharmacokinetics includes absorption, distribution, metabolism, and excretion of the drugs. Pharmacodynamics studies the effects of the administered drug on the body [14]. Pharmacodynamics includes the beneficial and harmful effects of the drugs on the body. Drugs may have stimulatory or inhibitory actions on the body. Additionally, they may have blocking or stabilizing actions. Furthermore, these drugs can cause their effects either by their depleting action on transmitters and enzymes or by their accumulation in the body [14]. It has been estimated that approximately 80% of adverse drug events (ADEs) occur due to elevated drug levels [13]. Multiple drug dosing and the rapid drug dose titrations can lead to increased drug levels in the body and the development of serious ADEs.

Table 25.1 describes important concepts in pharmacokinetics and the effect of aging on pharmacokinetics [15]. This data should assist clinicians in making appropriate dose adjustments when prescribing psychotropic medications for older adults.

The pharmacokinetic processes are catalyzed by different enzyme systems and are divided into phase I and phase II reactions [16]. Psychotropic drugs are initially exposed to phase I metabolism. The phase I reactions occur primarily in the endoplasmic reticulum of liver cells. These reactions may occur by either oxidation, cyclization, reduction, hydrolysis, or de-cyclization. The enzymes that carry out these reactions are called mixed-function oxidases and involve the cytochrome P450 (CYP450) monooxygenase and the nicotinamide adenine dinucleotide phosphate oxidase (NADPH). These reactions convert pharmacologically inactive compounds (a prodrug) to an active compound, e.g., the prodrug codeine is metabolized to its active metabolite morphine. During phase I reactions, psychotropic drugs (antidepressants and antipsychotics) may lose their pharmacological activity by the action of the CYP450 enzymes. The CYP450 enzymes also make these drugs more hydrophilic, thus rendering them partially or completely inactive. Most psychotropic drugs still need to be made more hydrophilic before they can be excreted by the kidneys.

Phase II reactions involve conjugation and take place in the cytoplasm of liver cells [16]. These involve interactions between polar functional groups of phase I metabolites. The sites on the drugs where conjugation reactions tend to occur include the carboxyl (COOH), hydroxyl (OH), amino (NH2), and the sulfhydryl (SH) groups. The products of conjugation reactions are less active than their substrates. Phase II conjugation makes phase I metabolites more hydrophilic and readily excretable, e.g., morphine is converted to its inactive metabolite morphine 3-0-glucuronide.

TABLE 25-1. Pharmacokinetics

Term	Description	Importance in older adults
Absorption	The rate of absorption of the drug from the gastrointestinal (GI) tract after oral administration influences the time course and the intensity of initial drug action The completeness of absorption (absolute bioavailability) influences the plasma concentration of the drug	The extent of absorption of psychotropic drugs is not significantly altered by the aging process unless there is overt GI pathology
Bioavailability	It describes the fraction of the drug that is available systemically	The greater the bioavailability of the drug, the greater its potency
Elimination half-life (t1/2)	It indicates the time that is required for the concentration of the drug in the body to reach half of its original value	Older adults have slower rates of metabolism and hence have longer drug half-lives Higher doses and multiple drug doses result in the accumulation of the drug in the body and cause toxicity and higher rates of adverse events
Maximum concentration (C_{max})	It denotes the peak plasma concentration of a drug after its administration	The greater the C_{max} of the drug, the greater the effect of the drug on the body
Maximum time (t_{max})	It indicates the time for the drug to reach C_{max}	The shorter the t_{max} of the drug, the faster is its onset of action
Plasma protein binding	Drugs when they enter the body are often bound to plasma proteins especially serum albumin and to a lesser extent lipoproteins, glycoproteins, and α-, β-, and γ-globulins The less protein bound the drug, the more efficiently it can cross the cell membranes The unbound fraction of the drug is the one that exhibits its pharmacological effects Most psychotropic medications except lithium are moderate to extensively protein bound	The less protein bound the drug, the more pharmacologically active it is The greater the protein binding of the drug, the longer the t1/2
Steady state	It indicates the time to when the drug is in dynamic equilibrium, i.e., there is no net change in the concentration of the drug in the body Drugs reach their steady state after four or five times their half-lives after regular dosing	Due to their longer t1/2 in older adults, the steady state for the drug is reached at a later time
Therapeutic window	It describes the range of drug dosages at which it can effectively treat the condition without causing adverse events	The wider the therapeutic window, the safer is the drug for clinical use
Volume of distribution (Vd)	It denotes the hypothetical volume in which a drug is distributed in the body It is also an indicator of the concentration of the drug in the body	As we age, lean muscle mass and total body water decrease, while total body fat tends to increase relative to the total body weight Older adults have a lower volume of distribution, thus the same dose of the drug will produce a higher concentration of the drug in an older adult when compared to a younger adult

The most significant enzymatic family that carries out the phase II reactions is the uridine 5′-diphosphate glucuronosyltransferases (UGTs). Lamotrigine, olanzapine, and many narcotic analgesics are metabolized by the UGTs.

Pharmacodynamics

Older adults tend to have greater susceptibility than younger individuals to different effects of the drug [15]. These include anticholinergic effects, extrapyramidal effects, orthostatic hypotension, and sedation. Many of these adverse effects of older adults occur even when the drug is present at the same concentration as in younger adults. Current data indicates that older adults may have greater sensitivity to anticholinergic activity, orthostatic hypotension, and sedation from psychotropic medications even at moderate plasma drug levels.

Cytochrome P450 (CYP450) System

Cytochrome P450 (CYP450) enzyme system is a collection of different enzymes that are responsible for the oxidative phase I metabolism of different medications. These enzymes influence the bioavailability and the pharmacological activity of medications [17]. The CYP450 enzymes are found at their highest concentrations in the liver and the small intestine. Although there are more than 50 isoforms of these enzymes (isozymes) in the system, six of them metabolize approximately 90% of drugs with the two most significant ones being the CYP2D6 and the CYP3A4 [18].

The drugs that are acted on by the CYP enzymes are called the "substrates" [16]. Many of the psychotropic drugs are also substrates for the CYP450 enzymes [17]. Certain drugs may increase the activity of the CYP enzymes and are called the "inducers," whereas certain other drugs can decrease the activity of the various CYP enzymes and are noted as "inhibitors" of the enzymes. Induction of the CYP enzymes by the drugs can result in reduced levels of the "substrate drugs," whereas inhibition of the CYP enzyme can cause elevated levels of the "substrate drugs". This induction and inhibition of enzymes can also result in serious drug-drug interactions and severe ADEs. For example, if an older adult is prescribed with aripiprazole, which is a substrate for the CYP3A4 isoenzyme along with fluoxetine, which is a CYP3A4 inhibitor, then the level of aripiprazole will become higher due to the inhibition of its metabolism and may cause significant ADEs. If, on the other hand, aripiprazole is co-administered with phenobarbital, which is a CYP3A4 inducer, then phenobarbital will induce the metabolism of aripiprazole, and its level will become lower resulting in lack of response to the drug at that particular dose.

A specific gene encodes for each of the CYP450 enzymes [18]. Each individual inherits one genetic allele from each of their parent. Alleles are referred to as the "wild-type" or the "variant-type." The "wild-type" of allele occurs more commonly in the general population. A normal CYP metabolizer usually receives two copies of "wild-type" alleles. When an individual receives either one or two "variant-type" alleles instead of one or both "wild-type" alleles, then the "variant type" alleles encode a CYP450 enzyme that has reduced or no activity. These individuals are called "poor metabolizers," whereas those individuals with one "wild-type" and one "variant-type" allele have reduced enzyme activity. When an individual inherits multiple copies of "wild-type" alleles that cause excess enzyme activity, then the individual is called a "rapid metabolizer" or an "ultrarapid metabolizer." These polymorphisms of the CYP enzymes may influence an individual's response to commonly prescribed drug classes and are thought to be responsible for the observed variations in drug response among individuals of different ethnic origins [19]. Among clinicians caring for older adults with psychiatric disorders, knowledge of drugs that are metabolized by the CYP enzymes including the potent inhibitors and inducers will help optimize their use by minimizing the possibility of ADEs and maximizing their efficacy. Genotype testing can determine if an individual has a specific enzyme polymorphism, and this information can be used to provide appropriate medication selection to maximize the effectiveness of treatment. Table 25.2 describes the cytochrome P450 system and its relationship to the common psychotropic drugs.

TABLE 25-2. Cytochrome P450 (CYP450) system and psychotropic drugs [17–19]

Enzymes	Substrate drugs		Inhibitor drugs		Inducer drugs	
1A2	Amitriptyline	Imipramine	Cimetidine	Fluvoxamine	Modafinil	Primidone
	Caffeine	Olanzapine	Ciprofloxacin	Grapefruit juice	Nicotine	Rifampin
	Clomipramine	Propranolol	Diltiazem	Mexiletine	Omeprazole	
	Clozapine	Riluzole	Erythromycin	Norfloxacin	Phenobarbital	
	Fluvoxamine	Theophylline	Fluoroquinolones	Ritonavir		
	Haloperidol	Verapamil				
		Warfarin				
2D6	**Antidepressants**	**Others**	Amiodarone	Metoclopramide	Dexamethasone	
	Amitriptyline	Amphetamine	Bupropion	Methadone	Rifampin	
	Clomipramine	Atomoxetine	Celecoxib	Norfluoxetine		
	Desipramine	Clonidine	Chlorpromazine	Paroxetine		
	Duloxetine	Codeine	Cimetidine	Perphenazine		
	Fluvoxamine	Dextromethorphan	Clomipramine	Propafenone		
	Fluoxetine	Donepezil	Cocaine	Ranitidine		
	Imipramine	Ondansetron	Fluoxetine	Ritonavir		
	Nortriptyline	Oxycodone	Fluphenazine	Sertraline		
	Paroxetine	Promethazine	Fluvoxamine	Thioridazine		
	Venlafaxine	Propranolol	Haloperidol	Venlafaxine		
	Antipsychotics	Tramadol				
	Aripiprazole					
	Chlorpromazine					
	Haloperidol					
	Perphenazine					
	Risperidone					
	Thioridazine					
3A4	**Benzodiazepines**	Dextromethorphan	Amiodarone	Miconazole Nefazodone	Barbiturates	St. John's wort
	Alprazolam	Domperidone	Cimetidine	Nelfinavir	Carbamazepine	Sulfinpyrazone
	Diazepam	Fentanyl	Ciprofloxacin	Nevirapine	Dexamethasone	
	Midazolam	Haloperidol	Clarithromycin	Norfloxacin	Modafinil	
	Triazolam	Lidocaine	Clotrimazole	Norfluoxetine	Nevirapine	
	Steroids	Methadone	Diltiazem	Omeprazole	Phenobarbital	
	Estradiol	Ondansetron	Erythromycin	Paroxetine	Phenylbutazone	
	Hydrocortisone	Pimozide	Fluconazole	Propoxyphene	Phenytoin	
	Progesterone	Propranolol	Fluoxetine	Quinidine	Pioglitazone	
	Testosterone	Quetiapine	Fluvoxamine	Ranitidine	Primidone	
	Others	Risperidone	Grapefruit juice	Ritonavir	Rifabutin	
	Aripiprazole	Sildenafil	Indinavir	Saquinavir	Rifampin	
	Buspirone	Tamoxifen	Itraconazole	Sertindole		
	Caffeine	Taxol	Ketoconazole	Verapamil		
	Cocaine	Trazodone	Metronidazole			
	Dexamethasone	Zaleplon				
		Ziprasidone				
		Zolpidem				

Using Pharmacokinetic Data to Optimize Psychotropic Prescriptions Among Older Adults

Although the aging process does not significantly alter the absorption of orally prescribed psychotropic drugs, the absorption of these drugs may be delayed by the presence of food and other drugs like antacids in the GI tract [15]. This may not cause any problems in the case of standing doses of medications that have reached steady state. But this delay in absorption can cause problems if the drug has been given for an immediate clinical effect such as the treatment of agitation or aggression. Bioavailability of certain drugs may also be affected by absorption, and dose adjustments may need to be made in these cases.

Drug clearance decreases with age, and these result in higher steady-state concentrations (C_{ss}) of the drugs at any given dose [15]. As it takes longer among older adults to reach $C_{ss,}$ the onset of therapeutic benefits and/or toxicity may be delayed. Given that the metabolism of psychotropic drugs is altered not only by the process of aging but also by other factors like cardiac, hepatic, and renal diseases and co-administration of other drugs, clinician must consider all of these factors before prescribing psychotropic drugs to older adults.

Although there is reduced protein binding and an increase in the free fraction of a number of drugs in older adults, there is limited evidence that this change by itself modifies the pharmacodynamic effects of psychotropic drugs on older adults [15]. However, when the increase in the free fraction of the drug is due to reduced plasma albumin levels, then caution must be exercised as this may be a marker for the development of drug toxicity due to other conditions including impaired renal or hepatic functions. Additionally, reduced protein binding may alter the interpretation of total free and bound serum or plasma concentrations of the drug. When the clearance of the drug is limited by its protein binding, then an increase in the free fraction of the drug will result in a reciprocal reduction in the total plasma concentration. Hence reducing the protein binding of certain drugs in the older adults may reduce their therapeutic and toxic plasma concentration ranges when the total plasma drug concentrations are measured.

Clinicians caring for older adults should prescribe lower starting doses of drugs and provide smaller dose increments using a slower titration schedule to avoid adverse effects [15]. They also should monitor the drug effects closely to identify any adverse effects promptly. Additionally, clinicians should use longer-duration drug trials to evaluate the effectiveness of the drugs as the time to reach the steady-state concentration of most drugs is prolonged among the elderly. Finally injudicious polypharmacy should be avoided as it increases the risk for severe drug interactions in vulnerable individuals without improving their overall effectiveness.

Psychotropic Medications

In this section, we have included information regarding the common psychotropic medications that are used to treat psychiatric disorders among older adults [20–28]. Tables 25.3, 25.4, 25.5, 25.6, 25.7, 25.8, and 25.9 describe the common classes of psychotropic medications used among older adults with psychiatric disorders. Table 25.10 describes the long-acting antipsychotic injectable medications available in the United States. Table 25.11 describes the American Psychiatric Association guideline for using antipsychotic medications in individuals with dementia. Fig. 25.1 describes the algorithm for the treatment of psychiatric disorders among older adults.

TABLE 25-3. Antidepressants [20–25]

Medications	Half-life hours ($t_{1/2}$)	Dosage/levels	Common side effects
Bupropion	15–20 h	150–450 mg/day	Seizures, agitation, dry mouth, restlessness, diminished appetite, weight loss, headache, constipation, insomnia, anxiety, and GI distress. Rarely, blood pressure elevation, cognitive dysfunction, and dystonia
Mirtazapine	26–37 h	15–45 mg/day	Sedation, increased appetite, weight gain, dizziness, dry mouth, headache, nausea. Rarely, neutropenia
Monoamine oxidase inhibitors (MAOIs)			
Phenelzine	10–11 h	15–60 mg/day	Postural hypotension, insomnia, agitation, daytime somnolence, hyperadrenergic crises, weight gain, dry mouth, urinary retention, constipation, nausea, flushing, hepatotoxicity, edema
Tranylcypromine	4–8 h	10–40 mg/day	Same as above
Selegiline (EMSAM)	40 h	6 mg/24 h	No dietary restriction till 6 mg/24 h. Site irritation is the most common side effect. Other rare side effects are hypertensive crisis, depression, hallucinations, vivid dreams, postural hypotension, rash, urticaria, nausea, headache, dry mouth

TABLE 25-3 (continued)

Medications	Half-life hours ($t_{1/2}$)	Dosage/levels	Common side effects
Serotonin norepinephrine reuptake inhibitors (SNRIs)			
Desvenlafaxine	10–11 h	25–50 mg/day	Nausea, dizziness, insomnia, hyperhidrosis, constipation, somnolence, decreased appetite, anxiety, and specific male sexual function disorders
Duloxetine	10–13 h	20–90 mg/day	Nausea, anxiety, dry mouth, insomnia, sedation, sexual dysfunction, headache, sweating, dizziness
Levomilnacipran (more selective for norepinephrine reuptake inhibition than serotonin reuptake inhibition)	12 h	40–120 mg/day	Nausea, constipation, hyperhidrosis, heart rate increase, erectile dysfunction, tachycardia, vomiting, and palpitations
Venlafaxine	5–11 h	37.5–375 mg/day	Nausea, insomnia, anxiety, nervousness, sedation, sexual dysfunction, headache, tremor, dizziness, constipation, sweating, tachycardia, palpitations, blood pressure elevation
Selective serotonin reuptake inhibitors (SSRIs)			
Citalopram	24–30 h	5–20 mg/day	Nausea, reduced appetite, weight loss, sweating, tremor, flushing, agitation, anxiety, jitteriness, sedation, insomnia, headache, sexual dysfunction, diarrhea, SIADH, hyponatremia, galactorrhea, hyperprolactinemia, dry mouth, prolonged bleeding time, bleeding tendencies, bruxism, hair loss, cognitive impairment, serotonin syndrome, weight gain with long-term treatment
Escitalopram	5–20 mg/day		Same as above
Fluoxetine	2–4 days fluoxetine and 7–9 days for metabolite	5–60 mg/day	Same as above
Fluvoxamine	15 h	25–300 mg/day	Same as above but greater weight gain, sedation, constipation, GI disturbance
Paroxetine	24 h	5–50 mg/day	Same as other SSRIs
SSRI and 5-hydroxytryptamine-1A (5-HT_{1A}) receptor partial agonist			
Vilazodone	25 h	10–40 mg/day	Diarrhea, nausea, vomiting, and insomnia
Tricyclic antidepressants (TCAs)			
Amitriptyline	12–24 h	50–200 mg/day Therapeutic plasma level 100–250 ng/mL	Sedation, orthostatic hypotension, anticholinergic effects (dry mouth, constipation, urinary retention, blurred vision, diminished working memory, dental cavities), cardiac conduction defects, significant weight gain, sexual dysfunction (erectile), cardiotoxicity, seizures, and respiratory arrest in overdose
Clomipramine	20–50 h	50–250 mg/day Therapeutic plasma level 150–300 ng/mL	Same as above
Nortriptyline	60–90 h	25–150 mg/day Therapeutic plasma level 50–150 ng/mL	Same as above
Serotonin (5-HT) transporter inhibitor, antagonism of 5-HT3A and 5-HT7 receptors and partial agonism of 5-HT1B receptors			
Vortioxetine (may improve cognition in depression)	57–66 h	10–20 mg/day	Nausea, constipation, and vomiting

Table 25-4. Antipsychotics [20, 21]

Medications	Half-life hours ($t_{1/2}$)	Dosage/levels	Side effects
Atypicals			
Aripiprazole	75 h	10–20 mg/day	Agitation, insomnia
Asenapine	24 h	5–20 mg/day	Somnolence, dizziness, dysgeusia, oral paresthesia, nausea, increased appetite, fatigue, increased weight
Clozapine	6–26 h	12.5–300 mg/day	Agranulocytosis, weight gain, seizures, postural hypotension, sedation, tachycardia, transient hyperthermia eosinophilia, rebound psychosis
Lurasidone	18 h	40–160 mg/day	Somnolence, akathisia, extrapyramidal symptoms, and nausea
Olanzapine	35 h	10–20 mg/day	Sedation, dizziness, weight gain associated with new-onset diabetes mellitus
Paliperidone (major active metabolite of risperidone)	23 h	3–12 mg/day	Extrapyramidal symptoms, akathisia, somnolence, dyspepsia, constipation, weight increase, and tachycardia
Risperidone	3–20 h	1–4 mg/day	Insomnia, postural hypotension, dizziness, hypotension, dizziness, galactorrhea, sexual dysfunction, weight gain, extrapyramidal symptoms (EPS) at higher doses
Quetiapine	6–8 h	25–300 mg/day in divided doses	Sedation, weight gain, orthostatic hypotension, insomnia, dry mouth
Ziprasidone	4–5 h	80–160 mg/day	Sedation, dry mouth, constipation
Typicals			
Chlorpromazine	18–40 h	10–200 mg/day	Urinary retention, weight gain, rash, leukopenia, agranulocytosis, cholestasis, decreased seizure threshold, EPS (tremor, parkinsonism, akathisia, tardive dyskinesia), and neuroleptic malignant syndrome (NMS), QTc prolongation, torsades de pointes
Fluphenazine	10–20 h	0.5–6 mg/day	Same as above
Haloperidol	10–20 h	0.5–10 mg/day	Same as above
Perphenazine	10–20 h	2–32 mg/day	Same as above and closed angle glaucoma
Trifluoperazine	10–20 h	1–15 mg/day	Same as above and hepatotoxicity

Table 25-5. Anxiolytics [20, 21]

Medications	Half-life hours ($t_{1/2}$)	Dosage/levels	Side effects
Benzodiazepines			
Alprazolam	6–20 h	0.25–3 mg/day	Sedation, drowsiness, fatigue, memory disturbance, muscle weakness, respiratory depression. Sudden withdrawal causes agitation, anxiety, insomnia, seizures, and hallucinations
Clonazepam	20–50 h	0.25–2 mg/day	
Diazepam	30–100 h	5–15 mg/day	
Lorazepam	10–20 h	1–3 mg/day	
Non-benzodiazepines			
Buspirone	2–11 h	10–60 mg/day in divided doses	Dizziness, headache, syncope, GI disturbance, nausea, paresthesia, restlessness, drowsiness
Hydroxyzine	7–20 h	50–100 mg/day	Anticholinergic toxicity, dry mouth, urinary retention. Use with caution in elderly

TABLE 25-6. Cognitive enhancers [20, 21]

Medications	Half-life hours ($t_{1/2}$)	Dosage/levels	Side effects
Cholinesterase inhibitors			
Donepezil	70 h	5–10 mg/day	Nausea, diarrhea, anorexia, insomnia, fatigue, muscle cramps
Galantamine	7 h	8–24 mg/day	Same as above
Rivastigmine	1.5 h	1.5–12 mg/day	Same as above
Rivastigmine patch	3.7 h	4.6 mg–9.5 mg/day	Irritation at the placement site
NMDA antagonist			
Memantine	60–100 h	7–28 mg/day	Sedation, agitation, urinary incontinence, urinary tract infection, insomnia

TABLE 25-7. Hypnotics [20, 21]

Medications	Half-life hours ($t_{1/2}$)	Dosage/levels	Side effects
Benzodiazepines			
Temazepam	8–20 h	7.5–30 mg qhs	Sedation, drowsiness, memory difficulties, fatigue, muscle weakness
Triazolam	1.5–5.5 h	0.125–0.2 mg qhs	Drowsiness, dizziness, unpleasant taste, memory difficulties
Non-benzodiazepines			
Eszopiclone	6 h	1–2 mg qhs	Drowsiness, GI disturbances, headache, dizziness
Zaleplon	1–2 h	5 mg qhs	Same as above
Zolpidem	2–3 h	5 mg qhs	Somnolence, fatigue, nausea, headache, dizziness, cognitive dysfunction, angioedema
Melatonin receptor agonist			
Ramelteon	1–2.5 h	8 mg qhs	Fatigue, nausea, headache, dizziness
Highly selective orexin receptor antagonist			
Suvorexant	12 h	10–20 mg qhs	Somnolence, headaches, abnormal dreams, dry mouth, cough

TABLE 25-8. Mood stabilizers [20, 21]

Medications	Half-life hours ($t_{1/2}$)	Dosage/levels	Side effects
Carbamazepine	12–17 h	100–600 mg/day in divided doses Therapeutic level 8–12 μg/mL	Dizziness, ataxia, clumsiness, sedation, dysarthria, diplopia, GI disturbance, blood dyscrasias, abnormal liver function test, tremor, memory disturbance, confusional state, conduction defect, SIADH, rash, lenticular opacities
Divalproex sodium	8–12 h	250–1000 mg/day Therapeutic level 50–100 μg/mL	GI disturbance, thrombocytopenia, platelet dysfunction, sedation, tremor, ataxia, alopecia, weight gain, hepatotoxicity, pancreatitis, rash, erythema multiforme
Lamotrigine	25 h	50–400 mg/day	Rash, Stevens-Johnson syndrome, headache, diplopia, ataxia, blurred vision, nausea, and vomiting
Lithium	20 h	150–1200 mg/day Therapeutic level 0.4–1.0 meq/l	Thirst, polyuria, weight gain, tremor, GI disturbance, interstitial nephritis, nephrotic syndrome, edema, benign intracranial hypertension, thyroid dysfunction, cardiac arrhythmias, acne, psoriasis, exfoliative dermatitis, alopecia, rash, relative leukocytosis
Topiramate	21 h	50–400 mg/day	Sedation, ataxia, somnolence, paresthesia, nystagmus, cognitive impairment, non-anion gap metabolic acidosis leading to kidney stones and osteoporosis
Gabapentin	5–7 h	300–1600 mg/day	Nausea, diplopia, glaucoma, hypotension, cardiac conduction defects, drowsiness, dizziness, unsteadiness, headache, tremor, edema, diplopia, nausea, vomiting
Oxcarbazepine	2–9 h	150–1200 mg/day	Drowsiness, dizziness, unsteadiness, headache, tremor, edema, diplopia, nausea, vomiting. Hyponatremia, photosensitivity, rash, Stevens-Johnson syndrome

TABLE 25-9. Medications used to treat substance use disorders [20, 21]

Medications	Half-life hours ($t_{1/2}$)	Dosage/levels	Side effects
Alcohol use disorder			
Acamprosate	20–30 h	1333 mg/day if weight < 60 kg 1998 mg/day if weight > 60 kg Given in three divided doses	Nausea, diarrhea and flatulence, insomnia, headache, confusion sexual dysfunction, pruritus Contraindicated in pregnancy, lactation, liver and kidney dysfunction
Disulfiram	60–120 h	250–500 mg/day	Fatigue, drowsiness, halitosis, body odor, tremor, headache, impotence, dizziness, hepatotoxicity, neuropathies, psychosis, catatonia
Naltrexone	4–13 h	50 mg/day	GI disturbance, abnormal liver function tests, anorexia, insomnia, anxiety, arthralgia, myalgia and rarely rhabdomyolysis
Nicotine use disorder			
Bupropion	11–14 h	200–450 mg/day	Seizure, agitation, dry mouth, anorexia, insomnia, weight loss, anxiety, constipation, GI disturbance, blood pressure elevation, cognitive dysfunction, and dystonias
Varenicline	17–24 h	1 mg twice daily	Nausea, headache, insomnia, dreams, abnormal taste, GI disturbance, suicidal ideation
Opioid use disorder			
Buprenorphine	37 h	8–16 mg/day or 32 mg three times a week	Dizziness, sedation, constipation, vertigo, nausea, vomiting, respiratory depression
Methadone	25 h	60–100 mg/day	Nausea, vomiting, constipation, bowel obstruction, euphoria, sedation, coma, bradycardia, hypotension, sexual dysfunction, gynecomastia, hyperprolactinemia

TABLE 25-10. Long-acting antipsychotic injectable medications available in the United States [27]

Medication	Half-life (t1/2) days	Starting dose (mg)	Second dose (mg)	Maintenance dose (mg)
Aripiprazole extended release	29.9–46.5 days	400 mg	400 mg after 4 weeks	300–400 mg every 4 weeks
Fluphenazine decanoate	61 days	20 mg	12.5–25 mg after 1–2 weeks	12.5–50 mg every 2–3 weeks
Haloperidol decanoate	21 days	50 mg	50–100 mg after 1–4 weeks	50–200 mg every 3–4 weeks
Paliperidone palmitate	25–49 days	234 mg	156 mg after 1 week	39–234 mg every 4 weeks
Olanzapine pamoate	30 days	210 mg	210–404 every 2–4 weeks for first 8 weeks	150–405 every 2–4 weeks

TABLE 25-11. American Psychiatric Association guideline for using antipsychotic medications in individuals with dementia [28]

1. If the risks and benefits assessment favors the use of an antipsychotic for behavioral/psychological symptoms in individuals with dementia, the treatment should be initiated at a low dose and to be titrated up to the minimum effective dose as tolerated
2. If the individual with dementia experiences a clinically significant adverse effect due to the antipsychotic medication, the potential risks and benefits of the antipsychotic medication should be reviewed by the clinician to determine if tapering and discontinuing of the medication are indicated
3. In individuals with dementia and agitation or psychosis, if there is no clinically significant response after a 4-week trial of an adequate dose of an antipsychotic, then the medication should be tapered and discontinued
4. Among individuals who show a positive response to treatment, the decision to possibly taper the antipsychotic medication should be discussed with the patient, the patient's family, and/or the surrogate decision-maker
5. Among the individuals who show an adequate response to treatment with an antipsychotic, an attempt to taper and withdraw the medication should be made within 4 months of initiation of treatment unless the individual experiences a recurrence of symptoms with previous attempts at tapering the antipsychotic medication
6. While the antipsychotic medication is being tapered, assessment of symptoms should occur at least every month during the taper and for at least 4 months after the medication is discontinued to identify signs of recurrence and, if there is a recurrence of symptoms, the reevaluation of the benefits and risks of antipsychotic treatment
7. In the absence of delirium, if non-emergency antipsychotic medication treatment is indicated, then haloperidol should not be used as a first-line agent
8. In individuals with dementia and agitation or psychosis, a long-acting injectable antipsychotic medication should not be utilized unless it is otherwise indicated for a co-occurring chronic psychotic illness

Conclusions

Psychiatric disorders are common among older adults. The aging process brings special challenges in the treatment of these disorders. The physiological changes associated with an aging human body greatly affect the pharmacokinetic properties of psychotropic medications. Additionally, the pharmacodynamic effects of the psychotropic medications on the aging body are often pronounced. Clinicians caring for older adults with psychiatric disorders must have sufficient knowledge of the pharmacokinetic changes associated with aging and the pharmacodynamic properties of the drug, if they want to optimize the treatment outcomes for these disorders. Knowledge of the CYP450 enzyme systems will aid clinicians in using judicious combination of psychotropic medications in cases of refractory psychiatric disorders or with comorbid conditions. Careful treatment planning with close monitoring of outcomes including efficacy and adverse effects will improve the quality of care of the vulnerable elderly with psychiatric disorders.

Obtain a thorough history
(Course of illness, medical, psychiatric, medications, pre-morbid personality, cognition and functions)

↓

Complete a focused physical examination

(Rule out underlying medical or neurological disorders)

↓

Order appropriate investigations

(Blood tests, urine examination, vitamin B 12 & folate levels, VDRL, neuroimaging)

↙ ↘

Treat comorbid medical/neurological disorder(s) Remove offending drug(s)

↓

Complete standardized rating scales and/or neuropsychological testing

↓

Assess patient's cognition

*(MMSE, MOCA, SLUMS)

↙ ↘

Treat with AchEIs*← Mild/Moderate MND* Moderate to Severe MND → Treat with AChEIs & memantine

↓

Define symptomatology and arrive at a diagnosis

↓

Initiate psychotherapy and/or pharmacotherapy (After informed consent)

↓

If monotherapy fails use judicious combination of medications
Use medications within prescribed dosage ranges
Initiate judicious dose titration(s)
Frequently assess for efficacy and side-effects of these medications
Maintain minimum effective doses of medications to optimize outcomes
Reduce and/or taper off medications that are causing side-effects or if medication(s) are ineffective

**MMSE: Mini Mental State Examination; MoCA: Montreal Cognitive Assessment; SLUMS: Saint Louis Mental Status; AchEIs: Acetylcholinesterase Inhibitor;s MND: Major Neurocognitive Disorder*

FIGURE 25-1. Algorithm for the treatment of psychiatric disorders among older adults [20–27]

References

1. Mental health and older adults. http://www.who.int/mediacentre/factsheets/fs381/en/. Accessed 10 Dec 2016.
2. Aging Statistics. https://aoa.acl.gov/Aging_Statistics/index.aspx. Accessed 10 Dec 2016.
3. Reynold K, Pietrzak RH, El-Gabalawy R, Mackenzie CS, Sareen J. Prevalence of psychiatric disorders in U.S. older adults: findings from a nationally representative survey. World Psychiatry. 2015;14(1):74–81.
4. Aparasu RR, Mort JR, Brandt H. Psychotropic prescription use by community-dwelling elderly in the United States. J Am Geriatr Soc. 2003;51(5):671–7.
5. Molinari VA, Chiriboga DA, Branch LG, et al. Reasons for psychiatric medication prescription for new nursing home residents. Aging Ment Health. 2011;15(7):904–12.
6. García-Gollarte F, Baleriola-Júlvez J, Ferrero-López I, Cruz-Jentoft AJ. Inappropriate drug prescription at nursing home admission. J Am Med Dir Assoc. 2012;13(1):83.e9–15.
7. Gurwitz JH, Field TS, Avorn J, et al. Incidence and preventability of adverse drug events in nursing homes. Am J Med. 2000;109(2):87–94.
8. Hartikainen S, Lönnroos E, Louhivuori K. Medication as a risk factor for falls: critical systematic review. J Gerontol A Biol Sci Med Sci. 2007;62(10):1172–81.
9. Peron EP, Gray SL, Hanlon JT. Medication use and functional status decline in older adults: a narrative review. Am J Geriatr Pharmacother. 2011;9(6):378–91.
10. Tampi RR, Williamson D, Mittal V, et al. Behavioral and psychological symptoms of dementia: part I—epidemiology, neurobiology, heritability, and evaluation. Clin Geriatr. 2011;19(5):41–6.
11. Tampi RR, Williamson D, Mittal V, et al. Behavioral and psychological symptoms of dementia: part II—treatment. Clin Geriatr. 2011;19(6):31–40.
12. By the American Geriatrics Society 2015 Beers Criteria Update Expert Panel. American Geriatrics Society 2015 updated beers criteria for potentially inappropriate medication use in older adults. J Am Geriatr Soc. 2015;63(11):2227–46.
13. Pollock B, Forsyth C, Bies R. The critical role of clinical pharmacology in geriatric psychopharmacology. Clin Pharmacol Ther. 2009;85(1):89–93.
14. Golan DE, Tashjian AH, Armstrong AJ, Armstrong AW, editors. Principles of pharmacology: the pathophysiologic basis of drug therapy. 2nd ed. Philadelphia: Lippincott Williams & Wilkins; 2007. p. 19–49.
15. von Moltke LL, Abernethy DR, Greenblatt DJ. Kinetics and dynamics of psychotropic drugs in the elderly. In: Salzman C, editor. Clinical geriatric psychopharmacology. 4th ed. Philadelphia, PA: Lippincott Williams & Wilkins; 2004. p. 87–114.
16. Madhusoodanan S, Velama U, Parmar J, Goia D, Brenner R. A current review of cytochrome P450 interactions of psychotropic drugs. Ann Clin Psychiatry. 2014;26(2):120–38.
17. Caley CF. Interpreting and applying CYP450 genomic test results to psychotropic medications. J Pharm Pract. 2011;24(5):439–46.
18. Lynch T, Price A. The effect of cytochrome P450 metabolism on drug response, interactions, and adverse effects. Am Fam Physician. 2007;76(3):391–6.
19. Eap CB. Personalized prescribing: a new medical model for clinical implementation of psychotropic drugs. Dialogues Clin Neurosci. 2016;18(3):313–22.
20. Albers LJ, Hahn RK, Reist C. Handbook of psychiatric drugs. Blue Jay: Current Clinical Strategies Publishing; 2011. p. 8–110.
21. Labbate LA, Fava M, Rosenbaum JF, Arana GW. Handbook of psychiatric drug therapy. 6th ed. Philadelphia: Lippincott Williams & Wilkins; 2010. p. 1–254.
22. Perry R, Cassagnol M. Desvenlafaxine: a new serotonin-norepinephrine reuptake inhibitor for the treatment of adults with major depressive disorder. Clin Ther. 2009;31(Pt 1):1374–404.
23. Asnis GM, Henderson MA. Levomilnacipran for the treatment of major depressive disorder: a review. Neuropsychiatr Dis Treat. 2015;11:125–35.
24. McCormack PL. Vilazodone: a review in major depressive disorder in adults. Drugs. 2015;75(16):1915–23.
25. Connolly KR, Thase ME. Vortioxetine: a new treatment for major depressive disorder. Expert Opin Pharmacother. 2016;17(3):421–31.
26. Jacobson LH, Callander GE, Hoyer D. Suvorexant for the treatment of insomnia. Expert Rev Clin Pharmacol. 2014;7(6):711–30.
27. Castillo EG, Stroup TS. Effectiveness of long-acting injectable antipsychotics: a clinical perspective. Evid Based Ment Health. 2015;18(2):36–9.
28. Reus VI, Fochtmann LJ, Eyler AE, Hilty DM, Horvitz-Lennon M, Jibson MD, Lopez OL, Mahoney J, Pasic J, Tan ZS, Wills CD, Rhoads R, Yager J. The American Psychiatric Association practice guideline on the use of antipsychotics to treat agitation or psychosis in patients with dementia. Am J Psychiatry. 2016;173(5):543–6.

26 Electroconvulsive Therapy

Ali Ahsan Ali, Garima Garg, Deena J. Tampi, and Rajesh R. Tampi

Introduction

The world is on the verge of a demographic milestone. For the first time in human history, the number of people aged 65 years or older will soon outpace the number of children under the age of 5 years [1]. Between 2015 and 2050, the proportion of the world's population over 60 years will nearly double from 12 to 22%. This changing population structure has led to an increased burden of noncommunicable diseases.

Neurological and psychiatric disorders are the leading causes of disability in the elderly, accounting for 17.4% of the total years lived with disability (YLDs) [1]. Approximately 15% of adults aged 60 years and older have a psychiatric disorder. Researchers and health-care professionals are aware of this growing public health issue and continue to seek effective treatment modalities for psychiatric disorders. Electroconvulsive therapy (ECT) has been proven to be a safe, effective, and rapid therapeutic intervention for the treatment of many neuropsychiatric disorders among older adults. In this chapter, we discuss the use of ECT among older adults with psychiatric disorders.

The Origins and Mechanism of Action of Electroconvulsive Therapy

Nominated for the Nobel Prize in the 1930s, the two Italian physicians, Cerletti and Bini, first used ECT to successfully treat catatonia in a patient suffering from schizophrenia [2]. In the 1940s and 1950s, ECT was used widely to treat many disorders but was slowly withdrawn after the advent of a wide variety of psychopharmacological agents. ECT has resurfaced in the last two decades with improvements in procedural safety, and the evidence for its efficacy among older adults with psychiatric disorders has grown significantly.

The exact neurobiological and therapeutic mechanisms of ECT remains unclear. One theory proposes that ECT attenuates the hypothalamic–pituitary axis [3], while another suggests that it boosts the levels of neurotransmitters in the central nervous system [4]. It is also postulated that ECT modulates neurotransmitter receptor activity and density [5]. Although the mechanism of action of ECT is still unclear, its antidepressant, antipsychotic, anti-catatonic, neuroendocrine, and neurotransmitter effects, as well as its strong effect on neurogenesis, have been clearly demonstrated [6].

Physiology of ECT

Normally, there are asynchronous electric waveforms generated throughout the brain at rest [7]. ECT is an electrically elicited synchronized waveform or a seizure that is induced in an individual while under the supervision of a skilled group of psychiatrists, anesthesiologists, and nurses in a controlled environment, either in an inpatient or outpatient setting [7]. The anesthesi-

R. R. Tampi et al. (eds.), *Psychiatric Disorders Late in Life*, https://doi.org/10.1007/978-3-319-73078-3_26

TABLE 26-1. Interaction between the brain, heart and the produced motor seizure

Cerebral physiology	Cardiovascular physiology	Correlating motor activity
EEG—variable, low-voltage fast activity, and polyspike rhythms	Increase in vagal tone that can cause bradycardia or brief period of asystole	Tonic/irregular clonic movements
EEG—hypersynchronous polyspikes and waves	Activation of sympathetic nervous system that causes tachycardia, hypertension, and increased myocardial oxygen demand EKG—may show ST and T wave changes	Clonic motor movements
EEG—abrupt termination of the seizure followed by a flat line	Second period of increase in vagal tone that can cause bradycardia and variable dysrhythmias (including ectopic beats)	No movement

ologist continuously monitors the airway, vitals, and the cardiac rhythm on an electrocardiography (EKG) strip and watches out for episodes of bradycardia or asystole. The ECT machine is calibrated to the desired convulsive stimulus intensity. This stimulus intensity can be determined before the procedure, and it varies among different individuals. Continuous electroencephalographic (EEG) monitoring is also obtained to determine the seizure adequacy and duration. The interaction between the brain, heart, and the produced motor seizure is summarized in Table 26.1.

Pre-ECT Evaluation

During the pre-ECT evaluation, it is very important to obtain an informed consent from the individual for both anesthesia and the electrical procedure. In emergency cases, probate court approval is required to conduct the ECT treatment [8].

A multidisciplinary team including a psychiatrist and anesthesiologist evaluates candidates for possible ECT treatment. Basic laboratory tests like complete blood count (CBC), basic metabolic profile (BMP), and EKG are obtained. The individual's past medical, psychiatric histories and current medications are reviewed as they may affect the safety, efficacy, and recovery after the procedure. Since some older adults may exhibit neurocognitive decline, it is also necessary to assess their baseline neurocognitive functioning, as inter-ictal amnesia may impact post-ECT cognitive functioning [9]. Depending on the severity of the neurocognitive decline, a careful assessment weighing the benefits versus risks for ECT treatments in each of these individuals is required.

Electrode Placements, Stimulus Dosing, and Treatment Schedule

Electrode placement, stimulus dosing, and treatment schedule influence the efficacy of therapy and determine the magnitude of subsequent cognitive side effects [10]. Hence, it is important to consider the various options individually especially if there is preexisting neurocognitive impairment.

The most commonly used electrode placement is bitemporal (BT), followed by the right unilateral (RUL) and the less studied bifrontal (BF) placements. Evidence supports the use of RUL ECT over BT ECT among older adults as it is associated with less cognitive effects [11], even when a significantly higher stimulus dose is used [10]. Bilateral ECT is used for medical or psychiatric emergencies or when looking to minimize the duration of the course in medically high-risk patients. BF placement is not superior to RUL placement when comparing the cognitive side effect profile [10].

Ultra-brief pulse stimulation has less short- and long-term cognitive side effects when compared to standard brief pulse treatments which initially replaced the use of sine-wave stimulation [8, 12]. Ultra-brief RUL ECT applied at markedly supra-seizure thresholds has similar efficacy to standard pulse width, bilateral or RUL ECT. In comparison, ultra-brief pulse bilateral ECT has lower efficacy when compared to unilateral electrode placements [13]. The use of ultra-brief pulse RUL ECT is associated with significantly fewer cognitive side effects without compromising on efficacy when compared to other electrode placements and is considered as first-line method of ECT among older adults.

Table 26-2. Electrode placements, their efficacy, and associated cognitive side effects

Electrode placement	Bitemporal	Right unilateral	Bifrontal
Anatomical placement	Both the electrodes are placed over the frontotemporal region about 1 in. above the midpoint of a line transecting the external canthus of the eye and the tragus of the ear	One electrode is placed over the right frontotemporal area and the other over the right centro-parietal area to the right of the vertex of the scalp	Both the electrodes are placed 2 in. above the external canthus of each eye
Preference	Least preferred	Most preferred	May be preferred in some cases
Cognitive side effects	Most side effects	Less side effects	Similar to right unilateral

The seizure threshold is dependent on the electrode placement, age, and gender [8, 14]. Seizure threshold is higher with bilateral electrode placement, advanced age, and among males. There is paucity of evidence to calculate the stimulus dosage based on these factors alone and requires further research.

The number of treatments administered depends on the clinical improvement noted and the degree of cognitive side effects. ECT is generally administered three times a week in the United States although preempting a fixed number of treatments is not advised. It can be reduced to twice or once a week if side effects are pronounced and should be stopped when a therapeutic plateau occurs.

The three primary types of electrode placements, their efficacy, and cognitive side effects are summarized in Table 26.2 [15].

Anesthesia Management for ECT

ECT is performed either as an inpatient or outpatient treatment under general anesthesia. All patients are required to have a full pre-anesthetic evaluation to assess its risks and optimize therapy [16]. The goal of anesthesia management is to have rapid induction and recovery time, minimize associated cardiovascular effects and musculoskeletal injury associated with the induced seizure [16]. Many anesthetic agents have anticonvulsant properties that need to be taken into consideration in order to optimize seizure duration. Similarly, doses of benzodiazepines and antiepileptic medications should be reduced prior to every ECT session as they may raise the seizure threshold causing difficulty in inducing the seizure.

Most commonly used anesthetics agents include methohexital (gold standard), etomidate, and propofol [16]. Succinylcholine is the most commonly used muscle relaxant to minimize musculoskeletal injury. Although the relationship between seizure duration and efficacy remains unclear, any seizure lasting less than 15 s is considered abortive [17]. Seizures greater than 20 s do not correlate with clinical response [18]. The mean seizure duration for all induction agents is greater than 17 s, including methohexital, etomidate, propofol, and thiopental, and hence these induction agents are suitable for ECT [19].

In the instance of an abortive seizure, increasing seizure duration is recommended by adding short-acting opioids to reduced doses of methohexital and propofol [20] or by switching to ketamine [21]. Etomidate can be particularly useful in elderly with high seizure thresholds or among seizure-resistant individuals [22]. For individuals with preexisting cardiac disease, propofol should be considered as the agent of choice as it attenuates the hemodynamic response during treatment [23].

The advantages and disadvantages of commonly used anesthetics agents are summarized in Table 26.3. Individual patient's characteristics may guide the selection of appropriate agent.

Evidence for Using ECT Among the Older Adults

The evidence for using ECT among older adults is promising and robust [7–9, 12, 30]. ECT has

TABLE 26-3. Comparison of commonly used anesthetic agents

Anesthetic agent and dosage[a]	Seizure quality	Advantages	Disadvantages
Methohexital 0.75–1.0 mg/kg	Gold standard	Long history of use Seizure duration can be attenuated using short-acting opioids (alfentanil)	Limited commercial availability Greater risk of adverse cardiac events when compared with propofol [19]
Propofol 0.75 mg/kg	Progressively shortens seizure duration [24]	Reduced risk of adverse cardiac events and sympathetic response [19, 25] Safer in patients with risk of cerebral hemorrhage [26] Seizure duration can be attenuated using short-acting opioids (alfentanil)	Shortened seizure duration in turn requiring higher electrical discharge leading to greater cognitive side effects [24]
Etomidate 0.15–0.3 mg/kg	Comparable to methohexital Increased duration when compared with propofol and thiopental [27]	Possible first-line for high seizure threshold [22] Minimal effect on seizure threshold overtime [22] Seizure duration can be attenuated using short-acting opioids (alfentanil)	Emergence of myoclonic movements Painful injection site [27] Hyperdynamic response when compared to propofol [28]
Thiopental 1.5–2.5 mg/kg		Increased response rates after six treatments and better cognitive functioning when compared to propofol [29]	
Ketamine 0.5–2.0 mg/kg	Similar to etomidate (high-quality seizures)	Lesser cognitive side effects Has an antidepressant potential of its own	Hyperdynamic response and temporary cardiac side-effects

[a]Recommended dose of agent for ECT by the American Psychiatric Association.

been studied to be safe, and effective for the treatment for depressive, psychotic, and manic disorders. Its use in the treatment of catatonia and neuromuscular syndrome can be lifesaving and can significantly improve functioning in patients with Parkinson's disease and dementia. Its utility is even more pronounced given the limitations of using psychotropics among older adults including severe side effects, increased probability to drug–drug interactions, issues with compliance, and increased risk of mortality [31]. The remission of illness when using ECT among older adults is equal to, if not better than when compared to its use among younger adults with only a slight decrease in tolerability [32].

Unipolar Depression

Multiple studies have indicated that the antidepressant effect of ECT is superior to pharmacological interventions [33–37]. The Prolonging Remission in Depressed Elderly (PRIDE) is a recently conducted multisite two-phase study [12]. This study showed that older adults with depression remitted when treated with ECT and venlafaxine in the phase 1 of the trial (55% of 60–69-year-olds and 69.7% of ≥70-year-old individuals, odds ratio (OR) 1.89, $P = 0.02$). The individuals who did not report suicidal ideation (SI) had higher odds of remitting than those who did (71.4% vs. 55.7%, OR 2.00, $P = 0.021$). The phase 2 of the trial studied the effects of continuation ECT plus medication (venlafaxine and lithium) when compared to medications (venlafaxine and lithium) alone [30]. This phase concluded that not only were there significant improvements in the depressive symptoms depicted by a reduction in the HAM-D scores at the end of 24 weeks in the ECT plus medication group when compared to the medication-only group ($P = 0.004$), but the time taken to produce an effect in former group was significantly lower ($P < 0.001$). While evaluating the safety and tolerability of ECT, the odds of being rated as "not ill at all" on the CGI-S score in the ECT plus medication group were 5.2 times greater than that in the medication-only group ($P = 0.009$). Approximately 16.7% of the individuals in the study had a relapse in their symptoms of depression, 13.1% in the ECT plus medication group, and 20.3% in the medication-only group (OR = 1.7). Additionally, the time taken to relapse was 7.5 weeks in the former group and 6.0 weeks in the latter group. Another study showed that the speed of remission of symptoms in severely depressed older adults was higher in the group treated with ECT versus medication-alone group [38]. Mean time to remission in the ECT group was 3.1 weeks, whereas it was 4.0 weeks in the medication-alone group.

The presence of psychotic features in depressed older adults is a positive predictor of bilateral ECT response. The response is often rapid and decreases the psychopathology significantly [36, 39].

Bipolar Depression

ECT has been shown to be effective in treating bipolar depression. ECT may be preferred over pharmacological management in cases of refractory bipolar depression and mania and in cases where the risk of hypomanic and manic switches is considered to be higher [34, 35, 40]. Data suggests that ECT is equally effective for both unipolar and bipolar depression [41–45]. A meta-analysis consisting of data from 2001 to 2009 showed that out of five major prospective studies and one chart review that were evaluated, five studies showed equal efficacy for ECT in the treatment of unipolar and bipolar depression, whereas one study showed ECT to be more efficacious among unipolar depressed patients [46].

ECT is an effective treatment for acute mania with a reported efficacy equal to or superior to that of lithium among younger individuals [47, 48]. Its evidence for utility among older adults with mania is based on a number of reports in the literature [44]. ECT is often recommended for use among individuals who have failed adequate psychopharmacological treatment. ECT is the treatment of choice when rapid relief of symptoms is required and in cases where the manic episode is severe enough to cause a significant risk of harm to self or others. It is also the treatment of choice among individuals who are intolerant to medications. As the acute episode subsides following the ECT treatment, maintenance on psychopharmacological agents is recommended, although a few individuals may require maintenance ECT to continue the euthymic state [49].

Psychotic Disorders

Damm et al. retrospectively studied the use of ECT among 380 individuals including older adults (30% were >60 years in age) who had a diagnosis of schizophrenia and depression [50]. The investigators reported considerable clinical improvement across all age groups with ECT treatment. Liu et al. reviewed the evidence from six prospective studies and one case series that was available between 1991 and 2012 on the utility of ECT in the treatment of schizophrenia, schizoaffective disorder, and related psychotic disorders [51]. They concluded that ECT was effective for both the acute and maintenance treatment for psychosis among individuals with schizophrenia, treatment-resistant catatonic schizophrenia, and schizoaffective disorder. ECT has not been found to have any significant utility among individuals with late-onset and very-late-onset psychosis due to structural brain changes noted on neuroimaging [52–55].

Catatonia

Catatonia can be seen among older adults and generally has a multifactorial etiology—due to general medical conditions, substance or medication induced, due to schizophrenia, or due to mood disorders [56]. Initial management is supportive including intravenous fluid administration. First-line treatment for mild to moderate catatonia is benzodiazepine administration. For benzodiazepine unresponsive individuals or individuals presenting with malignant (severe catatonia) or lethal catatonia, ECT is recommended [57]. Hatta et al. examined 50 individuals with a mean age of 50 years ± 17.9 years with catatonic symptoms who were treated with ECT [58]. The investigators reported a 100% remission rate among individuals who received ECT. High rates of response of catatonic symptoms to ECT have been reported in other studies [59–65]. It is important to note that ECT is effective in resolving catatonic symptoms despite different etiologies.

Neuroleptic Malignant Syndrome

Neuroleptic malignant syndrome (NMS) is not an uncommon presentation among older adults [66]. General medical, psychiatric, and neurological conditions can also mimic NMS and can frequently coexist [67]. Catatonia frequently mimics symptoms of NMS, and a lorazepam challenge test can be useful in differentiating the two conditions [68]. Initial management is supportive with the cessation of neuroleptics, followed by trials of dantrolene, bromocriptine, or amantadine for rigidity, hyperthermia, and tachycardia.

The literature supporting the use of ECT in NMS is sparse. Trollor et al. reviewed 55 cases that evaluated the use of ECT for NMS across different age groups including older adults [69]. ECT was administered as a primary treatment for NMS in 40 (73%) cases, as combined management of NMS and psychosis in ten (18%) cases and in five (9%) cases ECT was used primarily for psychiatric symptoms during active or resolving NMS. Twenty cases (63%) were noted to achieve full recovery, while the remaining cases (37%) achieved partial recovery.

Although ECT is safe for use among individuals with NMS, vigilance is needed regarding cardiovascular complications, as there is autonomic instability among individuals with NMS. ECT can be used as a primary treatment when there is difficulty in distinguishing NMS from catatonia, when the risk of leaving the NMS untreated is dangerous or when NMS is noted among individuals with psychotic depression [69, 70].

Behavioral Disturbances in Dementia

Behavioral disturbances are frequently seen among individuals with dementia and pose a challenge in management [71]. The management includes ruling out a medical etiology for the behaviors followed by non-pharmacological interventions that include behavior therapy, nursing/medical interventions, and patient/family education [72]. If these interventions fail, then a trial of pharmacotherapy is recommended. From the SSRI class, sertraline and citalopram are recommended [73]. From the antipsychotic group, risperidone and olanzapine have demonstrated modest utility but are associated with adverse side effects including cerebrovascular accidents and increased risk of mortality [74, 75].

Those individuals not responding to psychopharmacological intervention alone can be referred for ECT [76, 77]. A recent prospective study by Acharya et al. included 23 individuals with dementia who exhibited symptoms of agitation and aggression who responded well to ECT [78]. A significant decrease in scores on the Cohen–Mansfield Agitation Inventory (CMAI, $P = 0.006$) and the Neuropsychiatric Inventory (NPI, $P < 0.001$) was noted from baseline to discharge. There were no statistically significant changes in scores on the Cornell Scale for Depression in Dementia (CSDD) and the Alzheimer's Disease Cooperative Study Group–Activities of Daily Living (ADCS-ADL) scales. ECT was discontinued in three participants due to adverse events and two participants for poor treatment response.

Parkinson's Disease

Parkinson's disease (PD) is a common progressive neurodegenerative disorder among older adults [79]. It is estimated that between 2.7 and 90% of individuals with PD also have comorbid depression. Although the motor symptoms of PD are primarily treated using levodopa–carbidopa, dopamine agonists, and anticholinergics, their use is limited as individuals with PD may develop adverse side effects to these medications over time. ECT should be considered in such patients.

Fregni et al. pooled the results of five studies in their meta-analysis that studied the effects of ECT on the motor function among individuals with PD [80]. Their results supported the use of ECT in improving global motor function among these individuals. ECT improves the motor symptoms of

PD independent of its effects on comorbid psychiatric illness like depression. These findings are consistent with the conclusions of an earlier review of literature by Kennedy et al. which suggested independent improvements in both motor and psychiatric manifestations of PD with ECT [81].

Individuals with PD may develop delirium when treated with ECT. The use of right unilateral ECT, withholding the dose of levodopa on the morning of ECT, administering ECT treatments every 3–4 days and lowering electrical charge are some ways to curb this phenomenon [82].

Other Disorders

There is some evidence supporting the use of ECT for the treatment of depressive symptoms, psychotic symptoms, and chorea among individuals with Huntington's disease [83]. Seven individuals aged 20–56 years with Huntington's disease who were identified as having severe depression or psychosis were given RUL ECT with significant improvements in mood, psychotic symptoms, cognition, motor symptoms, and remission of suicidal ideation. The treatment was also well tolerated among these individuals.

Side Effect Profile and Contraindications for Using ECT

ECT is a very safe procedure with mortality rates of 1 death per 80,000 treatments [17]. Additionally, there are no "absolute" contraindications for using ECT. The relative contraindications for ECT are summarized in Table 26.4. The treatment teams need to judiciously evaluate the risk versus benefit of administering ECT in each case.

TABLE 26-4. Relative contraindications for ECT

1. Unstable or severe cardiovascular conditions such as recent myocardial infarction, unstable angina, poorly compensated congestive heart failure, and severe valvular cardiac disease
2. Aneurysms or vascular malformations that might be susceptible to rupture with increased blood pressure
3. Increased intracranial pressure due to some brain tumors or other space-occupying cerebral lesions
4. Recent cerebral infarction
5. Pulmonary conditions such as severe chronic obstructive pulmonary disease, asthma, or pneumonia
6. Patient status rated as ASA (American Society of Anesthesiologists) level 4 or 5

The older adult population often includes individuals with multiple cardiovascular, neurovascular, and respiratory comorbidities. Additionally, they often receive polypharmacy increasing their risk of developing medical complications and side effect from ECT. With thorough evaluation of preexisting medical comorbidities, the ECT techniques can be modified to minimize the side effects.

Cognitive side effects may limit the use of ECT among older adults [84]. They can be further divided into acute state of confusion (delirium), anterograde amnesia (most common), and retrograde amnesia (most serious). The delirium usually lasts less than 1 h. Those individuals having a seizure of >80 s tend to develop post-ECT delirium. Anterograde amnesia typically resolves between 1 and 3 weeks, whereas retrograde amnesia may take several months to recover. Retrograde amnesia is to a certain degree dependent on the extent of pre-ECT cognitive impairment and on post-ECT delirium [85]. The use of right, unilateral electrode placement with ultra-brief pulse ECT has been shown to substantially reduce the acute, short, and long-term cognitive side effects without compromising on therapeutic efficacy when compared to bilateral electrode placement with standard pulse treatment [13].

Between 0 and 77% of all individuals undergoing ECT may suffer from medical side effects [14]. Common side effects include tachycardia, fluctuations in hemodynamics, and transient arrhythmias. Elderly individuals with a recent myocardial infarction or intracerebral hemorrhage, volatile cardiac function, unstable vascular aneurysm, increased intracranial pressure, and space-occupying cerebral lesions are at an increased risk of developing side effects from ECT [14]. It is recommended that the benefit versus relative risk analysis of using ECT should be considered on a case by case basis in such scenarios.

Cardiovascular complications are the leading cause of morbidity and mortality with the use of ECT [32]. Cardiovascular risks can be modified using beta-blockers like labetalol, nitrates, or calcium channel blockers prior to therapy [86–88]. Propofol can be used in cases where the individual has cardiovascular risk factors as propofol is known to cause less cardiovascular adverse effects when compared with other anesthetic agents. Individuals with arrhythmias or thrombophlebitis are at an increased risk for embolic events. A mural thrombus should be ruled out using echocardiography prior to ECT, and use of anticoagulants should be considered. The risk of bone fractures in the older adults with osteoporosis can be reduced by the judicious use of the muscle relaxant, succinylcholine.

Conclusions

Psychiatric illness is a leading cause of disability among older adults. There are various options available for treating psychiatric disorders among older adults including psychotherapy, pharmacotherapy, and neuromodulation of which ECT is the most widely accepted procedure. ECT has been proven to be a safe and effective therapeutic intervention for the treatment of various psychiatric disorders among older adults. Ultra-brief right unilateral electrode placement is considered the standard initial ECT treatment for psychiatric disorders among this population. The most commonly used anesthetics for ECT are methohexital, etomidate, and propofol, and succinylcholine is the most commonly used muscle relaxant. Propofol is the most appropriate anesthetic for use among individuals with preexisting cardiac conditions. Cognitive and cardiovascular side effects are the most common side effects from the ECT with cardiovascular side effects being the leading cause of mortality. With adequate pre-ECT preparation, these side effects can be minimized.

References

1. Mental health and older adults. Word Health Organization. 2016. http://www.who.int/mediacentre/factsheets/fs381/en/. Accessed 19 Dec 2016.
2. Fink M. A clinician-researcher and ECDEU: 1959–1980. In: Ban T, et al., editors. The triumph of psychopharmacology and the story of CINP. Budapest: Animula; 2000. p. 82–92.
3. Aperia B, Bergman H, Engelbrektson K, et al. Effects of electroconvulsive therapy on neuropsychological function and circulating levels of ACTH, cortisol, prolactin, and TSH in patients with major depressive illness. Acta Psychiatr Scand. 1985;72:536–41.
4. Glue P, Costello J, Pert A, et al. Regional neurotransmitter responses after acute and chronic electroconvulsive shock. Psychopharmacology. 1990;100:60–5.
5. Lerer B. Electroconvulsive shock and neurotransmitter receptors: implications for mechanisms of action and adverse effects of electroconvulsive therapy. Biol Psychiatry. 1984;19:361–83.
6. McCall WV, Andrade C, Sienaert P. Searching for the mechanism(s) of ECT's therapeutic effect. J ECT. 2014;30(2):87–9.
7. Coffery CE, Kellner CH. Electroconvulsive therapy. In: Coffey CE, Cumming JL, editors. The American psychiatric press textbook of geriatric neuropsychiatry. 2nd ed. Washington, DC: American Psychiatric Press, Inc; 2000. p. 829–60.
8. Weiner RD, Krystal AD. Chapter 5: Electroconvulsive therapy. In: Blazer DG, Steffens DC, Busse EW, editors. The American Psychiatric Publishing textbook of geriatric psychiatry. 3rd ed. Washington, DC: American Psychiatric Press, Inc; 2004.
9. Kerner N, Prudic J. Current electroconvulsive therapy practice and research in the geriatric population. Neuropsychiatry (London). 2014;4(1):33–54.
10. Dybedal GS, Bjolseth TM, Benth JS, Tanum L. Cognitive effects of Bifrontal versus right unilateral electroconvulsive therapy in the treatment of major depression in elderly patients: a randomized controlled trial. J ECT. 2016;32:151–8.
11. Sackeim HA, Prudic J, Devanand DP, et al. A prospective, randomized, double-blind comparison of bilateral and right unilateral electroconvulsive therapy at different stimulus intensities. Arch Gen Psychiatry. 2000;57:425–34.
12. Kellner CH, Husain MM, Knapp RG, et al. Right unilateral ultrabrief pulse ECT in geriatric depression: phase 1 of the PRIDE study. Am J Psychiatry. 2016;173:1101–9.
13. Sackeim HA, Prudic J, Nobler MS, Fitzsimons L, Lisanby SH, Payne N, et al. Effects of pulse width and electrode placement on the efficacy and cognitive effects of electroconvulsive therapy. Brain Stimul. 2008;1(2):71–83.
14. Sackheim HA. The use of electroconvulsive therapy in late-life depression. In: Salzman C, editor. Geriatric psychopharmacology. 3rd ed. Baltimore, MD: Williams & Wilkins; 2004. p. 385–422.
15. McDonald W. Neuromodulation treatments for geriatric mood and cognitive disorders. Am J Geriatr Psychiatry. 2016;24:1130–41.

16. Tripathi P. Anesthetic management for ECT. In: Barnett SR, editor. Manual of geriatric anesthesia. New York, NY: Springer; 2013. p. 293–303.
17. Weiner R. American Psychiatric Association Committee on electroconvulsive therapy. Practice of electroconvulsive therapy recommendations for treatment, training and privileging: a task force report of the American Psychiatric Association. 2nd ed. Washington, DC: American Psychiatric Association; 2001.
18. Sackeim HA, Decina P, Portnoy S, Neeley P, Malitz S. Studies of dosage, seizure threshold, and seizure duration in ECT. Biol Psychiatry. 1987;22(3):249–68.
19. Hooten WM, Rasmussen KG Jr. Effects of general anesthetic agents in adults receiving electroconvulsive therapy: a systematic review. J ECT. 2008;24:208–23.
20. Akcaboy ZN, Akcaboy EY, Yigitbasł B, et al. Effects of remifentanil and alfentanil on seizure duration, stimulus amplitudes and recovery parameters during ECT. Acta Anaesthesiol Scand. 2005;49:1068–71.
21. Krystal AD, Weiner RD, Dean MD, et al. Comparison of seizure duration, ictal EEG, and cognitive effects of ketamine and methohexital anesthesia with ECT. J Neuropsychiatry Clin Neurosci. 2003;15(1):27–34.
22. Khalid N, Atkins M, Kirov G. The effects of etomidate on seizure duration and electrical stimulus dose in seizure-resistant patients during electroconvulsive therapy. J ECT. 2006;22(3):184–8.
23. Bailine SH, Petrides G, Doft M, Lui G. Indications for the use of propofol in electroconvulsive therapy. J ECT. 2003;19(3):129–32.
24. Bauer J, Hageman I, Dam H, et al. Comparison of propofol and thiopental as anesthetic agents for electroconvulsive therapy: a randomized, blinded comparison of seizure duration, stimulus charge, clinical effect, and cognitive side effects. J ECT. 2009;25(2):85–90.
25. Martin BA, Cooper RM, Parikh SV. Propofol anesthesia, seizure duration, and ECT: a case report and literature review. J ECT. 1998;14(2):99–108.
26. Saito S, Kadoi Y, Nara T, et al. The comparative effects of propofol versus thiopental on middle cerebral artery blood flow velocity during electroconvulsive therapy. Anesth Analg. 2000;91:1531–6.
27. Singh PM, Arora S, Borle A, Varma P, Trikha A, Goudra BG. Evaluation of etomidate for seizure duration in electroconvulsive therapy: a systematic review and meta-analysis. J ECT. 2015;31(4):213–25.
28. Gazdag G, Kocsis N, Tolna J, Iványi Z. Etomidate versus propofol for electroconvulsive therapy in patients with schizophrenia. J ECT. 2004;20(4):225–9.
29. Ingram A, Schweitzer I, Ng CH, Saling MM, Savage G. A comparison of propofol and thiopentone use in electroconvulsive therapy: cognitive and efficacy effects. J ECT. 2007;23(3):158–62.
30. Kellner CH, Husain MM, Knapp RG, et al. A novel strategy for continuation ECT in geriatric depression: phase 2 of the PRIDE study. Am J Psychiatry. 2016;173:1110–8.
31. Gill S, Bronskill S, Normand S, et al. Antipsychotic drug use and mortality in older adults with dementia. Ann Intern Med. 2007;146:775–86.
32. Wojcinska AA, Swiecicki L. The efficacy and safety of ECT in population before and after 60 years of age. Psychiatr Pol. 2016;50(5):1015–26.
33. McDonald IM, Perkins M, Marjerrison G, et al. Controlled comparison of amitriptyline and electroconvulsive therapy in the treatment of depression. BJP. 1966;122(12):1427–31.
34. Nemeroff CB, Evans DL, Gyulai L, et al. Double blind, placebo controlled comparison of imipramine and paroxetine in the treatment of bipolar depression. Am J Psychiatry. 2001;158(6):906–12.
35. Aziz R, Lorberg B, Tampi RR. Treatments of late life bipolar disorder. Am J Geriatr Pharmacother. 2006;4(4):347–64.
36. O'Connor MK, Knapp R, Husain MM, et al. The influence of age on the response of major depression to electroconvulsive therapy: a CORE report. Am J Psychiatry. 2001;9:382–90.
37. Tew JD, Mulsant BH, Haskett RF, et al. Acute efficacy of ECT in the treatment of major depression in the old-old. Am J Psychiatry. 1999;156:1865–70.
38. Spaans HP, Sienaert P, Bouckaert F, et al. Speed of remission in elderly patients with depression: electroconvulsive therapy v. medication. Br J Psychiatry. 2015;206:67–71.
39. Petrides G, Fink M, Husain MM, et al. ECT remission rates in psychotic versus nonpsychotic depressed patients: a report from CORE. J ECT. 2001;17(4):244–53.
40. Gijsman HJ, Geddes JR, Rendell JM, et al. Antidepressants for bipolar depression: a systematic review of randomized, controlled trials. Am J Psychiatry. 2004;161(9):1537–47.
41. Daly JJ, Prudic J, Devanand DP, et al. ECT in bipolar and unipolar depression: differences in speed of response. Bipolar Disord. 2001;3:95–104.
42. Agarkar S, Hurt S, Lisanby S, et al. ECT use in unipolar and bipolar depression. J ECT. 2012;28:e39–40.

43. Sienaert P, Vansteelandt K, Demyttenaere K, et al. Ultrabrief pulse ECT in bipolar and unipolar depressive disorder: differences in speed of response. Bipolar Disord. 2009;11(4):418–24.
44. Bailine S, Fink M, Knapp R, et al. Electroconvulsive therapy is equally effective in unipolar and bipolar depression. Acta Psychiatr Scand. 2010;121(6):431–6.
45. Grunhaus L, Schreiber S, Dolberg OT, et al. Response to ECT in major depression: are there differences between unipolar and bipolar depression? Bipolar Disord. 2002;4(1):91–3.
46. Dierckx B, Heijnen WT, van den Broek WW, Birkenhager TK. Efficacy of electroconvulsive therapy in bipolar versus unipolar major depression: a meta-analysis. Bipolar Disord. 2012;14:146–50.
47. Mukherjee S, Sackheim HA, Schnur DB. Electroconvulsive therapy of acute manic episodes: a review of 50 years' experience. Am J Psychiatry. 1994;151:169–76.
48. Small JG, Klapper MH, Kellams JJ, et al. Electroconvulsive treatment compared with lithium in the management of manic states. Arch Gen Psychiatry. 1988;45(8):727–32.
49. Salzman C. Clinical geriatric psychopharmacology. 4th ed. Philadelphia, PA: Lippincott Williams & Wilkins; 2005.
50. Damm J, Eser D, Schüle C, et al. Influence of age on effectiveness and tolerability of electroconvulsive therapy. J ECT. 2010;26(4):282–8.
51. Liu AY, Rajji TK, Blumberger DM, Daskalakis ZJ, Mulsant BH. Brain stimulation in the treatment of late-life severe mental illness other than unipolar nonpsychotic depression. Am J Geriatr Psychiatry. 2014;22(3):216–40.
52. Kramer BA. ECT in elderly patients with schizophrenia. Am J Geriatr Psychiatry. 1999;7(2):171–4.
53. Botteron K, Figiel GS, Zorumski CF. Electroconvulsive therapy in patients with late-onset psychoses and structural brain changes. J Geriatr Psychiatry Neurol. 1991;4:44–7.
54. Figiel GS, Botteron K, Zorumski CF, et al. The treatment of late age onset psychoses with electroconvulsive therapy. Int J Geriatr Psychiatry. 1992;7:183–9.
55. Howard R, Rabins P, Seeman M, et al. Late-onset schizophrenia and very-late-onset schizophrenia like psychosis: an international consensus. The international late-onset schizophrenia group. Am J Psychiatry. 2000;157:172–8.
56. American Psychiatric Association. Diagnostic and statistical manual of mental disorders: DSM-5. Washington, DC: American Psychiatric Association; 2013.
57. Aloysi AS, Popeo DM, Kellner CH. Cases of catatonia on an academic electroconvulsive therapy service: lessons to learn. J ECT. 2011;27(3):259–61.
58. Hatta K, Miyakawa K, Ota T, Usui C, Nakamura H, Arai H. Maximal response to electroconvulsive therapy for the treatment of catatonic symptoms. J ECT. 2007;23(4):233–5.
59. Bush G, Fink M, Petrides G, et al. Catatonia II. Treatment with lorazepam and electroconvulsive therapy. Acta Psychiatr Scand. 1996;93:137–43.
60. Hawkins J-M, Archer K-J, Strowski S-M, et al. Somatic treatment of catatonia. Int J Psychiatry Med. 1995;25:345–69.
61. Suzuki K, Awata S, Matsuoka H. Short-term effect of ECT in middle-aged and elderly patients with intractable catatonic schizophrenia. J ECT. 2003;19:73–80.
62. Suzuki K, Awata S, Matsuoka H. One-year outcome after response to ECT in middle-aged and elderly patients with intractable catatonic schizophrenia. J ECT. 2004;20:99–106.
63. Suzuki K, Awata S, Takano T, et al. Adjusting the frequency of continuation and maintenance electroconvulsive therapy to prevent relapse of catatonic schizophrenia in middle-aged and elderly patients who are relapse-prone. Psychiatry Clin Neurosci. 2006;60(4):486–92.
64. Suzuki K, Awata S, Takano T, et al. Continuation electroconvulsive therapy for relapse prevention in middle-aged and elderly patients with intractable catatonic schizophrenia. Psychiatry Clin Neurosci. 2005;59:481–9.
65. Rohland BM, Carroll BT, Jacoby RG. ECT in the treatment of the catatonic syndrome. J Affect Disord. 1993;29:255–61.
66. Lindsey PL. Psychotropic medication use among older adults: what all nurses need to know. J Gerontol Nurs. 2009;35:28–38.
67. Oruch R, Pryme IF, Engelsen BA, Lund A. Neuroleptic malignant syndrome: an easily overlooked neurologic emergency. Neuropsychiatr Dis Treat. 2017;13:161–75.
68. Carroll BT. Catatonia on the consultation-liaison service. Psychosomatics. 1992;33:310–5.
69. Trollor JN, Sachdev PS. Electroconvulsive treatment of neuroleptic malignant syndrome: a review and report of cases. Aust N Z J Psychiatry. 1999;33(5):650–9.
70. Scheftner WA, Shulman RB. Treatment choice in neuroleptic malignant syndrome. Convuls Ther. 1992;8:267–79.

71. International Psychogeriatric Association. Behavioral and psychological symptoms of dementia (BPSD): a clinical and research update. Int Psychogeriatr. 2000;12(Suppl 1):1–424.
72. Tariot PN. Treatment of agitation in dementia. J Clin Psychiatry. 1999;60(Suppl 8):11–20.
73. Seitz DP, Adunuri N, Gill SS, Gruneir A, Herrmann N, Rochon P. Antidepressants for agitation and psychosis in dementia. Cochrane Database Syst Rev. 2011;16(2):CD008191.
74. Sink KM, Holden KF, Yaffe K. Pharmacological treatment of neuropsychiatric symptoms of dementia: a review of the evidence. JAMA. 2005;293(5):596–608.
75. Lenzer J. FDA warns about using antipsychotic drugs for dementia. BMJ. 2005;330(7497):922.
76. Grant JE, Mohan SN. Treatment of agitation and aggression in four demented patients using ECT. J ECT. 2001;17(3):205–9.
77. Ujkaj M, Davidoff DA, Seiner SJ, Ellison JM, Harper DG, Forester BP. Safety and efficacy of electroconvulsive therapy for the treatment of agitation and aggression in patients with dementia. Am J Geriatr Psychiatry. 2012;20(1):61–72.
78. Acharya D, Harper DG, Achtyes ED, et al. Safety and utility of acute electroconvulsive therapy for agitation and aggression in dementia. Int J Geriatr Psychiatry. 2015;30(3):265–73.
79. Reijnders JS, Ehrt U, Weber WE, Aarsland D, Leentjens AF. A systematic review of prevalence studies of depression in Parkinson's disease. Mov Disord. 2008;23(2):183–9.
80. Fregni F, Simon DK, Wu A, Pascual-Leone A. Non-invasive brain stimulation for Parkinson's disease: a systematic review and meta-analysis of the literature. J Neurol Neurosurg Psychiatry. 2005;76(12):1614–23.
81. Kennedy R, Mittal D, O'Jile J. Electroconvulsive therapy in movement disorders: an update. J Neuropsychiatry Clin Neurosci. 2003;15:407–21.
82. McDonald WM, Meeks WT, McCall WV, Zorumski CF. Electroconvulsive therapy. In: Schatzberg AF, Nemeroff CB, editors. The American Psychiatric Publishing textbook of psychopharmacology. 4th ed. Arlington, VA: American Psychiatric Publishing; 2009.
83. Cusin C, Franco FB, Fernandez-Robles C, DuBois CM, Welch CA. Rapid improvement of depression and psychotic symptoms in Huntington's disease: a retrospective chart review of seven patients treated with electroconvulsive therapy. Gen Hosp Psychiatry. 2013;35(6):678.e3–5.
84. Reti IM, Krishnan A, Podlisky A, et al. Predictors of electroconvulsive therapy postictal delirium. Psychosomatics. 2014;55(3):272–9.
85. Sobin C, Sackeim HA, Prudic J, et al. Predictors of retrograde amnesia following ECT. Am J Psychiatry. 1995;152:995–1001.
86. Stoudemire A, Knos G, Gladson M, et al. Labetalol in the control of cardiovascular responses to electroconvulsive therapy in high-risk depressed medical patients. J Clin Psychiatry. 1990;51:508–12.
87. Ciraulo D, Lind L, Salzman C, et al. Sodium nitroprusside treatment of ECT-induced blood pressure elevations. Am J Psychiatry. 1978;135:1105–6.
88. Wajima Z, Yoshikawa T, Ogura A, et al. Intravenous verapamil blunts hyperdynamic responses during electroconvulsive therapy without altering seizure activity. Anesth Analg. 2002;95:400–2.

27 Psychotherapy

Brandon C. Yarns

Introduction

Psychotherapy is a treatment modality conducted by a trained therapist based on psychological principles whereby the interaction with the patient is the vehicle through which the therapeutic components are delivered [1]. Psychotherapy is also offered in the form of an available manual or treatment protocol [1].

In the early twentieth century, psychotherapy was assumed to be ineffective in older adults, based on assumptions that older adults were in a period of decline and incapable of new learning [2, 3]. However, the work of Erik Erikson in the latter half of the twentieth century changed many of these assumptions when he included phases of older adulthood in his model of psychosocial development, noting that even those nearing the end of life still have life tasks, potential virtues, and opportunities for growth, as well as possibilities for maladaptation and "malignancy," and are thus appropriate for psychotherapy [4].

More recently, neuroscience research has investigated how neuroplasticity, including brain growth and development, increases in synapses and dendritic spines and even growth of new neurons can continue into old age if there is sufficient physical and psychosocial stimulation [5–7]. This provides evidence that new learning is possible in older adults, and, in fact "psychosocial stimulation" such as psychotherapy may enhance it. Additionally, socio-emotional selectivity theory posits that older adults are even more likely to seek meaningful and positive social experiences to gain emotional nourishment, such as one would receive in psychotherapy, than younger adults [8].

This research and theory has been supported by recent findings that older adults may prefer psychotherapy to pharmacologic treatments in depression and anxiety care. The IMPACT investigators asked older primary care study participants about treatment preferences in depression care and depressed older adults preferred counseling to pharmacologic treatments 57–43% [9]. In a study of depressed patients' treatment preferences across multiple age groups, depressed patients chose individual psychotherapy over antidepressant medication (70–30%) and anticipated that psychotherapy would be more helpful for their depression than medications [10]. Finally, a survey of older adults recruited from the community endorsed a preference for psychotherapy as opposed to pharmacologic interventions in the event that they had anxiety sufficient to interfere with daily activities and were seeking mental health treatment [11].

In addition to research on patient preference, empirical studies have found various forms of psychotherapy to be effective for older adults when compared to pharmacotherapy. A 2006 meta-analytic comparison of pharmacotherapy and psychotherapy for depressed older adults indicated that both were effective with moderate to large effect sizes [12]. Although effect sizes were larger in psychotherapy studies than in pharmacotherapy studies, the authors cautioned against reading too much into this, as pharmacologic trials could more

R. R. Tampi et al. (eds.), *Psychiatric Disorders Late in Life*, https://doi.org/10.1007/978-3-319-73078-3_27

effectively produce an active placebo than psychotherapy trials, which may have decreased their effect sizes in the results. The authors concluded that the choice of pharmacotherapy or psychotherapy should be based on criteria apart from efficacy, such as contraindications, treatment access, or patient preference. It should be noted that psychotherapy may also be used in combination with antidepressant medication, and providers may want to consider both medication and psychotherapy in treating older adults with mental health needs.

Need, Access, and Utilization

Despite theoretical and empirical evidence that psychotherapy is a sensible treatment option for older adults in need of mental health services, psychotherapy still appears to be greatly underutilized. The US Census Bureau projects that the number of individuals 65 years and older in the United States will nearly double, to exceed 98 million by 2050 [13] and 20% of older adults experience some type of mental health concern, most commonly anxiety, severe cognitive impairment, and depression [14]. In a 2010 survey by Connor and colleagues, although rates of depression symptoms reached as high as 88%, more than half of the respondents had never seen a health professional for depression treatment and only 16% were currently in treatment for depression. Additionally, African American respondents had significantly less positive attitudes toward seeking mental health care when compared to their older White counterparts [15]. Finally, a 2005 study using Medicare claims data from the 1990s indicated that among depressed older adults, psychotherapy was used in only 25% of cases and only 33% of those who received treatment remained in "consistent treatment," defined a priori by the authors [16]. In this study, patients' socioeconomic and demographic characteristics did not affect the odds of receiving consistent psychotherapy, but the availability of local providers was positively correlated with consistent psychotherapy use [16]. Thus, although older depressed or anxious patients might prefer psychotherapy, there is a significant shortage of trained psychotherapists that limits patients' access to the treatment.

Nonetheless, new approaches in collaborative care have been shown to improve access to mental health services including IMPACT, which used problem-solving therapy, and PROSPECT, which used interpersonal psychotherapy, making psychotherapy more feasible for older adults in primary care [17, 18]. In fact, IMPACT improved access to counseling services, with 74% access in a collaborative care model versus only 33% access in care as usual [9].

A 2016 study showed that older adults are just as likely to receive treatment for depression as the younger adults in ambulatory care clinics but was far less likely to receive psychotherapy than antidepressant medication. Using data from the 2012 National Ambulatory Medical Care Survey, it was found that 65% of depressed patients received antidepressant medication and 19% psychotherapy [19]. Although it is unknown if this discrepancy was, in part, due to patient preference, it can be hypothesized from these findings that even more work is needed to improve access to psychotherapy.

Indications for Psychotherapy

Psychotherapeutic interventions have most commonly been studied in older adults for the treatment of depression, with a recent systematic review and meta-analysis citing 27 randomized trials using control groups that showed that psychotherapy was effective for depression in older adults [20]. Psychotherapy has also been studied for late-life anxiety disorders, including for generalized anxiety disorder, panic disorder, social phobia, and subjective anxiety [21–23]. The most recent review of interventions for generalized anxiety disorder in older adults pointed to 13 trials with parallel group designs [21].

Another indication for psychotherapy is for treating subsyndromal or subthreshold depressive symptoms, with scholars arguing that many older patients with clinically significant depressive symptoms do not reach the minimum diagnostic criteria for depression or dysthymic disorder [24]. Psychotherapy, in contradistinction to pharmacotherapy, has shown to have significant effects on subthreshold depression and may prevent the onset of major depression [25, 26], and individual psychotherapy has shown benefits in older adults [27, 28]. A systematic review and meta-analysis published in 2013 described four trials using group cognitive-behavior therapy for subthreshold depression in older adults that showed short-term but not long-term benefit [29]. A 2012 systematic review by Lee and colleagues describes psychotherapy interventions to prevent depression in older adults, including studies focused on cognitive-behavior therapy or problem-solving therapy interventions [30].

Two recent well-designed randomized clinical trials have shown that a chronic grief therapy (CGT) based on principles from cognitive-behavior therapy and interpersonal therapy strongly outperformed placebo, interpersonal therapy, and citalopram, making complicated grief an indication for a specific therapy protocol [31, 32].

A recent area of interest is psychotherapy to promote well-being in older adults. Studies have investigated art therapy, reminiscence, and mindfulness training for promoting well-being in older adults [33–35].

Insomnia is another area in which psychotherapy may be appropriate for older adults. According to a recent review, cognitive-behavior therapy and sleep hygiene are regarded as first-line treatments for insomnia in older adults, given the safety concerns with benzodiazepines and increased risk of dementia, injury, and falls with non-benzodiazepine receptor antagonists [36].

Traditional psychotherapies, such as cognitive-behavior therapy, have shown little promise so far in treating substance use disorders in the outpatient setting, mostly due to high dropout rates [37]. Additionally, 12-step models have been understudied in older populations [38]. One specific intervention, the Florida Brief Intervention and Treatment for Elders (BRITE) project, consisting of one to five sessions of motivational interviewing, education on substance misuse, and reasons to quit drinking and an offer of a 16-session cognitive-behavior therapy treatment for individuals at risk for licit and illicit substance misuse, showed a significant reduction in alcohol and prescription misuse, depressive symptoms, and suicide risk [39].

Most of the research on personality disorders in older adults have emphasized that personality disorders may be as prevalent as in younger adults, although they differ by specific diagnosis, and that personality disorders, when comorbid with other conditions, such as depression, contribute to poorer response to both pharmacotherapy and psychotherapy [40, 41]. Dialectical behavior therapy, based on Linehan's original 1993 manual, has been the only specific type of psychotherapy that has been studied specifically in treatment of personality disorders in older adults to date [42, 43].

Traditional forms of psychotherapy (described in detail below) are also not indicated to treat dementia, although several psychotherapy studies for depressed or anxious older adults have included individuals with cognitive impairment or executive dysfunction, and a number of behavioral interventions—most focusing on both patient and caregiver—as well as music and art therapy, have been studied to target mood and behavior symptoms of dementia [44–48].

Which Psychotherapy to Choose

Selection of a specific modality of psychotherapy for the depressed or anxious older adult is a complicated task. A 2016 systematic review and meta-analysis of 27 randomized controlled trials of psychotherapy for treatment of depression indicated that all bona fide psychotherapies, including cognitive-behavior and behavior therapies, problem-solving therapy, brief psychodynamic therapy, interpersonal therapy, reminiscence therapy and life review therapy, were effective for depression, although the effect sizes differed by the control group used in each study [20]. A 2008 Cochrane review on psychotherapy for older adults focused on comparisons of cognitive-behavior therapies and brief psychodynamic therapies and found no differences between the two treatments [49]. A 2007 meta-analysis that included 57 studies also concluded that several forms of psychotherapy for depressed, older adults were effective with variably medium to large effect sizes, although heterogeneity among the included studies' designs was high [50].

Although there are few comparative effectiveness trials of psychotherapies for older adults with depression and no systematic reviews or meta-analyses in this population, meta-analyses of comparative effectiveness trials in depressed adults show that there are no differences in the effectiveness of psychotherapies for depression, including cognitive-behavior therapies, behavioral activation, problem-solving therapy, brief psychodynamic therapy, interpersonal therapy, social skills training, and nondirective supportive treatment [25, 51].

So how does one decide? Evidence suggests that individual patient preference is an important consideration in choosing a treatment approach among depressed older individuals. In a study of depressed patients across multiple age groups, those patients assigned to a treatment congruent with their treatment preference had superior adherence to treatment and superior depression outcomes [10]. Similarly, in an interview study of 22 depressed older adults who had participated in a larger psychotherapy trial, patient preference was cited by the authors as an important consideration for treatment selection [52]. Finally, a 2011 systematic review by Kiosses and colleagues investigated predictors of treatment outcome and moderators of treatment effects; although evidence on predictors or moderators was preliminary, the authors argued for more attention to personalized psychotherapy interventions, congruent with a recent National Institute of Mental Health Report on future directions for interventions research [53].

Nonetheless, Dakin and Areán's work showed that most older patients have few expectations coming into psychotherapy [52]. Therefore, other possible considerations for treatment selection and special issues in the psychotherapy of older adults exist. As previously mentioned, the psychoanalyst Erik Erikson described psychosocial stages in the lives of older adults which are still relevant to treatment today [4]. Especially as older adults are working and living longer, some older adult therapy patients may be struggling with Erikson's seventh stage, called generativity versus stagnation, in which the individual struggles to pass on knowledge and skills to future generations to leave behind a legacy; if they do not succeed, they will feel that nothing will remain of theirs after they pass. Movement into Erikson's final stage of development, ego integrity versus despair, may also prompt the older person to seek psychotherapy, as she begins a process of looking back and evaluating her life to see if it has been a success by her own measure (integrity) or a failure (despair) [4]. Identification of these specific phase-of-life issues may affect treatment choice.

In addition to psychological factors, generational or cohort-based differences may be relevant to treatment selection for the older patient. Cohort differences, based on membership in a group defined by birth years, involve differences in beliefs, attitudes, and personality dimensions that remain stable as the group ages [54]. Little yet has been written on how psychotherapy with older adults may change as Baby Boomers continue to age.

Although it must be stressed that many older adults are healthy, active, and cognitively normal, common sense must be used to evaluate potential physical health barriers to engaging in psychotherapy, including physical limitations, cognitive impairment, and sensory impairment such as decreased visual acuity or hearing loss. If a patient's mobility hinders attendance at psychotherapy appointments, tele-psychotherapy is also gaining an evidence base and may be an appropriate treatment option to consider [55].

Finally, there is also some evidence to suggest that older adults tend to be more satisfied with mental health services delivered in their primary care physician's offices [9, 56–58].

Evidence for and Descriptions of Bona Fide Psychotherapies for Older Adults

What follows is a description of bona fide therapy modalities that have been studied in older adults and were part of recent meta-analyses [20, 22, 25, 50].

Cognitive-Behavior Therapies

A 2007 review by Pinquart and colleagues showed that more studies of depression in older adults using a cognitive-behavior therapy treatment arm have been conducted than with any other type of psychotherapy [50]. Additionally, a systematic review and meta-analysis revealed seven trials studying cognitive-behavior therapy for late-life anxiety disorders [22].

Cognitive-behavior therapy is a broad category of psychotherapies which includes cognitive therapy, behavior therapy, combined cognitive-behavior therapy, and "third-wave" therapies such as acceptance and commitment therapy (ACT), cognitive processing therapy (CPT), and dialectical behavior therapy (DBT) that tend to combine cognitive and behavioral techniques with mindfulness practices.

Cognitive-behavior therapy has its origins in the studies on classical and operant conditioning of the early twentieth century. Cognitive therapy is premised on the idea that maladaptive cognitions perpetuate and may even cause emotional and behavioral problems and that these cognitions may be modified through conditioning [59, 60]. Cognitive therapy procedures involve challenging maladaptive cognitions through "Socratic questioning" in session either verbally or by completion of worksheets and nearly always requires ongoing practice through the assignment of homework. When "behavioral experiments" or other behavioral techniques supplement cognitive therapy, the result is usually referred to as cognitive-behavior therapy. Behavioral therapy, such as systematic desensitization or behavioral activation, involves modifying behavior through classical or operant conditioning rather than changing cognitions in order to achieve lowering of emotional distress or other symptoms. Cognitive-behavior therapy techniques may also be used in a group format, and self-study cognitive bibliotherapy is also available and has a growing evidence base [61, 62].

Brief Dynamic Psychotherapy

Brief psychodynamic psychotherapy has been evaluated with positive results in several older studies involving treatment of depression in older adults [63–65]. It was also shown to be superior to cognitive-behavior therapy in a recent meta-analysis of nine comparative effectiveness trials for depression in Parkinson's disease patients with a mean age of 62 years [66].

A number of distinct yet overlapping approaches for brief dynamic psychotherapy have been developed, all of which are rooted in some aspects of psychoanalytic theory and consider the underlying personality structure and interpersonal relationships as having critical roles in the development and maintenance of a variety of symptoms, including depression [67]. In a comparison of the therapy process in 30 brief dynamic and 32 cognitive-behavior therapies, dynamic therapy was easily distinguished based on the relative emphasis of the evocation of affect and bringing troublesome feelings into awareness, integrating current difficulties with previous life experience and using the therapist-patient relationship as a change agent [68].

Brief dynamic therapy manuals are directive but often lack specific schedules, agendas, or detailed scripts for sessions to allow for flexibility, and brief dynamic therapy training was found equally feasible to cognitive-behavior therapy training in a large comparative effectiveness study for treatment of depression in adults that involved training of community therapists in these two modalities [69]. Training is usually conducted in group settings and is often augmented with discussion of video recordings of trainees' therapy sessions [70]. Several adherence scales have been developed along with training manuals to encourage further research in modern iterations of dynamic therapy [71, 72].

Problem-Solving Therapy

Problem-solving therapy or the similar problem adaptation therapy has been studied in depressed cognitively normal and cognitively impaired elders in mental health clinics and primary care and at home and also has several published studies that compare the treatment to supportive therapy [46, 73–76]. Some have written that because of the strength of study designs and selection of comparison groups in problem-solving therapy trials, problem-solving therapy currently has the best evidence for treating late-life depression [20, 53]. Problem-solving therapy was also used as the psychotherapy intervention in IMPACT [18].

Problem-solving therapy is based upon a specific theory of depression in which coping with stress leads to breakdown in problem-solving skills and resultant depression [77]. Treatment is therefore directed toward helping the patient identify concrete, tangible problems in her current life and working with the therapist to develop practical, immediately applicable behavioral solutions in order to reduce stress and resolve depression [75]. For example, if a problem is identified in which the patient forgets to take her bedtime medications, a stress-reducing solution might be to place a sticky note on the mirror reminding her to do so.

Interpersonal Therapy

Interpersonal therapy has been studied in depressed older adults as monotherapy, combination therapy with antidepressant medication and for maintenance following depression remission [28, 78–80]. Interpersonal therapy was also selected as the psychotherapy intervention in PROSPECT, which utilized a collaborative care model to decrease suicidal ideation and depressive symptoms in depressed older primary care patients [17].

Developed in the 1980s and adapted for older adults with depression in the 1990s, interpersonal therapy is a manualized, prescriptive modality lasting 12–16 sessions that is based upon the social psychology of Harry Stack Sullivan and Adolf Meyer and the premise that interpersonal relationships are "the stage on which depression is set" [81]. Both an instructional manual and treatment video on interpersonal therapy in older adults are available [82]. In contradistinction to dynamic therapy, interpersonal therapy focuses exclusively on relationships in the patient's current life rather than relationships of the past or the transference. In the beginning of treatment, the patient is assigned the "sick role," an interpersonal inventory is completed, and the patient's central problem is categorized into one of four broad categories: unresolved grief, role transition, role disputes, or interpersonal deficits [83]. Treatment is divided into three phases, the first establishing the focus of treatment, the second exploring new behaviors in current interpersonal relationships, and the third consolidating gains. Discussion is often supplemented with completion of depression scales and other written work [81].

Reminiscence and Life Review Therapies

Reminiscence therapy has been studied in depressed older adults and in older adults with dementia in either structured or unstructured formats [74, 84–87]. Frequently conducted in a group setting, reminiscence therapy encourages patients to look back over life in order to achieve Erikson's ego integrity [88]. When structured, the therapy may encourage patients to bring in photographs or objects or focus on certain themes such as smells that were important in one's life [87]. Theoretically related to reminiscence, life review therapy also has been studied for depressed older adults [89].

Conclusion

Psychotherapy is a useful and empirically justified, although underutilized, treatment option for older adults with depression and subthreshold depressive symptoms, chronic grief, anxiety, insomnia, and mood and behavioral symptoms of dementia. Specific modalities are also relevant for substance use disorders and personality disorders in older adults. Psychotherapy can be applied in a number of settings, including the patient's home, primary care clinic, or mental health clinic. Older depressed and anxious patients, in particular, tend to prefer psychotherapy over pharmacotherapy. Selection of a specific psychotherapy modality for an individual patient will mostly depend on what is available in a given system, patient preference, and other practical considerations rather than the evidence base, given the dearth of available research with high-quality study designs and sample sizes across psychotherapies.

Acknowledgments Dr. Yarns was supported by the VA Office of Academic Affiliations through the VA National Clinician Scholars Program.

References

1. Baskin TW, Tierney SC, Minami T, Wampold BE. Establishing specificity in psychotherapy: a meta-analysis of structural equivalence of placebo

controls. J Consult Clin Psychol. 2003;71(6):973–9. https://doi.org/10.1037/0022-006x.71.6.973.
2. Freud, S. (1905). On psychotherapy. Standard edition, London, Hogarth Press 7(267), 64–145.
3. Hepple J. Psychotherapies with older people: an overview. Adv Psychiatr Treat. 2004;10(5):371–7.
4. Erikson EH. Identity and the life cycle: selected papers. In: Psychological issues. New York: International Universities Press; 1959.
5. Gage FH. Neurogenesis in the adult brain. J Neurosci. 2002;22(3):612–3.
6. Jeste DV, Palmer BW, Rettew DC, Boardman S. Positive psychiatry: its time has come. J Clin Psychiatry. 2015;76(6):675–83. https://doi.org/10.4088/JCP.14nr09599.
7. Pascual-Leone A, Amedi A, Fregni F, Merabet LB. The plastic human brain cortex. Annu Rev Neurosci. 2005;28:377–401. https://doi.org/10.1146/annurev.neuro.27.070203.144216.
8. Carstensen LL, Isaacowitz DM, Charles ST. Taking time seriously. A theory of socioemotional selectivity. Am Psychol. 1999;54(3):165–81.
9. Gum AM, Areán PA, Hunkeler E, Tang L, Katon W, Hitchcock P, et al. Depression treatment preferences in older primary care patients. The Gerontologist. 2006;46(1):14–22.
10. Raue PJ, Schulberg HC, Heo M, Klimstra S, Bruce ML. Patients' depression treatment preferences and initiation, adherence, and outcome: a randomized primary care study. Psychiatr Serv. 2009;60(3):337–43. https://doi.org/10.1176/appi.ps.60.3.337.
11. Mohlman J. A community based survey of older adults' preferences for treatment of anxiety. Psychol Aging. 2012;27(4):1182–90. https://doi.org/10.1037/a0023126.
12. Pinquart M, Duberstein PR, Lyness JM. Treatments for Later-Life Depressive Conditions: A Meta-Analytic Comparison of Pharmacotherapy and Psychotherapy. Am J Psychiatry. 2006;163(9):1493–501. https://doi.org/10.1176/ajp.2006.163.9.1493.
13. U.S. Census Bureau. National population projections: summary tables. US Census Web site. 2014. http://www.census.gov/population/projections/data/national/2014/summarytables.html. Accessed 25 Oct 2016.
14. American Association of Geriatric Psychiatry. Geriatrics and mental health—the facts. 2008. http://www.aagponline.org/prof/facts_mh.asp. Accessed 23 June 2008.
15. Conner KO, Copeland VC, Grote NK, Koeske G, Rosen D, Reynolds CF, Brown C. Mental health treatment seeking among older adults with depression: the Impact of stigma and race. Am J Geriatr Psychiatry. 2010;18(6):531–43. https://doi.org/10.1097/JGP.0b013e3181cc0366.
16. Wei W, Sambamoorthi U, Olfson M, Walkup JT, Crystal S. Use of psychotherapy for depression in older adults. Am J Psychiatry. 2005;162(4):711–7. https://doi.org/10.1176/appi.ajp.162.4.711.
17. Bruce ML, Ten Have TR, Reynolds CF 3rd, Katz II, Schulberg HC, Mulsant BH, et al. Reducing suicidal ideation and depressive symptoms in depressed older primary care patients: a randomized controlled trial. JAMA. 2004;291(9):1081–91. https://doi.org/10.1001/jama.291.9.1081.
18. Unützer J, Katon W, Callahan CM, et al. Collaborative care management of late-life depression in the primary care setting: a randomized controlled trial. JAMA. 2002;288(22):2836–45. https://doi.org/10.1001/jama.288.22.2836.
19. Choi NG, DiNitto DM, Marti CN, Kunik ME. When depression is diagnosed, older adults are as likely as younger adults to be prescribed pharmacotherapy and psychotherapy. Gen Hosp Psychiatry. 2016;43:6–11. https://doi.org/10.1016/j.genhosppsych.2016.08.002.
20. Huang AX, Delucchi K, Dunn LB, Nelson JC. A systematic review and meta-analysis of psychotherapy for late-life depression. Am J Geriatr Psychiatry. 2016;23(3):261–73. https://doi.org/10.1016/j.jagp.2014.04.003.
21. Goncalves DC, Byrne GJ. Interventions for generalized anxiety disorder in older adults: systematic review and meta-analysis. J Anxiety Disord. 2012;26(1):1–11. https://doi.org/10.1016/j.janxdis.2011.08.010.
22. Hendriks GJ, Oude Voshaar RC, Keijsers GP, Hoogduin CA, van Balkom AJ. Cognitive-behavioural therapy for late-life anxiety disorders: a systematic review and meta-analysis. Acta Psychiatr Scand. 2008;117(6):403–11. https://doi.org/10.1111/j.1600-0447.2008.01190.x.
23. Wetherell JL, Sorrell JT, Thorp SR, Patterson TL. Psychological interventions for late-life anxiety: a review and early lessons from the CALM study. J Geriatr Psychiatry Neurol. 2005;18(2):72–82. https://doi.org/10.1177/0891988705276058.
24. Lavretsky H, Kumar A. Clinically significant non-major depression: old concepts, new insights. Am J Geriatr Psychiatry. 2002;10(3):239–55.
25. Cuijpers P, Smit F, van Straten A. Psychological treatments of subthreshold depression: a meta-analytic review. Acta Psychiatr Scand. 2007;115(6):434–41. https://doi.org/10.1111/j.1600-0447.2007.00998.x.
26. Fournier JC, DeRubeis RJ, Hollon SD, Dimidjian S, Amsterdam JD, Shelton RC, Fawcett J. Antidepressant

drug effects and depression severity: a patient-level meta-analysis. JAMA. 2010;303(1):47–53. https://doi.org/10.1001/jama.2009.1943.
27. Haringsma R, Engels GI, Cuijpers P, Spinhoven P. Effectiveness of the coping with depression (CWD) course for older adults provided by the community-based mental health care system in the Netherlands: a randomized controlled field trial. Int Psychogeriatr. 2006;18(2):307–25. https://doi.org/10.1017/s104161020500253x.
28. Mossey JM, Knott KA, Higgins M, Talerico K. Effectiveness of a psychosocial intervention, interpersonal counseling, for subdysthymic depression in medically ill elderly. J Gerontol A Biol Sci Med Sci. 1996;51((4):M172–8.
29. Krishna M, Honagodu A, Rajendra R, Sundarachar R, Lane S, Lepping P. A systematic review and meta-analysis of group psychotherapy for sub-clinical depression in older adults. Int J Geriatr Psychiatry. 2013;28(9):881–8. https://doi.org/10.1002/gps.3905.
30. Lee SY, Franchetti MK, Imanbayev A, Gallo JJ, Spira AP, Lee HB. Non-pharmacological prevention of major depression among community-dwelling older adults: a systematic review of the efficacy of psychotherapy interventions. Arch Gerontol Geriatr. 2012;55(3):522–9. https://doi.org/10.1016/j.archger.2012.03.003.
31. Shear MK, Reynolds CF 3rd, Simon NM, Zisook S, Wang Y, Mauro C, et al. Optimizing treatment of complicated grief: a randomized clinical trial. JAMA Psychiat. 2016;73(7):685–94. https://doi.org/10.1001/jamapsychiatry.2016.0892.
32. Shear MK, Wang Y, Skritskaya N, Duan N, Mauro C, Ghesquiere A. Treatment of complicated grief in elderly persons: a randomized clinical trial. JAMA Psychiat. 2014;71(11):1287–95. https://doi.org/10.1001/jamapsychiatry.2014.1242.
33. Bennington R, Backos A, Harrison J, Etherington Reader A, Carolan R. Art therapy in art museums: promoting social connectedness and psychological well-being of older adults. Arts Psychother. 2016;49:34–43. https://doi.org/10.1016/j.aip.2016.05.013.
34. Choy JCP, Lou VWQ. Effectiveness of the modified instrumental reminiscence intervention on psychological well-being among community-dwelling Chinese older adults: a randomized controlled trial. Am J Geriatr Psychiatry. 2016;24(1):60–9. https://doi.org/10.1016/j.jagp.2015.05.008.
35. Mallya S, Fiocco AJ. Effects of mindfulness training on cognition and well-being in healthy older adults. Mindfulness. 2016;7(2):453–65. https://doi.org/10.1007/s12671-015-0468-6.
36. Schroeck JL, Ford J, Conway EL, Kurtzhalts KE, Gee ME, Vollmer KA, Mergenhagen KA. Review of safety and efficacy of sleep medicines in older adults. Clin Ther. 2016;38(11):2340–72. https://doi.org/10.1016/j.clinthera.2016.09.010.
37. Schonfeld, L., Dupree, L. W., Dickson-Euhrmann, E., Royer, C. M., McDermott, C. H., Rosansky, J. S.,. .et al. (2000). Cognitive-behavioral treatment of older veterans with substance abuse problems. J Geriatr Psychiatry Neurol, 13(3), 124–129.
38. Wu LT, Blazer DG. Illicit and nonmedical drug use among older adults: a review. J Aging Health. 2011;23(3):481–504. https://doi.org/10.1177/0898264310386224.
39. Schonfeld L, Hazlett RW, Hedgecock DK, Duchene DM, Burns LV, Gum AM. Screening, brief intervention, and referral to treatment for older adults with substance misuse. Am J Public Health. 2015;105(1):205–11. https://doi.org/10.2105/ajph.2013.301859.
40. Kool S, Dekker J, Duijsens IJ, de Jonghe F, Puite B. Efficacy of combined therapy and pharmacotherapy for depressed patients with or without personality disorders. Harv Rev Psychiatry. 2003;11(3):133–41.
41. Zweig RA. Personality disorder in older adults: assessment challenges and strategies. Prof Psychol Res Pract. 2008;39(3):298–305. https://doi.org/10.1037/0735-7028.39.3.298.
42. Linehan M. Cognitive-behavioral treatment of borderline personality disorder. New York: Guilford Press; 1993.
43. Lynch TR, Cheavens JS, Cukrowicz KC, Thorp SR, Bronner L, Beyer J. Treatment of older adults with co-morbid personality disorder and depression: a dialectical behavior therapy approach. Int J Geriatr Psychiatry. 2007;22(2):131–43. https://doi.org/10.1002/gps.1703.
44. Bruer RA, Spitznagel E, Cloninger CR. The temporal limits of cognitive change from music therapy in elderly persons with dementia or dementia-like cognitive impairment: a randomized controlled trial. J Music Ther. 2007;44(4):308–28.
45. Cornejo R, Brewer R, Edasis C, Piper AM. Vulnerability, sharing, and privacy: analyzing art therapy for older adults with dementia. Paper presented at the Proceedings of the 19th ACM Conference on Computer-Supported Cooperative Work & Social Computing, San Francisco, California, USA. 2016. http://delivery.acm.org/10.1145/2820000/2819960/1572_cornejo.pdf?ip=149.142.80.32&id=2819960&acc=ACTIVE%20SERVICE&key=CA367851C7E3CE77%2E79535EF926D6BC05%2E4D4702B0C3E38B35

%2E4D4702B0C3E38B35&CFID=685912815-&CFTOKEN=32148404&__acm__=1477369346_0f0f0859d27959cd58853b7ea754a118.
46. Gustavson KA, Alexopoulos GS, Niu GC, McCulloch C, Meade T, Areán PA. Problem-solving therapy reduces suicidal ideation in depressed older adults with executive dysfunction. Am J Geriatr Psychiatry. 2016;24(1):11–7. https://doi.org/10.1016/j.jagp.2015.07.010.
47. Vernooij-Dassen M, Draskovic I, McCleery J, Downs M. Cognitive reframing for carers of people with dementia. Cochrane Database Syst Rev. 2011;11:CD005318. https://doi.org/10.1002/14651858.CD005318.pub2.
48. Wilkins CH, Mathews J, Sheline YI. Late life depression with cognitive impairment: evaluation and treatment. Clin Interv Aging. 2009;4:51–7.
49. Wilson KC, Mottram PG, Vassilas CA. Psychotherapeutic treatments for older depressed people. Cochrane Database Syst Rev. 2008;1:CD004853. https://doi.org/10.1002/14651858.CD004853.pub2.
50. Pinquart M, Duberstein PR, Lyness JM. Effects of psychotherapy and other behavioral interventions on clinically depressed older adults: a meta-analysis. Aging Ment Health. 2007;11(6):645–57. https://doi.org/10.1080/13607860701529635.
51. Barth, J., Munder, T., Gerger, H., Nüesch, E., Trelle, S., Znoj, H.,. . et al. (2016). Comparative efficacy of seven psychotherapeutic interventions for patients with depression: a network meta-analysis. Focus, 14(2), 229–243. doi:https://doi.org/10.1176/appi.focus.140201.
52. Dakin EK, Areán P. Patient perspectives on the benefits of psychotherapy for late-life depression. Am J Geriatr Psychiatry. 2013;21(2):155–63. https://doi.org/10.1016/j.jagp.2012.10.016.
53. Kiosses DN, Leon AC, Arean PA. Psychosocial interventions for late-life major depression: evidence-based treatments, predictors of treatment outcomes, and moderators of treatment effects. Psychiatr Clin North Am. 2011;34(2):377–401., viii. https://doi.org/10.1016/j.psc.2011.03.001.
54. Ryder NB. The cohort as a concept in the study of social change. Am Sociol Rev. 1965;30(6):843–61. https://doi.org/10.2307/2090964.
55. Egede LE, Gebregziabher M, Walker RJ, Payne EH, Acierno R, Frueh BC. Trajectory of cost overtime after psychotherapy for depression in older veterans via telemedicine. J Affect Disord. 2017;207:157–62. https://doi.org/10.1016/j.jad.2016.09.044.
56. Bartels, S. J., Coakley, E. H., Zubritsky, C., Ware, J. H., Miles, K. M., Arean, P. A.,. . et al. (2004). Improving access to geriatric mental health services: a randomized trial comparing treatment engagement with integrated versus enhanced referral care for depression, anxiety, and at-risk alcohol use. Am J Psychiatry, 161(8), 1455–1462. doi:https://doi.org/10.1176/appi.ajp.161.8.1455.
57. Chen H, Coakley EH, Cheal K, Maxwell J, Costantino G, Krahn DD, et al. Satisfaction with mental health services in older primary care patients. Am J Geriatr Psychiatry. 2006;14(4):371–9. https://doi.org/10.1097/01.JGP.0000196632.65375.b9.
58. Gum AM, Ayalon L, Greenberg JM, Palko B, Ruffo E, Areán PA. Preferences for professional assistance for distress in a diverse sample of older adults. Clin Gerontol. 2010;33(2):136–51. https://doi.org/10.1080/07317110903551901.
59. Beck AT. Cognitive therapy: nature and relation to behavior therapy. Behav Ther. 1970;1(2):184–200.
60. Ellis A. Reason and emotion in psychotherapy. Oxford: Lyle Stuart; 1962.
61. Krishna M, Jauhari A, Lepping P, Turner J, Crossley D, Krishnamoorthy A. Is group psychotherapy effective in older adults with depression? A systematic review. Int J Geriatr Psychiatry. 2011;26(4):331–40. https://doi.org/10.1002/gps.2546.
62. Naylor EV, Antonuccio DO, Litt M, Johnson GE, Spogen DR, Williams R, et al. Bibliotherapy as a treatment for depression in primary care. J Clin Psychol Med Settings. 2010;17(3):258–71. https://doi.org/10.1007/s10880-010-9207-2.
63. Gallagher-Thompson D, Steffen AM. Comparative effects of cognitive-behavioral and brief psychodynamic psychotherapies for depressed family caregivers. J Consult Clin Psychol. 1994;62(3):543–9.
64. Jarvik LF, Mintz JIM, Steuer J, Gerner R. Treating geriatric depression: a 26-week interim analysis. J Am Geriatr Soc. 1982;30(11):713–7. https://doi.org/10.1111/j.1532-5415.1982.tb01987.x.
65. Thompson LW, Gallagher D, Breckenridge JS. Comparative effectiveness of psychotherapies for depressed elders. J Consult Clin Psychol. 1987;55(3):385.
66. Xie CL, Wang XD, Chen J, Lin HZ, Chen YH, Pan JL, Wang WW. A systematic review and meta-analysis of cognitive behavioral and psychodynamic therapy for depression in Parkinson's disease patients. Neurol Sci. 2015;36(6):833–43. https://doi.org/10.1007/s10072-015-2118-0.
67. Driessen E, Cuijpers P, de Maat SC, Abbass AA, de Jonghe F, Dekker JJ. The efficacy of short-term psychodynamic psychotherapy for depression: a meta-analysis. Clin Psychol Rev. 2010;30(1):25–36. https://doi.org/10.1016/j.cpr.2009.08.010.

68. Jones EE, Pulos SM. Comparing the process in psychodynamic and cognitive-behavioral therapies. J Consult Clin Psychol. 1993;61(2):306–16. https://doi.org/10.1037/0022-006X.61.2.306.
69. Connolly Gibbons MB, Gallop R, Thompson D, Luther D, Crits-Christoph K, Jacobs J, et al. Comparative effectiveness of cognitive therapy and dynamic psychotherapy for major depressive disorder in a community mental health setting: a randomized clinical noninferiority trial. JAMA Psychiat. 2016;73(9):904–11. https://doi.org/10.1001/jamapsychiatry.2016.1720.
70. Abbass A. Small-group videotape training for psychotherapy skills development. Acad Psychiatry. 2004;28(2):151–5. https://doi.org/10.1176/appi.ap.28.2.151.
71. Abbass A, Sheldon A, Gyra J, Kalpin A. Intensive short-term dynamic psychotherapy for DSM-IV personality disorders: a randomized controlled trial. J Nerv Ment Dis. 2008;196(3):211–6. https://doi.org/10.1097/NMD.0b013e3181662ff0.
72. Barber J, Critis-Christoph P. Development of a therapist adherence/competence rating scale for supportive-expressive dynamic psychotherapy: a preliminary report. Psychother Res. 1996;6(2):81–94. https://doi.org/10.1080/10503309612331331608.
73. Alexopoulos GS, Raue P, Arean P. Problem-solving therapy versus supportive therapy in geriatric major depression with executive dysfunction. Am J Geriatr Psychiatry. 2003;11(1):46–52.
74. Arean PA, Perri MG, Nezu AM, Schein RL, Christopher F, Joseph TX. Comparative effectiveness of social problem-solving therapy and reminiscence therapy as treatments for depression in older adults. J Consult Clin Psychol. 1993;61(6):1003–10.
75. Areán PA, Raue P, Mackin RS, Kanellopoulos D, McCulloch C, Alexopoulos GS. Problem-solving therapy and supportive therapy in older adults with major depression and executive dysfunction. Am J Psychiatry. 2010;167(11):1391–8. https://doi.org/10.1176/appi.ajp.2010.09091327.
76. Kiosses DN, Arean PA, Teri L, Alexopoulos GS. Home-delivered problem adaptation therapy (PATH) for depressed, cognitively impaired, disabled elders: a preliminary study. Am J Geriatr Psychiatry. 2010;18(11):988–98. https://doi.org/10.1097/JGP.0b013e3181d6947d.
77. Nezu AM. A problem-solving formulation of depression: a literature review and proposal of a pluralistic model. Clin Psychol Rev. 1987;7(2):121–44.
78. Miller MD, Frank E, Cornes C, Houck PR, Reynolds CF 3rd. The value of maintenance interpersonal psychotherapy (IPT) in older adults with different IPT foci. Am J Geriatr Psychiatry. 2003;11(1):97–102.
79. Reynolds CF 3rd, Frank E, Perel JM, Imber SD, Cornes C, Miller MD, et al. Nortriptyline and interpersonal psychotherapy as maintenance therapies for recurrent major depression: a randomized controlled trial in patients older than 59 years. JAMA. 1999;281(1):39–45.
80. van Schaik A, van Marwijk H, Ader H, van Dyck R, de Haan M, Penninx B, et al. Interpersonal psychotherapy for elderly patients in primary care. Am J Geriatr Psychiatry. 2006;14(9):777–86. https://doi.org/10.1097/01.JGP.0000199341.25431.4b.
81. Miller MD. Using interpersonal therapy (IPT) with older adults today and tomorrow: a review of the literature and new developments. Curr Psychiatry Rep. 2008;10(1):16–22. https://doi.org/10.1007/s11920-008-0005-6.
82. Hinrichsen GA, Clougherty KF. Interpersonal psychotherapy for depressed older adults. Washington, DC: American Psychological Association; 2006.
83. Hinrichsen GA. Interpersonal psychotherapy as a treatment for depression in later life. Prof Psychol Res Pract. 2008;39(3):306.
84. Fry P. Structured and unstructured reminiscence training and depression among the elderly. Clin Gerontol. 1983;1(3):15–37.
85. Gallagher DE, Thompson LW. Treatment of major depressive disorder in older adult outpatients with brief psychotherapies. Psychotherapy. 1982;19(4):482.
86. Watt LM, Cappeliez P. Integrative and instrumental reminiscence therapies for depression in older adults: intervention strategies and treatment effectiveness. Aging Ment Health. 2000;4(2):166–77.
87. Woods B, Spector A, Jones C, Orrell M, Davies S. Reminiscence therapy for dementia. Cochrane Database Syst Rev. 2005;2:CD001120.
88. Boylin W, Gordon SK, Nehrke MF. Reminiscing and ego integrity in institutionalized elderly males. The Gerontologist. 1976;16(2):118–24. https://doi.org/10.1093/geront/16.2.118.
89. Serrano JP, Latorre JM, Gatz M, Montanes J. Life review therapy using autobiographical retrieval practice for older adults with depressive symptomatology. Psychol Aging. 2004;19(2):272.

28 Multidisciplinary Approaches

Jennifer Jacobson, Ashley Trust, Erica C. Garcia-Pittman, and Gayle Ayers

Introduction

A multidisciplinary approach to geriatric patient management involves coordination between the treating psychiatrist and all other members of the medical healthcare team involved in the patient's care [1–4]. Such a multidisciplinary team may include any number of providers, each of whom shares the common goal of providing comprehensive care to each patient. In addition to the treating psychiatrist, the team could include the patient's primary care physician; other medical specialists, such as a neurologist or palliative care team; a clinical pharmacist or social worker; therapist; home health nurse; or nursing home staff. Each of these potential team members and their contributions to care will be discussed separately in the coming text. Providers should keep in mind that each member of a multidisciplinary team plays an important role in providing geriatric patients with the individualized care they need to treat their complicated clinical problems. Coordination of care between multiple providers in various fields improves patient outcomes. This section will first delineate common interdisciplinary approaches to patient care in an outpatient setting and will then discuss inpatient collaborative care models.

Multidisciplinary Treatment Programs in Outpatients

Multidisciplinary treatment programs help to coordinate care between providers and can be used in treating physical as well as psychiatric illnesses [1–4]. They may also help decrease the all-cause mortality in geriatric patients struggling with depressive illnesses [5]. A few different techniques can be used in outpatient treatment settings to integrate different providers or specialties into the care of each patient. One such technique is to adopt a specialized team management structure. In a specialized team management structure, the primary care physician is assisted in the clinic by a nurse specializing in outpatient geriatric care. The nurse helps the primary care physician manage complex cases and evaluates geriatric patients. This allows the physician to focus on the general aspects of wellness, while the nurse targets common geriatric problems, which saves time and prevents problems from slipping through the cracks. Another available treatment option is to assign each clinic provider a specific set of criteria on which to focus during the management of each patient's care in an assembly line-like design. Each provider,

R. R. Tampi et al. (eds.), *Psychiatric Disorders Late in Life*, https://doi.org/10.1007/978-3-319-73078-3_28

whether it is a physician, physician's assistant, nurse practitioner, or nurse, has a specific role to play in each patient's assessment. To ease the assessment process, staff members have access to screening questionnaires, structured note outlines, and additional office staff to whom community outreach and program enrollment can be delegated [1]. For complicated or time-consuming problems that would traditionally prolong appointment times, the designated support staff can provide assistance and streamline care.

Research supports the use of the two aforementioned clinical treatment designs in the assessments and management of geriatric patients. Two community-based studies revealed that patients receiving standardized, practice-based management of common geriatric issues allowed physicians to provide better quality of care for incontinence and falls [6]. These common geriatric issues could easily be missed during a more traditional medical evaluation without the needed time for a more thorough investigation of geriatric-specific issues. Allowing providers to co-manage geriatric care results in better quality of care in the treatment of common geriatric ailments, including dementia, falls, and incontinence [2, 3]. Dividing clinical duties allows each provider to focus more closely on the aspects of care specific to their individual assessment.

This approach is formally designated as the Comprehensive Geriatric Assessment (CGA) and has been noted to be beneficial in several research studies [4, 6–8]. One study evaluated treatment outcomes in geriatric patients receiving care through either a CGA program or typical outpatient care through health maintenance organizations (HMOs) [4]. The study revealed that guided integrative care results in fewer admissions to skilled nursing facilities and decreases days of admission. Another randomized controlled trial investigated the efficacy of the CGA intervention when used to evaluate elderly patients living independently in the community [7]. The patient participants suffered from some combination of functional impairment, urinary incontinence, repeated falls, and/or depressive symptoms. Compared with patients in the control limb, those patients randomly assigned to the CGA treatment limb exhibited improvement in functional status, energy level, and social interactions at 15 months. A third trial evaluated patients with complex cases and randomly assigned them to receive either CGA care or usual care [8]. Results indicated that patients receiving interdisciplinary treatment exhibited improved functionality, lower rates of depression, and less frequent home healthcare referrals at 6 months. CGA programs utilize multiple providers to improve geriatric patient outcomes by helping each provider focus on individual issues while maintaining an overall broad scope of the patient as a whole.

Geriatric patients often present to outpatient psychiatric clinics with multiple medical comorbidities and complicating psychosocial factors [1, 6]. Integrating social work support into the outpatient setting can be vital to maintaining a standard of excellence in outpatient care. Several programs have been developed in order to help facilitate social work involvement within the treatment team. One such program is the Geriatric Resources for Assessment and Care of Elders (GRACE) [5]. This program focuses on an integrated team approach of geriatric patients in the outpatient setting. Each patient's long-term care plan is developed and managed by a nurse practitioner and a social worker, both of whom coordinate treatment plans with the patient's primary care physician and an interdisciplinary team specializing in geriatric patients. Similar collaborative care programs employ non-physician mental health professionals (nurse practitioners, social workers, etc.) to provide psychoeducation to patients and help incorporate psychiatric health maintenance into primary care settings. These programs are alternatively referred to as integrative care or care management programs [9].

Another area in which integrative care has been employed is in regard to depressed patients seeking both medication management and psychotherapy [10]. In these instances, the geriatric psychiatrist must coordinate care with the psychologist or clinical social worker providing therapy. Geriatric psychiatrists also work closely with neuropsychologists, to help providers differentiate between neurocognitive disorders and primary affective disorders which can be difficult to distinguish in the elder population. In order to facilitate communication between providers and investigate the effectiveness of integrated care in a clinical setting, the University of Washington developed the Improving Mood-Promoting Access to Collaborative Treatment [IMPACT] program [10]. The IMPACT program utilizes psychologists as depression care managers in a collaborative care model with physicians. The psychologists' responsibilities as part of the collaborative care team consist of calling patients to provide education about their depression and monitoring symptoms and treatment response. They offer six to eight counseling sessions during which they coach patients in behavioral activation during treatment and schedule each additional visit. The geriatric psychiatrist collaborates with the psychologist to manage each patient's care.

Employing integrative programs such as the IMPACT program can improve outcomes for geriatric patients [9]. One randomized controlled trial compared symptom remission rates over 4 months in 208 African American patients with depression who received either social worker support or a wait list control condition [11]. The social worker in each case placed referrals for medical and social services, provided psychoeducation about depression and stress reduction techniques, and also provided behavioral activation. Remission was achieved by 44% of patients in the treatment group versus 27% of those receiving usual care. Another randomized controlled trial followed patients with minor depression or dysthymia for 1 year and compared remission rates in patients receiving home social work support to patients receiving usual care [12]. The social workers in each case conducted eight in-home problem-solving therapy (PST) sessions and behavioral activation sessions and provided psychoeducation to the patient about antidepressant use. The usual care consists of a letter sent to each patient's primary care physician informing them of the depression diagnosis. Remission was achieved by 36% of patients in the treatment group versus on 12% of those receiving usual care [12].

Several other studies have assessed the efficacy of similar programs, all of which revealed improved outcomes for patients receiving collaborative care [13–15]. One such study investigated treatment outcomes in 1226 geriatric patients who were randomly assigned to receive either collaborative care or usual care [5]. Of the patients studied, 396 suffered from unipolar major depression, 203 suffered from minor depression, and 627 had no depressive diagnoses. Collaborative care decreased mortality by 24% in patients with major depression when compared with usual care. This decreased mortality rate was comparable to the risk of death in patients without any depressive diagnoses. Conversely, patients with major depression who received usual care had mortality rates almost twice as high as patients without any depressive diagnoses. Collaborative care did not impact mortality rates of patients with minor depression [5]. Another randomized controlled trial studied 57 geriatric patients being treated in a psychiatric clinic for depressive disorders over 6 months [16]. It investigated outcomes in patients who received usual care (pharmacotherapy) with those who received collaborative care in addition to pharmacotherapy. Geriatric patients who received a combination of collaborative care plus pharmacotherapy exhibited the best outcomes. A randomized controlled study involving the GRACE program revealed that geriatric patients treated via the collaborative intervention enjoyed a better quality of life, improved overall health, and fewer emergency department visits when compared to geriatric patients receiving general care [17]. High-risk patients in the GRACE program also had fewer hospitalizations compared with control subjects.

The collaboration of care between psychotherapy and psychiatry has been proven to be useful, although it is frequently underutilized in the treatment of elderly depressed patients [18, 19]. As part of a national study investigating the effects of collaborative versus usual care in the treatment of depressed patients, researchers discovered that patients in the collaborative care models experienced better outcomes. More patients who received care management plus pharmacotherapy achieved remission of depressive symptoms when compared to those individuals who only received pharmacotherapy (55 vs. 29%) [5]. Similarly, in investigations of patients already receiving either individual, couple, or group therapy, the addition of pharmacotherapy improved patient outcomes. Even in patients suffering from only minor depressive symptoms, integrating psychotherapy into collaborative care models can provide additional help for patients [20, 21].

Coordinating care between the primary treating physician and other specialists is an invaluable tool for optimizing the quality of care that patients receive, in regard to both patients' physical and emotional health. A "clinical specialist" can refer to another physician, but often "specialists" are non-physician experts in a particular field. For instance, clinical or community pharmacists can be an important resource to help guide patient care and improve outcomes. Involving community pharmacists in patient care helps reduce medication-related errors [22–27]. One vital role filled by pharmacists is assisting with medication reconciliation for patients. Based upon the safety goals set forth by the Joint Commission, all providers are required to perform comprehensive medication reconciliations at every transition point in care, including hospital admissions, transfers, discharges, and outpatient clinic appointments [28]. Pharmacists can be an invaluable resource for maintaining an accurate medication list to accomplish this goal and limit medication-related errors [22–27]. The reason that medication reconciliation is so important is that the most common cause of adverse drug events for patients living independently is incorrect or inconsistent adherence to the prescribed medication regimen. This issue accounts for 21% of all preventable adverse drug events in the ambulatory Medicare population [29]. Employing assistance from clinical pharmacists can help patients to clarify medication dosing instructions and limit the potential for these types of errors.

Polypharmacy is a common issue in the geriatric population, and the potential for medication-related errors increases with the number of medications a patient is taking. Compared with patients prescribed two or fewer medications, those individuals taking three or greater medications are more likely to incur dosing errors, increasing their risk for adverse drug reactions [30]. Adverse drug reactions can occur even in patients on two or fewer medications. As an example, anticholinesterase inhibitors can potentially exacerbate or mimic depressive symptoms, and their effects should be closely monitored. By routinely involving a clinical pharmacist in each patient's care, each case is more closely reviewed specifically for possible drug interactions, thereby limiting the potential for adverse events [31]. Pharmacist involvement with the treatment team can not only clarify dosing schedules and amounts but can also simplify the organizational process for the patient. For instance, blister packs for medications can be individually prepared by the pharmacist to assist the patient [26]. By confirming that medications are being taken as prescribed and clarifying instructions when discrepancies occur, pharmacists improve patient adherence to medication regimens and thus improve the quality of care each patient receives.

Not only does pharmacist participation in treatment improve patient care, but it reduces costs placed on the healthcare system addressing otherwise preventable drug-related errors. The Institute of Medicine published a report in 2007 estimating than an average of between 380,000 and 450,000 preventable adverse drug events occur each year in the United States [32]. Each adverse drug event cost hospitals an average of $5857. Based on these figures, in 2006, the US healthcare system was estimated to have spent approximately $3.5 billion related to managing preventable adverse drug events [33]. Integrating pharmacists into the treatment team could potentially save the healthcare system billions of dollars annually by preventing these needless errors from occurring.

Another way in which a multidisciplinary treatment approach reduces costs is by shifting the treatment focus to illness prevention. Preventing illnesses saves significant costs that would otherwise be expended either on the management of chronic illnesses or the treatment of acute illnesses. In order to transition from illness management and treatment to illness prevention in the elderly population, the healthcare system must increase access to care in an aging population with increasing mobility and transportation limitations. One way to accomplish this goal is through the use of home geriatric assessment programs. Such programs retain focus on maintaining patient independence, and visits are often conducted at home or via telephone. The treatment team typically consists of a geriatric home nurse, physical therapist, social worker, and psychologist, all working collaboratively. Specialty referrals are also available for patients when necessary [5]. Home assessment programs allow elderly patients the opportunity to receive the same healthcare services available in outpatient clinics without requiring these patients to leave their homes.

These home assessment programs have been proven to be beneficial in multiple meta-analyses in preserving functionality and reducing mortality in geriatric patients [34–37]. One such meta-analysis reviewed 21 randomized controlled trials comparing patient outcomes in different multidimensional home assessment programs [37]. This study concluded that the home assessment programs can effectively reduce functional decline if clinical examinations are performed at each visit and reduce mortality in patients younger than 77 years in age. Home assessment programs allow functionally impaired patients to receive care without the challenge of leaving home. Improved elderly patient access to care then shifts the healthcare focus toward preventative medicine and helps preserve functioning among older adults.

One practical benefit of implementing CGA treatment programs and maintaining a focus on illness prevention is a decrease in the rate of hospital readmissions, which decreased the financial burden on patients, families, and the healthcare system [38]. CGA programs implement many of the same initiatives as care transition programs designed to reduce hospital readmissions and emergency department visits [39]. By doing so, CGA programs have effectively lowered readmission rates in at least two studies on patients recently discharged from the emergency department [40, 41]. In patients recently discharged from the hospital, CGA programs have helped prevent readmission for up to 1 year, drastically reducing hospital costs [38]. If collaborative, home-based care models were to be universally adopted, the United States could potentially save billions of dollars per year on hospital readmission costs.

It is important to note that although several studies have indicated great benefits to applying a multidisciplinary treatment approach to geriatric care, some studies have produced less compelling results. For instance, a few randomized trials evaluating patient outcomes when treated with a multidisciplinary approach compared with usual care have uncovered no differences between the two treatment arms in terms of mortality, hospital admission rates, or quality of life [42, 43]. Home assessment programs, while beneficial in multiple domains, have not been proven effective in preventing nursing home admissions [5]. CGA programs have demonstrated inconsistent benefit for patients participating as part of a post-hospitalization discharge program [34, 38, 40, 41, 44]. One randomized trial compared CGA programs in the home with usual care in post-hospitalization follow-up appointments. Rates of functional decline, hospital readmission, and mortality were no different between the two groups after 60 days [44]. A similar randomized trial investigated the difference in outcomes for patients receiving comprehensive discharge planning and home follow-up and patient receiving usual care [40]. At 24 weeks, no difference had emerged in functional status, post-discharge acute care visits, depressions, or patient satisfaction.

Multidisciplinary Treatment Programs in Inpatients

This chapter has thus far focused on outpatient treatment approaches to a collaborative care model. A multidisciplinary approach to treatment can also be applied in an inpatient setting. Geriatric patients often present with complicated clinical presentations with multiple confounding variables. Due to such complex presentations, geriatric patients admitted to inpatient units can especially benefit from applying an interdisciplinary approach to their care. Doing so helps all providers simultaneously maintain focus on multiple areas or problems at once.

A typical inpatient multidisciplinary team for geriatric patients includes the attending physician, geriatrician, nursing staff, physical/occupational/speech therapists, outpatient providers, social worker, and discharge staff, all of whom contribute daily to the global patient assessment and treatment recommendations. An effective interdisciplinary team will ideally help to facilitate communication between physicians and families, help to locate physicians when necessary, clarify daily goals of care, and perform interdisciplinary rounds on each patient. Interdisciplinary rounds allow for the discussion of all problems pertinent to a case in the presence of all the providers. This open discussion ensures that all active issues are adequately addressed in a timely manner and pitfalls in care are avoided. A collaborative care approach also facilitates communication between the treatment team and the patients' families. Open communication between the treatment team and the families of complex, elderly patients improves the quality of care for the patient [45]. Studies conducted on hospitalized geriatric patients following hip fracture repairs revealed that those patients receiving a multidisciplinary approach to treatment had shorter hospitalizations and fewer complications, such as delirium [46, 47]. Involvement of geriatricians to assist general hospitalists in the care of elderly patients is especially beneficial in decreasing mortality, readmissions, delirium, and other complications [48, 49].

Some hospitals have designated specialized geriatric units for elderly patients. These units allow complex geriatric patients to receive care from a dedicated multidisciplinary staff, which reduces functional decline and discharges to long-term care facilities [50]. Each geriatric unit can be tailored to the location and setting of care, and multiple variations on this approach exist [51]. The Department of Veterans Affairs hospitals have created Geriatric Evaluation and Management Units (GEMUs) for this purpose. The civilian equivalent in academic hospital settings are referred to as Acute Care of the Elderly (ACE) units. ACE units were initially conceptualized as a brief recovery unit with an emphasis on postsurgical rehabilitation to enhance mobility and independent living. More recently, however, ACE units have been converted into more conventional geriatric wards. A multidisciplinary team approach is employed in both GEMUs and ACE units, and the wards are designed with structural modifications to assist with activities of daily living. These modifications help combat the common challenges faced by elderly patients during hospitalizations. One drawback to these units is that due to increased duration of admission to these units, availability cannot keep up with demand. Thus, these units are usually only available in the Department of Veterans Affairs hospitals [52].

Several studies have corroborated the finding that dedicated geriatric units improve patient outcomes through an interdisciplinary treatment approach. One meta-analysis of 22 randomized trials evaluated long-term patient outcomes at 6 and 12 months following hospital admission. In comparing patients who received collaborative, interdisciplinary care in specialized geriatric units with those who received general hospital admission, the study found that specialized geriatric units reduce patient mortality at both 6 and 12 months post-hospitalization [53]. Another meta-analysis of 17 randomized controlled trials involving patient outcomes in geriatric rehabilitation units revealed that these programs resulted in decreased mortality, fewer nursing home admissions, and improved functional status at discharge [54]. Over 80 individual randomized controlled trials and numerous meta-analyses conducted in the United States have consistently demonstrated that collaborative care increases patient and provider satisfaction and preserves patient functioning as well as improving patient outcomes and lowering costs [10].

Other hospitals without the resources to create a dedicated geriatric unit have attempted to provide patients in different units with an interdisciplinary approach to care, though with mixed results [55]. A significant barrier to success in these models is the lack of a specialized geriatric-focused staff and inconsistent nursing staff between the different units. Some hospitals have created a mobile geriatric care team to assist the attending hospitalist physician in the management of elderly patients [56]. One trial investigated the differences in outcome between hospitalized patients over 70 years old treated by a geriatric multidisciplinary team (though not in specialized geriatric units) versus those receiving usual care. No changes were found in duration of hospital stay, readmission rates, falls, restraint use, or use of sleeping medications. Observed improvements included that patients were more likely to engage in end-of-life discussions and their functional impairments were more readily identified [48]. An alternative to dedicated geriatric units or a mobile geriatric unit is the Hospital Elder Life Program (HELP). It includes training staff and volunteers to work with elderly hospitalized patients and to provide basic assistance during hospitalization. These interventions include reorienting patients, providing intellectual stimulation, and improving sleep hygiene [49]. The HELP has been shown to facilitate swifter hospital discharge, improve patient satisfaction, reduce delirium rates, and decrease the financial burden of the hospital [57–59].

Multidisciplinary Treatment Programs in Nursing Home or Skilled Nursing Facility

This multidisciplinary model can be applied to patients in nursing home or skilled nursing facility (SNF) settings with similar benefits. Nursing homes and skilled nursing facilities provide patients with residential care for both acute and chronic illnesses. Ninety-five percent of SNFs provide both long- and short-term care [60]. The overall goal for short-term care is for the patient to return to the community; however, some patients may require short-term end-of-life care, while others will need long-term nursing home care. Long-term facilities provide assistance with activities of daily living, such as bathing, eating, toileting, etc. SNF staff members include registered nurses, medical directors, licensed vocational nurses, physical and occupational therapists, speech-language pathologists, as well as dietary counselors [61]. Members of the SNF and nursing home medical staff must be able to manage medically complex geriatric patients as well as handle any potentially difficult ethical issues that could arise [62].

Nursing facilities must be equipped to provide the complex care needed to address multiple medical comorbidities and polypharmacy associated with most members of the geriatric population. The average nursing home resident is taking up to eight different medications, and one-third of the residents are taking nine or more medications [63]. Family caregivers lack the time and skill to handle the needs of these elderly patients, and professional medical expertise is often required to avoid medication-associated adverse events. The utility of applying a multidisciplinary approach to treatment in a SNF or nursing home lies in each provider's ability to target specific areas of treatment without sacrificing any other aspects of care in the process. Dividing 12 problems between several providers decreases the workload on each provider and decreases the likelihood of missing details in each case.

In a nursing home or SNF inpatient setting, one important way to facilitate collaborative care is by integrating psychiatric and medical treatment. The addition of a psychiatrist to the medical treatment team offers an invaluable perspective on managing common issues such as delirium, dementia, depression, and behavioral issues. These problems are pervasive throughout the nursing home and SNF resident population. One nationwide study in 2005 investigated the prevalence of depression in the nursing home population. It revealed that 55% of the 634,060 residents involved in the study suffered from depression during the first year at the facility [64]. Another study conducted in an Ohio nursing home found that 23% of those diagnosed with depression were untreated [65]. Depression in nursing home patients is a significant problem and one that has been under-recognized and undertreated. Applying a multidisciplinary approach to treatment of nursing home patients would allow both their medical and psychiatric issues to be more readily addressed and treated. One multicenter trial compared the ability of skilled nursing facility treatment teams to identify depression in non-demented residents [66]. The trial randomized participants into either typical care by the facility staff or into management by a multidisciplinary team. The study revealed that the multidisciplinary team was more readily able to identify and treat depression in this patient population and the prevalence of depression decreased in units with such teams. Studies like this one provide evidence that implementing a collaborative care approach to treating nursing home patients would improve outcomes.

Multidisciplinary Treatment Programs in Palliative Care and Hospice

Another important consideration as the elderly patient population ages is the integration of palliative care and hospice into the treatment model. Both palliative care and hospice care are integral to the management of the nursing home population, as one-quarter of all US deaths take place in a SNF [67]. There has been a gradual increase in the palliative and hospice care in skilled nursing facilities, rising from 14% in 1999 to 33% in 2006 [68]. In 2014, hospice care programs were caring for up to 1.7 million individuals in the United States [69]. Hospice care is designed to provide palliative care through an interdisciplinary care team approach. It requires the collaboration between nurses, social workers, chaplains, bereavement counselors, and hospice physicians in addition to primary care physicians to help control symptoms such as pain, anorexia, and depression. An important consideration is the inclusion of a psychiatrist in the hospice treatment team, as depressive symptoms often co-occur with pain in patients near the end of life. Such a multidisciplinary approach is necessary to address the complicated issues that arise at the end of life.

Evidence confirms that collaborative end-of-life care is beneficial in easing the transition from life to death, not only for the patient but also for the patients' families. One large national study that found family members of recently deceased nursing home patients reported a superior quality of care when hospice was involved (70.7%) compared to when they were not (41.6%). Another study showed that families of dying nursing home patients reported improved control of psychical symptoms with palliative care involvement, with satisfaction ratings improving from 64 to 93% [70]. Palliative care involvement also reduces the number of unnecessary medical interventions, such as diagnostics, imaging, and intensive care unit and emergency department visits. In addition, these teams can help reduce polypharmacy by eliminating drugs that are unlikely to provide benefit at the end of life, such as lipid-lowering agents. By integrating palliative care into the medical treatment of patients near the end of life, patients receive an improved quality of care. Reducing unnecessary procedures and medications also reduces the healthcare costs placed on patients, families, hospitals, and the healthcare system as a whole [71–77].

Conclusions

As patients age, a major goal of care is to preserve functioning and quality of life. Implementing collaborative care models to outpatient, inpatient, and end-of-life treatment is a vital change necessary to accomplish this goal. Multidisciplinary approaches to care have been proven to improve patient and provider satisfaction, as well as quality of care. As the elderly population increases, integrative care models should be implemented across all treatment settings to ensure that patients receive the highest quality of care.

References

1. Ward KT, Reuben DB. Comprehensive geriatric assessment. 2016. http://www.uptodate.com. Accessed 6 Feb 2016.
2. Ganz DA, Koretz BK, Bail JK, et al. Nurse practitioner comanagement for patients in an academic geriatric practice. Am J Manag Care. 2010;16:e343.
3. Reuben DB, Ganz DA, Roth CP, et al. Effect of nurse practitioner comanagement on the care of geriatric conditions. J Am Geriatr Soc. 2013;61:857.
4. Burns R, Nichols LO, Martindale-Adams J, Graney MJ. Interdisciplinary geriatric primary care evaluation and management: two-year outcomes. J Am Geriatr Soc. 2000;48:8.
5. Gallo JJ, Morales KH, Bogner HR, et al. Long term effect of depression care management on mortality in older adults: follow-up of cluster randomized clinical trial in primary care. BMJ. 2013;346:f2570.
6. Wenger NS, Roth CP, Shekelle PG, et al. A practice-based intervention to improve primary care for falls, urinary incontinence, and dementia. J Am Geriatr Soc. 2009;57:547.
7. Reuben DB, Frank JC, Hirsch SH, et al. A randomized clinical trial of outpatient comprehensive geriatric assessment coupled with an intervention to increase adherence to recommendations. J Am Geriatr Soc. 1999;47:269.
8. Boult C, Boult LB, Morishita L, et al. A randomized clinical trial of outpatient geriatric evaluation and management. J Am Geriatr Soc. 2001;49:351.

9. Unützer J, Park M. Older adults with severe, treatment-resistant depression. JAMA. 2012;308: 909.
10. University of Washington Psychiatry and Behavioral Sciences Division of Integrated Care and Public Health. Impact: improving mood- promoting access to collaborative treatment. 2016. http://www.aims-uw.edu. Accessed 23 Feb 2016.
11. Gitlin LN, Harris LF, McCoy MC, et al. A home-based intervention to reduce depressive symptoms and improve quality of life in older African Americans: a randomized trial. Ann Intern Med. 2013;159:243.
12. Ciechanowski P, Wagner E, Schmaling K, et al. Community-integrated home-based depression treatment in older adults: a randomized controlled trial. JAMA. 2004;291:1569.
13. Bruce ML, Ten Have TR, Reynolds CF 3rd, et al. Reducing suicidal ideation and depressive symptoms in depressed older primary care patients: a randomized controlled trial. JAMA. 2004;291:1081.
14. Alexopoulos GS, Katz IR, Bruce ML, et al. Remission in depressed geriatric primary care patients: a report from the PROSPECT study. Am J Psychiatry. 2005;162:718.
15. Alexopoulos GS, Reynolds CF 3rd, Bruce ML, et al. Reducing suicidal ideation and depression in older primary care patients: 24-month outcomes of the PROSPECT study. Am J Psychiatry. 2009;166:882.
16. Jeong H, Yim HW, Jo SJ, et al. The effects of care management on depression treatment in a psychiatric clinic: a randomized controlled trial. Int J Geriatr Psychiatry. 2013;28:1023.
17. Counsell SR, Callahan CM, Clark DO, et al. Geriatric care management for low-income seniors: a randomized controlled trial. JAMA. 2007;298:2623.
18. Areán PA, Cook BL. Psychotherapy and combined psychotherapy/pharmacotherapy for late life depression. Biol Psychiatry. 2002;52:293.
19. Morgan AC. Practical geriatrics: psychodynamic psychotherapy with older adults. Psychiatr Serv. 2003;54:1592.
20. Lyness JM, Heo M, Datto CJ, et al. Outcomes of minor and subsyndromal depression among elderly patients in primary care settings. Ann Intern Med. 2006;144:496.
21. Gould RL, Coulson MC, Howard RJ. Cognitive behavioral therapy for depression in older people: a meta-analysis and meta-regression of randomized controlled trials. J Am Geriatr Soc. 2012;60:1817.
22. Cochrane RA, Mandal AR, Ledger-Scott M, Walker R. Changes in drug treatment after discharge from hospital in geriatric patients. BMJ. 1992;305:694.
23. Gurwitz J. Case and commentary. Spotlight case. Double trouble. Medicine. 2005. www.webmm.ahrq.gov/case.aspx?caseID=104. Accessed 27 Mar 2016.
24. The Institute for Safe Medication Practices. How to take your medications safely. 2016. http://www.ismp.org/Newsletters/consumer/alerts/Brochure.asp. Accessed 27 Mar 2016.
25. Cramer JA. Enhancing patient compliance in the elderly. Role of packaging aids and monitoring. Drugs Aging. 1998;12:7.
26. Milton JC, Hill-Smith I, Jackson SH. Prescribing for older people. BMJ. 2008;336:606.
27. Bell CM, Fischer HD, Gill SS, et al. Initiation of benzodiazepines in the elderly after hospitalization. J Gen Intern Med. 2007;22:1024.
28. National Patient Safety Goal on Reconciling Medication Information (NPSG.3.06.01). The Joint Commission. 2010. http://www.jointcommission.org/npsg_reconciling_medication. Accessed 23 Feb 2016.
29. Field TS, Mazor KM, Briesacher B, et al. Adverse drug events resulting from patient errors in older adults. J Am Geriatr Soc. 2007;55:271.
30. Forster AJ, Clark HD, Menard A, et al. Adverse events among medical patients after discharge from hospital. CMAJ. 2004;170:345.
31. Espinoza RT, Unutzer J. Diagnosis and management of late-life unipolar depression. 2016. http://www.uptodate.com. Accessed 6 Feb 2016.
32. Aspden P, Wolcott JA, Bootman JL, Cronenwett LR. Preventing medication errors: quality chasm series. Washington, DC: The National Academic Press; 2007.
33. Bates DW, Spell N, Cullen DJ, et al. The costs of adverse drug events in hospitalized patients. Adverse drug events prevention study group. JAMA. 1997;277:307.
34. Stuck AE, Siu AL, Wieland GD, et al. Comprehensive geriatric assessment: a meta-analysis of controlled trials. Lancet. 1993;342: 1032.
35. Stuck AE, Egger M, Hammer A, et al. Home visits to prevent nursing home admission and functional decline in elderly people: systematic review and meta-regression analysis. JAMA. 2002;287:1022.
36. Elkan R, Kendrick D, Dewey M, et al. Effectiveness of home based support for older people: systematic review and meta-analysis. BMJ. 2001;323:719.
37. Huss A, Stuck AE, Rubenstein LZ, et al. Multidimensional preventive home visit programs for community-dwelling older adults: a systematic review and meta-analysis of randomized

controlled trials. J Gerontol A Biol Sci Med Sci. 2008;63:298.
38. Naylor MD, Aiken LH, Kurtzman ET, et al. The care span: the importance of transitional care in achieving health reform. Health Aff (Millwood). 2011;30:746.
39. Hesselink G, Schoonhoven L, Barach P, et al. Improving patient handovers from hospital to primary care: a systematic review. Ann Intern Med. 2012;157:417.
40. Naylor MD, Brooten D, Campbell R, et al. Comprehensive discharge planning and home follow-up of hospitalized elders: a randomized clinical trial. JAMA. 1999;281:613.
41. Caplan GA, Williams AJ, Daly B, Abraham K. A randomized, controlled trial of comprehensive geriatric assessment and multidisciplinary intervention after discharge of elderly from the emergency department--the DEED II study. J Am Geriatr Soc. 2004;52:1417.
42. Kuo HK, Scandrett KG, Dave J, Mitchell SL. The influence of outpatient comprehensive geriatric assessment on survival: a meta-analysis. Arch Gerontol Geriatr. 2004;39:245.
43. Fletcher AE, Price GM, Ng ES, et al. Population-based multidimensional assessment of older people in UK general practice: a cluster-randomised factorial trial. Lancet. 2004;364:1667.
44. Siu AL, Kravitz RL, Keeler E, et al. Postdischarge geriatric assessment of hospitalized frail elderly patients. Arch Intern Med. 1996;156:76.
45. O'Leary KJ, Sehgal NL, Terrell G, et al. Interdisciplinary teamwork in hospitals: a review and practical recommendations for improvement. J Hosp Med. 2012;7:48.
46. Vidán M, Serra JA, Moreno C, et al. Efficacy of a comprehensive geriatric intervention in older patients hospitalized for hip fracture: a randomized, controlled trial. J Am Geriatr Soc. 2005;53:1476.
47. Marcantonio ER, Flacker JM, Wright RJ, Resnick NM. Reducing delirium after hip fracture: a randomized trial. J Am Geriatr Soc. 2001;49:516.
48. Wald HL, Glasheen JJ, Guerrasio J, et al. Evaluation of a hospitalist-run acute care for the elderly service. J Hosp Med. 2011;6:313.
49. Inouye SK, Bogardus ST Jr, Baker DI, et al. The hospital elder life program: a model of care to prevent cognitive and functional decline in older hospitalized patients. Hospital elder life program. J Am Geriatr Soc. 2000;48:1697.
50. Landefeld CS, Palmer RM, Kresevic DM, et al. A randomized trial of care in a hospital medical unit especially designed to improve the functional outcomes of acutely ill older patients. N Engl J Med. 1995;332:1338.
51. Jayadevappa R, Bloom BS, Raziano DB, Lavizzo-Mourey R. Dissemination and characteristics of acute care for elders (ACE) units in the United States. Int J Technol Assess Health Care. 2003;19:220.
52. Mattison M. Hospital management of older adults. 2015. http://www.uptodate.com. Accessed 10 Apr 2016.
53. Ellis G, Whitehead MA, O'Neill D, et al. Comprehensive geriatric assessment for older adults admitted to hospital. Cochrane Database Syst Rev. 2017;9:CD006211.
54. Bachmann S, Finger C, Huss A, et al. Inpatient rehabilitation specifically designed for geriatric patients: systematic review and meta-analysis of randomised controlled trials. BMJ. 2010;340:c1718.
55. Arbaje AI, Maron DD, Yu Q, et al. The geriatric floating interdisciplinary transition team. J Am Geriatr Soc. 2010;58:364.
56. Farber JI, Korc-Grodzicki B, Du Q, et al. Operational and quality outcomes of a mobile acute care for the elderly service. J Hosp Med. 2011;6:358.
57. Rubin FH, Neal K, Fenlon K, et al. Sustainability and scalability of the hospital elder life program at a community hospital. J Am Geriatr Soc. 2011;59:359.
58. Mouchoux C, Rippert P, Duclos A, et al. Impact of a mulifaceted program to prevent postoperative delirium in the elderly: the CONFUCIUS stepped wedge protocol. BMC Geriatr. 2011;11:25.
59. Hshieh TT, Yue J, Oh E, et al. Effectiveness of multicomponent nonpharmacological delirium interventions: a meta-analysis. JAMA Intern Med. 2015;175:512.
60. Medicare Payment Advisory Committee. Report to the Congress: Medicare payment policy. Chapter 8: Skilled nursing facilities, Washington, DC. 2014. www.medpac.gov/documents/reports/mar14_entirereport.pdf?sfvrsn=0. Accessed 4 Feb 2015.
61. Gillick MR, Yurkofsky M. Medical care in skilled nursing facilities (SNFs) in the United States. 2016. http://www.uptodate.com. Accessed 6 Feb 2016.
62. Zweig SC, Popejoy LL, Parker-Oliver D, Meadows SE. The physician's role in patients' nursing home care: "She's a very courageous and lovely woman. I enjoy caring for her". JAMA. 2011;306:1468.
63. Gurwitz JH, Field TS, Avorn J, et al. Incidence and preventability of adverse drug events in nursing homes. Am J Med. 2000;109:87.

64. Hoover DR, Siegel M, Lucas J, et al. Depression in the first year of stay for elderly long-term nursing home residents in the USA. Int Psychogeriatr. 2010;22:1161.
65. Levin CA, Wei W, Akincigil A, et al. Prevalence and treatment of diagnosed depression among elderly nursing home residents in Ohio. J Am Med Dir Assoc. 2007;8:585.
66. Leontjevas R, Gerritsen DL, Smalbrugge M, et al. A structural multidisciplinary approach to depression management in nursing-home residents: a multicentre, stepped-wedge cluster-randomised trial. Lancet. 2013;381:2255.
67. Aragon K, Covinsky K, Miao Y, et al. Use of the Medicare posthospitalization skilled nursing benefit in the last 6 months of life. Arch Intern Med. 2012;172:1573.
68. Miller SC, Lima J, Gozalo PL, Mor V. The growth of hospice care in U.S. nursing homes. J Am Geriatr Soc. 2010;58:1481.
69. NHPCO Facts and Figures on Hospice. 2015. http://www.nhpco.org/hospice-statistics-research-press-room/facts-hospice-and-palliative-care. Accessed 10 Apr 2016.
70. Baer WM, Hanson LC. Families' perception of the added value of hospice in the nursing home. J Am Geriatr Soc. 2000;48:879.
71. Morrison RS, Penrod JD, Cassel JB, et al. Cost savings associated with US hospital palliative care consultation programs. Arch Intern Med. 2008;168:1783.
72. Bakitas M, Lyons KD, Hegel MT, et al. Effects of a palliative care intervention on clinical outcomes in patients with advanced cancer: the project ENABLE II randomized controlled trial. JAMA. 2009;302:741.
73. Wright AA, Zhang B, Ray A, et al. Associations between end-of-life discussions, patient mental health, medical care near death, and caregiver bereavement adjustment. JAMA. 2008;300:1665.
74. Wright AA, Keating NL, Balboni TA, et al. Place of death: correlations with quality of life of patients with cancer and predictors of bereaved caregivers' mental health. J Clin Oncol. 2010;28:4457.
75. Jang RW, Krzyzanowska MK, Zimmermann C, et al. Palliative care and the aggressiveness of end-of-life care in patients with advanced pancreatic cancer. J Natl Cancer Inst. 2015;107(3).
76. Wang L, Piet L, Kenworthy CM, Dy SM. Association between palliative case management and utilization of inpatient, intensive care unit, emergency department, and hospice in Medicaid beneficiaries. Am J Hosp Palliat Care. 2015;32:216.
77. May P, Garrido MM, Cassel JB, et al. Prospective cohort study of hospital palliative care teams for inpatients with advanced cancer: earlier consultation is associated with larger cost-saving effect. J Clin Oncol. 2015;33:2745.

29 Setting-Specific Treatment Issues

Azziza Oluwakemi Bankole and Mamta Sapra

Introduction

As the population ages, the medical community is facing new dilemmas on how we can provide needed and appropriate care to the aging population. Aging affects individuals differently based on genetics and our multifaceted environment. A proportion of the older adult population goes through the process of healthy aging with minimal impact on day-to-day function. The majority of older adults have differing levels of mental and physical health problems that negatively impact healthy aging.

Traditionally we tend to envision setting-specific care for older adults as just nursing homes. However, older adults require varying levels of support ranging from little or no support in independent living in its different guises to full care in nursing homes. Such settings include hospitals, inpatient rehabilitation units, independent living facilities, long-term care (LTC) facilities, and in-community programs.

The diagnosis and treatment of mental health disorders are integral to the improvement of the overall health of the individuals in LTC facilities. Managing psychiatric disorders in LTC facilities is associated with several challenges because of complex medical needs of LTC residents, polypharmacy, and limited presence of mental health services in many of these facilities.

Epidemiology

The likelihood of requiring care in a LTC facility increases with age. Kemper et al. [1] estimated that greater than two-thirds of adults ≥ 65 years of age will require care in such settings. In 2010, an estimated 40.2 million older adults resided in LTC facilities [2]. According to the 2004 National Nursing Home Survey (NNHS), 4% of Americans 65 years and older are living in nursing homes [3]. In the 2004 NNHS sample, 44% of individuals had one psychiatric disorder diagnosis (n = 5931), and 26% (n = 3543) had a dual diagnosis, with two or more psychiatric disorder diagnoses [4]. Dementia was the most common psychiatric diagnosis in long-term care. A total of 687,581 LTC residents aged 65 years or older were identified as having dementia accounting for 52% of all LTC residents in this age group. Among those with dementia, 36.9% had some current behavioral symptom associated with dementia. Depressive symptoms were identified in over 35% of all LTC residents. Anxiety disorders were also common in NNHS with over 11% of all residents having an anxiety disorder. The prevalence of schizophrenia, bipolar disorder, and alcohol use disorder was much less common being diagnosed in 3.6%, 1.5%, and 1% of all residents, respectively.

R. R. Tampi et al. (eds.), *Psychiatric Disorders Late in Life*, https://doi.org/10.1007/978-3-319-73078-3_29

More recently, the National Study of Long-Term Care Providers [5] showed a decline from 1.5 million older adults 65 years and older living in 16,100 nursing homes [3] to 1.4 million living in 15,600 facilities. The availability of mental health care varies with the setting. Approximately 52% of residential care communities provided mental health services when compared with 87% of the nursing homes [5]. Residents of LTC facilities tend to have higher levels of cognitive and physical dysfunction.

The population of older adults living in LTC facilities is an especially vulnerable one. The 2004 NNHS [3] revealed that 75% of residents required assistance in three or more activities of daily living and 50% had dementia. Communication may be a barrier as a result of deficits from strokes, dementia, or other neurological disorders. Few nursing homes have access to a geriatric specialist. Residents are susceptible to social isolation and inactivity [6] contributing to insomnia, depression, and loss of strength with the greatest rate of decline in those with dementia [7]. Research suggests that a multifaceted approach when compared to a single-domain intervention is better for overall function among residents living at LTC facilities [8, 9].

In the next section, we describe various common psychiatric disorders seen in nursing homes and their treatments.

Depression

Depressive disorders are among the most common psychiatric diagnoses among nursing home residents. The prevalence of major depressive disorder in nursing home residents is approximately 14.4% with a higher prevalence rate for minor or clinically significant depression of up to 20% [10]. Depression among nursing home residents is usually persistent and is complicated by concurrent medical illnesses, disability, and pain. Depression in nursing home residents is also associated with a number of negative health outcomes including weight loss, dehydration, decline in activities of daily living, and mortality. Depression is also common in hospitalized older adults with prevalence ranging from 11 to 29% [11]. Early identification and treatment are of the utmost importance regardless of setting.

Depression screening is an integral part of ensuring optimal mental health among older adults. Older adults may not voluntarily provide this information, and their ability to communicate this information may be impaired by a number of deficits. Facilities may choose to screen all residents at certain intervals or train staff to identify at-risk residents. Regardless of which method is used in a particular facility, providing staff with appropriate screening tools and training them to use these tools well are essential. Nursing home staff needs to be aware of factors that contribute to the development of depression. Recognition is a vital step in the management of depression in such settings. Various screening instruments have been recommended including the Geriatric Depression Scale (GDS) (long and short forms) [12, 13, 14], the Cornell Scale for Depression in Dementia (CSDD) [15], and the Hamilton Depression Rating Scale (HAM-D) [16]. One study found that nursing home staff use of instruments such as the CSDD and HAM-D increased the sensitivity of depression diagnoses by staff from approximately 32 to 50% [17]. Screening tools must be short and uncomplicated such that they can be used by staff with no substantial mental health training. The CSDD [15], a 19-item scale, although widely accepted and highly sensitive and specific in detecting depression, failed to discriminate between depressed and non-depressed nursing home residents when administered by unlicensed staff [18]. Jeon et al. [19] showed that a shortened version (CDDS-4) had clinical utility in the nursing home setting when used by the nursing home staff. Different versions of the GDS [13, 14] have been utilized in nursing homes with GDS-15 [14] having a sensitivity of 84.3% and specificity of 73.8%. Validity and reliability of the GDS [13, 14] are limited in patients with dementia, and the CSDD [15] should be used in residents with moderate to severe cognitive impairment. The clinical utility of screening tools also depends on the setting in which they are used [20].

A systematic review by Simning and Simons [21] examined the treatment of depression in nursing home residents without cognitive impairment and looked at psychotherapeutic and pharmacological interventions. Evidence for cognitive behavior therapy (CBT) effectiveness is mixed.

Few studies involving reminiscence therapy have been done in both group and individual treatments and have shown treatment effect favoring reminiscence and life review when compared to standard care as usual [22, 23]. Other psychosocial interventions that have been tested include exercise programs, individually provided avian therapy, and group visitations with dog companion which are associated with reductions in depressive symptoms when compared to care as usual.

In the last 15 years, there has been an increase in the use of antidepressants in nursing home residents. Most studies looking at pharmacological interventions in nursing home settings are limited by their small sample size and lack of controls. There are a limited number of studies that evaluated the effectiveness of antidepressants in the nursing home setting. A review of antidepressant medications in nursing homes by Boyce et al. [10] examined four randomized trials—two compared the effectiveness of treatment with a selective serotonin reuptake inhibitor (SSRI) to placebo, one compared the effectiveness of an SSRI to a serotonin-norepinephrine reuptake inhibitors (SNRIs), and one compared the effectiveness of the tricyclic antidepressant (TCA) nortriptyline at two different dose regimens. All four were heterogeneous in terms of participant characteristics and study outcome measures. Another trial comparing paroxetine to placebo in nursing home residents with depression found that paroxetine was not more effective than placebo and may have been associated with delirium and worsening mini-mental state examination (MMSE) scores [24]. Another trial comparing venlafaxine and sertraline found that venlafaxine might not be as well tolerated in nursing home residents as sertraline [25]. The antidepressant effect of nortriptyline was greater at high doses for nursing home residents with intact cognition and might indicate variation in antidepressant response based on cognitive status [26]. The limited amount of evidence from randomized and non-randomized clinical trials suggests that depressed nursing home residents have a modest response to antidepressant medications. Majority of clinically depressed nursing home residents who have neither dementia nor significant medical comorbidity respond better to antidepressants. Most depressed nursing home residents with dementia and significant physical comorbidity do not show lasting improvements when treated with antidepressants. Katz and Parmelee [27] had suggested a treatment-resistant group with self-care deficits who showed failure to thrive and diminished treatment response. Based on the guidelines applicable to older adults in general, SSRIs are the first-line, SNRIs the second-line, and TCAs the third-line treatments for depression among nursing home residents. Of the TCAs, nortriptyline is often preferred because of better tolerance, less orthostatic hypotension, and more predictable pharmacodynamics.

There is a need for more studies that combine antidepressants with non-pharmacological interventions for examining the benefits of combined approaches along with more randomized controlled trials with some of the newer antidepressants in the nursing home population.

Anxiety

Anxiety is often overlooked in LTC facility residents with symptoms being ascribed to other things. Prevalence rates for anxiety disorders vary from 3 to 20% [28] with generalized anxiety disorder and specific phobias being the most common types seen in LTC population. Anxiety in LTC facilities is associated with pain, antidepressant use, depression, and lower perceived quality of life [29]. As with depression, the standardized clinical tools have limitations when used among this population. The Brief Anxiety and Depression Scale [30] and the Geriatric Anxiety Inventory-short form [31] have been shown to be useful tools in assessing anxiety in the nursing home population.

Optimal treatment of anxiety in LTC facilities should consist of both non-pharmacological and pharmacological interventions. CBT has been shown to be better than treatment as usual for older adults in the community setting [32, 33] but with less robust results when compared to younger adults [34]. Studies have also shown benefit from supportive therapy [32] and preferential music therapy in residents with dementia and anxiety [35].

Benzodiazepines are frequently prescribed for anxiety in LTC facilities. Stevenson et al. [36]

showed that 13% of residents were prescribed a benzodiazepine, of which 42% had no appropriate or potentially appropriate diagnosis associated with the benzodiazepine prescription. Benzodiazepine use in older adults is associated with impaired cognition, falls, hip fractures, daytime sedation, gait problems, and developing dependence on the medication [37]. They have also been found to be associated with impaired nighttime sleep quality [38]. SSRIs and SNRIs are most commonly prescribed for anxiety in the residential settings as anxiety often coexists with depression. Buspirone is another pharmacological option, but providers should be aware of the possibility of reduced efficacy in residents who have been on benzodiazepines in the past [39, 40].

Pain

Pain is a common symptom in older adults with rates in residential settings ranging from 28 to 73% [41]. The concept of normalizing pain highlights the process in which experienced or reported pain is seen as being expected in this population [42]. Untreated or undertreated pain is common [43] and is a source of unnecessary suffering to individuals. Residents who were able to communicate their pain were more likely to receive an intervention [44, 45]. Standardized pain assessments tailored to cognitive function may improve the recognition and treatment of pain [45]. Psychiatric disorders can act as barrier to effective pain care for a substantial segment of the nursing home population. Residents who had psychiatric disorders were less likely to be noted as having pain, were rated as having less severe pain, and were more likely to have "missing"/"don't know" pain severity ratings than were residents without psychiatric disorders [3]. This was found to be true for all four of the most prevalent psychiatric disorders in nursing homes and occurred independent of residents' age, gender, racial background, and physical functioning. Residents with psychiatric disorders were less likely to be provided opioids and more likely to be provided only non-opioid medications for pain. This association is also seen in residents with cognitive impairment [46]. The Checklist of Nonverbal Pain Indicators (CNPI) [47] was developed for use in the cognitively impaired population in mind. It is an observational tool that relies on eliciting verbal and nonverbal cues or behaviors that have been reported to be highly associated with pain, e.g., groans, grimacing, rubbing, etc. The US Department of Health and Human Services guidelines for pain management includes recognition of pain, characterization, appropriate interim treatment, using a patient-centered interdisciplinary care plan, setting treatment goals, and monitoring and adjusting plan as necessary [48].

Behavioral Disturbances in Dementia

Behavioral disturbances, also called neuropsychiatric symptoms, are common in nursing home patients with dementia and can range from psychosis, anxiety, depression, and sleep disorders to agitation and aggression. Behavioral symptoms have significant negative impact on the quality of life and are one of the most common predictors of nursing home placement [49]. Behavioral symptoms associated with dementia are usually recognized by the staff, but having a valid instrument can help assess the behavior better as well as plan for intervention. The Minimum Data Set (MDS), a standardized screening and assessment tool, is routinely used to assess behavior problems in LTC facilities. It contains items that measure physical, psychological, and psychosocial functioning. Studies comparing the MDS with research instruments [50, 51] demonstrated good inter-rater reliability coefficients (0.63) and concurrent validity correlations of 0.51–0.58 [52].

Assessment and management of dementia-related behavioral symptoms often require evaluation of social, environmental, and acute medical problems. In the nursing home setting, studies of non-pharmacological interventions outnumbered studies of pharmacological interventions. A review by Conn and Seitz [53] looked at pharmacological and non-pharmacological interventions in the LTC setting. This paper highlighted three major systematic reviews. The one by O'Connor et al. [54] examined experimental studies of psychosocial treatments of behavioral disturbances in dementia. Treatments with moderate or large effect sizes included aromatherapy, ability-focused caregiver education, bed baths, preferred music, and muscle relaxation training and suggested modifying intervention based on individual preferences. Kong et al. [55] carried out both a systematic review and a meta-analysis which concluded that only sensory interventions including aromatherapy, thermal bath, calming music, and hand massage were effective in reducing agitation. Vernooij-Dassen et al. [56] also reviewed psychosocial interventions in dementia care specific to nursing home residents. The authors synthesized 27 literature reviews as well as guidelines from Europe, the USA, and Canada. They concluded that the most effective interventions utilized behavioral management techniques, cognitive stimulation, or physical activity interventions. Some of the interventions included reality orientation, physical exercise, and positive behavior therapy highlighting pleasant events. Several other interventions specific to the nursing home setting that might be promising in reducing neuropsychiatric symptoms associated with neurocognitive disorder include music therapy, massage and touch therapy, and Snoezelen. The Agency for Healthcare Research and Quality: Advancing Excellence in Health Care (AHRQ) 2012 guidelines emphasizes limited evidence supporting the use of antipsychotics in the management of behavioral symptoms in dementia among nursing home residents. At the same time, guidelines still state that antipsychotics may be considered for patients not responding to other treatments [57]. Before initiating an antipsychotic medication in persons with dementia, an assessment of the risks and benefits should be done with ongoing collaboration and discussion with the patient and their family/caregiver.

In the next section, we discuss the use of pharmacological agents in long-term care.

Psychopharmacology in Long-Term Care

Given the high prevalence of psychiatric disorders in LTC facilities, the resident population has a high percentage of psychotropic medication usage. Estimates in Canadian LTC facilities show that antipsychotics, antidepressants, and benzodiazepines are prescribed in 30%, 12%, and 23% of residents, respectively [58]. Approximately 30% of US LTC residents with dementia receive treatment with cholinesterase inhibitors [59]. It was also noted that approximately 73% of these individuals on cholinesterase inhibitors were also being treated with antipsychotics, antidepressants, or benzodiazepines [59]. With the Omnibus Budget Reconciliation Act of 1987 (OBRA-87) [60], there have been changes in the trend of psychotropic drug use in nursing homes in the USA. The data suggest that after the OBRA regulations were issued, psychotropic drug use has been more appropriate and risk of adverse effects is lower [61].

Although psychotropic medications are frequently prescribed to LTC facility residents, there have been few randomized controlled trials of medication interventions in residents with psychiatric disorders. Complex comorbid medical disorders and the need for functional assistance make this population more vulnerable to adverse effects from psychotropics. Drug interactions also are common when psychotropics are prescribed in combination with medications used to treat medical illnesses. Studies in LTC facilities have demonstrated higher risk for falls, increased risk of fractures with benzodiazepines, extrapyramidal symptoms with antipsychotics, and cognitive impairment along with anticholinergic side effects with the use of psychotropics. Gurwitz and colleagues [62] examined the incidence and prevalence of adverse drug events in a large nursing home cohort and found that antipsychotics were associated with high incidence of adverse effects followed by antibiotics, antidepressants, and sedative hypnotics. Neuropsychiatric symptoms like sedation, confusion, hallucinations, and delirium were the most frequent adverse events noted. Discontinuation of antipsychotic medications needs to be considered as part of the standard treatment plan among older adults with psychiatric disorders living at LTC facilities. Underlying factors that lead to behavioral symptoms along with medical conditions that can cause these symptoms should be assessed prior to initiation of treatment with antipsychotics. Guidelines recommend combining non-pharmacological interventions with antipsychotics for the management of behavioral symptoms refractory to non-pharmacological interventions. Current guidelines to limit antipsychotic prescriptions among nursing home residents are difficult to implement due to lack of staff training in non-pharmacological alternatives, the wishes of distressed relatives and caregivers, staffing issues, and the lack of expert geriatric mental health services at these facilities.

Adult Day Services

Adult day services (ADS) help support the health, nutritional, social, and daily living needs of adults with functional limitations in a group setting during daytime hours. Adult day care also supports family caregivers by enabling them to continue to work and receive respite. The National Study of Long-Term Care Providers [5] reported an estimate of 4800 ADS centers in the USA. Approximately 84% of ADS centers are located in metropolitan areas, leaving many suburban and rural older adults without this important option. Over 64% of ADS participants are 65 and older in age [5]. It has been difficult to measure the effectiveness of ADS due to lack of standard definition, type of interventions provided, the variability in attendance among participants, and the variation in size of different centers. Despite these challenges, ADS benefit caregivers, provide educational programs, and support group treatments. ADS have positive impact on the emotional well-being of participants [63, 64]. With the growing population of older adults and the fiscal challenges we face in providing them long-term care services, more research is needed to examine the ability of ADS to prevent or delay more costly long-term care for older adults with psychiatric disorders.

Conclusions

Aging is a complex process, and understanding its effect on our patients helps us provide better care to these individuals. Awareness of the higher rates of psychiatric disorders in LTC facilities and similar settings is essential for all staff involved in care of individuals in these facilities. Individuals living in these facilities have greater levels of physical, mental, and social vulnerabilities. The emphasis on care among these individuals should be on early identification of the various disorders and provision of treatment. Adequate training of staff including the use of standardized screening tools has been shown to help identify older adults in need of further interventions. Additionally, the use of a multifaceted approach in the management of psychiatric disorders among older adults receiving care at the various care facilities has been shown to result in better outcomes.

References

1. Kemper P, Komisar HL, Alecxih L. Long-term care over an uncertain future: what can current retirees expect? Inquiry. 2005–2006;42(4):335–50.
2. Vincent GK, Velkoff VA. The next four decades: the older population in the United States: 2010 to 2050. Current population reports. Washington, DC: US Census Bureau; 2010. p. 25–1138.
3. Jones AL, Dwyer LL, Bercovitz AR, Strahan GW. The National Nursing Home Survey: 2004 overview. Vital Health Stat 13. 2009;167:1–155.
4. Seitz D, Purandare N, Conn D. Prevalence of psychiatric disorders among older adults in long-term care homes: a systematic review. Int Psychogeriatr. 2010;22(7):1025–39.
5. Harris-Kojetin L, Sengupta M, Park-Lee E, Valverde R, Caffrey C, Rome V, Lendon J. Long-term care providers and services users in the United States: data from the National Study of long-term care providers, 2013–2014. Vital Health Stat 3. 2016;38(x–xii):1–105.
6. Forster A, Lambley R, Hardy J, Young J, Smith J, Green J, Burns E. Rehabilitation for older people in long-term care. Cochrane Database Syst Rev. 2009;1:CD004294.
7. Carpenter GI, Hastie CL, Morris JN, Fries BE, Ankri J. Measuring change in activities of daily living in nursing home residents with moderate to severe cognitive impairment. BMC Geriatr. 2006;6:7.
8. Lorenz RA, Gooneratne N, Cole CS, Kleban MH, Kalra GK, Richards KC. Exercise and social activity improve everyday function in long-term care residents. Am J Geriatr Psychiatry. 2012;20(6):468–76.
9. Owsley C, Sloane M, McGwin G Jr, Ball K. Timed instrumental activities of daily living tasks: relationship to cognitive function and everyday performance assessments in older adults. Gerontology. 2002;48(4):254–65.

10. Boyce RD, Hanlon JT, Karp JF, Kloke J, Saleh A, Handler SM. A review of the effectiveness of antidepressant medications for depressed nursing home residents. Am Med Dir Assoc. 2012;13(4):326–31.
11. Koenig HG, Meador KG, Cohen HJ, Blazer DG. Depression in elderly hospitalized patients with medical illness. Arch Intern Med. 1988;148(9):1929–36.
12. Mitchell AJ, Bird V, Rizzo M, Meader N. Which version of the geriatric depression scale is most useful in medical settings and nursing homes? Diagnostic validity meta-analysis. Am J Geriatr Psychiatry. 2010;18(12):1066–77.
13. Yesavage JA, Brink TL, Rose TL, Lum O, Huang V, Adey M, Leirer VO. Development and validation of a geriatric depression screening scale: a preliminary report. J Psychiatr Res. 1982–1983;17(1):37–49.
14. Yesavage JA, Brink TL, Rose TL, Lum O, Huang V, Adey MB, Leirer VO. Development and validation of a geriatric depression screening scale: a preliminary report. J Psychiatr Res. 1983;17:37–49.
15. Alexopoulos GS, Abrams RC, Young RC, Shamoian CA. Cornell scale for depression in dementia. Biol Psychiatry. 1988;23(3):271–84.
16. Hamilton M. A rating scale for depression. J Neurol Neurosurg Psychiatry. 1960;23:56–62.
17. Teresi J, Abrams R, Holmes D, et al. Prevalence of depression and depression recognition in nursing homes. Soc Psychiatry Psychiatr Epidemiol. 2001;36:613–20.
18. Watson LC, Zimmerman S, Cohen LW, Dominik R. Practical depression screening in residential care/assisted living: five methods compared with gold standard diagnoses. Am J Geriatr Psychiatry. 2009;17(7):556–64.
19. Jeon YH, Liu Z, Li Z, Low LF, Chenoweth L, O'Connor D, Beattie E, Davison TE, Brodaty H. Development and validation of a short version of the Cornell scale for depression in dementia for screening residents in nursing homes. Am J Geriatr Psychiatry. 2016;24(11):1007–16.
20. Blank K, Gruman C, Robison JT. Case-finding for depression in elderly people: balancing ease of administration with validity in varied treatment settings. J Gerontol A Biol Sci Med Sci. 2004;59(4):378–84.
21. Simning A, Simons KV. Treatment of depression in nursing home residents without significant cognitive impairment: a systematic review. Int Psychogeriatr. 2017;29(2):209–26.
22. Wang JJ. The effects of reminiscence on depressive symptoms and mood status of older institutionalized adults in Taiwan. Int J Geriatr Psychiatry. 2005;20(1):57–62.
23. Chiang KJ, Chu H, Chang HJ, Chung MH, Chen CH, Chiou HY, Chou KR. The effects of reminiscence therapy on psychological well-being, depression, and loneliness among the institutionalized aged. Int J Geriatr Psychiatry. 2010;25(4):380–8.
24. Burrows AB, Salzman C, Satlin A, Noble K, Pollock BG, Gersh T. A randomized, placebo-controlled trial of paroxetine in nursing home residents with non-major depression. Depress Anxiety. 2002;15(3):102–10.
25. Oslin DW, Ten Have TR, Streim JE, Datto CJ, Weintraub D, DiFilippo S, Katz IR. Probing the safety of medications in the frail elderly: evidence from a randomized clinical trial of sertraline and venlafaxine in depressed nursing home residents. J Clin Psychiatry. 2003;64(8):875–82.
26. Streim JE, Oslin DW, Katz IR, Smith BD, DiFilippo S, Cooper TB, Ten Have T. Drug treatment of depression in frail elderly nursing home residents. Am J Geriatr Psychiatry. 2000;8(2):150–9.
27. Katz IR, Parmelee PA. Overview. In: Rubinstein RL, Lawton MP, editors. Depression in long term and residential care. New York: Springer; 1997. p. 1–25.
28. Creighton AS, Davison TE, Kissane DW. The prevalence of anxiety among older adults in nursing homes and other residential aged care facilities: a systematic review. Int J Geriatr Psychiatry. 2016;31(6):555–66.
29. Creighton AS, Davison TE, Kissane DW. The correlates of anxiety among older adults in nursing home and other residential aged care facilities: a systematic review. Int J Geriatr Psychiatry. 2017;32(2):141–54.
30. Mansbach WE, Mace RA, Clark KM. The Brief Anxiety and Depression Scale (BADS): a new instrument for detecting anxiety and depression in long-term care residents. Int Psychogeriatr. 2015;27(4):673–81.
31. Gerolimatos LA, Gregg JJ, Edelstein BA. Assessment of anxiety in long-term care: examination of the Geriatric Anxiety Inventory (GAI) and its short form. Int Psychogeriatr. 2013;25(9):1533–42.
32. Stanley MA, Beck JG, Novy DM, Averill PM, Swann AC, Diefenbach GJ, Hopko DR. Cognitive-behavioral treatment of late-life generalized anxiety disorder. J Consult Clin Psychol. 2003;71(2):309–19.
33. Wetherell JL, Gatz M, Craske MG. Treatment of generalized anxiety disorder in older adults. J Consult Clin Psychol. 2003;71(1):31–40.

34. Flint AJ. Generalised anxiety disorder in elderly patients: epidemiology, diagnosis and treatment options. Drugs Aging. 2005;22(2):101–14.
35. Sung HC, Chang AM, Lee WL. A preferred music listening intervention to reduce anxiety in older adults with dementia in nursing homes. J Clin Nurs. 2010;19(7–8):1056–64.
36. Stevenson DG, Decker SL, Dwyer LL, Huskamp HA, Grabowski DC, Metzger ED, Mitchell SL. Antipsychotic and benzodiazepine use among nursing home residents: findings from the 2004 National Nursing Home Survey. Am J Geriatr Psychiatry. 2010;18(12):1078–92.
37. American Psychiatric Association. Benzodiazepine dependence, toxicity and abuse. Washington, DC: American Psychiatric Association; 1990.
38. Chen L, Bell JS, Visvanathan R, Hilmer SN, Emery T, Robson L, Hughes JM, Tan EC. The association between benzodiazepine use and sleep quality in residential aged care facilities: a cross-sectional study. BMC Geriatr. 2016;16(1):196.
39. Schweizer E, Rickels K, Lucki I. Resistance to the anti-anxiety effect of buspirone in patients with a history of benzodiazepine use. N Engl J Med. 1986;314:719–20.
40. DeMartinis N, Rynn M, Rickels K, et al. Prior benzodiazepine use and buspirone response in the treatment of generalized anxiety disorder. J Clin Psychiatry. 2000;61:91–4.
41. Abdulla A, Adams N, Bone M, Elliott AM, Gaffin J, Jones D, Knaggs R, Martin D, Sampson L, Schofield P. British geriatric society. Guidance on the management of pain in older people. Age Ageing. 2013;42(Suppl 1):i1–57.
42. Vaismoradi M, Skär L, Söderberg S, Bondas TE. Normalizing suffering: a meta-synthesis of experiences of and perspectives on pain and pain management in nursing homes. Int J Qual Stud Health Well-being. 2016;11(1):31203.
43. Liu JY, Leung DY. Pain treatments for nursing home residents with advanced dementia and substantial impaired communication: a cross-sectional analysis at baseline of a cluster randomized controlled trial. Pain Med. 2016;18(9):1649–57. pii: pnw242
44. Bauer U, Pitzer S, Schreier MM, Osterbrink J, Alzner R, Iglseder B. Pain treatment for nursing home residents differs according to cognitive state—a cross-sectional study. BMC Geriatr. 2016;16:124.
45. Won A, Lapane K, Gambassi G, Bernabei R, Mor V, Lipsitz LA, Nygaard HA, Jarland M. Correlates and management of nonmalignant pain in the nursing home. SAGE study group. Systematic assessment of geriatric drug use via epidemiology. J Am Geriatr Soc. 1999;47(8):936–42.
46. Nygaard HA, Jarland M. Are nursing home patients with dementia diagnosis at increased risk for inadequate pain treatment? Int J Geriatr Psychiatry. 2005;20(8):730–7.
47. Feldt KS. The checklist of nonverbal pain indicators (CNPI). Pain Manag Nurs. 2000;1(1):13–21.
48. US Department of Health and Human Services. https://www.guideline.gov/summaries/summary/45524
49. Sansoni J, Anderson KH, Varona LM, et al. Caregivers of Alzheimer's patients and factors influencing institutionalization of loved ones: some considerations on existing literature. Ann Ig. 2013;25(3):235–46.
50. Hawes C, Morris JN, Phillips CD, Mor V, Fries BE, Nonemaker S. Reliability estimates for the minimum data set for nursing home resident assessment and care screening (MDS). Gerontologist. 1995;35(2):172–8.
51. Frederiksen K, Tariot P, De Jonghe E. Minimum Data Set Plus (MDS+) scores compared with scores from five rating scales. J Am Geriatr Soc. 1996;44(3):305–9.
52. Snowden M, McCormick W, Russo J, Srebnik D, Comtois K, Bowen J, Teri L, Larson EB. Validity and responsiveness of the minimum data set. J Am Geriatr Soc. 1999;47(8):1000–4.
53. Conn DK, Seitz DP. Advances in the treatment of psychiatric disorders in long-term care homes. Curr Opin Psychiatry. 2010;23(6):516–21.
54. O'Connor DW, Ames D, Gardner B, King M. Psychosocial treatments of psychological symptoms in dementia: a systematic review of reports meeting quality standards. Int Psychogeriatr. 2009;21(2):241–51.
55. Kong EH, Evans LK, Guevara JP. Nonpharmacological intervention for agitation in dementia: a systematic review and meta-analysis. Aging Ment Health. 2009;13(4):512–20.
56. Vernooij-Dassen M, Vasse E, Zuidema S, Cohen-Mansfield J, Moyle W. Psychosocial interventions for dementia patients in long-term care. nt Psychogeriatr. 2010;22(7):1121–8.
57. Sorbi S, Hort J, Erkinjuntti T, Fladby T, Gainotti G, Gurvit H, Nacmias B, Pasquier F, Popescu BO, Rektorova I, Religa D, Rusina R, Rossor M, Schmidt R, Stefanova E, Warren JD, Scheltens P, EFNS Scientist Panel on Dementia and Cognitive Neurology. EFNS-ENS guidelines on the diagnosis and management of disorders associated with dementia. Eur J Neurol. 2012;19(9):1159–79.
58. Conn DK, Ferguson I, Mandelman K, Ward C. Psychotropic drug utilization in long-term-care facilities for the elderly in Ontario, Canada. Int Psychogeriatr. 1999;11(3):223–33.

59. Seitz DP, Gruneir A, Conn DK, Rochon PA. Cholinesterase inhibitor use in U.S. nursing homes: results from the national nursing home survey. J Am Geriatr Soc. 2009;57(12):2269–74.
60. Hawes C, Mor V, Phillips CD, Fries BE, Morris JN, Steele-Friedlob E, Greene AM, Nennstiel M. The OBRA-87 nursing home regulations and implementation of the resident assessment instrument: effects on process quality. J Am Geriatr Soc. 1997;45(8):977–85.
61. Ryan JM, Kidder SW, Daiello LA, Tariot PN. Psychopharmacologic interventions in nursing homes: what do we know and where should we go? Psychiatr Serv. 2002;53(11):1407–13.
62. Gurwitz JH, Field TS, Avorn J, McCormick D, Jain S, Eckler M, Benser M, Edmondson AC, Bates DW. Incidence and preventability of adverse drug events in nursing homes. Am J Med. 2000;109(2):87–94.
63. Fields NL, Anderson KA, Dabelko-Schoeny H. The effectiveness of adult day services for older adults: a review of the literature from 2000 to 2011. J Appl Gerontol. 2014;33(2):130–63.
64. Gaugler JE, Jarrott SE, Zarit SH, Stephens MP, Townsend A, Greene R. Adult day service use and reductions in caregiving hours: effects on stress and psychological well-being for dementia caregivers. Int J Geriatr Psychiatry. 2003;18(1):55–62.

30 Special Management Problems

Rosanne M. Radziewicz and Cheryl Bradas

Introduction

Special management problems in geriatrics are common among individuals with dementia. These problems have been termed "Behavioral and Psychological Symptoms of Dementia (BPSD)," a term designated by the International Psychogeriatric Association as "symptoms of disturbed perception, thought content, mood or behavior that frequently occurs in patients with dementia" [1]. If left untreated, these behavioral disturbances can lead to increased mortality [2], greater healthcare resource utilization [3], high rates of admission to psychiatric or residential settings [4], early institutionalization [5], higher use of psychotropic medications [4, 6, 7], and caregiver burden [8].

Epidemiology

Estimates are that at any one point of time as many as two-thirds (67%) of individuals with dementias will exhibit behavioral disturbances that are considered disruptive and unsafe [9]. Agitation and behavioral disturbances can occur in as many as half of community dwellers [10, 11] and 64–80% of residents in long-term care (LTC) settings [11–14].

Individuals with psychosis also pose special management problems. Hallucinations and illusions occur in 10–28% of patients with Alzheimer's disease (AD) [15, 16]. Estimates of the prevalence of delusions in AD have ranged from 10 to 73% [17], with an average of approximately 35% [15]. Prevalence rates of hallucinations range from 3 to 49% [16].

The most common BPSD are wandering, sundowning, shadowing, hoarding, aggression, stubbornness and uncooperativeness with care, inappropriate sexual behavior, and repetitive and vocally disruptive behaviors.

In this next section we review some of the common BPSD in more detail.

Wandering

Up to 60% of persons with dementia will wander [18]. Of the BPSD, wandering is the most unsafe behavior [19]. The phenomenon of wandering is a multidimensional concept which has been defined in various ways including dementia-related locomotion [19]; aimless locomotion with lapping and/or pacing [20]; aimless movement [21]; attempting to go "home," entering other's rooms, and attempting to leave an institution [22]; missing in the community [20]; and a collection of behavioral abnormalities [23]. Wandering can lead to increased morbidity and mortality primarily from accidents, falls, and getting lost [24]. In the most global sense, wandering is viewed from dichotomous perspectives, either as a derogatory term to those with dementia or as a normal human activity [25]. At present for wandering, there is no scientifically agreed upon operational definition, mutually accepted

R. R. Tampi et al. (eds.), *Psychiatric Disorders Late in Life*, https://doi.org/10.1007/978-3-319-73078-3_30

understanding of the concept, or clear understanding of the etiology [25]. However, two universal characteristics of wandering do appear in every description of wandering: being cognitively impaired and walking [25].

The vast majority of research in dementia-related wandering has been completed by Algase and her team with their most current proposed definition as:

"A syndrome of dementia-related locomotion behavior having a frequent, repetitive, temporally disordered and/or spatially disoriented nature is manifested in lapping, random and/or pacing patterns, some of which are associated with eloping, eloping attempts or getting lost unless accompanied [19]."

The gap which remains is the distinction between wandering to enhance the wanderer's sense of well-being and wandering which may have adverse effects, leaving the healthcare professional or caregiver to interpret the wanderer's motivation for wandering and the potential consequences which may exist [25].

Three wandering typologies have been identified by Algase and her research team: classic, moderate, and subclinical [26]. Classic wanderers exhibited the most wandering in terms of both frequency and duration and also tend to wander earlier in the day. Furthermore, classic wanderers were the most cognitively impaired and were the most independent in mobility. However, their overall health was the poorest. Moderate wanderers tended to wander about half the time of the classic wanderers and had less cognitive impairment, decreased mobility, and better overall health status than classic or subclinical wanderers. Subclinical wanderers had low levels of wandering often being identified by staff as non-wanderers. They were the least cognitively impaired and had a level of mobility similar to the moderate wanderers, and their overall health status was between the classic and moderate wanderers [26]. While three typologies were identified, variation within groups was high. Wandering may occur during the day or in the evening which, often times, creates semantic confusion between wandering and sundowning [25]. However, sundowning also includes agitated behaviors [27]. While there is no definite time for wandering, it does occur throughout the day with direct wandering primarily early in the day and random wandering increasing as the day goes on [28]. However, some authors have identified peak times to be between 2:00 pm and 4:00 pm [29] or 7:00 am and 7:00 pm [25].

Based on a systematic literature review, Robinson et al. [23] identified a lack of robust evidence to recommend the use of any specific non-pharmacological interventions to reduce or prevent dementia-related wandering. However, options to consider include physical barriers, physical restraints, distraction therapies, sensory therapies, behavioral therapies, caregiver interventions, and environmental modifications [23, 24]. Non-pharmacological interventions should remain the first choice of intervention as they are relatively low risk. As with non-pharmacological interventions, there are no clear indications of which type of specific pharmacological therapy should be used for wandering [24]. Furthermore, the use of atypical antipsychotics such as risperidone and olanzapine increased mortality 60–70% primarily from heart failure, sudden death, and pneumonia in addition to being associated with increased risk of falls [24].

Sundowning

The prevalence rates of sundowning among individuals with dementia range from 2.4% to as high as 66% [27, 30, 31]. Sundowning is thought to be the second most disruptive BPSD after wandering by some authors [27], and it causes significant caregiver burden often resulting in premature institutionalization [27, 32–36]. Sundown syndrome in persons with dementia is a collection of behaviors representing multiple symptoms such as confusion, agitation, anxiety, wandering, hallucinations (auditory and visual), suspiciousness, and screaming which tend to begin in the late afternoon and often continue into the evening and night hours [27, 37]. While it occurs primarily among the cognitively impaired, those exhibiting sundown syndrome characteristics may or may not have dementia [27]. "Sundowning" is not a psychiatric diagnosis but rather a descriptive term. What distinguishes sundowning from late afternoon or evening wandering are the associated disruptive behaviors [27]. As with wandering, there is not an agreed upon consensus of a conceptual definition or clear underlying etiology of sundowning [27, 32, 37, 38].

The etiology of sundowning has generally been divided into three major categories: physiological, psychological, and environmental. Proposed theories have focused on sensory deprivation, circadian rhythm disorders, sleep disorders, maladaptive responses to environmental stimuli, temporal changes in body temperature, medication side effects or "wearing off" often from antidepressants and antipsychotics, and medical and psychiatric conditions [27, 32, 39, 40]. In a qualitative study by Nowak and Davis, six behavioral characteristics of sundowning were identified: physical aggression, resistiveness, disconcerted verbalizing, nighttime sleeplessness, wandering, and daytime sleepiness [41]. Diagnosis of sundowning is strictly clinical as there are no lab tests or imaging to confirm diagnosis. There is also semantic confusion between sundowning and delirium as sundowning is often called nocturnal delirium [37]. However, delirium is characterized by altered behavior and mental status with an acute onset, fluctutating course, inattention, and either disorganzied thinking or an altered level of consciousness which is considered a medical emergency [37, 42]. The majority of authors argue sundowning, unlike delirium, is not associated with an acute medical illness or high mortality [27, 36, 40, 42]. Yet, some authors have identified delirium as a precursor to sundowning [27] and is considered a marker of frailty [39, 40, 43].

Treatments for sundowning consist of both non-pharmacological and pharmacological interventions. Effective interventions have included light therapy to improve quality of sleep, music therapy, aromatherapy, caregiver education, the use of melatonin in those with circadian rhythm disruptions, acetylcholinesterase inhibitors (AChEIs) (although no strong evidence exists for their use), and the use of antipsychotics (the most widely used for symptoms of sundowning) with risperidone being one of the most commonly used medications. There is a paucity of research on prognosis of persons experiencing sundowning syndrome. In addition, there is limited data on prevention measures [27].

Shadowing

A common BPSD is shadowing or the following closely of another person contributing to significant caregiver burden from stress, lack of privacy, anger, and anxiety [44, 45]. Prevalence is difficult to determine as shadowing is often grouped within other measurement tools such as the anxiety subscale of the Neuropsychiatric Inventory (NPI) [46], the Revised Memory and Behavior Problems Checklist (RMBPC) [47], and in "other" categories [45]. When examining the relationship between results of the Mini-Mental State Examination (MMSE) and Clinical Dementia Rating (CDR) scale, an inverse relationship was noted with an increase in anxiety and shadowing to a decrease in cognitive function [48, 49]. Prevalence rates of 14% at baseline and as high as 62% at 5 years were noted by researchers administering the anxiety subscale of the NPI in community-dwelling older adults in Cache County, Utah [50].

It has been suggested that shadowing is a result of fear, uncertainty, or feelings of insecurity [44] and is considered the most intrusive BPSD occurring in the later stages of dementia [44]. In AD, progressive neurodegeneration occurs over a period of years with the temporal lobes and limbic areas being the regions experiencing the greatest changes [45]. A relationship has been suggested between persons with dementia who had genetic variation in the serotonin transporter gene with short alleles and activation of the amygdala [51] as well as short alleles and risk for unresolved attachment issues [52]. While the temporal lobes and limbic areas are impacted by Alzheimer's, the orbitofrontal cortex does not appear to be impacted to the same degree, an area which contains survival-based instinctual behaviors such as proximity seeking [45, 53]. Like sundowning, shadowing is more frequent in the late afternoon or early evening [44], and shadowing may precede sundowning in some persons with dementia. Psychoeducational interventions are primarily focused on the caregiver and are centered on disease-based changes, distraction, caregiver self-efficacy, environmental modifications, and journaling [45, 54].

Hoarding

Hoarding disorder (HD) is a chronic condition with symptoms being described along a continuum of collecting items to self-neglect, with prevalence rates among persons with dementia ranging from 1 to 22% [55, 56]. Not only do persons with HD collect an excessive amount of objects, but they also have intense difficulty discarding or separating with items to the point rooms cannot be used for their original purpose [55–58]. It has long been suggested that hoarding resulted from obsessive-compulsive disorder (OCD) and obsessive-compulsive personality disorder (OCPD); however, recent evidence over the past two decades suggests that hoarding is a new diagnostic category and was recognized in the *Diagnostic and Statistical Manual*, 5th edition (DSM-5), as a distinct disord Hoarding disorder (HD)er: hoarding disorder (HD) [55, 57]. While hoarding can occur in OCD, 60–80% of the cases are independent of OCD with differing neurocognitive profiles as well as treatment outcomes [55, 58]. Obsessive-compulsive disorder symptoms fluctuate over time yet remain relatively consistent. Hoarding symptoms, on the other hand, tend to be progressive, slowly increasing over time, and appear to be related to deficits in executive function [58]. Hoarding behaviors in dementia are more common when individuals are less severely impaired, and while persons with HD may develop dementia in late life, persons with dementia can develop hoarding symptoms creating investigative chal Hoarding disorder (HD)lenges for researchers [55].

Once considered a low-severity behavior, HD is now recognized to contribute substantially to caregiver burden and, for the hoarder, social isolation, health risks, functional impairment, and distress [56, 58]. Selective serotonin reuptake inhibitors (SSRIs) are commonly used for hoarding in OCD; however, there is no empirical support regarding specific medications for hoarding in dementia. Yet, SSRIs as well as serotonin-norepinephrine reuptake inhibitors (SNRIs) remain the most commonly used pharmacologic treatment for HD [56, 58]. Additionally, while behavioral interventions have shown promise for hoarding in persons with developmental disabilities, previous samples had not included persons with dementia [56]. Current literature identifies cogni Hoarding disorder (HD)tive behavioral therapy (CBT) as the key feature of psychotherapy for persons with HD [55, 58].

Aggression

Aggression occurs between 25 and 87% of elderly residents living in nursing homes with cognitive decline [59–63]. Aggression has been linked to atrophy of the frontal, insular, amygdala, cingulate, and hippocampal regions of the brain [64]. Evidence varies on whether behavioral symptomatology emerges with a decline in cognition [7, 64, 65]. Genetic studies in AD show a significant association between the number of apolipoprotein E (APOE) epsilon 4 alleles present, with delusions and more severe agitation and aggression being seen among homozygous APOE epsilon 4 carriers [66]. Aggression is also associated with psychosis, depression, and agitation [67]. Among individuals with AD, psychosis is associated with low education (mild/moderate stages) and African American race (moderate/severe stages) [67]. Other studies show aggression as more likely if the individual has a history of conduct disorder [61], requires more assistance with personal care [4], and has pain [8, 68–71] and disruptions in sleep [72].

Aggressive behavior can be physical or verbal and contribute to burnout among caregivers. One study revealed that 27% of geriatric patients displayed verbal assaults, and 20% of these elderly patients engaged in physical assaults [73]. As staff and others withdraw from aggressive patients, the result can lead to an increase in the patient's disorientation and frustration and lowering of self-esteem [74]. Frequently, team meetings to review triggers to aggression can be useful in limiting this behavior in residential settings.

It is estimated that approximately 77% of the challenging behaviors are psychosocial in nature and are modifiable with non-pharmacological strategies [75–77]. Helpful strategies include limiting unnecessary stimulation [6] and person-centered care (e.g., considering the person over the task, approach of gentleness, verbal support) [77–84]. Individualizing music has been effective in providing short-term reductions in agitation [85, 86]. Training caregivers in models of care such as the progressively lowered stress threshold (PLST) model [81, 87, 88]; the Antecedent, Behavior, Consequence Model [89]; bathing without a battle training [78]; or other behavioral management training programs [90] has shown a reduction of aggression behaviors with performing activities of daily living (ADLs).

Psychotropic medications have had some value in treating aggression in individuals with dementia, but none are indicated for aggression in dementia [91]. Caution is indicated when using these medications due to the risk of adverse effects, particularly the increased risk of cardiovascular events and early mortality [91]. A systematic review showed that off-label use of atypical antipsychotics for treating AD-related agitation showed only modest efficacy or no benefits when compared with placebo [92].

Antipsychotics [olanzapine, risperidone] have been found to be useful for short-term use (6–12 weeks) for the management of anger, aggression, and paranoia among individuals with AD [some clinical improvement] [93, 94]. Short-term use of propranolol has shown efficacy in improving agitation/aggression including uncooperativeness and anxiety in nursing home residents with probable or possible AD [95].

Electroconvulsive therapy has shown promise in a few descriptive studies to be a safe treatment option for reducing symptoms of agitation and aggression among individuals with dementia whose behaviors are refractory to medication management [96, 97].

Stubbornness and Uncooperativeness with Care

Stubbornness and uncooperativeness with care among individuals with dementia has been shown to be related to unmet needs with pain control [98, 99], communication deficits with deteriorating cognitive status [67], and declining functional status [65]. One study of self-destructive behavior in a nursing home environment showed that uncooperativeness with care was associated with LTC settings in which there were fewer policies and training for staff on dealing with difficult behaviors [100].

In a systematic review of RCTs and quasi-experimental studies, playing patient-preferred music [101, 102] and person-centered care significantly reduced uncooperative behavior [101]. Education of the caregivers on managing behaviors has been successful in reducing behavioral symptoms and promoting positive affect among individuals with dementia [103]. Intervention protocols that showed positive effect included complex guideline-based interventions [104], education to modify antecedents and consequences of the behavior [105], and individualized interventions for the resident [106]. For verbal aggression, an individualized protocol for managing behavior that includes addressing needs for comfort, social interaction, and sensory stimulation was significant in reducing disrupted behavior during the actual intervention [107].

Despite the value of person-centered care managing disruptive behaviors, it is not often implemented. A study of older adults living in a rural area showed that caregivers had a good understanding of possible underlying causes of behaviors among individuals with dementia, but a poor understanding of appropriate methods of management and resources available to assist them. Time constraints were frequently cited by respondents as being problematic in managing behavioral problems [108].

Uncooperative behaviors are often amenable to pharmacological management strategies. Short-term use of propranolol may be helpful specifically for aggression and uncooperativeness; however, its usefulness in the very old and frail population is limited by the high frequency of relative contraindications to beta-adrenergic antagonist treatment and diminution of initial behavioral improvements over time [95].

Low-dose antipsychotics have been useful in treating behaviors [109] but are limited by extrapyramidal effects, anticholinergic effects, sedation, postural hypotension, risk of falls, cardiovascular accidents, torsade de pointes, and death [110].

Carbamazepine used to treat agitation, hostility, and uncooperativeness in severely demented individuals with AD who had failed antipsychotic treatment showed significant improvements in factor score activation and hostility after 4 weeks [111].

Inappropriate Sexual Behavior

Normal aging slows the sexual cycle, but does not take away the elder's capacity to enjoy sex as a way of expressing closeness. With cognitive decline, it can be difficult for the older adult to appropriately express their need for intimacy. Inappropriate sexual behavior (ISB) with dementia occurs between 2 and 25% of individuals with cognitive decline and is defined as any verbal or physical action of a sexual nature that is displayed in an inappropriate social context, causes distress to all those involved, and impairs the care of the patient in that environment [10, 112, 113]. Types of ISBs include sexual talk, acts, implied sexual acts (pornography) [114], or false sexual allegations (delusions, hallucinations, delusional obsessions). Sexual behaviors can be further defined as intimacy seeking or disinhibition [115].

Sexual behavior is natural and those with dementia have the same right as others to express their sexual feelings. Assessment of a person's competency to engage in a sexual relationship is necessary to avoid a violation of rights, protect vulnerability to exploitation, and minimize risk of harm. For proper diagnosis and to determine appropriate intervention strategies, a thorough assessment must include the type and frequency of behavior, the context and contributing factors, whether the behavior is problematic or poses risk and if so to whom, whether the patient is competent, or whether behavior is a sign of self-care deficit rather than an ISB [113, 116].

Assessments and evaluations should be carefully documented to support the use of management strategies. The St. Andrew's Sexual Behaviour Assessment (SASBA) instrument was developed as a valid and reliable tool to measure and record ISB [117]. This scale allows observation and determination of severity of four categories of ISB (verbal comments, noncontact, exposure, and touching others) which can help standardize behavioral outcomes.

In a review of literature, ISBs occur from a relationship between the neurological, physical, psychological, and environmental factors [118]. The most prominent change in frontotemporal dementia is hypo-sexual behavior [119]. ISBs can be the result of damage to four different brain regions: the frontal lobes, the temporolimbic system, the striatum, and the hypothalamus [112]. Damage to the frontal system can result in disinhibition as seen in various dementias, multiple sclerosis and frontal tumors, and stroke [112, 120, 121]. Disruption of the temporolimbic system may result in hypersexual behaviors such as those observed in strokes, tumors or epilepsy involving the temporal lobes, or the Kluver-Bucy syndrome (i.e., bilateral medial temporal lobe dysfunction characterized by hypersexuality, hyperorality, emotional placidity, and an inability to recognize objects or faces) [122, 123]. Pathology involving the striatum (seen in cases of Parkinson's disease, Tourette's syndrome, and Huntington's disease) may produce obsessive-compulsive features, including sexual fixations. Lesions of the hypothalamus can provoke hypersexual behavior. An example of such hypothalamic damage is the uncommon Kleine-Levin syndrome, which is typically seen in adolescent males and involves alternating episodes of hypersomnia and hyperphagia [112].

Sensory impairments, delusions, and misidentifications may be a factor in ISBs. Premorbid behaviors and mood disorders can affect sexual interest and misinterpretation of cues. Social factors include lack of usual sexual partner, lack of privacy, understimulating, or unfamiliar environments. Alcohol and benzodiazepines can produce disinhibition, and L-dopa can cause hypersexuality in people with Parkinson's disease [113]. The sudden emergence of ISB can herald delirium, and a comprehensive approach is needed to rule out underlying medical illness [124].

Treatment should involve clarifying the differential diagnoses such as psychosis, mood disorders, and delirium and the use of agents that can trigger disinhibition or hypersexuality (levodopa, benzodiazepines, alcohol, and stimulants).

First-line treatment for ISBs is the use of nonpharmacological strategies and the involvement of the caregiver or family for support. Treatment strategies include the removal of precipitating factors (e.g., overstimulating television or radio programs), modifying triggers (monitoring if another resident reminds the patient of his/her spouse), distraction, providing consistent and gentle redirection, avoiding confrontation, reducing communication barriers [121], involvement of geriatric medicine specialists [125], and creative strategies to help release sexual urges [126]. Modifications to clothing (e.g., trousers that open in the back or have zippers removed) may also be helpful.

Suggested pharmacological management strategies for ISBs in dementia are based on case reports and uncontrolled studies [124] and must be used with caution in view of their possible adverse effects among the older adult population. Pharmacologic treatments include (1) antidepressants including sertraline [127], paroxetine [128], citalopram [129, 130], clomipramine [131], and trazodone [132]; (2) antiandrogens including medroxyprogesterone acetate [133–136], cyproterone, [137, 138], and finasteride [139]; (3) LHRH agonists including leuprolide [140]; (4) estrogens including diethylstilbestrol [138, 141] and oral or transdermal estrogen [142]; (5) antipsychotics including haloperidol [143, 144] and quetiapine [145–147]; (6) anticonvulsants including gabapentin [148–150] and carbamazepine [151–153]; (7) cholinesterase inhibitors including rivastigmine [154] and donepezil [155]; (8) cimetidine [156]; (9) beta blockers including propranolol [140] and pindolol [157]; and (10) other drugs including ketoconazole and spironolactone [156]. Based on a link identified between the cannabinoid pathway and dementia [158, 159], a case report showed nabilone, a synthetic cannabinoid, improved sexual disinhibition associated with dementia in a patient who was refractory to other treatment modalities [160].

Algorithms have been proposed based on severity of behaviors [142, 161]. Unless the patient is engaging in or theatening dangerous acts involving physical contact, serotoninergics (first choice, SSRIs; second choice, TCAs) are first-line agents followed by antiandrogens (cyproterone acetate or medroxyprogesterone acetate) as second-line agents. LHRH agonists (first choice) and estrogens (second choice) are considered third-line agents. Combination therapy is reasonable if the individual fails to respond to monotherapy.

Repetitive Behaviors

Repetitive behaviors, including repetitive questioning and repetitive actions, are thought to be amnestic behaviors among BPSD [162, 163] (old 2–3). While repetitive questioning (the most frequent repetitive behavior) is common in the early stages of dementia, repetitive actions are often not seen until the person's dementia is more advanced [162–164]. Among individuals with dementia, repetitive behaviors are often due to anxiety, frustration, challenges with coping from multiple stimuli, environmental deprivation, and unmet needs [165]. Repetitive behaviors are also hypothesized to be a result of disruption in the basal ganglia or corticostriatal structures [164] as well as an increase or preservation of regional cerebral blood flow in the left pericallosal region [162]. While typically not harmful, repetitive behaviors can add to caregiver burden (AA). Suggestions for managing repetitive behaviors tend to focus around diversions, redirection, reassurance, and behavioral interventions such as purposeful activities and memory books [165].

Vocally Disruptive Behavior

Vocally disruptive behavior (VDB) includes repetitive questions, frequent requests for attention, complaining, whining, making strange noises, screaming, using abusive language, moaning, perseveration, and repetitive and inappropriate requests. It is estimated that vocally disruptive behaviors occur in approximately 11–30% of nursing home residents [166, 167].

VDB is often related to vulnerability, suffering, and a loss of meaning [99, 168–170]. The most prevalent unmet needs identified as causes of VDB include boredom/sensory deprivation, loneliness/need for social interaction, and the need for meaningful activity. Discomfort is also commonly associated with VDB [99, 170]. In one study, negative vocalizations were associated with infantilizing communication (elderspeak) [171].

VDB often occurs in advanced stages of dementia [172]. Other causes of VDB include physical discomfort, psychiatric illness (psychosis, hallucinations, delusions, self-stimulation, depression, anxiety/panic, prior history of loss, abuse, or stress), and social factors (social isolation or sensory deprivation) [166]. Case studies of VDB have shown this behavior is reinforced by contingent attention by the nursing staff [173].

Consequences of VDB include aggression by other residents in nursing home (NH) settings [174], caregiver burden, early NH placement, overuse of polypharmacy, and increased healthcare costs [175].

McMinn et al. suggest interventions targeted toward treating neurological causes of VDB, addressing unmet needs, increase stimulation to address possible deprivation or loneliness, and the use of behavioral approaches including reinforcing more adaptive behaviors [166]. It is realistic to expect a residual level of VDB even after interventions [176]. In addition, targeted training to the caregivers and providing consultation to support patient-centered care may reduce caregiver burden with this challenging behavior [177].

Treatment of VDB has limited efficacy. The type of intervention chosen should be guided by the assessment and be included in the patient's care plan to ensure consistency. Addressing sensory deprivation, social isolation, disorientation, communication deficits, discomfort, and pain in nursing care plan was effective when followed [178]. In one study, preferred music, one-to-one social interactions, and watching a family-generated videotape were effective in decreasing VDB over nonintervention controls [179]. The value of case conferences to manage VDB has mixed results [180]. Communication skills training and behavioral management of nursing assistants demonstrated a positive reduction of VDB [181]. Operant treatments and contingent attention to quiet behavior had limited success and appear to be more acceptable to nursing staff and elderly individuals [181, 182].

Evidence indicates that treatment with antidepressants may reduce VDB [166]. Treatment with risperidone has also shown benefit in the management of VDB, particularly if the VDB is associated with psychosis or aggression [183]. A few case reports also indicate the value of using ECT for managing VDB [184].

Restraints

Evidence indicates that restraints are often used among older adults who exhibit poor participation with activities of daily living (ADL), who demonstrated severe cognitive and mobility impairments, who had repeated verbal and physical agitation, and among those with a history of previous fall and/or fracture [185–188]. Restraints are often used with the goal of protecting the patient or others from harm or to permit necessary care or treatment [188] with the mistaken belief that they are necessary to ensure safety, provide postural support, or prevent falls. Despite its common use, there is no literature that indicates that restraints actually protect patients [189] or prevent falls [190–194]. Restraints can also result in fractures [194], can worsen psychological well-being [195], and can promote the negative effects of immobility including functional and cognitive decline [196, 197], incontinence, pressure ulcers, weakening, increased dependency and regressive behaviors, and even death [198]. Older adults in restraint had longer lengths of stay in the hospital [199] and demonstrated decreased quality of life [200]. The use of restraints may also contradict the older individual's right to freedom, autonomy, and respect [201].

Evidence indicates that there are inconsistencies regarding the nursing staff's definition of restraints [202] and the mistaken belief that the utilization of restraints among the elderly benefits the institution [201]. Due to the dangers associated with the use of restraints among the elderly, the Omnibus Budget Reconciliation Act (OBRA) of 1987 places strict regulations on their use among this vulnerable population [203]. These regulations have helped reduce the use of restraint among older adults [204].

Physical restraints include any method or device that limits a person's freedom to move or access his or her body and/or cannot be easily removed. It is the intent of the method or device on the person that causes it to be a restraint. Examples of physical restraints include:

- Side rails on beds used to prevent the patient from leaving the bed
- Limb and waist restraints
- Hand mitts that restrict movement in the fingers/wrist

- Geri chairs
- Over-the-bed tables and trays that cannot be removed without help
- Chairs or recliners that do not let a person get up on his or her own
- Keeping a person in a closed or locked area for long periods of time
- Positioning a wheelchair so that the person cannot move it or get out of it

Chemical restraint includes any medication that is used involuntarily with the intent of restricting a person's behavior or function [205].

Restraint alternatives must be attempted and found to be unsuccessful before using restraints [206]. Programs that are successful in reducing restraint include a person-centered approach, assessing and monitoring for changes in behavior, environmental modifications, flexibility, team dialogue, and respect for patient's needs and rights [207]. Education to staff and families has been found successful in promoting restraint reduction [208–210] and the use of psychotropic drugs [211].

Conclusions

Evidence indicates that BPSD are not uncommon and worsen outcomes among individuals with dementia. Additionally, BPSD poses a significant risk for harm to the older adult with dementia and their caregivers. Often the etiology for many of these behaviors is multifactorial with close interactions between the biological, psychological, and social factors. Current evidence does not indicate which type of non-pharmacological or pharmacological therapies is most effective in the treatment of these behaviors. But, non-pharmacological strategies are preferred given the significant risks associated with the use of pharmacological agents among individuals with dementia. Individualized treatment approaches are recommended, and in most cases psychoeducation to caregivers and staff to increase understanding of underlying causes of these behaviors and options for management has been found to be helpful.

References

1. International Psychogeriatric Association. Behavioral and Psychological Symptoms of Dementia (BPSD) educational pack – module 1. http://dbmas.org.au/uploads/resources/IPA_BPSD_Educational_Pack.pdf. Published 1998, Updated 2002, Accessed 12 May 2016.
2. Finkel SI, Costa e Silva J, Cohen G, Miller S, Sartorius N. Behavioral and psychological symptoms of dementia: a consensus statement on current knowledge and implication for research and treatment. Int Psychogeriatr. 1996;8(3 Suppl):497–500.
3. Steele C, Rovner B, Chase GA, Folstein M. Psychiatric symptoms and nursing home placement patients with Alzheimer's disease. Am J Psychiatry. 1990;147:1049–51.
4. Gibbons P, Gannon M, Wrigley M. A study of aggression among referrals to a community-based psychiatry of old age service. Int J Geriatr Psychiatry. 1997;12(3):384–8.
5. O'Donnell BF, Drachman DA, Barnes HJ, Peterson KE, Swearer JM, Lew RA. Incontinence and troublesome behaviors predict institutionalization in dementia. J Geriatr Psychiatry Neurol. 1992;5:45–52.
6. Isaksson U, Graneheim UH, Åström S, Karlsson S. Physically violent behaviour in dementia care: characteristics of residents and management of violent situations. Aging Ment Health. 2011;15(5):573–9.
7. Majic T, Pluta JP, Mell T, Treusch Y, Gutzmann H, Rapp MA. Correlates of agitation and depression in nursing home residents with dementia. Int Psychogeriatr. 2012;24(7):1779–89.
8. Morgan RO, Sail KR, Snow AL, Davila JA, Fouladi NN, Kunik ME. Modeling causes of aggressive behavior in patients with dementia. Gerontologist. 2013;53(5):738–47.
9. Lyketsos CG, Steinberg M, Tschanz JT, Norton MC, Steffens DC, Breitner JC. Mental and behavioral disturbances in dementia: findings from Cache County Study on Memory and Aging. Am J Psychiatry. 2000;157:708–14.
10. Stubbs B. Displays of inappropriate sexual behaviour by patients with progressive cognitive impairment: the forgotten form of challenging behaviour? J Psychiatr Ment Health Nurs. 2011;18(7):602–7.
11. Folstein M, Anthony IC, Parhad I, Duffy B, Gruenberg EM. The meaning of cognitive impairment in the elderly. J Am Geriatr Soc. 1985;33:228–35.
12. Margallo-Lana M, Swann A, O'Brien J, et al. Prevalence and pharmacological management of behavioral and psychological symptoms amongst dementia sufferers living in care environments. Int J Geriatr Psychiatry. 2001;16:39–44.
13. Zimmer JG, Watson N, Treat A. Behavioral problems among patients in skilled nursing facilities. Am J Public Health. 1984;74(10):1118–24.
14. Jackson M, Drugovich M, Fretwell M, Spector W, Steinberg J, Rosenstein R. Prevalence and correlates

of disruptive behavior in the nursing home. J Aging Health. 1989;1:349–69.
15. Burns A, Jacoby R, Levy R. Psychiatric phenomena in Alzheimer's disease, IV: disorders of behaviour. Br J Psychiatry. 1990;157:86–94.
16. Wragg RE, Jeste DV. Overview of depression and psychosis in Alzheimer's disease. Am J Psychiatry. 1989;146:577–87.
17. Leuchter AF, Spar JE. The late-onset psychosis. J Nerv Ment Dis. 1985;173:488–94.
18. Alzheimer's Association. Wandering and getting lost. http://www.alz.org/care/alzheimers-dementia-wandering.asp. Updated 2016, Accessed 17 May 2016.
19. Algase DL, Moore DH, Vandeweerd C, Gavin-Dreschnackb DJ. Mapping the maze of terms and definitions in dementia-related wandering. Aging Ment Health. 2007;11(6):686–98. https://doi.org/10.1080/13607860701366434.
20. Rowe MA, Vandeveer SS, Greenblum CA, List CN, Fernandex RM, Mixson NE, Ahn HC. Persons with dementia missing in the community: is it wandering or something unique? BMC Geriatr. 2011;5:11–28. https://doi.org/10.1186/1471-2318-11-28.
21. Rasquin SMC, Willems C, De Villegar S, Geers S, Soede M. The use of technical devices to support outdoor mobility of dementia patients. Technol Dementia. 2007;19(2–3):113–20.
22. Lai CK, Arthur DG. Wandering behavior in people with dementia. J Adv Nurs. 2003;44(2):173–82.
23. Robinson L, Hutchings D, Corner L, Beyer F, Dickinson H, Vanoli A, Finch T, Hughes J, Ballard C, May C, Bond J. A systematic literature review of the effectiveness of non-pharmacological interventions to prevent wandering in dementia and evaluation of the ethical implications and acceptability of their use. Health Technol Assess. 2006;10(26):1–108.
24. Nelson A, Algase DL. Evidence-based protocols for managing wandering behavior. New York: Springer Publishing Company; 2007.
25. Halek M. Description of the behavior of wandering in people with dementia living in nursing homes-review of the literature. Scand J Caring Sci. 2012;26:404–13. https://doi.org/10.1111/j.1471-6712.2011.00932.x.
26. Algase DL, Antonakos C, Beattie ER, Beel-Bates CA, Yao L. Empirical derivation and validation of a wandering typology. JAGS. 2009;57:2037–45. https://doi.org/10.1111/j.1532-5415.2009.02491.x.
27. Khachiyants N, Trinkle D, Son SJ, Kim KY. Sundown syndrome in persons with dementia: an update. Psychiatry Investig. 2011;8:275–87. https://doi.org/10.4306/pi.2011.8.4.275.
28. Silverstein NM, Flaherty G, Tobin S. Dementia and wandering behavior. New York: Springer Publishing Company; 2006.
29. Algase DL, Antonakos C, Beattie ER, Beel-Bates CA, Yao L. New parameters for daytime wandering. Res Gerontol Nurs. 2009;2(1):58–68.
30. Alzheimer's Association. Sleep issues and sundowning. http://www.alz.org/care/alzheimers-dementia-sleep-issues-sundowning.asp. Updated 2016, Accessed 17 May 2016.
31. Bliwise D. What is sundowning? J Am Geriatr Soc. 1994;42:1009–11.
32. Bachman D, Rabins P. "Sundowning" and other temporary associated agitation states in dementia patients. Annu Rev Med. 2006;57:499–511.
33. Bedrosian TA, Nelson RJ. Sundowning syndrome in aging and dementia: research in mouse models. Exp Neurol. 2013;243:67–73.
34. Cohen-Mansfield J. Temporal patterns of agitation in dementia. Am J Geriatr Psychiatry. 2007;15:395–405.
35. Gallagher-Thompson D, Brooks JO, Bliwise D, Leadr J, Yesavage JA. The relationship among caregivers stress, 'sundowning' symptoms and cognitive decline in Alzheimer's disease. J Am Geriatr Soc. 1992;40:807–10.
36. Skjerve A, Nygaard HA. Improvement in sundowning in dementia with Lewy bodies after treatment with donepezil. Int J Geriatr Psychiatry. 2000;15:1147–51.
37. Cipriani G, Lucetti C, Carlesi C, Danti S, Nuti A. Sundown syndrome and dementia. Eur Geriatr Med. 2015;6:375–80.
38. Rindlisbacher P, Hopkins RM. An investigation of the sundowning syndrome. Int J Geriatr Psychiatry. 1991;7:15–23.
39. Exum ME, Phelps BJ, Nabers LE, Osborne JG. Sundown syndrome: is it reflected in the use of PRN medications for nursing home residents? Gerontologist. 1993;33:756–61.
40. Little JT, Satlin A, Sunderland T, Volicer L. Sundown syndrome in severely demented patients with probable Alzheimer's disease. J Geriatr Psychiatry Neurol. 1995;8:103–6.
41. Nowak L, Davis JE. A qualitative examination of the phenomenon of sundowning. J Nurs Scholarsh. 2007;39(3):256–8.
42. Inouye SK, Westendrop RG, Saczynski JS. Delirium in elderly people. Lancet. 2014;383:911–22. https://doi.org/10.1016/S0140-6736(13)60688-1.
43. Ferrazzoli D, Sica F, Sancesario G. Sundowning syndrome: a possible marker of frailty in Alzheimer's disease? CNS Neurol Disord Drug Targets. 2013;12:525–8.
44. Fisher Center for Alzheimer's Research Foundation. Shadowing: The challenge of never being alone. https://www.alzinfo.org/pym/feature/shadowing-2/. Updated 2016, Accessed 17 May 2016.
45. Lilly M, Hermanns M, Beckstrand J, Booth A, Farlow M. Illumination of shadowing behavior in individuals with Alzheimer's disease: Proximity-Seeking? As life becomes the "strange situation". Internet J Neurol. 2010;13(2). http://ispub.com/IJN/13/2/11657. Updated 2013, Accessed 12 May 2016.
46. Cummings J. Behavioral and neuropsychiatric outcomes in Alzheimer's disease. CNS Spectr. 2005;10(11 Suppl 18):22–5.

47. Johnson MMS, Wackerbarth SB, Schmitt FA. Revised memory and behavior checklist. Clin Gerontol. 2001;22(3–4):87–108.
48. Porter V, Buxton W, Fairbanks L, Strickland T, O'Connor S, Rosenberg-Thompson S, Cummings J. Frequency and characteristics of anxiety among patients with Alzheimer's disease and related dementias. J Neuropsychiatry Clin Neurosci. 2003;15(2):180–6.
49. Fuh JL, Wang SJ, Cummings JL. Neuropsychiatric profiles in patients with Alzheimer's disease and vascular dementia. J Neurol Neurosurg Psychiatry. 2005;76:1337–41.
50. Steinberg M, Shao H, Zandi P, Lyketsos C, Welsh-Bohmer K, Norton M, Breitner J, Steffens D, Tschanz J, Cache County Investigators. Point and 5-year period prevalence of neuropsychiatric symptoms in dementia: The Cache County Study. Int J Geriatr Psychiatry. 2008;23(2):170–7. https://doi.org/10.1002/gps.1858.
51. Bertolinio A, Arciero G, Rubino V, Latorre V, DeCandida M, Mazzola V, Blasi G, Caforio G, Hariri A, Kolachana B, Nardini M, Weinberger D, Scarabino T. Variation of human amygdala response during threatening stimuli as a function of 5′HTTLPR genotype and personality style. Biol Psychiatry. 2005;57:1517–25.
52. Caspers K, Paradiso S, Yucuis R, Troutman B, Arndt S, Philibert R. Association between the serotonin transporter promoter polymorphism (5-HTTLPR) and adult unresolved attachment. Dev Psychol. 2009;45(1):64–76.
53. Kringelbach M. The human orbitofrontal cortex: linking reward to hedonic experience. Nat Rev Neurosci. 2005;6:691–702.
54. Gitlin LN, Kales H, Lyketsos MHS. Managing behavioral symptoms in dementia using non-pharmacologic approaches: an overview. JAMA. 2012;308(19):2020–9. https://doi.org/10.1001/jama.2012.36918.
55. Ayers CR, Najimi S, Mayes TL, Dozier ME. Hoarding disorder in older adulthood. Am J Geriatr Psychiatry. 2014;23(4):416–22. https://doi.org/10.1016/j.jagp.2014.05.009.
56. Baker JC, LeBlanc LA, Raetz PB, Hilton LC. Assessment and treatment of hoarding in an individual with dementia. Behav Ther. 2011;42:135–42.
57. Fontenelle LF, Grant JE. Hoarding disorder: a new diagnostic category in ICD-11? Revista Brasileria de Psiquiatria. 2014;36:S28–39. https://doi.org/10.1590/1516-4446-2013-1269.
58. Mathews CA. Hoarding disorder: more than just a problem of too much stuff. J Clin Psychiatry. 2014;75(18):893–4. https://doi.org/10.4088/JCP.14ac09325.
59. Schreiner AS. Aggressive behaviors among demented nursing home residents in Japan. Int J Geriatr Psychiatry. 2001;16(2):209–15.
60. Ryden MB, Bossenmaier M, McLachlan C. Aggressive behavior in cognitively impaired nursing home residents. Res Nurs Health. 1991;14(2):87–95. https://doi.org/10.1002/nur.4770140203.
61. O'Leary D, Jyringi D, Sedler M. Childhood conduct problems, stages of Alzheimer's disease, and physical aggression against caregivers. Int J Geriatr Psychiatry. 2005;20(5):401–5.
62. Sampson EL, White N, Leurent B, Scott S, Lord K, Round J, Jones L. Behavioural and psychiatric symptoms in people with dementia admitted to the acute hospital: prospective cohort study. Br J Psychiatry. 2014;205(3):189–96.
63. Ryden MB. Aggressive behavior in persons with dementia who live in the community. Alzheimer Dis Assoc Disord. 1988;2:342–55.
64. Trzepacz PT, Yu P, Bhamidipati PK, et al. Frontolimbic atrophy is associated with agitation and aggression in mild cognitive impairment and Alzheimer's disease. Alzheimers Dement. 2013;9(5 Suppl):S95–S104.
65. Tractenberg RE, Weiner MF, Patterson MB, Gamst A, Thal LJ. Emergent psychopathology in Alzheimer's disease patients over 12 months associated with functional, not cognitive, changes. J Geriatr Psychiatry Neurol. 2002;15(2):110–7.
66. van der Flier WM, Staekenborg S, Pijnenburg YAL, et al. Apolipoprotein E genotype influences presence and severity of delusions and aggressive behavior in Alzheimer disease. Dement Geriatr Cogn Disord. 2006;23(1):42–6.
67. Lopez OL, Becker JT, Sweet RA, et al. Psychiatric symptoms vary with the severity of dementia in probable Alzheimer's disease. J Neuropsychiatry Clin Neurosci. 2003;15(3):346–53.
68. Ahn H, Horgas A. Does pain mediate or moderate the effect of cognitive impairment on aggression in nursing home residents with dementia? Asian Nurs Res (Korean Soc Nurs Sci). 2014;8(2):105–9. https://doi.org/10.1016/j.anr.2014.03.003.
69. Ahn H, Garvan C, Lyon D. Pain and aggression in nursing home residents with dementia: Minimum Data Set 3.0 Analysis. Nurs Res. 2015;64(4):256–63.
70. van Dalen-Kok AH, Pieper MJ, de Waal MW, Lukas A, Husebo BS, Achterberg WP. Association between pain, neuropsychiatric symptoms, and physical function in dementia: a systematic review and meta-analysis. BMC Geriatr. 2015;15:49.
71. Ahn H, Horgas A. The relationship between pain and disruptive behaviors in nursing home residents with dementia. BMC Geriatr. 2013;13:14.
72. Cohenmansfield J, Marx MS. The relationship between sleep disturbances and agitation in a nursing home. J Aging Health. 1990;2(1):42–57.
73. Burgio LD, Jones LT, Butler F, Engel BT. The prevalence of geriatric behavior problems in an urban nursing home. J Gerontol Nurs. 1988;14:31–4.
74. Winger J, Schirm V, Stewart D. Aggressive behavior in long-term care. J Psychosoc Nurs Ment Health Serv. 1987;25(4):28–33.

75. Caspi E. Aggressive behaviors between residents with dementia in an assisted living residence. Dementia (London). 2015;14(4):528–46.
76. Panza F, Solfrizzi V, Seripa D, Imbimbo BP, Santamato A, Lozupone M, Prete C, Greco A, Pilotto A, Logroscino G. Progresses in treating agitation: a major clinical challenge in Alzheimer's disease. Expert Opin Pharmacother. 2015;16(17):2581–8.
77. Bird M, Llewellyn-Jones RH, Korten A. An evaluation of the effectiveness of a case-specific approach to challenging behaviour associated with dementia. Aging Ment Health. 2009;13(1):73–83.
78. Gozalo P, Prakash S, Qato DM, Sloane PD, Mor V. Effect of the bathing without a battle training intervention on bathing-associated physical and verbal outcomes in nursing home residents with dementia: a randomized crossover diffusion study. J Am Geriatr Soc. 2014;62(5):797–804.
79. Hoeffer B, Talerico KA, Rasin J, Mitchell CM, Stewart BJ, McKenzie D, Barrick AL, Rader J, Sloane PD. Assisting cognitively impaired nursing home residents with bathing: effects of two bathing interventions on caregiving. Gerontologist. 2006;46(4):524–32.
80. Sloane PD, Hoeffer B, Mitchell CM, et al. Effect of person-centered showering and the towel bath on bathing-associated aggression, agitation, and discomfort in nursing home residents with dementia: a randomized, controlled trial. J Am Geriatr Soc. 2004;52(11):1795–804.
81. Huang HL, Kuo LM, Chen YS, Liang J, Huang HL, Chiu YC, Chen ST, Sun Y, Hsu WC, Shyu YIL. A home-based training program improves caregivers' skills and dementia patients' aggressive behaviors: a randomized controlled trial. Am J Geriatr Psychiatry. 2013;21:1060–70.
82. Wolf DM, Lehman L, Quinlin R, Zullo T, Hoffman L. Effect of patient-centered care on patient satisfaction and quality of care. J Nurs Care Qual. 2008;23(4):316–21.
83. Enmarker I, Olsen R, Hellzen O. Management of person with dementia with aggressive and violent behaviour: a systematic literature review. Int J Older People Nursing. 2011;6(2):153–62.
84. Skovdahl K, Kihlgren AL, Kihlgren M. Dementia and aggressiveness: video recorded morning care from different care units. J Clin Nurs. 2003;12:888–98.
85. Ledger AJ, Baker FA. An investigation of long-term effects of group music therapy on agitation levels of people with Alzheimer's disease. Aging Ment Health. 2007;11(3):330–8.
86. Clark ME, Lipe AW, Bilbrey M. Use of music to decrease aggressive behaviors in people with dementia. J Gerontol Nurs. 1998;24:10.
87. Hall GR, Buckwalter KC. Progressively lowered stress threshold: a conceptual model for care of adults with Alzheimer's disease. Arch Psychiatr Nurs. 1987;1:399–406.
88. Gerdner LA, Buckwalter KC, Reed D. Impact of a psychoeducational intervention on caregiver response to behavioral problems. Nurs Res. 2002;51(6):363–74.
89. Skinner BF. Science and human behavior. New York: Free Press; 1953.
90. Gormley N, Lyons D, Howard R. Behavioural management of aggression in dementia: a randomized controlled trial. Age Ageing. 2001;30(2):141–5.
91. Mittal V, Kurup L, Williamson D, Muralee S, Tampi RR. Risk of cerebrovascular adverse events and death in elderly patients with dementia when treated with antipsychotic medications: a literature review of evidence. Am J Alzheimers Dis Other Demen. 2011;26(1):10–28.
92. Nardell M, Tampi RR. Pharmacological treatments for frontotemporal dementias: a systematic review of randomized controlled trials. Am J Alzheimers Dis Other Demen. 2014;29(2):123–32.
93. Sultzer DL, Davis SM, Tariot PN, et al. Clinical symptom responses to atypical antipsychotic medications in Alzheimer's disease: phase 1 outcomes from the CATIE-AD effectiveness trial; CATIE-AD Study Group. Am J Psychiatry. 2008;165(7):844–54.
94. Powell A, Flynn P, Rischbieth S, McKellar D. Managing severe aggression in frontotemporal dementia. Australas Psychiatry. 2014;22(1):86–9.
95. Peskind ER, Tsuang DW, Bonner LT, et al. Propranolol for disruptive behaviors in nursing home residents with probable or possible Alzheimer disease: a placebo-controlled study. Alzheimer Dis Assoc Disord. 2005;19(1):23–8.
96. Acharya D, Harper DG, Achtyes ED, et al. Safety and utility of acute electroconvulsive therapy for agitation and aggression in dementia. Int J Geriatr Psychiatry. 2015;30(3):265–73.
97. Ujkaj M, Davidoff DA, Seiner SJ, Ellison JM, Harper DG, Forester BP. Safety and efficacy of electroconvulsive therapy for the treatment of agitation and aggression in patients with dementia. Am J Geriatr Psychiatry. 2012;20(1):61–72.
98. Ahn A, Horgas A. Understanding the relationship between pain and disruptive behaviours in residents with dementia. Can Nurs Home. 2013;24(4):19–24.
99. Cohen-Mansfield J, Dakheel-Ali M, Marx MS, Thein K, Regier NG. Which unmet needs contribute to behavior problems in persons with advanced dementia? Psychiatry Res. 2015;228(1):59–64. https://doi.org/10.1016/j.psychres.2015.03.043. Epub 2015 Apr 14
100. Low LF, Draper B, Brodaty H. The relationship between self-destructive behaviour and nursing home environment. Aging Ment Health. 2004;8(1):29–33.
101. Konno R, Kang HS, Makimoto K. A best-evidence review of intervention studies for minimizing resistance-to-care behaviours for older adults with dementia in nursing homes. J Adv Nurs. 2014;70(10):2167–80.
102. Han P, Kwan M, Chen D, Yusoff SZ, Chionh HL, Goh J, Yap P. A controlled naturalistic study on a weekly music therapy and activity program on disruptive and depressive behaviors in dementia. Dement Geriatr Cogn Disord. 2011;30(6):540–6.

103. McCabe MP, Bird M, Davison TE, Mellor D, MacPherson S, Hallford D, Seedy M. An RCT to evaluate the utility of a clinical protocol for staff in the management of behavioral and psychological symptoms of dementia in residential aged-care settings. Aging Ment Health. 2015;19(9):799–807. https://doi.org/10.1080/13607863.2014.967659.
104. Rapp MA, Mell T, Majic T, et al. Agitation in nursing home residents with dementia (VIDEANT Trial): effects of a cluster-randomized, controlled, guideline implementation trial. J Am Med Dir Assoc. 2013;14(9):690–5.
105. Nogales-González C, Losada-Baltar A, Márquez-González M, Zarit SH. Behavioral intervention for reducing resistance in care recipients to attending adult day care centers: a pilot study. Clin Gerontol. 2014;37(5):493–505.
106. Van Haitsma KS, Curyto K, Abbott KM, Towsley GL, Spector A, Kleban M. A randomized controlled trial for an individualized positive psychosocial intervention for the affective and behavioral symptoms of dementia in nursing home residents. J Gerontol B Psychol Sci Soc Sci. 2015;70(1):35–45. https://doi.org/10.1093/geronb/gbt102.
107. Bédard A, Landreville P, Voyer P, Verreault R, Vézina J. Reducing verbal agitation in people with dementia: evaluation of an intervention based on the satisfaction of basic needs. Aging Ment Health. 2011;15(7):855–65.
108. Ervin K, Finlayson S, Cross M. The management of behavioural problems associated with dementia in rural aged care. Collegian. 2012;19(2):85–95.
109. Reus VI, Fochtmann LJ, Eyler AE. The American Psychiatric Association Practice Guideline on the use of antipsychotics to treat agitation or psychosis in patients with dementia. Am J Psychiatry. 2016;173(5):543–6.
110. Tremolizzo L, Tironi M, Ferrarese C, Appollonio I. Neuroleptic equivalent dose differences and behavioral and psychological symptoms of dementia. Dement Geriatr Cogn Disord. 2013;35(1/2):118–20.
111. Lemke MR. Effect of carbamazepine on agitation in Alzheimer's inpatients refractory to neuroleptics. J Clin Psychiatry. 1995;56(8):354–7.
112. Ozkan B, Wilkins K, Muralee S, Tampi RR. Pharmacotherapy for inappropriate sexual behaviors in dementia: a systematic review of literature. Am J Alzheimers Dis Other Demen. 2008;23(4):344–54.
113. Series H, Dégano P. Hypersexuality in dementia. Adv Psychiatr Treat. 2005;11(6):424–31.
114. Szasz G. Sexual incidents in an extended care unit for aged men. J Am Geriatr Soc. 1983;31(7):407–11.
115. De Medieros K, Rosenberg PB, Baker AS, Onyike CU. Improper sexual behaviors in elders with dementia living in residential care. Dement Geriatr Cogn Disord. 2008;26:370–7. https://doi.org/10.1159/000163219.
116. Lichtenberg PA, Strzepek DM. Assessments of institutionalized dementia patients' competencies to participate in intimate relationships. Gerontologist. 1990;30:117–20.
117. Knight C, Alderman N, Johnson C, Green S, Birkett-Swan L, Yorstan G. The St Andrew's Sexual Behaviour Assessment (SASBA): development of a standardized recording instrument for the measurement and assessment of challenging sexual behaviour in people with progressive and acquired neurological impairment. Neuropsychol Rehabil. 2008;18(2):129–59.
118. Cipriani G, Ulivi M, Danti S, Lucetti C, Nuti A. Sexual disinhibition and dementia. Psychogeriatrics. 2016;16(2):145–53. https://doi.org/10.1111/psyg.12143.
119. Ahmed RM, Kaizik C, Irish M, Mioshi E, Dermody N, Kiernan MC, Piguet O, Hodges JR. Characterizing sexual behavior in frontotemporal dementia. J Alzheimers Dis. 2015;46(3):677–86. https://doi.org/10.3233/JAD-150034.
120. Lishman WA. Organic psychiatry: the psychological consequences of cerebral disorder. 3rd ed. Oxford: Blackwell Science; 1998.
121. Bardell A, Lau T, Fedoroff JP. Inappropriate sexual behavior in a geriatric population. Int Psychogeriatr. 2011;23(7):1182–8.
122. Kluver H, Bucy P. "Psychic blindness" and other symptoms following bitemporal lobectomy in rhesus monkeys. Am J Phys. 1937;119:352–3.
123. Mendez MF, Shapira JS. Hypersexual behavior in frontotemporal dementia: a comparison with early-onset Alzheimer's disease. Arch Sex Behav. 2013;42(3):501–9. https://doi.org/10.1007/s10508-012-0042-4.
124. Joller P, Gupta N, Seitz DP, Frank C, Gibson M, Gill SS. Approach to inappropriate sexual behaviour in people with dementia. Can Fam Physician. 2013;59(3):255–60.
125. Bird M, Jones RH, Korten A, Smithers H. A controlled trial of a predominantly psychosocial approach to BPSD: treating causality. Int Psychogeriatr. 2007;19(5):874–91.
126. Tune LE, Rosenberg J. Nonpharmacological treatment of inappropriate sexual behavior in dementia: the case of the pink panther. Am J Geriatr Psychiatry. 2008;16(7):612–3.
127. Anneser JM, Jox RJ, Borasio GD. Inappropriate sexual behaviour in a case of ALS and FTD: successful treatment with sertraline. Amyotroph Lateral Scler. 2007;8(3):189–90.
128. Stewart JT, Shin KJ. Paroxetine treatment of sexual disinhibition in dementia. Am J Psychiatry. 1997;154(10):1474.
129. Raji M, Liu D, Wallace D. Case report: sexual aggressiveness in a patient with dementia: sustained clinical response to citalopram. Ann Longterm Care. 2000;8:81–3.
130. Chen ST. Treatment of a patient with dementia and inappropriate sexual behaviors with citalopram. Alzheimer Dis Assoc Disord. 2010;24(4):402–3.

131. Leo RJ, Kim KY. Clomipramine treatment of paraphilias in elderly demented patients. J Geriatr Psychiatry Neurol. 1995;8(2):123–4.
132. Simpson DM, Foster D. Improvement in organically disturbed behavior with trazodone treatment. J Clin Psychiatry. 1986;47(4):191–3.
133. Cooper AJ. Medroxyprogesterone acetate (MPA) treatment of sexual acting out in men suffering from dementia. J Clin Psychiatry. 1987;48(9):368–70.
134. Weiner MF, Denke M, Williams K, Guzman R. Intramuscular medroxyprogesterone acetate for sexual aggression in elderly men. Lancet. 1992;339(8801):1121–2.
135. Light SA, Holroyd S. The use of medroxyprogesterone acetate for the treatment of sexually inappropriate behaviour in patients with dementia. J Psychiatry Neurosci. 2006;31(2):132–4.
136. Cross BS, DeYoung GR, Furmaga KM. High-dose oral medroxyprogesterone for inappropriate hypersexuality in elderly men with dementia: a case series. Ann Pharmacother. 2013;47(1):e1. https://doi.org/10.1345/aph.1R533.
137. Haussermann P, Goecker D, Beier K, Schroeder S. Low-dose cyproterone acetate treatment of sexual acting out in men with dementia. Int Psychogeriatr. 2003;15(2):181–6.
138. Kyomen HH, Nobel KW, Wei JY. The use of estrogen to decrease aggressive physical behavior in elderly men with dementia. J Am Geriatr Soc. 1991;39(11):1110–2.
139. Na HR, Lee JW, Park SM, Ko SB, Kim S, Cho ST. Inappropriate sexual behaviors in patients with vascular dementia: possible response to finasteride. J Am Geriatr Soc. 2009;57(11):2161–2.
140. Ott BR. Leuprolide treatment of sexual aggression in a patient with dementia and the Klüver-Bucy syndrome. Clin Neuropharmacol. 1995;18(5):443–7.
141. Levitsky AM, Owens NJ. Pharmacologic treatment of hypersexuality and paraphilias in nursing home residents. J Am Geriatr Soc. 1999;47:231–4.
142. Lothstein LM, Fogg-Waberski J, Reynolds P. Risk management and treatment of sexual disinhibition in geriatric patients. Conn Med. 1997;61:609–18.
143. Rosenthal M, Berkman P, Shapira A, Gil I, Abramovitz J. Urethral masturbation and sexual disinhibition in dementia: a case report. Isr J Psychiatry Relat Sci. 2003;40(1):67–72.
144. Kobayashi T. Effect of haloperidol on a patient with hypersexuality following frontal lobe injury. Psychogeriatrics. 2004;4(2):49–52.
145. Prakash R, Pathak A, Munda S, Bagati D. Quetiapine effective in treatment of inappropriate sexual behavior of Lewy body disease with predominant frontal lobe signs. Am J Alzheimers Dis Other Demen. 2009;24(2):136–40.
146. MacKnight C, Rojas-Fernandez C. Quetiapine for sexually inappropriate behavior in dementia. J Am Geriatr Soc. 2000;48(6):707.
147. Schneider LS, Dagerman K, Insel PS. Efficacy and adverse effects of atypical antipsychotics for dementia: meta-analysis of randomized, placebo-controlled trials. Am J Geriatr Psychiatry. 2006;14(3):191–210.
148. Sheldon LJ, Ancill RJ, Holliday SG. Gabapentin in geriatric psychiatry patients. Can J Psychiatr. 1998;43(4):422–3.
149. Alkhalil C, Hahar N, Alkhalil B, Zavros G, Lowenthal DT. Can gabapentin be a safe alternative to hormonal therapy in the treatment of inappropriate sexual behavior in demented patients? Int Urol Nephrol. 2003;35(2):299–302.
150. Alkhalil C, Tanvir F, Alkhalil B, Lowenthal DT. Treatment of sexual disinhibition in dementia: case reports and review of the literature. Am J Ther. 2004;11(3):231–5.
151. Löfgren E, Tapanainen JS, Koivunen R, Pakarinen A, Isojärvi JI. Effects of carbamazepine and oxcarbazepine on the reproductive endocrine function in women with epilepsy. Epilepsia. 2006;47(9):1441–6.
152. Freymann N, Michael R, Dodel R, Jessen F. Successful treatment of sexual disinhibition in dementia with carbamazepine – a case report. Pharmacopsychiatry. 2005;38(3):144–5.
153. Alagiakrishnan K, Sclater A, Robertson D. Role of cholinesterase inhibitor in the management of sexual aggression in an elderly demented woman. J Am Geriatr Soc. 2003;51(9):1326.
154. Chemali Z. Donepezil and hypersexuality: a report of two cases. Prim Psychiatry. 2003;10(7):78–9.
155. Lo Coco D, Cannizzaro E. Inappropriate sexual behaviors associated with donepezil treatment: a case report. J Clin Psychopharmacol. 2010;30(2):221–2.
156. Wiseman SV, McAuley JW, Freidenberg GR, Freidenberg DL. Hypersexuality in patients with dementia: possible response to cimetidine. Neurology. 2000;54:2024.
157. Jensen CF. Hypersexual agitation in Alzheimer's disease. J Am Geriatr Soc. 1989;37(9):917.
158. Campbell VA, Gowran A. Alzheimer's disease; taking the edge off with cannabinoids? Br J Pharmacol. 2007;152(5):655–62. https://doi.org/10.1038/sj.bjp.0707446.
159. Orgado JM, Fernández-Ruiz J, Romero J. The endocannabinoid system in neuropathological states. Int Rev Psychiatry. 2009;21(2):172–80. https://doi.org/10.1080/09540260902782828.
160. Zajac DM, Sikkema SR, Chandrasena R. Nabilone for the treatment of dementia-associated sexual disinhibition. Prim Care Companion CNS Disord. 2015;17(1). https://doi.org/10.4088/PCC.14l01695.
161. Guay DR. Inappropriate sexual behaviors in cognitively impaired older individuals. Am J Geriatr Pharmacother. 2008;6(5):269–88.
162. Kishimoto Y, Terada S, Sato S, Yoshida H, Honda H, Takeda N, Oshima E, Ishihara T, Kuroda S. Repetitive questioning behavior in Alzheimer's disease: relationship to regional cerebral blood flow. Psychiatry Res. 2010;184:151–6.
163. Wellbery C. Repetitive behaviors: a clue to early dementia. Am Fam Physician. 2016;68(2):371–2.

164. Cipriani G, Vedovello M, Ulivi M, Nuti A, Lucetti C. Repetitive and stereotypic phenomena and dementia. Am J Alzheimers Dis Other Demen. 2013;28(3):223–7.
165. Alzheimer's Association. Repetition and Alzheimer's. http://www.alz.org/care/alzheimers-dementia-repitition.asp. Updated 2016, Accessed 17 May 2016.
166. McMinn B, Draper B. Vocally disruptive behaviour in dementia: development of an evidence based practice guideline. Aging Ment Health. 2005;9(1):16–24.
167. Cohen-Mansfield J, Werner P, Marx M. Screaming in nursing home residents. J Am Geriatr Soc. 1990;38:785–92.
168. Bourbonnais A, Ducharme F. The meanings of screams in older people living with dementia in a nursing home. Int Psychogeriatr. 2010;22(7):1172–84. https://doi.org/10.1017/S1041610209991670.
169. Hydén LC. Non-verbal vocalizations, dementia and social interaction. Commun Med. 2011;8(2):135–44.
170. Sloane PD, Davidson S, Buckwalter K, et al. Management of the patient with disruptive vocalization. Gerontologist. 1997;37(5):675–82.
171. Herman RE, Williams KN. Elderspeak's influence on resistiveness to care: focus on behavioral events. Am J Alzheimers Dis Other Demen. 2009;24(5):417–23. https://doi.org/10.1177/1533317509341949.
172. Koopmans RT, van der Molen M, Raats M, Ettema TP. Neuropsychiatric symptoms and quality of life in patients in the final phase of dementia. Int J Geriatr Psychiatry. 2009;24(1):25–32. https://doi.org/10.1002/gps.2040.
173. Buchanan JA, Fisher JE. Functional assessment and non-contingent reinforcement in the treatment of disruptive vocalization in elderly dementia patients. J Appl Behav Anal. 2002;35(1):99–103.
174. Rosen T, Lachs MS, Bharucha AJ, Stevens SM, Teresi JA, Nebres F, Pillemer K. Resident-to-resident aggression in long-term care facilities: insights from focus groups of nursing home residents and staff. J Am Geriatr Soc. 2008;56(8):1398–408. https://doi.org/10.1111/j.1532-5415.2008.01808.x.
175. Lantz MS. Verbally disruptive behavior in a patient with vascular dementia. Clin Geriatr. 2009;17(2):20–3.
176. Meares S, Draper B. Treatment of vocally disruptive behaviour of multifactorial aetiology. Int J Geriatr Psychiatry. 1999;14(4):285–90.
177. Turner S. Behavioural symptoms of dementia in residential settings: a selective review of non-pharmacological interventions. Aging Ment Health. 2005;9(2):93–104.
178. Lindgren C, Hallberg IR. Diagnostic reasoning in the care of a vocally disruptive severely demented patient. Scand J Caring Sci. 1992;6(2):97–103.
179. Cohen-Mansfield J, Werner P. Management of verbally disruptive behaviors in nursing home residents. J Gerontol A Biol Sci Med Sci. 1997;52A(6):M369–77.
180. Reuther S, Dichter MN, Buscher I, et al. Case conferences as interventions dealing with the challenging behavior of people with dementia in nursing homes: a systematic review. Int Psychogeriatr. 2012;24(12):1891–903. https://doi.org/10.1017/S1041610212001342.
181. Burgio LD, Hardin JM, Sinnott J, Janosky J, Hohman MJ. Nurses' acceptance of behavioral treatments and pharmacotherapy for behavioral disturbances in older adults. Appl Nurs Res. 1995;8(4):174–81.
182. Burgio LD, Cotter EM, Stevens AB, Hardin JM, Sinnott J, Hohman MJ. Elders' acceptability ratings of behavioral treatments and pharmacotherapy for the management of geriatric behavioral disturbances. Gerontologist. 1995;35(5):630–6.
183. Kopala LC, Honer WG. The use of risperidone in severely demented patients with persistent vocalizations. Int J Geriatr Psychiatry. 1997;12(1):73–7.
184. Carlyle W, Killick L. ECT: an effective treatment in the screaming demented patient. J Am Geriatr Soc. 1991;39(6):637.
185. Sloane PD, Mathew LJ, Scarborough M, Desai JR, Koch GG, Tangen C. Physical and pharmacologic restraint of nursing home patients with dementia. Impact of specialized units. JAMA. 1991;265(10):1278–82.
186. Hofmann H, Hahn S. Characteristics of nursing home residents and physical restraint: a systematic literature review. J Clin Nurs. 2014;23(21/22):3012–24.
187. Bredthauer D, Becker C, Eichner B, Koczy P, Nikolaus T. Factors relating to the use of physical restraints in psychogeriatric care: a paradigm for elder abuse. Z Gerontol Geriatr. 2005;38(1):10–8.
188. Kirkevold Ø, Engedal K. A study into the use of restraint in nursing homes in Norway. Br J Nurs. 2004;13(15):902–5.
189. Wang WW, Moyle W. Physical restraint use on people with dementia: a review of the literature. Aust J Adv Nurs. 2005;22(4):46–52.
190. Kröpelin TF, Neyens JC, Halfens RJ, Kempen GI, Hamers JP. Fall determinants in older long-term care residents with dementia: a systematic review. Int Psychogeriatr. 2013;25(4):549–63. https://doi.org/10.1017/S1041610212001937.
191. Tilly J, Reed P. Falls, wandering, and physical restraints: a review of interventions for individuals with dementia in assisted living and nursing homes. Alzheimers Care Today. 2008;9(1):45–50.
192. Huabin L, Lin M, Castle N. Physical restraint use and falls in nursing homes: a comparison between residents with and without dementia. Am J Alzheimers Dis Other Demen. 2011;26(1):44–50.
193. Talerico KA, Evans LK. Responding to safety issues in frontotemporal dementias. Neurology. 2001;56(11 Suppl 4):S52–5.
194. Luo H, Lin M, Castle N. Physical restraint use and falls in nursing homes: a comparison between residents with and without dementia. Am J Alzheimers Dis Other Demen. 2011;26(1):44–50. https://doi.org/10.1177/1533317510387585. 11.
195. Flannery RB. Restraint procedures and dementia sufferers with psychological trauma. Am J Alzheimers Dis Other Demen. 2003;18(4):227–30.

196. Foebel AD, Onder G, Finne-Soveri H, et al. Physical restraint and antipsychotic medication use among nursing home residents with dementia. J Am Med Dir Assoc. 2016;17(2):184.e9–184.e14. https://doi.org/10.1016/j.jamda.2015.11.014.
197. Scherder EJ, Bogen T, Eggermont LH, Hamers JP, Swaab DF. The more physical inactivity, the more agitation in dementia. Int Psychogeriatr. 2010;22(8):1203–8. https://doi.org/10.1017/S1041610210001493.
198. Cotter VT. Restraint free care in older adults with dementia. Keio J Med. 2005;54(2):80–4.
199. Gerace A, Mosel K, Oster C, Muir-Cochrane E. Restraint use in acute and extended mental health services for older persons. Int J Ment Health Nurs. 2013;22(6):545–57. https://doi.org/10.1111/j.1447-0349.2012.00872.x.
200. Te Boekhorst S, Depla MF, Francke AL, Twisk JW, Zwijsen SA, Hertogh CM. Quality of life of nursing-home residents with dementia subject to surveillance technology versus physical restraints: an explorative study. Int J Geriatr Psychiatry. 2013;28(4):356–63. https://doi.org/10.1002/gps.3831.
201. Weiner C, Tabak N, Bergman R. Use of restraints on dementia patients: an ethical dilemma of a nursing staff in Israel. JONAS Healthc Law Ethics Regul. 2003;5(4):87–93.
202. Zwijsen SA, Depla MF, Niemeijer AR, Francke AL, Hertogh CM. The concept of restraint in nursing home practice: a mixed-method study in nursing homes for people with dementia. Int Psychogeriatr. 2011;23(5):826–34. https://doi.org/10.1017/S1041610210002267.
203. Federal Nursing Home Reform Act from the Omnibus Budget Reconciliation Act of Developed by Hollis Turnham, Esquire. http://www.ncmust.com/doclib/OBRA87summary.pdf. Published 1987, Accessed 15 May 2016.
204. Capezuti E. Minimizing the use of restrictive devices in dementia patients at risk for falling. Nurs Clin North Am. 2004;39(3):625–47.
205. Pies R. Pharmacologic restraint vs therapeutic intent. JAMA. 1991;266(2):216. https://doi.org/10.1001/jama.1991.03470020042021.
206. Gastmans C, Milisen K. Use of physical restraint in nursing homes: clinical-ethical considerations. J Med Ethics. 2006;32(3):148–52. https://doi.org/10.1136/jme.2005.012708.
207. Evans LK, Cotter VT. Avoiding restraints in patients with dementia: understanding, prevention, and management are the keys. Am J Nurs. 2008;108(3):40–9; quiz 50.
208. Testad I, Aasland AM, Aarsland D. The effect of staff training on the use of restraint in dementia: a single-blind randomised controlled trial. Int J Geriatr Psychiatry. 2005;20(6):587–90.
209. Testad I, Ballard C, Brønnick K, Aarsland D. The effect of staff training on agitation and use of restraint in nursing home residents with dementia: a single-blind, randomized controlled trial. J Clin Psychiatry. 2010;71(1):80–6. https://doi.org/10.4088/JCP.09m05486oli.
210. Testad I, Mekki TE, Førland O, et al. Modeling and evaluating evidence-based continuing education program in nursing home dementia care (MEDCED)—training of care home staff to reduce use of restraint in care home residents with dementia. A cluster randomized controlled trial. Int J Geriatr Psychiatry. 2016;31:24–32. https://doi.org/10.1002/gps.4285.
211. Zwijsen SA, Smalbrugge M, Eefsting JA, et al. Coming to grips with challenging behavior: a cluster randomized controlled trial on the effects of a multidisciplinary care program for challenging behavior in dementia. J Am Med Dir Assoc. 2014;15(7):531.e1–10. https://doi.org/10.1016/j.jamda.2014.04.007.

Part VI

Medico-Legal Issues in Geriatric Psychiatry

31 Policy, Ethical, and Legal Issues

Aarti Gupta and Meera Balasubramaniam

The Role of the Geriatric Psychiatrist in Health-Care Systems

The process of aging involves the intersection of physical, mental, and emotional health, personal values and beliefs, and individual's role in the immediate family and the society at large. Each of these factors influences the others with consequences for the overall well-being of an older adult. Optimal care of geriatric mental health patients can never be isolated from the above domains. It requires the collaboration of multiple specialized disciplines, in a setting that is best suited to deliver health care to an individual in question, against the background of finite resources. The latter includes financial resources as well as the limited availability of clinicians with specialized training in geriatric mental health.

In 2008, the Institute of Medicine (IOM) released a report titled "Retooling for an Aging America: Building The Health Care Workforce," highlighting the workforce crisis in the care of older adults. The proportion of the population over age 65 is expected to increase from 12.4% of the total US population in 2000 to 20% by the year 2030 [1]. During the same time period, the number of older adults with psychiatric illness is expected to increase twofold to a total of 15 million [2]. Presently, there are about 1700 board-certified geriatric psychiatrists in the United States—one for every 23,000 older Americans. That ratio is estimated to diminish to one geriatric psychiatrist for every 27,000 individuals 65 and older by 2030 [3]. Clearly, there will be a growing need for an increased number of physicians with this training as well as the judicious use of the existing mental health-care workforce.

Older adults are found in a variety of clinical and residential settings: homeless shelters, personal homes, ambulatory care services, acute care and partial hospitals, adult day care, subacute care facilities, nursing homes, assisted living facilities, subsidized senior housing, naturally occurring retirement communities (NORCs), and hospice care settings. Each of these is governed by different systems of organization and sources of funding. The diversity of the settings and the multitude of issues facing older adults make it imperative that the geriatric psychiatrist partners with providers from other disciplines. These include internists, geriatricians, neurologists, nurses, social workers, discharge planners, elder law attorneys, psychologists, and occupational and physical therapists. The geriatric psychiatrist is expected to be familiar with the structure and complexity of each of these settings to be able to provide good quality of care to patients and families.

The field is evolving in terms of novel service delivery approaches suited to serve older adults. For example, the collaborative care model is gaining ground across institutions. The Improving Mood-Promoting Access to Collaborative

R. R. Tampi et al. (eds.), *Psychiatric Disorders Late in Life*, https://doi.org/10.1007/978-3-319-73078-3_31

Treatment (IMPACT) collaborative care management program is the most frequently cited model in this regard. Patients in the study who received the IMPACT intervention had access to a depression care manager (trained nurse or psychologist) who was supervised by a psychiatrist and a primary care liaison [4]. The care manager offered psychoeducation, care management, support of antidepressant management (prescribed by the primary care physician), or brief psychotherapy. The psychiatrists supervised every patient's treatment plan and offered in-person consultations to patients with diagnostic challenges or unsatisfactory improvement. At the end of the follow-up period, patients who received this intervention were found to have greater reduction in depressive symptoms, more satisfaction with their care, less functional impairment, and a higher quality of care, when compared to those who received the usual treatment by their primary care physicians. This model is an example of a successful multidisciplinary approach that utilized the psychiatrist as a consultant in a judicious manner to achieve effective outcomes. This model also recognizes the chronicity of medical and psychiatric conditions constituting geriatric syndromes, the impact of mental health on compliance with medical treatment, the need for medical monitoring for the side effects of psychotropic medications, the challenges of making multiple clinic visits for the frail older adult, and the stigma around seeking specific mental health care.

Home-based mental health care of older adults is also gaining momentum. Reifler and Bruce reviewed existing programs across the nation, in which they highlighted the clinical focus, staffing, and budget of each program. The authors drew attention to the complex needs of homebound adults and recommended partnering with health, social, or aging service organizations. They also called for incorporating services for transportation, meals, financial counseling, and legal advice into the model [5]. The role of a geriatric psychiatrist in the hospital and long-term care settings similarly encompass clinical care of the individual patient and areas of collaboration with allied disciplines. They are covered in the corresponding sections of the book, to which readers are referred.

The geriatric psychiatrist is required to simultaneously play the roles of an individual clinician, a team member, a leader, and an educator. This necessitates an in-depth understanding of psychiatric, medical, social, ethical, and legal challenges that the process of aging thrusts upon older adults and their families. The next few sections of this chapter will provide an overview of the interplay between clinical, ethical, and legal challenges in the care of the older adult and the role of the geriatric psychiatrist in helping patients and families work through these situations.

Ethical Issues in Geriatric Psychiatry

The Case of Mr. B

Mr. B is a 75-year-old man who was brought to the emergency room (ER) of a tertiary care hospital with shortness of breath. His medical history included Type 2 diabetes, hypertension, and aortic stenosis. He also had a diagnosis of major depression for which he had been in treatment. He was diagnosed with acute decompensation of congestive heart failure and admitted to the medical inpatient unit where he received treatment for his congestive heart failure. Echocardiogram indicated severe aortic stenosis, for which the consulting cardiology team recommended aortic valve replacement surgery. Mr. B declined the option of surgery, expressing that he had lived "a long and full life" and that he did not wish to undergo any surgical intervention. The medical team was concerned that Mr. B was depressed and that this was influencing his decision. Therefore, they requested psychiatric consultation to evaluate his capacity to make a decision regarding aortic valve replacement surgery.

At the time of the evaluation, Mr. B demonstrated mild depressive symptoms but without an active death wish. However, significant deficits in memory and language were observed. His three adult children, all of whom lived in different cities, visited him in the hospital. They shared with the psychiatrist that the patient's home condition had significantly deteriorated from the last time they visited him. They found numerous unpaid bills and unopened medication bottles that lay scattered. Mr. B scored 18/30 on the Montreal Cognitive Assessment Test (MOCA), corresponding to moderate dementia [6].

On psychiatric evaluation, Mr. B was found to have the capacity to refuse surgery. Within a few days, he was medically stabilized and deemed ready for discharge from the hospital. He wished to return home, said that he "valued" his independence greatly and did not think he needed any assistance. The medical treatment team consulted psychiatry once again to assist in determining if Mr. B had the capacity to live independently. His family wished to know if they should take over the management of finances.

The vignette described above raises important questions that relate to the care of Mr. B. Does he have the capacity to refuse aortic valve replacement surgery? How does his dementia impact this capacity? Is he safe to go home and continue to live independently? Can he manage his finances? More importantly, does he have the capacity to make those choices for himself?

Geriatric psychiatrists frequently find themselves in the position of sorting through clinical and ethical dilemmas in their work with older patients. Clinicians must have a solid understanding of these concepts as scenarios such as the case of Mr. B are common. They impact the care of older adults and even form the basis of legal implications for them. The Belmont Report developed by the National Commission for the Protection of Human Subjects of Biomedical and Behavioral Research identified four ethical principles vital to health care, namely, autonomy (the act of self-determination), beneficence (the act of doing good), nonmaleficence (the act of doing no harm), and justice (act of appropriate use of scarce healthcare resources) [7]. Ethical issues arise in the clinical setting, such as the case of Mr. B, when one or more of these principles are in conflict with each other.

This section will provide an overview of common ethical challenges that arise in the care of elderly patients and offer a practical approach to understanding and managing them. We will first examine how age and the process of aging influence decision-making and introduce unique ethical dimensions to clinical care. This will be followed by a discussion of the concepts of informed consent and capacity evaluation, with focus on common clinical situations encountered by geriatric psychiatrists.

Aging and Decision-Making

Aging, in itself, introduces multiple layers to the process of decision-making. Firstly, the increase in life expectancy is associated with simultaneous increases in the incidence of medical and psychiatric illnesses and cognitive and functional impairments. The influence of medical technology and the availability of life-support measures such as ventilation and artificial feeding have made it possible to externally control the time of death, practices that may be in conflict with the concept of health and death for some individuals. The changing landscape of increasing life expectancy and advances in the healthcare system serves to increase the overall frequency of medical decision-making that older adults and their families find themselves in.

Secondly, societies vary widely in their perception of aging, a factor that might have both explicit and implicit influences on the health care of their oldest members. On one hand, Daniel Callahan called for age-based rationing of health care, a concept that values social justice above other ethical principles. He stated that under economic constraints, scarce resources ought to be preferentially allocated to younger members of the society. He argued that maintaining a high quality of life within a finite life span was a more reasonable goal than longevity alone [8, 9]. On the other hand, some groups accord a superior and more respected status to the elderly, a viewpoint that values autonomy and beneficence [9]. Thirdly, individuals and societies differ in their preference for autonomy versus reliance on family members for joint decision-making [9]. Lastly, elderly individuals, by virtue of extensive life experiences, have well-formed perspectives on quality of life, longevity, and losses. These values impact their decision-making [9].

Autonomy and Informed Consent

Medical ethics stresses on the principle of autonomy which implies that individuals should be allowed to make independent choices and act in accordance to them without coercion [10, 11]. The concept of informed consent was born out of the necessity to honor autonomy. Informed consent is based on the availability of relevant information, decisional capacity, and voluntarism [11, 12]. Older adults are vulnerable to several conditions that may affect their ability to provide informed consent. Visual and hearing impairment and incorrect assumption on the part of younger providers about an older adult's level of knowledge about existing medical treatments are some of the conditions that hinder the availability of adequate information. Voluntarism is the ability to make choices without coercion. It may be affected by cognitive impairment, specifically executive dysfunction [11, 13]. The presence of apathy which may be an accompanying feature of dementia and psychotic or mood disorders are factors that could affect the ability to make a free choice, independent of whether the individual possesses decisional capacity or not [14]. The possibility of coercion on the part of caregivers is something all geriatric psychiatrists must be sensitive to [11].

Decisional Capacity

Decisional capacity entails the ability to understand information relevant to a clinical situation and about the available choices, to understand how the situation at hand is applicable to them, to reason about the information and choices available, and to also make and express a consistent choice [10, 11, 15]. Decisional capacity is specific to the context, the task at hand, and the time of the evaluation. For example, an individual may possess the capacity to make a decision about a specific diagnostic test (such as colonoscopy) but lack the capacity to make a decision about living independently.

Capacity may be adversely affected by several medical and psychiatric conditions. Delirium, which is common in the elderly and contributed to by several medical conditions, is a common cause of impaired capacity. Decisional capacity impaired by delirium may fluctuate with time. Dementia, by impacting memory, judgment, and problem-solving, is another important contributor to decisional incapacity in older adults. A cross-sectional study focusing on the capacity to participate in research found that greater than 60% of individuals with mild to moderate Alzheimer's disease (AD) were found to lack decisional capacity [16]. Huthwaite et al. conducted a 2-year follow-up study and found that even at baseline, individuals with AD demonstrated impaired decisional capacity across domains of understanding information, appreciating its relevance and reasoning. On follow-up, the AD group had experienced further decline across all four domains, with the greatest impairments being in the understanding and reasoning functions [17]. Parkinson's disease (PD) was found to be associated with impaired decisional capacities, even among individuals who did not have accompanying dementia, with further decline after they developed dementia [11, 18]. Depressed individuals, especially those with pronounced hopelessness have been reported to overestimate risks and underestimate benefits from medical interventions [11, 19]. When compared with individuals with depression- and age-matched controls, a higher proportion of individuals diagnosed with schizophrenia lacked the capacity to make medical decisions. They demonstrated poorer understanding, appreciation, and reasoning abilities [10, 20]. Poor insight, i.e., lack of awareness of their illness, is found to be a strong predictor of impaired decisional capacity among individuals with psychiatric illnesses [21].

Capacity Versus Competence

Competence is a term that is frequently encountered in the context of capacity to make decisions [22]. Although capacity and competence are used interchangeably, competence is by definition a legal construct determined by the court of law, while capacity is a clinical construct determined by clinicians. Competence is dichotomous and fixed—an individual is either competent to perform a task or not. Capacity, on the other hand, can fluctuate with time. A "sliding scale" approach is considered acceptable while evaluating capacity: for a high-benefit and low-risk intervention, the standard required for consent is lower; for a high-risk or low-benefit intervention, more stringent standards are expected [22].

Assessment of Capacity

Psychiatrists are frequently consulted to assess the capacity of patients to make medical decisions [22]. Although this consultation is most commonly requested in the hospital setting when a patient refuses a recommended intervention, a psychiatrist may also be called upon to assess capacity if it is suspected that a patient is consenting to an intervention without adequate understanding.

Firstly, clinicians must be sensitive to the possibility of decisional incapacity among older adults. While no specific diagnosis automatically amounts to incapacity, it is important for clinicians to be aware of the illnesses described in the previous section, which have been frequently associated with impaired capacity. The next step is to clarify the referral question and become familiar with the situation at hand. For example, an assessment of the capacity to make medical decisions would entail adequate familiarity on the part of the consulting psychiatrist regarding the patient's illness and the choices being offered to them. The psychiatrist must then ensure that the patient has received adequate information about their illness as well as the risks and benefits of the intervention recommended to the patient. A consultant may additionally request that the treating medical or other specialty team be present at the time of the capacity evaluation to provide the patient with the necessary information to aid their decision-making.

There are several validated instruments available to assess decisional capacity, the most commonly used tools being the MacArthur Competence Assessment Tool for Treatment (MacCAT-T) [23], the Hopemont Capacity Assessment Interview (HCAI) [24], and the Competency to Consent to Treatment Interview (CCTI) [25]. During the interview, the clinician must initiate a general discussion about the patient's clinical situation and evaluate the patient's understanding and appreciation of their illness and the treatment choices that they are being offered. The clinical interview must also include an exploration of the patient's values and goals, as these may impact the choices an individual makes. Table 31-1 describes the process of assessing the capacity of Mr. B to refuse the aortic valve replacement surgery, using the model described by Grisso and Appelbaum [26].

While structured cognitive assessments such as the Montreal Cognitive Assessment (MOCA) [6] may help with clarification of the diagnosis that is contributing to incapacity, no specific cutoff scores have been reported that directly predicts the presence or absence of incapacity [22]. Collateral information from family and caregivers may be helpful in understanding the patient's overall values, general pattern of decision-making, and their prior experience with the task that they are being evaluated for. For example, an individual who has historically made decisions in collaboration with family may need to be evaluated through a slightly different angle than someone with a history of making decisions independently.

Careful documentation of the capacity evaluation is essential. The rationale for whether a patient is believed to have or lack decisional capacity must be elucidated. In the case of individuals found to lack capacity, the psychiatrist should opine on whether the incapacity is reversible and suggest ways to restore capacity. The "legal" section of the chapter will focus on activation of a health-care power of attorney or guardianship for individuals in whom decisional capacity for a specific task is found to be irreversibly lacking.

Capacity to Manage Finances

Financial capacity is a medicolegal concept that defines the ability of an individual to independently manage their finances, in a manner that is consistent with their values, belief systems, and self-interests [27, 28]. Assessment of financial capacity has clinical, ethical, and legal implications for the older adult. It is a key determinant of the ability to live independently. Impairment of

TABLE 31-1. Clinical assessment of medical decision-making capacity in older adults

Decisional ability	Assessment approach
Understanding	Mr. B is informed about his illness. This would entail information about what is aortic stenosis, how it has resulted in congestive heart failure, and how his current symptoms of shortness of breath are related to it He would then need to be informed the reasons why his medical team is recommending aortic valve replacement surgery and how the surgery is likely to improve his condition. This would be followed by details of the benefits, risks of the procedure, and alternative treatment options, and this information would need to be provided, preferably by a medical expert, in the language best understood by the patient Mr. B is then asked to repeat the above information provided in his own words and his comprehension is assessed Examples of questions: • What problems do you have right now? • Do you think you have a problem with your heart? • What treatment is your doctor recommending? • What are the risks and benefits of the surgery that you have been recommended? • Have any alternative treatment options be discussed?
Appreciation	The clinician tests if Mr. B is able to apply the information provided, to his own life and condition. S/he has to look for the impact of psychosis and mood symptoms in how Mr. B appraises the benefits and risks of treatment • What, according to you, is wrong with your health at the present time? • Why do you believe you're experiencing shortness of breath? • Do you believe you need any treatment? • What according to you is the aortic replacement surgery going to do for your symptoms? • Can the surgery improve your shortness of breath? Help you live longer? • Can the surgery have side effects or cause new problems? • What do you believe may happen if you don't receive the surgery?
Reasoning	The clinician assesses how Mr. B arrived at the decision to not have the aortic valve replacement surgery. She/he must look for the presence or absence of distortions in his thought process • Can you walk me through your thought process of deciding to not have the surgery? • Can you share with me why not having the surgery is a better option for you than having it?
Expressing a choice	The clinician must determine if Mr. B is able to communicate in a consistent manner, his decision to not have the aortic valve replacement surgery (or have the surgery, if the patient has changed his decision) • Have you made a decision about your treatment? • What is your decision about the aortic valve replacement surgery?

the ability to manage finances will result in decreased access to medical care, housing, and social services and make the individual susceptible to abuse and exploitation.

Adults over the age of 65 years constitute approximately 13% of the US population [29] and own 34% of the total wealth [30]. It has been reported that a whopping $18.1 trillion is managed by older adult households in the country. Financial ability is adversely affected by neurodegenerative illnesses such as Alzheimer's disease (AD), Parkinson's disease (PD), frontotemporal dementia (FTD), as well as disorders like schizophrenia which may compromise judgment and problem-solving skills. As the life expectancy and incidence of dementing illnesses continue to increase, clinicians will frequently find themselves in positions of determining a patient's financial capacity.

Financial capacity comprises of a broad range of functions, from simple tasks such as naming and counting currency to complex tasks such as maintaining a checkbook and tipping, understanding, and prioritizing bills and to more sophisticated tasks such as making investment decisions [30, 31]. Allied aspects of this capacity are donative capacity and testamentary capacity. Marson conceptualized financial capacity as having two components, namely, performance and judgment components [30]. The performance aspect is the ability to execute financial tasks such as tipping or paying bills. The judgment aspect is an assessment of whether an individual possesses appropriate judgment and problem-solving skills when it comes to their finances. This distinction is important because individuals may be impaired in one domain but not the other. For example, an individual with frontotemporal dementia (FTD) may have preserved abilities to perform tasks such as paying bills and maintaining checkbooks. However, disinhibition and poor judgment resulting from their illness may cause them to make impulsive donations and investment decisions, which could hamper their overall financial well-being.

Widera et al. outlined the role of a clinician relating to finances into five categories [27]. These include:

1. Education: This involves a basic introduction of the concept of financial incapacity to patients and families, encouraging advance financial planning, recommendation for the appointment of a durable power of attorney. Readers are referred to the "legal" section of this chapter for details on durable power of attorney.
2. Recognizing signs of impairment in financial capacity: It is recommended that clinicians working with older adults be attuned to subtle signs which might indicate financial incapacity. Marson described "warning signs" of impairment such as missed bills, paying bills more than once, misplacing documents, missing tax deadlines, deterioration of mathematical skills reflecting in regular activities such as tipping, and investments that reflect poor judgment [30, 32]. Other signs of impairment and exploitation include addition of new names to financial accounts, unexplained disappearance of money, and a sudden involvement of relatives claiming interest in a patient's financial affairs.
3. Assessment of capacity to manage finances: This step requires a patient-centered approach, rather than mere reliance on standardized cognitive evaluations. It is imperative that the clinician first familiarize themselves with an individual's baseline level of financial functioning, so as to be able to assess for decline [31]. The second step involves a clear understanding of the financial skills the individual needs to possess in order to manage safely and independently in their current environment. For example, financial skill sets required of a retired 75-year-old man living in an assisted living facility where meals are provided would be significantly different from those required of a 65-year-old breadwinner who is working at a managerial level in an organization. Thirdly, the clinician is required to assess a patient's current financial ability by way of patient interviews, cognitive and neuropsychological evaluations, and collateral sources. Following this, the clinician should determine the level of congruence or incongruence between an individual's current financial abilities and the demands of their immediate environment [31].
4. Help support financial independence: It is recommended that the clinician work toward optimizing the patient's financial independence to the extent that is feasible and safe. Advocating for appointment of a durable power of attorney is one such step. Families may also be encouraged to work with banks and other financial institutions in bringing about provisions such as overdraft protection, auto-deposits, and need for dual signatures for transactions involving higher amounts [27].
5. Make appropriate referrals: The assessment of financial capacity is complex, and clinicians possess varying levels of experience and expertise in this area. In complex cases such as those involving family disputes or suspected abuse, it is recommended that clinicians make appropriate referrals to colleagues such as neuropsychologists, forensic psychologists and psychiatrists, and occupational therapists, all of whom possess the training to supplement this assessment. In suspected cases of abuse or exploitation, referral to the Adult Protective Services (APS) is also strongly recommended [27].

As an extension of the assessment of financial capacity, a geriatric psychiatrist may also be called upon to assess a patient's ability to write a will. In some instances, this may be a retrospective evaluation, to determine if the individual possessed testamentary capacity at the time of writing the will. In order to possess testamentary capacity, it is believed that a testator must possess adequate understanding of the concept and purpose of the will and know the nature of their assets and the available beneficiaries. However, accurate and detailed knowledge of their assets is not a prerequisite [22, 33]. Another consideration is whether the execution of the will is wholly voluntary or driven by undue influence. While undue influence can occur even in an individual who has financial and testamentary capacity, conditions, such as dementia, physical and sensory impairments, and dependence on the exploiter for assistance or companionship, increase the susceptible for victimization [22, 33, 34]. It is recommended that clinicians who conduct evaluations of testamentary capacity obtain medical, financial, and legal records as relevant as well as collateral information from family members and other clinicians involved in a patient's care.

Capacity to Live Independently

The ability to live safely and independently is an important life goal for many older adults [35, 36]. Medical, psychiatric, cognitive impairments or a combination thereof can adversely impact one's ability to do so. It is imperative to perform a detailed assessment of capacity for independent living in patients who are felt to be vulnerable to either self-neglect or abuse and exploitation by others [35]. These requests may be initiated by family members or friends, other clinicians, discharge planners in hospitals, and agencies such as Adult Protective Services, to name a few. Accurate assessment of this capacity has key implications for patients. It forms the basis for allocation of in-home resources, guardianship proceedings, and referral to assisted living facilities or skilled nursing facilities. Underestimating a patient's capacity to live independently will result in some loss of autonomy for them [37]. It will also lead to inappropriate channeling of already limited community resources. On the other hand, an overestimation of a patient's ability to live independently is likely to increase their risks for medical and psychiatric deterioration as well as abuse and exploitation by others [35].

Five domains of safe and independent living have been described, namely, (1) personal needs and hygiene, including bathing, toileting, dressing, and feeding; (2) condition of the home environment, including basic repair and maintenance; (3) activities for independent living, such as shopping, preparing meals, cleaning, and transportation; (4) medical self-care, such as medication management and illness monitoring; and (5) financial affairs, which includes paying bills and making financial decisions [36, 38]. Each domain relies on medical, psychiatric, cognitive, and functional abilities to different extents. The ability to make everyday decisions and live independently may be jeopardized by partial deficits across many domains or significant deficits across one or few domains. Common clinical situations that call for assessment of capacity are older adults in whom there is concern about their ability to perform tasks (such as taking medications regularly) but who refuse assistance in performing them (e.g., using a pillbox or having a visiting nurse).

Clinical assessment of the capacity for independent living entails two components, namely, decisional capacity and executive capacity. *Decisional capacity* implies that an individual is able to understand and articulate their personal, medical, and environmental needs, that they are aware of their limitations, and that they are able to describe how they will accomplish their needs in the context of their limitations. *Executive capacity* implies the ability to maintain of an individual to fulfill their personal, medical, and environmental needs. It accounts for physical impairments. If an individual is able to execute necessary tasks by asking for assistance and delegating responsibilities suitably, they are deemed to possess executive capacity for independent living [35, 37].

Naik et al. described a two-step Articulate-Demonstrate approach to assess capacity for independent living. It includes inputs from the patients, family members, or other caregivers. The "Articulate" step, which is often done in the office setting, comprises of an *individualized* approach which focuses on the specific needs and deficits of the patient in question and a *standardized* approach which utilizes structured assessments [35]. In the *individualized* approach, the psychiatrist first performs a clinical assessment to identify common causes of self-neglect such as cognitive impairment and depression. For example, is dementia or depression contributing to their poor compliance with medications? The clinician then assesses the patient's decision-making capacity across the five domains of safe and independent living as described above. The Assessment of Capacity for Everyday Decision-Making (ACED), a semi-structured interview developed by Lai and Karlawish, is a useful tool to make this assessment [37]. This instrument is guided by the Mac-CAT-T, and its objective is to assess a patient's ability to understand a problem; to appreciate its relevance to their circumstances; to understand available solutions, benefits, and risks of each available solution; and to be able to reason each choice, make a choice, and express it consistently [37]. For example, is the abovementioned patient able to understand why they need to take medications regularly, are they aware of their difficulties with taking medications, are they able to articulate the relative benefits and risks of maintaining their current independence versus using a pillbox versus having a visiting nurse, and are they able to make a consistent choice about what they would like to do? The standardized approach supplements the assessment by performing relevant evaluations with validated instruments such as the Executive Interview (EXIT), the Montreal Cognitive Assessment (MOCA), and the Geriatric Depression Scale (GDS) [35].

The Demonstrate step is an assessment of whether an individual is able to put to action their understanding of their problem and the choice they have made. This includes multidisciplinary assessments in the home setting, collateral information from caregivers, and occupational therapy assessments in the clinic or home setting. The Kohlman Evaluation of Living Skills (KELS) is a useful tool in this regard [35]. For the patient who has elected to use a pillbox, this step will include an assessment of whether they are able to appropriately fill the pillbox, observational information from family members who have seen the older adult fill their pillboxes, examination of medication bottles, and medication refill information from the pharmacy.

Capacity to Drive Safely

For many older adults, driving is an important means to independent living and social connectedness. Loss of this ability may affect their ability to obtain health care, engage with their local community, and lead to social isolation and even clinical depression [39, 40]. However, old age and in particular cognitive impairment are frequently associated with reduction in one's capacity to drive safely. Motor vehicle accident injuries were identified as the most common cause of injury-related deaths among individuals between the ages of 65 and 74 years [41]. Elderly drivers were reported to have a higher rate of accidents, when compared to other demographic groups, with the exception of cognitively intact drivers below the age of 25 years [22]. Drivers with dementia have a higher accident rate when compared to age-matched controls across many studies [39, 41, 42]. Individuals with mild cognitive impairment were also found to have impairments in their driving skills [43]. However, a vast majority of drivers with mild dementia have been able to pass formal driving tests [39, 44].

In light of these statistics, geriatric psychiatrists are often faced with the responsibility of appropriate identification and prompt referral of patients who are at high risk for unsafe driving. Self-reports are considered unhelpful in determining safety for driving. Brown et al. reported that while 94% of patients rated themselves as safe drivers, only 41% passed the on-road driving test [45]. Caregiver ratings are considered more reliable, especially in instances when the caregiver identified the patient as unsafe to drive [46]. Among the structured measures of rating dementia, the Clinical Dementia Rating (CDR) tool has been established as a useful measure to assess severity of cognitive impairment. A CDR score of 1, corresponding to mild dementia, has been reported as a sensitive measure to identify unsafe drivers. There is poor correlation between MMSE scores and driving ability [46]. A history of crash in the last 1–5 years or traffic citations in the last 2–3 years were identified as more useful means to predict future crashes, than the presence of dementia alone [46].

It is recommended that at the time of initial diagnosis of dementia, clinicians discuss with patients and families the association of cognitive impairment with unsafe driving. A multidisciplinary approach is recommended in making a decision regarding future driving. Although it is clearly established that individuals with severe dementia should no longer drive, there is no consensus about whether and when individuals with mild cognitive impairment or mild dementia should relinquish their driving privileges [22, 46]. However, in the event of any concern about an older adult's driving ability, it is the responsibility of the clinician to promptly refer them for a formal driving assessment. A good therapeutic relationship, a firm but gentle approach in helping the patient and family consider the safety of themselves and others, and appropriate involvement of caregivers are recommended. It is important that physicians be aware of their individual state laws regarding the obligation to report dangerous driving.

Capacity for Sexual Relations

A large proportion of older adults, including those with cognitive impairment and those domiciled in supervised living arrangements such as nursing homes, remain sexually active [11, 47]. Sexual activity can be a source of comfort to many older adults. It has also been established that many institutionalized elderly individuals remain capable of deriving sexual pleasure [47]. However, it is important to weigh this against the very real potential for exploitation of vulnerably elderly individuals with dementia. This is no established consensus on ways to evaluate the capacity of the older to consent to a sexual act. Lichtenberg and Strzepek [47] proposed a model for capacity assessment which includes the following:

1. Awareness of the relationship: Specifically if the person is aware of who is initiating the sexual contact. It also requires careful assessment to determine if the consent is stemming from delusional beliefs about the identity of the other individual.
2. The ability to avoid exploitation: Especially the ability to say no in the event of undesired sexual contact. Another aspect to consider is if the behavior is consistent with one's premorbid values.
3. Awareness of the potential risks: The risks include awareness of the possibly time-limited nature of the relationship.

The authors have provided an overview of the ethical issues most commonly encountered in the clinical setting. Disclosing the diagnosis of dementia to patients, assessing the capacity to vote, making decisions about the potential benefits versus risks of continuing cognition enhancing medications in severely demented individuals, and assessing the capacity to consent to research are some of the other issues where geriatric psychiatrists may be called upon to provide an expert opinion. For these topics, interested readers are referred to the professional literature [48, 49].

Medicolegal Issues in Geriatric Psychiatry

Health-care providers working with older adults are often faced with situations that need legal involvement. Physicians may be the first ones to identify some of these issues such as lack of decision-making capacity, while other issues such as elderly abuse may incidentally come to their attention. Health-care providers need to be aware of these issues as they are often entrusted with the responsibility of guiding their patients through these complex matters.

Advance Health-Care Planning

Mental health illnesses in elderly can lead to loss of decision-making capacity. Health-care decision-making and delivery can become challenging under such circumstances and threaten the doctrines of informed consent and autonomy. The process and basis of decision-making for a person who has lost decision-making capacity have been debated over the last few decades, and though the process has evolved overtime, there continue to be ethical dilemmas and differing opinions. The level of ethical complexity can be even higher when the decisions involve end-of-life situations. In absence of knowledge of patient's wishes and choices about their health care, it's difficult to determine if use of aggressive life-saving measures will prolong their life or sufferings. Some of these difficulties can be circumvented if patients state their health-care choices to be implemented, should they lose capacity to make decisions in future, through the process of advance health-care planning.

Advance health-care planning (AHCP) "is a process whereby a patient, in consultation with health care providers, family members and important others makes decisions about his or her future health care" [50]. This is the process through which the health-care providers and families learn about patient's choice of treatments and end-of-life medical decisions that should be implemented in an event they are not able to speak for themselves at that time. The essential elements of AHCP are gaining an understanding of patient's values, beliefs, and wishes about their health-care treatment as opposed to focusing on specific hypothetical clinical scenarios [51]. Integrating patient's choices into routine, ongoing care helps better understand patient's wishes and plans for the future. Such discussions should include reviewing patient's current condition, prognosis, and future expectations. Working with patients in formulating their future health-care choices is a slow, iterative ongoing discussion over multiple visits and should be revisited every time there is a change in patient's medical conditions. Assessing patient's readiness to participate in AHCP and addressing barriers is crucial during this stressful and emotional process. Although traditionally AHCP is thought of in context with elderly, it is a process an individual can undertake at any time after 18 years of age. The specific laws governing AHCP vary from state to state, but they essentially serve the same purpose. A copy of state's advance directives can be obtained by contacting the local area Agency on Aging or state's health department.

AHCP can be recorded in a legal document called "advance directives." Health-care providers should encourage patients to formulate their advance directives to maintain a written record of their health-care choices. Data from the 2004 National Nursing Home Survey and the 2007 National Home and Hospice Care Survey shows that, overall, 28% of home health-care patients, 65% of nursing home residents, and 88% of discharged hospice care patients had at least one advance directive on record [52]. Another study found higher completion of advance directives for women, persons who were older, who identified themselves as White, and who had higher levels of income and education. Suffering from cancer, chronic illnesses and institutionalization at nursing home also increased rates of completion of advance directives [53].

There are two main types of advance directives—the "Living Will" and the "durable power of attorney," although there can be documents combining elements of both.

The Living Will is the oldest form of advance directive, which was first proposed by a Illinois human rights attorney, Luis Kutner, in 1969 [54]. A Living Will spells out a person's preferences for end-of-life medical care. It includes statements on life-sustaining treatments like resuscitation, intubation, tube feeding, dialysis, medication preferences, and organ and tissue donation. It may also document patient's wishes in regard to palliative care management including pain management and invasive tests and where the person wishes to die. To increase public awareness and improve completion of Living Will, Patient Self Determination Act [55] was passed which went into effect in December 1991. This act mandates that all Medicare-certified institutions provide written information regarding patients' right to formulate advance directives and explaining what right-to-die options are available under their state law [56]. In most states Living Will goes into effect when a person is diagnosed with a condition specified in their state's Living Will law and when two different physicians certify patient's loss of capacity.

Living Will often results in Physician Orders for Life-Sustaining Treatment (POLST), in which the doctor fills out a form, much like a medical order, based on patient's directives to ensure that the patient receives his preferred treatment in case of need [57]. POLST is an actionable palliative care tool, which is recognized by the whole medical community including first responders and informs them of the treatments the patient wishes to have. It is generally intended for people who have already received a terminal diagnosis. Certain states mandate POLST in certain patient populations such as assisted living and nursing facilities, hospices, home health agencies, dialysis centers, and hospital inpatients being transferred to long-term care [58].

Overtime it became evident that Living Wills were limited in stating patient's wishes as there were often clinical situations that were not addressed in the Living Will. This led to the development of another form of advance directives called "durable power of attorney." Power of attorney (PoA) is a legal authorization which lets one person to be appointed by another person to act on their behalf in matters of private affairs, business, or other legal matters. However, a PoA is revoked if the appointing person loses decision-making capacity. This prohibits the use of PoA for advance health-care planning and led to the development of durable power of attorney (DPoA), also known as "health-care proxy," "health-care surrogate," or "medical power of attorney." The DPoA is a document in which a person (Principle) appoints another trusted person (Agent) to make health-care decisions on their behalf if they are rendered incapacitated in the future. A DPoA can be appointed only while the principle still has capacity and is generally the spouse, next of kin, or a close friend. The decisional powers vested in the DPoA can be very limited or broad depending on what has been specified by the principal, and if the principle wants the agent to give their own input in making the decision, they can allow the agent a certain degree of leeway in the decision-making process. A DPoA has an advantage of decisions being made in keeping with the current circumstances as opposed to the hypothetical scenarios as in the Living Will.

Advance directives offer the advantages of maintaining an individual's autonomy and dignity at end of life and prevent use of aggressive life-prolonging measures. Studies show having advance directives in place significantly reduces stress, anxiety, and depression in the surviving caregivers [59, 60]. Advance directives not only decrease the decision-making burden on caregivers and doctors but also reduce legal burden of appointing conservators. However, there are several criticisms of the way advance directives are currently formulated. Writing down the choices in advance directives often occurs as a one-time process, and they are often not revisited overtime. However, patients may change their treatment choices as their health deteriorates and prognosis is more evident. In such circumstances, advance directives may violate the autonomy that it was designed to protect [61, 62]. Other shortcomings of advance directives are poor completion rates, unavailability of documentation in time of need, poor monitoring of their implementation, and unclear standards for agent's conduct, leading to a risk of abuse by DPoA. The risk of abuse can be reduced by seeking legal advice, choosing someone trustworthy, and building in periodic reviews and accounting into the document. A DPoA can also be revoked or changed as long as the person still has capacity. Patients should be encouraged to carry a wallet-sized card specifying that they have advance directives and give a copy of their advance directives to their doctors, hospitals, and family to ensure they are implemented when needed.

New models of advance directives have evolved to circumvent some of the shortcomings of traditional advance directives models. The best known such model is "Five Wishes" which addresses a person's personal, emotional, spiritual, and medical wishes and is more versatile and comprehensive than the traditional Living Will documents. It currently meets statutory criteria in 42 US states (https://www.agingwithdignity.org/five-wishes). Another program called "Respecting Choices" was started in Wisconsin, USA, in 1991 as a part of community-wide care planning system. Local health-care institutions devised ways to always have advance directives available in patient's medical records. Roles of health-care professionals in helping patients with AHCP were clear, trainings were offered, and quality improvement projects were undertaken if the outcomes were not as desired (http://www.gundersenhealth.org/respecting-choices/). Data from April 1995 to March 1996 shows that of 540 adult deaths in two hospitals, 85% had advance directives, 96% of which were available in medical records [63].

Surrogate Decision-Making

Many patients are faced with an incapacitating illness do not state their future treatment choices in advance. In the absence of advance directives, a surrogate decision-maker is chosen to make decisions on their behalf. Choosing a treatment option for any person is ethically and morally complex decision to make and is fraught with challenges of who to choose as a surrogate and

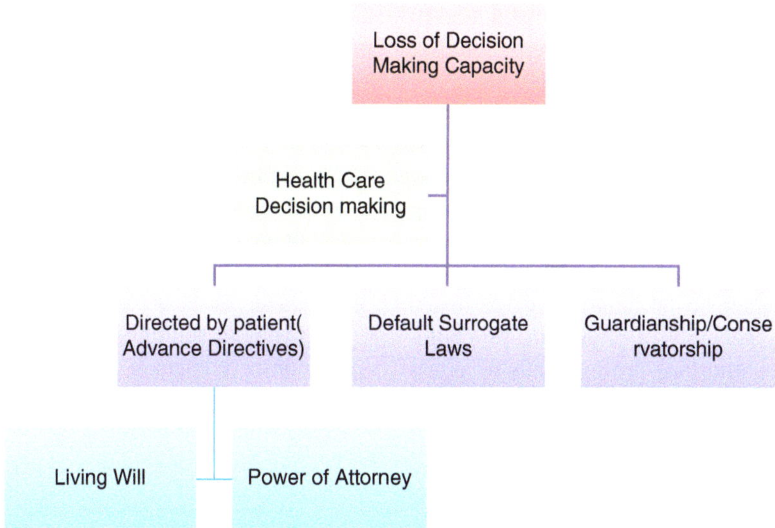

FIGURE 31-1. Surrogate decision-making

how to make surrogate decisions. Surrogates have been shown to suffer long-term psychological and physical outcomes from having to make decisions for their loved ones and should be supported by the clinicians and other family members [64, 65]. Help of hospital's ethical committees can be sought in reducing the decision-making burden on the surrogates and to ensure that a sound decision is made. The choice of a surrogate decision-maker, if not detailed in advance directives, is either made based on a hierarchy established by individual state's law, i.e., default surrogate laws or by a court-appointed party such as a guardian or conservator [66]. Figure 31-1 describes the various options available for surrogate decision-making.

Default Surrogate Laws

Most states specify a priority of surrogates in their state statutes in absence of advance directives [67]. These laws underline the importance of needing alternative forms of decision-making for an incapacitated adult while reducing the burden on court and families to go through a legal system of appointing a surrogate. Currently, 44 states in the United States have described default surrogate laws. Two types of surrogate laws are currently recognized: hierarchy surrogate consent laws and consensus surrogate consent laws. According to hierarchy surrogate consent laws, the next of kin and closest family members usually become the designated surrogate, while consensus statutes allow all reasonably available people to come to a consensus about who should act as the decision-maker [67]. These laws often:

1. Specify the limitations of surrogate decision-makers, often restricting areas of decision-making
2. Address disagreement process among equal priority surrogates
3. Provide standard for decision-making

In states that do not have default surrogate laws, the closest family members still make the decisions, but the absence of clearly defined laws can hamper the process of surrogate decision-making. In such instances, or if a patient does not have any family members, the court can appoint a guardian or a conservator to take care of patient's affairs and make decisions on their behalf.

Guardianship (Conservatorship)

Guardianship, also, referred to as conservatorship, is a legal process utilized when a person can no longer make or communicate safe or sound decisions about his/her person and/or property or has become susceptible to fraud or undue influence [68]. A guardian is a person or agency appointed by the probate court through a due process to oversee the financial and/or personal affairs of an adult person who is determined by the court to be incapable of managing their own affairs. The court must first determine if the prospective ward is incapacitated. Most states require a medical evaluation by designated professionals, generally a physician, psychologist, or other authorized professionals to assess for decision-making capacity. If the person is determined to have lost capacity, a due process ensues, wherein the prospective ward is notified of all proceedings and is allowed representation by counsel. The individual is allowed to cross-examine witnesses and present evidence and has the right to a jury trial. If the person is found to be incapacitated, the court determines the "the least restrictive alternative" for the prospective ward as it affects the ward's legal rights in those areas that he or she has been determined incapable of managing. The process can be initiated by families, health-care providers, government agencies, or other interested parties by petitioning the court. The chosen conservator may be a family member or a relative, or a court-appointed party, like attorneys, department of human services, or department of social services. It is a fiduciary role, i.e., the conservator has the responsibility to act as a faithful trustee and in the best interest of the ward. Conservatorship is often an involuntary process, but a conservator may also be appointed for the same purpose for a capable person who requests such assistance (voluntary conservator).

A conservatorship may be limited or unlimited in its scope and authorities of a conservator vary accordingly [69]. The court may appoint a limited guardian if there is one particular area of the older person's life that he or she is incapable of managing or may grant unlimited authorities to the conservator if the person is found incompetent in multiple areas. There are generally two types of conservators: conservator of person manages health and welfare and conservator of estate manages financial affairs. The conservators may have broad authorities over their wards specified by the court including decisions about their residence, medical treatment, and end-of-life decisions. However, a conservator needs to petition the court to obtain permission for [68]:

- Placing the conserved person in an institution or long-term care
- Changing residence of the conserved person
- Changing tenancy or lease of the conserved person
- Disposing or selling household furnishings of the conserved person
- Selling, mortgaging, or transfering real estate of the conserved person
- Making gifts from conserved person's income or assets
- Using portion of income to support someone who the conserved person is legally required to support
- Investing funds of the conserved person
- Consenting to psychiatric medications for the conserved person
- Executing a document to determine the manner in which the remains of a conserved person will be disposed after death

Conservatorship can lead to extensive curtailment of an individual's rights and should be chosen as a last resort [70]. Alternatives to conservatorship, such as trusts, case management, representatives or substitute payees, community agencies and services should be considered whenever possible [71].

Standards for Surrogate Decision-Making

Substituted Judgment Standard

This standard requires that the surrogate makes the decision that the person would have made for themselves if they could do so. The decision made using substituted judgment standard may not be the same that the surrogate or the health-care team would have made otherwise and is made in keeping with patient's values. This approach is widely practiced and is regarded the best way to safeguard a person's autonomy in absence of any guidelines from them and reduces the decision-making burden on the surrogate. However, some studies show that this is a flawed approach and does not protect patient's autonomy that it was designed to protect. Some of the arguments against substituted judgments are change in a person's wishes over time and inability of surrogates to accurately predict their loved ones wishes [72]. Despite best efforts, patient-designated and next-of-kin surrogates correctly predict patient's treatment preferences in about two-thirds of the cases. Moreover, though most decision-making standards lay emphasis on protecting a person's autonomy, it's found that most patients would want to make their decisions in collaboration with their surrogates and health-care providers as opposed to solely by themselves [73].

Best Interest Standard

This standard is used when there is no surrogate appointed or nothing is known about a patient's values and wishes. This standard requires the surrogate and/or health-care team to choose a treatment that would be in best interest of the patient. This standard is often criticized to be vague and liable to abuse by decision-makers [74].

Elder Abuse

Elder abuse refers to intentionally harmful or neglectful acts by caregiver that harms the vulnerable older adult. Elder abuse is common but often goes unrecognized. One study shows that diagnosis of elder abuse in emergency rooms is two times lower than its prevalence in the population [75]. Self-reported data from 2185 respondents over 70 years of age in a 2010 National Intimate Partner and Sexual Violence Survey (NISVS) showed that 14% of these individuals experienced some form of abuse in the past year, with 12.1% reporting psychological abuse and 1.7% experiencing physical abuse. Approximately 20.8% were abused by both intimate and non-intimate partners. Health-care insecurity was found to be the best correlate of elder abuse [76].

Studies show that majority of victims of elder abuse are over 75 years old, women, and White. Factors such as dependence for activities of daily living, cognitive deficits, guilt, fear of institutionalization, fear of retaliation, disabilities, and physical frailty make the elderly easy victims. Typically, perpetrators live close to the victim and are often close relatives, generally spouse or adult children. Substance use, mental illness, financial dependence on elderly, and history of violence make the perpetrators more likely to abuse the victim [77].

Older adults may be abused in home or institutions and suffer different forms of abuse as detailed in Table 31-2.

Assessment and Diagnosis of Elderly Abuse

Currently there are no screening guidelines for elderly abuse as there is no clear evidence of benefit from regular screening. It is suggested that physicians can detect elder abuse early if they maintain a general high suspicion for it [81]. Table 31-2 details important signs that may help in suspecting elderly abuse and helps with further investigations. An instrument used in primary care setting, such as the Elder Abuse Suspicion Index (EASI), was found to have a sensitivity and specificity of 0.47 and 0.75 [82], respectively, which can be used to detect elderly abuse in cognitively intact patients. Patients who present with injuries and suspected abuse should be evaluated carefully, and a detailed medical history should be obtained. Particular attention should be paid to medication review and noting any offending medications like anticoagulants, sedatives, and anticholinergic medications that can lead to signs and symptoms that mimic elderly abuse. Caution should also be used in detecting elder abuse when the signs and symptoms mimic those of medical conditions seen in old age. Table 31-3 outlines medical conditions that may mimic elderly abuse. In assessing for elder abuse, patient should be asked about their daily routine and their perception of safety of their environment. It's also important to interview the caregiver separately from the patient where elderly abuse is suspected.

In cases where physicians have a high suspicion of elderly abuse, patients should be

TABLE 31-2. Forms of elderly abuse [78–80]

Form	Examples	Red flags
Physical	Hitting, kicking, slapping, force feeding, and restraints	Unexplained bruises in unusual locations, fractures, cuts, sores, burns, intraoral soft tissue injuries, ligature marks, subconjunctival hemorrhage, scalp swelling, and delay in seeking help for injuries
Emotional	Yelling, threatening, humiliation, and social isolation	Unexplained changes in behavior like withdrawal from the environment
Neglect	Caregiver does not respond to the older person's needs	(a) Lack of basic hygiene, clothing, medical aids (glasses, hearing aid, medications, walker, dentures) (b) Untreated bed sores (c) Unexplained weight loss (d) Dehydration, fecal impaction (e) Missing medications (f) Delay in seeking help for injuries
Sexual	Touching, fondling an incompetent person, verbal sexual harassment, and forced sexual activity	Unexplained or new sexually transmitted diseases
Abandonment	Leaving an elderly alone without planning for their care	Unexplained deterioration in health, diaper rash/urine burns, unexplained weight loss, dehydration, and fecal impaction
Financial	Theft of money and coercing the elderly to give/transfer their assets	(a) Lack of amenities that person could easily afford (b) Caregiver with control of elder's money and failing to provide for their needs (c) Elderly person giving uncharacteristically expensive gifts to caregiver

TABLE 31-3. Conditions that mimic elderly abuse [77, 83, 84]

Neglect	Constipation from medications or hypercalcemia, fecal impaction, vaginitis, urinary tract infection (in women), poor wound healing, diabetes mellitus, dehydration secondary to medications
Burns and scalds	Stevens-Johnson syndrome from medications, contact dermatitis, toxic epidermal necrolysis
Sexual assault	Cystocele, uterine prolapse, fixed drug eruption, vaginal bleeding and excoriation from low estrogen, inflammatory bowel disease, vaginitis, perineal excoriation from incontinence or lichen sclerosus, decreased anal sphincter function
Blunt force trauma/ contusion	Fragile photo-aged skin, allergic reactions, fixed drug eruption, bleeding disorder secondary to medications, senile purpura, steroid purpura, fracture from osteoporosis or Paget disease of the bone, Cushing syndrome, thrombocytopenia, subdural hematoma secondary to a fall or coagulopathy
Chemical restraint	Iatrogenic polypharmacy or drug-drug interactions, increased drug levels secondary to decreased renal clearance
Starvation	Inflammatory bowel disease, anorexia caused by mental illness, weight loss from diabetes mellitus, malabsorption caused by hypothyroidism

referred for multidisciplinary assessment and treatment. Hospitalization may be warranted in some cases. A home visit could be requested from social workers or Adult Protective Services, and further actions are guided by state laws. Most states mandate physicians to report elderly abuse to Adult Protective Services [85]. A safety plan should be devised for an elderly patient who has been abused, which should advise patient on knowing their rights, safe places to go to, important phone numbers to keep at hand, regular follow-up appointments with doctors, and frequent home visits from case managers/social workers. Safety of returning to the same environment should be ascertained.

Forensic Issues in Geriatric Psychiatry

The US criminal justice system is aging at a remarkably more rapid rate when compared to the rest of the US population [86]. Incarcerated older adults have unique needs at the intersection of the geriatric and forensic services but are often marginalized by both services. It costs approximately $70,000 annually to accommodate an older adult in prison, an estimate that is three times higher when compared to younger inmates [87]. The combination of extremely poor quality of life and increasing costs makes the care of older adults in the criminal justice system and makes this topic an important public health concern. In this subsection, we will first examine this topic from an epidemiological perspective. The growing numbers of incarcerated older adults, their illness burden, and specialized needs will be elucidated. We will then discuss competence to stand trial with reference to elderly offenders.

Older Adults in the Criminal Justice System: A Growing Population

The time period between 1996 and 2008 saw over 500,000 older adults cycle in and out of US jails, reflecting a 250% increase [88, 89]. Between 1990 and 2009, the overall US population grew by more than a half, and the total prison population doubled while there was an astounding threefold increase in the population of older prisoners [86]. According to the Human Rights Watch, the number of sentenced federal and state prisoners above the age of 65 grew 94 times faster than the total sentenced prisoner population between 2007 and 2010 [90]. The US Department of Justice's Bureau of Justice statistics reported in May 2016 that 66% of state prisoners age 55 or older were serving time for a violent offense, when compared to 58% across other age groups. Elderly individuals are also serving significantly longer sentences than their younger counterparts. For new violent offenses, the sentence length for prisoners over the age of 55 was reported to be 182 months (15 years), remarkably higher, when compared to 116 months (10 years) for individuals between the ages of 40 and 54 and 55 months (5 years) for younger adults between the ages of 18 and 39 [91]. Elderly offenders constitute different subtypes: the first-time older offenders who find themselves in the criminal justice system late in life, the older chronic offenders who find themselves in and out of the system, and the inmate who has grown old in prison. In the next section, we will discuss the illness burden among this population of older adults and the need for concerted efforts on the part of the corrections, aging, and mental health systems.

The Burden of Illness

Poor physical health, comorbid mental illness, environmental risk factors, and exposure to violence lead to accelerated aging among inmates, such that "old age" is presumed to start at 50 in the prison population [90, 92]. Older incarcerated adults have a substantially higher burden of chronic medical illnesses such as hypertension, asthma, arthritis, cancer, and hepatitis when compared to younger prisoners and older non-prisoners [86, 93]. Information on the epidemiology of psychiatric illness among incarcerated older adults is limited by two factors. The first is underdiagnoses, and the second is an overall paucity of research focusing on this age group. A special report of the Bureau of Justice Statistics, the largest national census on the burden of mental illness in the criminal justice system till date, reported that the highest percentage of mental illness was found among older adults in county jails (52.4%), followed by state prisons (39.6%) and federal prisons (36.1%) [94]. Barry et al. reported the prevalence of depression to be approximately 25%, significantly higher than the numbers reported among community-dwelling adults. This group also identified older incarcerated adults as being particularly susceptible to depression and suicide [92]. Studies conducted in other western countries demonstrated varying rates: 30% [95] and 83.3% [96]. Poor vision, overall poor health, chronic pain and disability, but not the length of the sentence correlated with the severity of depression [92, 96]. Approximately 40% of older inmates in a county jail were found to have psychotic disorders [97]. Data from a state prison showed that the prevalence of schizophrenia and bipolar disorder is to be 25% and 18%, respectively, among elderly prisoners [98]. Older adults are at elevated risk for post-traumatic stress reactions due to a higher prevalence for early childhood trauma, ongoing exposure to violence and psychosocial stress, concern over ailing physical health [99], and the fear of dying in prison [100]. Being older and mentally ill places these individuals at higher risks for physical [101] and sexual victimization [102, 103]. Flatt et al. examined older adults in a county jail and reported that approximately 40% of their sample screened positive for PTSD [4]. History of substance use, especially alcohol use, is very high in this population, 67.7–70% [104, 105], although using patterns while being incarcerated has been difficult to discern.

Cognitive impairment is another area of increasing concern for older prisoners. Till date, there has been no national census on the prevalence of dementia in this population. It has been estimated that there were approximately 125,220 prisoners with dementia in 2010, a number that is expected to double in 2030 and triple by 2050 [87]. A combination of increasing burden of chronic illnesses, exposure to trauma, brain injury, chronic substance use, poor living conditions, and mental illnesses predisposes older incarcerated adults to dementia [87, 106]. The process of diagnosing dementia is challenging in this population. There is absence of a reliable and consistent informant, a factor that greatly aids the diagnosis of dementia in the community. Additionally, the standard definitions of activities of daily living (ADLs) and instrumental activities of daily living (IADLs) have limited utility in the context of incarceration. Williams et al. established the prison activities of daily living (PADLs), a list of activities specific to everyday living in the prison, to facilitate the diagnosis of cognitive impairment [107].

Prison activities of daily living
1. Dropping to the floor for alarms
2. Standing for head counts
3. Ambulating to the dining hall for meals
4. Hearing orders from staff
5. Climbing up and down from the top bunk

Dementia gravely impacts the quality of life among the incarcerated older adults. They struggle to follow rules due to impairments in memory, reasoning, and executive functioning as well as personality changes. This inability to comply with tasks makes them more vulnerable to receiving institutional charges, including solitary confinement [87, 108]. Wandering and pacing behaviors resulting from visuospatial impairment disrupt the living areas [87], making demented older adults more likely to become victims as well as perpetrators of violence [103].

There is no policy that requires jails and prisons to provide appropriate geriatric- specific medical and psychiatric care to incarcerated individuals. A few isolated programs focusing on geriatric care have been developed in correctional facilities across the country. The Unit for the Cognitively Impaired (UCI) in Fishkill, New York, consists of a 30-bed unit, with good lighting, an outdoor patio, and interdisciplinary staff trained in the care of cognitively impaired individuals [87]. The "True Grit" program in the Nevada Department of Corrections incorporates numerous activities such as physical activities and art therapy [87]. The California Men's Colony in San Luis Obispo, California, has a specialized dementia unit. This program operates around the principle of "peer support" whereby volunteer inmates with long-standing records of exemplary behavior receive specialized training and are responsible for making sure their elderly counterparts are safe and receive medical care and social support [87].

Experts across the world have also begun to question if the purposes of imprisonment, namely, deterrence, incapacitation, and rehabilitation as conceptualized by legal philosophers, are served in the context of physically and cognitively impaired older adults. They ask if imprisonment is indeed necessary to deter crime in an individual who is unable to recall the circumstances leading to their incarceration or to process the consequences of their previous criminal behavior due to advanced dementia. They have also argued against the need for continued incarceration of older adults who are already incapacitated by physical and cognitive impairments. The feasibility of rehabilitation in this subgroup has also been challenged [109].

The growing segment of elderly prisoners, their unique health-care needs, the lack of an established system to provide cost-effective care to them, and the rising costs have necessitated the identification of priorities to meet these needs. Nine priority areas were conceptualized by a group of experts in prison health care, geriatric medicine and psychiatry, palliative care, prison administration, and prison advocacy. The priority areas identified include defining the term "older prisoner," correctional staff training, defining functional impairment in prison, recognizing and assessing cognitive impairment and dementia, identifying the needs of older women prisoners, creating uniform policies for geriatric housing units, identifying challenges for older adults upon release, improving medical early release policy, and enhancing prison-based palliative care programs [110].

Geriatric Competence to Stand Trial

Competence to stand trial is defined as the legally determined capacity of a criminal defendant to proceed with criminal adjudication [111]. The Dusky Standard was outlined by the court after the landmark Dusky versus the United States, 362 US 402 case. It established that a defendant must be able to understand the objectives of the legal proceedings and be able to assist counsel in his defense in order to be deemed competent to stand trial [111]. With the rising number of geriatric arrests, forensic psychiatrists are being increasingly called upon to evaluate if these older adults are competent to stand trial. There are few studies focusing specifically on geriatric defendants. The rates of incompetence to stand trial vary from 32.3% [19] to 50% [112] in the reports available in the literature.

Among younger defendants, functional psychiatric impairments from psychosis are associated with incompetence [112]. However, dementia, rather than psychosis, is the most common diagnosis among elderly individuals found incompetent to stand trial [112, 113]. Frierson et al. further established alcohol-induced persisting dementia as the common subtype of dementia correlating with incompetence [113]. Disorientation and memory were found to be the most common predictors of incompetence. Defendants who are unable to comprehend a basic sense of person and place or retain information about the case are understandably unable to assist counsel in their defense. Abstraction is required to appreciate the right to legal representation and the right against self-incrimination, the lack of which may affect the competence to stand trial even among individuals with early stages of dementia [29].

Despite the strong association of dementia with incompetence, it is important to note that the diagnosis does not preclude the possibility of restoration of competence [30]. Morris et al. outlined some recommendations to restore competence among cognitively impaired defendants. They call for thorough evaluation to determine and describe the cognitive deficits that contributed to incompetence and initiating treatment geared toward the specific deficits. For example, a defendant who was unable to appropriately participate in court proceedings due to paranoia toward one's attorney may have a chance at being restored with antipsychotic treatment. In contrast, a defendant who was unable to assist counsel due to inability to recognize one's attorney resulting from a progressive dementing illness may be less responsive to treatment. Evaluation for reversible causes of cognitive impairment, management of medical comorbidities, and optimal treatment of comorbid depression are other essential steps toward restoring competence [114].

Treatment Setting Regulations in Geriatric Psychiatry

There are currently 15,600 nursing homes in the United States that house a total of 1.4 million residents. Of these residents 84.9% are over 65 years old, while 41.6% are over 85 years of age. A recent report from National Center for Health Statistics shows that prevalence of dementia in nursing home population is 50.4% while 48.7% of the residents suffer from depression. These rates are higher compared with any other long-term care facility [115]. It is thus imperative that the nursing homes be equipped to treat patients with mental health illnesses, while also being mindful of unique challenges that old age posits. Currently Medicaid pays for 62.9% of the nursing home residents, and the Center of Medicare and Medicaid services (CMS) requires that nursing homes maintain specific standards and follow certain regulations to receive their reimbursement.

Historical Perspective on Nursing Home Regulation and Reform

First federal regulations of long-term care facilities were introduced in Title 1 of the Social Security Act of 1935, which established an Old-Age Assistance program and mandated that its funds only go to the elderly living in nursing homes. This leads to a proliferation of private nursing homes in the United States. However, there was little regulatory oversight over the nursing homes which lead to poor quality of care and nonuniformity in care standards. Passage of Medicare and Medicaid acts in 1965 established some regulations but couldn't ensure better quality of care [116]. In 1970s there were incidents of multiple deaths due to fire and food poisoning in two different nursing homes, while a survey of nursing homes showed major certification deficiencies. The outrage from these cumulative incidences and reports leads to imposition of stricter regulations on nursing homes. Health Care Financing Administration (HCFA), which was established in 1977 to coordinate Medicare and Medicaid, was entrusted with the responsibility of overseeing regulation of these facilities. HCFA proposed changes to improve the certification process for these facilities and to improve quality of care of the residents by elevating their rights to a condition of participation in Medicare and Medicaid and by including resident assessment process. However, these reforms came to a halt with the change in the government and emphasis on universal deregulation by the Reagan government. After much opposition and debate to deregulate long-term care facilities, Institute of Medicine (IOM) was contracted in 1983 to conduct a study on nursing home regulations and quality of care being delivered. IOM released the report "Quality of Care in Nursing Homes" in 1986, which reported that many certified nursing homes provided very inadequate and shockingly deficient care. The report said that not only were the current regulatory system inadequate, deregulation of nursing homes would be inappropriate. Parallel to the study conducted by IOM, a Senate Special Committee on Aging also investigated the issue and reported similar dismal results. Based on the recommendations of IOM report, Congress passed the nursing home reform provisions in Subtitle C of Omnibus Budget Reconciliation Act of 1987 (OBRA 87) [117].

OBRA 87 brought about changes in three major arenas. It established higher quality of care standards for nursing home residents, revised the survey and enforcement system, and merged Medicaid and Medicare standards and certifications into a single system [118].

1. Higher Quality of Care

OBRA laid down specifications for quality of care to promote "maximum practicable functioning" for the nursing home residents. It requires:

(a) Nursing facilities to be responsible for assisting residents in maintaining their activities of daily living including bathing, dressing, eating, ambulating, transferring, and toileting.
(b) Preadmission screening and annual resident reviews (PASRR) should be conducted to make sure that the resident continued to meet the need for placement in nursing home. PASRR requires that (1) all applicants to a Medicaid-certified nursing facility be evaluated for serious mental illness an intellectual disability, (2) be offered the most appropriate setting for their needs (acute hospitalization, community, or nursing facility), and (3) receive the services they need in those settings.
(c) The residents should be assessed at the time of admission and periodically thereafter. These assessments should be used to develop a written plan of care that should be reviewed and revised periodically by an attending physician and a registered nurse. It specified the

creation of a comprehensive functional assessment tool used for clinical assessment and individualized care planning for each resident. Data collected from this tool is used by CMS as one of the measures of the facility's performance.

(d) Physical restraints are specifically prohibited as way for disciplining or convenience. Use of antipsychotic medication as a chemical restraint requires specific indications.

The law and regulations also established a number of quality-of-life rights including the right [119]:

(a) To freedom from abuse, mistreatment, and neglect
(b) To freedom from physical restraints
(c) To privacy
(d) To accommodation of medical, physical, psychological, and social needs
(e) Participation in resident and family groups
(f) To be treated with dignity
(g) To exercise self-determination
(h) To communicate freely
(i) To participate in the review of one's care plan and to be fully informed in advance about any changes in care, treatment, or change of status in the facility
(j) To voice grievances without discrimination or reprisal

OBRA laws also made provisions for better staffing of nursing homes and specified minimal training and credentialing needed by staff members, thus enhancing the quality of care delivered [120]. Nursing homes were required to have every resident be seen by a physician and to ensure availability of a physician at all times.

2. Revised Survey and Enforcement System

OBRA act is required for states to conduct unannounced surveys of nursing home facilities by a multidisciplinary team of professionals at least once every 15 months. The surveyors observed the delivery of care and interviewed residents and families. Sanctions were imposed on facilities that did not meet set standards [118].

3. Merger of Medicare and Medicaid Standards

and Processes

Until OBRA was enforced, skilled nursing facilities and intermediate care facilities needed to meet different standards and were regulated differently. However, OBRA established a unified set of higher standards for both type of facilities, thus removing the arbitrary difference between them. The new standards were substantially higher as detailed above [118].

Impact of OBRA on Psychiatric Care in Nursing Homes

There are few studies that evaluated the impact of OBRA, and the available studies cannot be generalized due to limitations in research methodology [121]. Nevertheless, they demonstrate an overall improved quality of care for nursing home residents in the post-OBRA era. Decreases in the use of physical and chemical restraints are the most widely demonstrated effects. Physical restraints include any device that limits the patient's movements like bedrails, chairs that prevent patients from getting up, belts, etc. Cognitive impairment, behavioral problems, psychiatric illness, and physical dependence have been shown to lead to most cases of restraints [122, 123]. Restraints in the elderly have shown to increase morbidity and mortality and should be avoided. Physical restraints can lead to increase falls, skin breakdown, incontinence, constipation, loss of dignity, and psychological effects like depression from being in restraints [124–126]. Under OBRA 87, residents have the right to be free from any kind of restraint that's not required to treat their medical symptoms. Restraint rates as high as 41% were observed pre OBRA [127]. A CMS survey shows decline in physical restraints from 21.1% in 1991 to less than 5% in 2007 [126].

Antipsychotic medications are often used off label in the elderly for management of behavioral problems due to dementia as a form of chemical restraint. However, the data shows that only one-third of patients may show improvement in their behavioral symptoms from antipsychotic use

[128]. Studies suggest the use of behavioral interventions, environmental interventions, and other safer medications to treat behavioral problems in dementia while reserving the use of antipsychotics for agitation and/or psychosis that is severe enough to warrant treatment [129]. There is an increased risk of stroke and death associated with the use of antipsychotics in patients with dementia, in addition to all their other side effects. Most nursing home residents who are currently prescribed antipsychotics are more than 85 years of age, females, and White. Most users of antipsychotics in nursing homes are diagnosed with dementia (70%) [130]. OBRA requires that nursing home facilities attempt to taper or discontinue antipsychotic drugs for their resident at least every 6 months, but if two trials of tapering have failed and patient has relapsed, another attempt to taper may be contraindicated. Studies showed that the use of antipsychotics in nursing home residents were between 20 and 40% before the enforcement for OBRA, following which the use of antipsychotics has declined by 30–36% since [131–133]. The 2004 National Nursing Home Survey report shows that the prevalence of anti-psychotic/anti-manic medications at 24.82% [134] with the use of typical antipsychotics being less than 1%. Despite an overall decrease in antipsychotic use in the nursing home population, the rate of its prescription remains high and needs further monitoring.

Nursing home regulations were necessary and have shown an overall benefit. However, there is limited data to show the cost-benefit ratio. Hence, more research is necessary to establish benefits of OBRA and to further inform regulatory and reform policies [135].

Conclusions

Aging process can cause alterations in physical and mental functioning of older adults rendering them vulnerable to exploitation. Treatment of older adults is thus fraught with unique ethical and legal challenges. Health-care professionals need to be cognizant of these issues in treatment of their elderly patients in an effort to maintain their autonomy and prevent abuse. Certain illnesses that are more common in older adults can affect their capacity to make decisions. However, loss of capacity should not be assumed due to old age but should be evaluated specific to the situation. Furthermore, every effort should be made to restore capacity in an event it is found to be lacking. Another way of protecting an older person's rights and facilitating a life based on their own decisions even after they lose decision-making capacity is Advanced Health Care Planning (AHCP). Health-care professionals should initiate a discussion about AHCP with their patients and their families and review it periodically. Advising patients to appoint a power of attorney (PoA) to make decisions on their behalf if they are ever not able to do so for themselves in future can help safeguard their autonomy. An important medicolegal issue that deserves consideration in older adults is that of elderly abuse. Signs and symptoms of elder abuse can masquerade as those of illnesses commonly seen in this age group and hence can easily be missed. A thorough assessment is necessitated if abuse is suspected. Most states mandate physicians to report elderly abuse. Lastly, the older adults in prisons are a lesser studied population, but there is a pressing need for better training of prison staff in issues of geriatric psychiatry as this population is growing and has its unique needs.

References

1. US Census Bureau. 2000. http://www.census.gov/main/www/cen2000.html.
2. Jeste DV, Alexopoulos GS, Bartels SJ, Cummings JL, Gallo JJ, Gottlieb GL, et al. Consensus statement on the upcoming crisis in geriatric mental health: research agenda for the next 2 decades. Arch Gen Psychiatry. 1999;56(9):848–53.
3. IOM report retooling for an aging America: building the health care workforce. http://www.nationalacademies.org/hmd/Reports/2008/Retooling-for-an-Aging-America-Building-the-Health-Care-Workforce.aspx.
4. Unutzer J, Katon W, Callahan CM, Williams JW Jr, Hunkeler E, Harpole L, et al. Collaborative care management of late-life depression in the primary care setting: a randomized controlled trial. JAMA. 2002;288(22):2836–45.
5. Reifler BV, Bruce ML. Home-based mental health services for older adults: a review of ten model programs. Am J Geriatr Psychiatry. 2014;22(3):241–7.
6. Nasreddine ZS, Phillips NA, Bedirian V, Charbonneau S, Whitehead V, Collin I, et al. The

Montreal Cognitive Assessment, MoCA: a brief screening tool for mild cognitive impairment. J Am Geriatr Soc. 2005;53(4):695–9.
7. The Belmont Report. http://www.hhs.gov/ohrp/regulations-and-policy/belmont-report/-xbasic.
8. Callahan D, Prager K. Medical care for the elderly: should limits be set? Virtual Mentor. 2008;10(6):404–10.
9. Rabins PV, Black BS. Ethical issues in geriatric psychiatry. Int Rev Psychiatry. 2010;22(3):267–73.
10. Appelbaum PS, Grisso T. The MacArthur treatment competence study. I: mental illness and competence to consent to treatment. Law Hum Behav. 1995;19(2):105–26.
11. Walaszek A. Clinical ethics issues in geriatric psychiatry. Psychiatr Clin North Am. 2009; 32(2):343–59.
12. Roberts LW. Informed consent and the capacity for voluntarism. Am J Psychiatry. 2002;159(5):705–12.
13. Workman RH Jr, McCullough LB, Molinari V, Kunik ME, Orengo C, Khalsa DK, et al. Clinical and ethical implications of impaired executive control functions for patient autonomy. Psychiatr Serv. 2000;51(3):359–63.
14. Grimes AL, McCullough LB, Kunik ME, Molinari V, Workman RH Jr. Informed consent and neuroanatomic correlates of intentionality and voluntariness among psychiatric patients. Psychiatr Serv. 2000;51(12):1561–7.
15. Karlawish J. Measuring decision-making capacity in cognitively impaired individuals. Neurosignals. 2008;16(1):91–8.
16. Kim SY, Caine ED, Currier GW, Leibovici A, Ryan JM. Assessing the competence of persons with Alzheimer's disease in providing informed consent for participation in research. Am J Psychiatry. 2001;158(5):712–7.
17. Huthwaite JS, Martin RC, Griffith HR, Anderson B, Harrell LE, Marson DC. Declining medical decision-making capacity in mild AD: a two-year longitudinal study. Behav Sci Law. 2006;24(4):453–63.
18. Martin RC, Okonkwo OC, Hill J, Griffith HR, Triebel K, Bartolucci A, et al. Medical decision-making capacity in cognitively impaired Parkinson's disease patients without dementia. Mov Disord. 2008;23(13):1867–74.
19. Ganzini L, Lee MA, Heintz RT, Bloom JD, Fenn DS. The effect of depression treatment on elderly patients' preferences for life-sustaining medical therapy. Am J Psychiatry. 1994;151(11):1631–6.
20. Jeste DV, Dunn LB, Palmer BW, Saks E, Halpain M, Cook A, et al. A collaborative model for research on decisional capacity and informed consent in older patients with schizophrenia: bioethics unit of a geriatric psychiatry intervention research center. Psychopharmacology. 2003;171(1):68–74.
21. Cairns R, Maddock C, Buchanan A, David AS, Hayward P, Richardson G, et al. Reliability of mental capacity assessments in psychiatric in-patients. Br J Psychiatry J Ment Sci. 2005;187:372–8.
22. Wettstein RM. Legal issues geriatric psychiatrists should understand. In: Pittsburgh pocket psychiatry series. New York: Oxford University Press; 2013.
23. von Uexkull T. Current problems and tasks of psychosomatic medicine. 2. Med Klin. 1973;68(43):1415–9.
24. Edelstein B. Hopemont capacity assessment interview manual and scoring guide. Morgantown: West Virginia University; 1999.
25. Marson DC, Ingram KK, Cody HA, Harrell LE. Assessing the competency of patients with Alzheimer's disease under different legal standards. A prototype instrument. Arch Neurol. 1995;52(10):949–54.
26. Appelbaum PS, Grisso T. Assessing patients' capacities to consent to treatment. N Engl J Med. 1988;319(25):1635–8.
27. Widera E, Steenpass V, Marson D, Sudore R. Finances in the older patient with cognitive impairment: "he didn't want me to take over". JAMA. 2011;305(7):698–706.
28. Marson D, Hebert T. Testamentary capacity. In: Encyclopedia of psychology and the law. Thousand Oaks, CA: Sage; 2008. p. 798–801.
29. American Psychological Assocation. Fact sheet: age and socioeconimic status. http://www.apa.org/pi/ses/resources/publications/age.aspx.
30. Marson DC. Clinical and ethical aspects of financial capacity in dementia: a commentary. Am J Geriatr Psychiatry. 2013;21(4):392–0.
31. Marson D. Commentary: a role for neuroscience in preventing financial elder abuse. Public Policy Aging Rep. 2016;26(1):12–24.
32. Facklemann K. Memory loss, money loss: early Alzheimer's patients flunk financial test. USA Today. 2008.
33. Shulman KI, Cohen CA, Kirsh FC, Hull IM, Champine PR. Assessment of testamentary capacity and vulnerability to undue influence. Am J Psychiatry. 2007;164(5):722–7.
34. Peisah C, Finkel S, Shulman K, Melding P, Luxenberg J, Heinik J, et al. The wills of older people: risk factors for undue influence. Int Psychogeriatr. 2009;21(1):7–15.
35. Naik AD, Lai JM, Kunik ME, Dyer CB. Assessing capacity in suspected cases of self-neglect. Geriatrics. 2008;63(2):24–31.
36. Skelton F, Kunik ME, Regev T, Naik AD. Determining if an older adult can make and execute decisions to live safely at home: a capacity assessment and intervention model. Arch Gerontol Geriatr. 2010;50(3):300–5.
37. Lai JM, Karlawish J. Assessing the capacity to make everyday decisions: a guide for clinicians and an agenda for future research. Am J Geriatr Psychiatry. 2007;15(2):101–11.
38. Moye J, Butz SW, Marson DC, Wood E. A conceptual model and assessment template for capacity evaluation in adult guardianship. The Gerontologist. 2007;47(5):591–603.

39. Wheatley CJ, Carr DB, Marottoli RA. Consensus statements on driving for persons with dementia. Occup Ther Health Care. 2014;28(2):132–9.
40. Marottoli RA, Mendes de Leon CF, Glass TA, Williams CS, Cooney LM Jr, Berkman LF, et al. Driving cessation and increased depressive symptoms: prospective evidence from the new haven EPESE. Established populations for epidemiologic studies of the elderly. J Am Geriatr Soc. 1997;45(2):202–6.
41. Carr DB, Ott BR. The older adult driver with cognitive impairment: "It's a very frustrating life". JAMA. 2010;303(16):1632–4.
42. Rizzo M, McGehee DV, Dawson JD, Anderson SN. Simulated car crashes at intersections in drivers with Alzheimer disease. Alzheimer Dis Assoc Disord. 2001;15(1):10–20.
43. Frittelli C, Borghetti D, Iudice G, Bonanni E, Maestri M, Tognoni G, et al. Effects of Alzheimer's disease and mild cognitive impairment on driving ability: a controlled clinical study by simulated driving test. Int J Geriatr Psychiatry. 2009;24(3):232–8.
44. Ott BR, Heindel WC, Papandonatos GD, Festa EK, Davis JD, Daiello LA, et al. A longitudinal study of drivers with Alzheimer disease. Neurology. 2008;70(14):1171–8.
45. Brown LB, Ott BR, Papandonatos GD, Sui Y, Ready RE, Morris JC. Prediction of on-road driving performance in patients with early Alzheimer's disease. J Am Geriatr Soc. 2005;53(1):94–8.
46. Iverson DJ, Gronseth GS, Reger MA, Classen S, Dubinsky RM, Rizzo M. Practice parameter update: evaluation and management of driving risk in dementia: report of the quality standards Subcommittee of the American Academy of neurology. Neurology. 2010;74(16):1316–24.
47. Lichtenberg PA, Strzepek DM. Assessments of institutionalized dementia patients' competencies to participate in intimate relationships. The Gerontologist. 1990;30(1):117–20.
48. American Bar Association/American Psychological Association Assessment of Capacity in Older Adults Working Group. Assessment of older adults with diminished capacity: a handbook for psychologists. Washington, DC: American Bar Association; 2008.
49. Klein E, Karlawish J. Ethical issues in the neurology of aging and cognitive decline. In: Aminoff M, Boller F, Swaab D, editors. Ethical and legal issues in neurology: handbook of clinical neurology. Amsterdam: Elsevier; 2014.
50. Singer PA, Robertson G, Roy DJ. Bioethics for clinicians: 6. Advance care planning. CMAJ. 1996;155(12):1689–92.
51. Lum HD, Sudore RL, Bekelman DB. Advance care planning in the elderly. Med Clin North Am. 2015;99(2):391–403.
52. Jones AL, Moss AJ, Harris-Koejtin JD. Use of advance directives in long-term care populations: centers for disease control and prevention, division of health care. Statistics. 2011. http://www.cdc.gov/nchs/products/databriefs/db54.htm.
53. Inoue M. The influence of sociodemographic and psychosocial factors on advance care planning. J Gerontol Soc Work. 2016;59(5):401–22.
54. Sabatino CP. Advance directives and advance care planning: legal and policy issues: office of the Assistant secretary for planning and evaluation. 2007. https://aspe.hhs.gov/basic-report/advance-directives-and-advance-care-planning-legal-and-policy-issues.
55. Patient Self Determination Act of 1990. 1990.
56. Kelley K. The patient self-determination act. A matter of life and death. Physician Assist. 1995;19(3):49. 53–6, 9–60 passim
57. Hickman SE, Keevern E, Hammes BJ. Use of the physician orders for life-sustaining treatment program in the clinical setting: a systematic review of the literature. J Am Geriatr Soc. 2015;63(2):341–50.
58. Pope TM, Hexum M. Legal briefing: POLST: physician orders for life-sustaining treatment. J Clin Ethics. 2012;23(4):353–76.
59. Detering KM, Hancock AD, Reade MC, Silvester W. The impact of advance care planning on end of life care in elderly patients: randomised controlled trial. BMJ. 2010;340:c1345.
60. Bischoff KE, Sudore R, Miao Y, Boscardin WJ, Smith AK. Advance care planning and the quality of end-of-life care in older adults. J Am Geriatr Soc. 2013;61(2):209–14.
61. Hickman SE, Hammes BJ, Moss AH, Tolle SW. Hope for the future: achieving the original intent of advance directives. The Hastings Center Report. 2005;Spec No:S26–30.
62. Spranzi M, Fournier V. The near-failure of advance directives: why they should not be abandoned altogether, but their role radically reconsidered. Med Health Care Philos. 2016;19(4):563–8.
63. Gunderson Lutheran Medical Foundation. Respecting choices. http://www.eutanasia.ws/hemeroteca/z9.pdf.
64. Meeker MA. Family surrogate decision making at the end of life: seeing them through with care and respect. Qual Health Res. 2004;14(2):204–25.
65. Meeker MA, Jezewski MA. Family decision making at end of life. Palliat Support Care. 2005;3(2):131–42.
66. Pope TM. Legal fundamentals of surrogate decision making. Chest. 2012;141(4):1074–81.
67. Wynn S. Decisions by surrogates: an overview of surrogate consent laws in the United States. Bifocal. 2014;36(1):10–4.
68. National Guardianship Association. About Guardianship. http://www.guardianship.org/what_is_guardianship.htm.
69. Kane MN. Legal guardianship and other alternatives in the care of elders with Alzheimer's disease. Am J Alzheimers Dis Other Demen. 2001;16(2):89–96.
70. Peters R, Schmidt WC Jr, Miller KS. Guardianship of the elderly in Tallahassee, Florida. The Gerontologist. 1985;25(5):532–8.

71. Wilber KH, Reynolds SL. Rethinking alternatives to guardianship. The Gerontologist. 1995;35(2):248–57.
72. Tunney RJ, Ziegler FV. Toward a psychology of surrogate decision making. Perspect Psychol Sci. 2015;10(6):880–5.
73. Torke AM, Alexander GC, Lantos J. Substituted judgment: the limitations of autonomy in surrogate decision making. J Gen Intern Med. 2008;23(9):1514–7.
74. Kopelman LM. The best interests standard for incompetent or incapacitated persons of all ages. J Law Med Ethics. 2007;35(1):187–96.
75. Evans CS, Hunold KM, Rosen T, Platts-Mills TF. Diagnosis of elder abuse in U.S. emergency departments. J Am Geriatr Soc. 2017;65(1):91–7.
76. Rosay ABP, Mulford CFP. Prevalence estimates and correlates of elder abuse in the United States: The National Intimate Partner and Sexual Violence Survey. J Elder Abuse Negl. 2017;29(1):1–14.
77. Collins KA. Elder maltreatment: a review. Arch Pathol Lab Med. 2006;130(9):1290–6.
78. Ahmad M, Lachs MS. Elder abuse and neglect: what physicians can and should do. Cleve Clin J Med. 2002;69(10):801–8.
79. National Institute of Aging. Elder abuse. 2015. http://www.nia.nih.gov/health/publication/elder-abuse.
80. National Center on Elder Abuse. Red flags of abuse. https://ncea.acl.gov/resources/docs/Red-Flags-Elder-Abuse-NCEA-2015.pdf.
81. Hoover RM, Polson M. Detecting elder abuse and neglect: assessment and intervention. Am Fam Physician. 2014;89(6):453–60.
82. Yaffe MJ, Wolfson C, Lithwick M, Weiss D. Development and validation of a tool to improve physician identification of elder abuse: the Elder Abuse Suspicion Index (EASI). J Elder Abuse Negl. 2008;20(3):276–300.
83. Switzer JA, Michienzi AE. Elder abuse: an update on prevalence, identification, and reporting for the orthopaedic surgeon. J Am Acad Orthop Surg. 2012;20(12):788–94.
84. Kruger RM, Moon CH. Can you spot the signs of elder mistreatment? Postgrad Med. 1999;106(2):169–73. 177–8, 183
85. Swagerty DL Jr, Takahashi PY, Evans JM. Elder mistreatment. Am Fam Physician. 1999;59(10):2804–8.
86. Williams BA, Goodwin JS, Baillargeon J, Ahalt C, Walter LC. Addressing the aging crisis in U.S. criminal justice health care. J Am Geriatr Soc. 2012;60(6):1150–6.
87. Maschi T, Kwak J, Ko E, Morrissey MB. Forget me not: dementia in prison. The Gerontologist. 2012;52(4):441–51.
88. Forbes MK, Crome E, Sunderland M, Wuthrich VM. Perceived needs for mental health care and barriers to treatment across age groups. Aging Ment Health. 2017;21(10):1072–8.
89. Beck AJ, Berzofsky M, Caspar R, Krebs C. Sexual victimization in prisons and jails reported by inmates, 2011–12. BJS. 2013.
90. Watch HR. Old behind bars: the aging prison population in the United States. 2012. http://www.hrw.org/sites/default/files/reports/usprisons0112webwcover_0.pdf.
91. Bureau of Justice Statistics. Prisoners aged 55 or older made up 10 percent of the state prison population in 2013, up from 3 percent in 1993. 2016. http://www.bjs.gov/content/pub/press/aspp9313pr.cfm.
92. Barry LC, Wakefield DB, Trestman RL, Conwell Y. Disability in prison activities of daily living and likelihood of depression and suicidal ideation in older prisoners. Int J Geriatr Psychiatry. 2017;32(10):1141–9.
93. Binswanger IA, Krueger PM, Steiner JF. Prevalence of chronic medical conditions among jail and prison inmates in the USA compared with the general population. J Epidemiol Community Health. 2009;63(11):912–9.
94. James D, Glaze L. Bureau of Justice Statistics Special Report: mental health problems of prison and jail inmates. 2006. http://www.bjs.gov/content/pub/pdf/mhppji.pdf.
95. Fazel S, Hope T, O'Donnell I, Jacoby R. Hidden psychiatric morbidity in elderly prisoners. Br J Psychiatry J Ment Sci. 2001;179:535–9.
96. Kingston P, Le Mesurier N, Yorston G, Wardle S, Heath L. Psychiatric morbidity in older prisoners: unrecognized and undertreated. Int Psychogeriatr. 2011;23(8):1354–60.
97. Paradis C, Broner N, Maher L-M, O'rourke T. Mentally ill elderly jail detainees: psychiatric, psychosocial and legal factors. J Offender Rehabil. 2011;31(1-2):77–86.
98. Caverley S. Older mentally ill inmates: a descriptive study. J Correct Health Care. 2006;12(4):262–8.
99. Maschi T, Morgen K, Zgoba K, Courtney D, Ristow J. Age, cumulative trauma and stressful life events, and post-traumatic stress symptoms among older adults in prison: do subjective impressions matter? The Gerontologist. 2011;51(5):675–86.
100. Aday R. Aging prisoners' concerns toward dying in prison. OMEGA-J Death Dying. 2006;52(3):199–216.
101. Blitz CL, Wolff N, Shi J. Physical victimization in prison: the role of mental illness. Int J Law Psychiatry. 2008;31(5):385–93.
102. Struckman-Johnson C, Struckman-Johnson D, Rucker L, Bumby K, Donaldson S. Sexual coercion reported by men and women in prison. J Sex Res. 1996;33(1):67–76.
103. Stojkovic S. Elderly prisoners: a growing and forgotten group within correctional systems vulnerable to elder abuse. J Elder Abuse Negl. 2007;19(3–4):97–117.
104. Lewis CF, Fields C, Rainey E. A study of geriatric forensic evaluees: who are the violent elderly? J Am Acad Psychiatry Law. 2006;34(3):324–32.
105. Arndt S, Turvey CL, Flaum M. Older offenders, substance abuse, and treatment. Am J Geriatr Psychiatry. 2002;10(6):733–9.

106. Maschi T, Dennis KS, Gibson S, MacMillan T, Sternberg S, Hom M. Trauma and stress among older adults in the criminal justice system: a review of the literature with implications for social work. J Gerontol Soc Work. 2011;54(4):390–424.
107. Williams BA, Lindquist K, Sudore RL, Strupp HM, Willmott DJ, Walter LC. Being old and doing time: functional impairment and adverse experiences of geriatric female prisoners. J Am Geriatr Soc. 2006;54(4):702–7.
108. Craig Haney University. The psychological impact of incarceration. 2001. https://aspe.hhs.gov/basic-report/psychological-impact-incarceration-implications-post-prison-adjustment.
109. Fazel S, McMillan J, O'Donnell I. Dementia in prison: ethical and legal implications. J Med Ethics. 2002;28(3):156–9.
110. Williams BA, Stern MF, Mellow J, Safer M, Greifinger RB. Aging in correctional custody: setting a policy agenda for older prisoner health care. Am J Public Health. 2012;102(8):1475–81.
111. Mossman D, Noffsinger SG, Ash P, Frierson RL, Gerbasi J, Hackett M, et al. AAPL practice guideline for the forensic psychiatric evaluation of competence to stand trial. J Am Acad Psychiatry Law. 2007;35(4 Suppl):S3–72.
112. Heinik J, Kimhi R, Ph. Hes. J. Dementia and crime: a forensic psychiatry study unit in Israel. Int J Geriatr Psychiatry. 1994;9:491–4.
113. Frierson RL, Shea SJ, Shea ME. Competence-to-stand-trial evaluations of geriatric defendants. J Am Acad Psychiatry Law. 2002;30(2):252–6.
114. Morris DR, Parker GF. Effects of advanced age and dementia on restoration of competence to stand trial. Int J Law Psychiatry. 2009;32(3):156–60.
115. National Center for Health Statistics. Long-term care providers and services users in the United States: data from the national study of long-term care providers, 2013–2014. 2016.
116. Elderly FAT. The history of nursing homes. http://www.4fate.org/history.pdf.
117. Emerzian AD, Stampp T. Nursing home reform: its legislative history and economic impact upon nursing homes. Benefits Q. 1993;9(1):19–28.
118. Wiener JM, Freiman MP, Brown D. Nursing home care quality: twenty years after the Omnibus Budget Reconciliation Act of 1987. 2007. http://www.allhealth.org/briefingmaterials/Wiener-1002.pdf.
119. Klauber M. The 1987 Nursing Home Reform Act: AARP. 2001. http://www.aarp.org/home-garden/livable-communities/info-2001/the_1987_nursing_home_reform_act.html.
120. Francese T, Mohler M. Long-term care nurse staffing requirements: has OBRA really helped? Geriatr Nurs. 1994;15(3):139–41.
121. Kumar V, Norton EC, Encinosa WE. OBRA 1987 and the quality of nursing home care. Int J Health Care Finance Econ. 2006;6(1):49–81.
122. Huizing AR, Hamers JP, de Jonge J, Candel M, Berger MP. Organisational determinants of the use of physical restraints: a multilevel approach. Soc Sci Med. 2007;65(5):924–33.
123. Sullivan-Marx EM, Strumpf NE, Evans LK, Baumgarten M, Maislin G. Predictors of continued physical restraint use in nursing home residents following restraint reduction efforts. J Am Geriatr Soc. 1999;47(3):342–8.
124. Mohler R, Richter T, Kopke S, Meyer G. Interventions for preventing and reducing the use of physical restraints in long-term geriatric care. Cochrane Database Syst Rev. 2011;2:CD007546.
125. Evans D, Wood J, Lambert L. Patient injury and physical restraint devices: a systematic review. J Adv Nurs. 2003;41(3):274–82.
126. Centers for Medicare and Medicaid Services. Freedom from unnecessary physical restraints: two decades of National Progress in Nursing Home Care. 2008.
127. Strumpf NE, Tomes N. Restraining the troublesome patient. A historical perspective on a contemporary debate. Nurs Hist Rev. 1993;1:3–24.
128. Wragg RE, Jeste DV. Neuroleptics and alternative treatments. Management of behavioral symptoms and psychosis in Alzheimer's disease and related conditions. Psychiatr Clin North Am. 1988;11(1):195–213.
129. Tariot PN, Profenno LA, Ismail MS. Efficacy of atypical antipsychotics in elderly patients with dementia. J Clin Psychiatry. 2004;65(Suppl 11):11–5.
130. Kamble P, Chen H, Sherer J, Aparasu RR. Antipsychotic drug use among elderly nursing home residents in the United States. Am J Geriatr Pharmacother. 2008;6(4):187–97.
131. Lantz MS, Giambanco V, Buchalter EN. A ten-year review of the effect of OBRA-87 on psychotropic prescribing practices in an academic nursing home. Psychiatr Serv. 1996;47(9):951–5.
132. Llorente MD, Olsen EJ, Leyva O, Silverman MA, Lewis JE, Rivero J. Use of antipsychotic drugs in nursing homes: current compliance with OBRA regulations. J Am Geriatr Soc. 1998;46(2):198–201.
133. Stoudemire A, Smith DA. OBRA regulations and the use of psychotropic drugs in long-term care facilities: impact and implications for geropsychiatric care. Gen Hosp Psychiatry. 1996;18(2):77–94.
134. Dwyer LL, Raofi S, Lees KA, Laulose R. Medication data from nationally representative provider-and population-based surveys. 2006. http://www.cdc.gov/nchs/ppt/duc2006/Dwyer_50.ppt.
135. Walshe K. Regulating U.S. nursing homes: are we learning from experience? Health Aff. 2001;20(6):128–44.

Part VII

Medical and Neurologic Aspects of Geriatric Psychiatry

32 Care of Patients with Neurologic Disease

Sophia Wang

Movement Disorders and Amyotrophic Lateral Sclerosis (ALS)

Parkinson's Disease

Parkinson's disease (PD) has a prevalence of 1% of people who are 60 and over [1]. The prevalence of PD increases until patients are in their 80s [2]. Although PD traditionally focuses on motor symptoms, there is growing recognition of the importance of the cognitive and psychiatric symptoms in the late stages of the disease. About 15–20% of patients have MCI at the time of diagnosis, and the prevalence of dementia is about 50% after 10 years from disease onset [3]. About 35% of patients have depression and about 40% of patients have anxiety [4]. The prevalence of impulsive control disorders is less than 15% [5].

PD dementia (PDD) and dementia with Lewy bodies (DLB) make up the class of the Lewy body dementias (LBD) [3].The classic hallmark of LBD is the deposition of α-synuclein (Lewy bodies) in neurons and associated neuronal loss. It is not well-known whether α-synuclein is neurotoxic or part of a neuroprotective reaction. Furthermore, proteins involved in other types of dementia (β-amyloid and tau) may also appear in idiopathic and familial PD. This suggests a synergistic interaction between pathophysiology of PD and other processes seen in AD. There is no significant co-occurrence between idiopathic PD and cerebrovascular disease [3].

Risk factors for PD include age, male sex, nonsmoking status, family history, pesticide exposure, and heavy metal exposure [1]. Only 15% of patients with PD have a family history of the illness. Mutations in *LRRK2* (leucine-rich repeat kinase 2) and *SNCA* (α-synuclein) are associated with autosomal dominant PD. Mutations in *PARK2* (parkin RBR E3 ubiquitin protein ligase), *PARK7* (Parkinson protein 7), or *PINK1* (PTEN-induced putative kinase 1) are associated with autosomal recessive PD. Certain genes such as *GBA* (glucosidase, beta, acid) and *UCHL1* (ubiquitin C-terminal hydrolase L1) may modify the risk for PD [6]. Risk factors for PDD include age, time of diagnosis, rigid-akinetic phenotype, severe impairment, impaired semantic fluency, genetic factors, low educational attainment, and postural instability [7].

The clinical diagnosis of Parkinson's disease is based on the Queen Square Brain Bank Criteria [8]. The first step is to diagnose parkinsonism syndromes, which are bradykinesia and at least one of the following: (1) muscular rigidity, (2) 4–6 Hz rest tremor, or (3) postural instability not caused by primary visual, vestibular, cerebellar, or proprioceptive dysfunction. The second step is to review the exclusion criteria which include neuroleptic use at onset, supranuclear gaze, more than one affected relative, and early severe dementia with disturbances of memory, lan-

R. R. Tampi et al. (eds.), *Psychiatric Disorders Late in Life*, https://doi.org/10.1007/978-3-319-73078-3_32

guage, and praxis. Clinicians should also consider antiemetics, antivertigo medications, and, less commonly, other non-dopaminergic medications such as lithium or valproic acid as possible causes for the symptoms. The third step is to determine whether the patient has three supportive features of PD, which include unilateral onset, rest tremor present, response to levodopa, and clinical course of 10 years. Note that in DLB, dementia develops within 1 year of onset of spontaneous parkinsonism, whereas in PDD, dementia develops as the disease progresses. In the late phase of PD, non-motor symptoms become the predominant issue, and this is often when psychiatrists are consulted [9]. Common non-motor symptoms include physical concerns such as falls, postural instability, urinary dysfunction, and dysarthria and choking. They also include a range of psychiatric issues including excessive daytime sleepiness, dementia, psychosis, apathy, depression, and anxiety.

Dopaminergic agents continue to be the initial treatment for motor symptoms from PD. Common drug classes are levodopa formulations (including carbidopa-levodopa), catechol-O-methyltransferase (COMT) inhibitors (including entacapone and tolcapone), dopamine agonists (including pramipexole and ropinirole), monoamine oxidase-B inhibitors, and amantadine. Deep brain stimulation (DBS) is effective for motor symptoms in advanced PD, but patients who underwent DBS of the subthalamic nucleus were found to have greater rates of both attempted and completed suicides [10]. The suicide rate for this population continued to be higher than expected for at least a year after the procedure [10]. Patients who undergo DBS of the subthalamic nucleus should be monitored carefully for suicide. On the other hand, patients who undergo pallidal stimulation have improved depressive symptoms, so this type of stimulation is preferred for patients with PD and comorbid psychiatric disorders.

Rivastigmine is FDA-approved for use among individuals with PDD. Depression should be managed among individuals with PD by reducing psychosocial stressors and increasing the dose of the dopamine agonist. If these approaches do not work, then depression can be treated with tricyclic antidepressants (TCAs), selective serotonin reuptake inhibitors (SSRIs), or serotonin-norepinephrine reuptake inhibitors (SNRIs) [10]. TCAs have anticholinergic effects, and the efficacy of SSRIs is questionable among individuals with PD. Venlafaxine and nortriptyline are thought to be the preferred antidepressants for depression among individuals with PD. Cognitive behavioral therapy (CBT) may also be helpful for depression among individuals with PD [10]. Electroconvulsive therapy (ECT) and repetitive transcranial magnetic stimulation (rTMS) may have efficacy in treating severe depression among individuals with PD.

The first step in treating psychosis in PD is to determine whether non-pharmacologic interventions can be used among these individuals. Hallucinations that do not bother the patient or create severe behavioral disturbances should not be treated unless requested by the patient or their family members. Caregivers should receive education about how to manage the psychotic symptoms in individuals with PD. Secondly the dose of levodopa-carbidopa should be reduced to the minimum effective dose to reduce the dopaminergic burden. In many cases, however, patients cannot tolerate a lower dose because of worsening parkinsonian symptoms. Antipsychotics such as quetiapine and clozapine can be used; clozapine has anticholinergic effects and requires close lab monitoring for neutropenia and agranulocytosis. Pimavanserin, a serotonin (2A) receptor inverse agonist, was approved by the FDA in 2016 for Parkinson's disease psychosis.

Essential Tremor

One of the most common pathologic tremors in older adults is essential tremor (ET). ET is often described as "benign," but as the disease progresses with age, it can become quite disabling. The diagnosis of ET relies on clinical examination. The classic presentation is bilateral, symmetric postural tremor that is visible and persistent [11]. It is present in the hands and forearms, but other parts of the body such as the voice and head may also be affected. Other symptoms such as dystonia, significant balance disturbance, cognitive decline, or isolated tremor of specific body part such as the head or jaw should raise concerns for other disorders. Essential tremor is generally treated with beta-blockers, trihexyphenidyl, primidone, and clonazepam [12]. Beta-blockers such as propranolol are first-line agents but can be contraindicated in patients with asthma. Trihexyphenidyl and clonazepam are on the Beers criteria list given their adverse effect profile and primidone can cause significant sedation among older individuals.

Huntington's Disease (HD)

HD is a rare movement disorder which initially presents as mild chorea (often a slight fidgetiness) but eventually progresses to complete physical disability, dementia, and death [13]. The estimated worldwide prevalence of HD is 2.71 per 100,000. This prevalence, however, ranges from an overall prevalence of 5.70 per 100,000 in North America, Europe, and Australia to 0.40 per 100,000 in Asia [14]. HD is caused by the trinucleotide CAG repeat expansion of the huntingtin (*HTT*) gene on chromosome 4. This repeat expansion results in a toxic gain of functional mutant huntingtin protein. Based on cell and animal models, the mutant huntingtin causes a number of pathogenic processes including oxidative stress, protein misfolding, neuronal dysfunction, and eventual cell death [15].

The degree of penetrance of HD depends on the number of trinucleotide repeats; variable penetrance occurs between 36 and 39 repeats and full penetrance occurs at ≥40 repeats [15]. HD is an autosomal dominant disorder, with each child having a 50/50 chance of inheriting the disorder. With each generation, however, HD can present with more severe symptoms and signs and have an earlier age of onset because of the process of "anticipation." Anticipation occurs due to an increase in the number of trinucleotide repeats with each generation as these can potentially increase during cell division [16].

The age of onset of HD is usually in their 40–50s but can range widely from childhood to old age [13]. The disease duration is about 20 years, and patients become wheelchair bound because of the severity of the chorea and eventually die from aspiration due to dysphagia and dysarthria [13]. Clinicians have traditionally focused on the motor features of HD (chorea, dystonia, and motor impersistence). However, there has been an increasing recognition of importance of the cognitive and psychiatric features of HD recently. The initial cognitive deficits are consistent with a subcortical dementia. Patients have difficulty with executive function, attention, working memory, and psychomotor speed, whereas semantic memory, language, and visuospatial functioning remain relatively intact [17]. Eventually, all patients progress to dementia. Psychiatric manifestations include depression, irritability, anxiety, mood lability, and suicidality. All patients who are at risk for HD or are coping with functional decline from HD should be carefully assessed for suicide. In a study over 4000 individuals in the Huntington Study Group database, the prevalence of suicide ideation in the group before a formal diagnosis had been made was 9.1%. In those patients who were diagnosed with HD, 16.7% had suicidal ideation in early stage and 21.6% had suicidal ideation as they started to lose their independence due to functional decline [18]. The PREDICT-HD group found that psychiatric symptoms develop more commonly during the prodrome period and symptoms worsened as the disease progressed [19]. The gold standard for diagnosis of HD is genetic testing; however, in cases of a clinical presentation and a clear family history of autosomal dominant transmission, genetic testing can be deferred. Approximately 10% of HD cases are sporadic and genetic testing should be done to confirm HD and rule out Huntington's-like diseases [13]. Neuroimaging, lumbar puncture, and other genetic or autoimmune tests can also be obtained to rule out other disorders.

The only FDA-approved treatment for HD is tetrabenazine. Tetrabenazine reduces synaptic monoamines (including dopamine) and has been shown to improve chorea [13]. However, it can also worsen neuropsychiatric symptoms, including suicidality, so it must be used cautiously. D2 blockers can be used off-label to symptomatically manage chorea. Olanzapine, SSRIs, and adjunct mood stabilizers (carbamazepine, valproic acid, and lamotrigine) can be useful for managing the common psychiatric symptoms in HD including depression, anxiety, irritability, mood lability, and suicidality [13]. Non-pharmacologic interventions are of limited use for psychiatric symptoms in HD, especially as the disease progresses.

Interdisciplinary teams, particularly with palliative care specialists are crucial in ensuring the optimal management and quality of life for HD patients.

Amyotrophic Lateral Sclerosis (ALS)

ALS is a motor neuron disease (MND) that causes degeneration of the upper and/or the lower motor neurons. It is the most commonly acquired MND with an estimated prevalence in the USA of 3.9 out of 100,000 individuals [20]. Sporadic ALS (about 90% of cases) occurs more commonly in those 60–69 years in age [21]. Patients with a familial history of ALS, however, have an average age of onset of approximately 46 years [22]. Common clinical features of ALS include both signs of upper motor neuron (UMN) disease such as spasticity, hyperreflexia, clonus, pathologic reflexes, and lower motor neuron (LMN) disease such as muscle wasting, flaccidity, hyporeflexia, and fasciculations. The diagnosis of ALS should fulfill the revised El Escorial criteria: (1) evidence of LMN degeneration by clinical, electrophysiological, or neuropathologic examination; (2) evidence of UMN degeneration by clinical examination; (3) progressive spread of symptoms or signs within a region or to other regions, as determined by history or examination; and (4) absence of any other disease processes as evidenced by electrophysiological, pathological, or neuroimaging studies which may explain these findings [23]. Patients have an average life expectancy of 2–5 years and usually die from respiratory failure.

Genetic studies of familial ALS suggest that ALS may be caused by pathological aggregation of various types of proteins in the motor neurons, and this aggregation then results in cell death [22]. Genetic studies suggest an overlap in the pathophysiology between some types of ALS and FTD, since they both share the expansion of chromosome 9 open reading frame 7 (C9orf72) and mutations in transactive response (TAR) DNA-binding protein 43 kDa (TDP-43) [24, 25].

The only FDA-approved treatment for ALS is riluzole, a modulator of glutamate neurotransmission. Comorbid depression and anxiety can be managed with pharmacologic interventions such as SSRIs, SNRIs, mirtazapine, or bupropion and with non-pharmacologic interventions such as psychological support and counseling. Pseudobulbar affect can be managed with dextromethorphan/quinidine, SSRIs, or amitriptyline. Non-pharmacologic measures for symptomatic management include adjustment of fluid and fiber intake for constipation; use of humidifier and reduction of dairy intake for phlegm; acupuncture, massage, and pool therapy for pain; and stretching, massage, and pool therapy for spasticity [22].

Multiple Sclerosis (MS)

Multiple sclerosis (MS) occurs due to the immune system inappropriately attacking myelin, a protein which covers the nerve fibers and is important for the conduction of electrical signal through the nerve fibers. The estimated prevalence of MS varies by geography. It is most prevalent in Western Europe and North America and lowest in Asia, Africa, and the Middle East. Recent studies indicate a prevalence ranging from 50 to 200 per 100,000 in Western Europe and North America [26]. About 9–14% of patients with MS are 65 and older, mainly due to increased survival times [27]. The onset of MS is usually in 20–40-year age group of adults. Late-onset MS (after 50 years of age) is rare but generally has a primary progressive course [27]. Females are at higher risk of developing MS. Latitudinal changes appear to make a difference in Australia and New Zealand but not North America and Europe. The neurobiology of MS is not well-understood. Genetics are known to play a role, but there is only a 25% concordance in twin studies, which suggests that environmental triggers such as a viral infection probably play a role in the pathophysiology of MS [26].

Typical presentations for MS are optic neuritis, internuclear ophthalmoplegia, or partial transverse myelitis [28]. These transient neurologic symptoms must last 24 or more hours and cannot be better explained by other etiologies such as infection. The McDonald criteria updated in 2010 specify the fulfillment of the criteria for dissemination in space and dissemination in time. In brief, a combination of clinical examination, clinical history corroborated by MRI findings, visual evoked potentials, and specific neuroradiological findings which meet the McDonald criteria can be used to confirm the diagnosis of MS. The new MRI criteria now allows for increased sensitivity for the diagnosis of MS. CSF oligoclonal bands are no longer used as a diagnostic criteria but rather as supportive evidence in possible cases [28]. About 80% of initial presentation is relapsing-remitting type, namely, the patient has a complete or partial resolution of neurologic symptoms from "an attack" during which prominent neurologic symptoms/signs are present. The other major type of initial presentation is the primary progressive type, which is characterized by a lack of resolution of neurologic symptoms from an attack. Eventually relapsing-remitting type progresses to the primary progressive type.

Steroids are a well-established treatment for the reduction of severity and duration of MS episodes. Since the early 2000s, several disease-modifying therapies for relapsing-remitting MS have been approved or are currently in clinical trials [29, 30]. First-line treatments for MS include the well-established injectables, β-interferon, and glatiramer acetate. Three oral medications have been approved by the FDA: fingolimod, teriflunomide, and dimethyl fumarate [30]. Their efficacy compared to the injectables needs to be studied further. Monoclonal antibodies have been another major area of study for MS therapeutics [30]. Natalizumab is FDA-approved for MS but requires careful monitoring for progressive multifocal leukoencephalopathy which is potentially fatal. Other monoclonal antibodies including alemtuzumab, daclizumab, and CD20 monoclonal antibodies (rituximab and ocrelizumab) are still under investigation for efficacy and adverse effects. Mitoxantrone (an immunosuppressant) is FDA-approved for the treatment of advanced or chronic MS. Dalfampridine is FDA-approved to improve walking in patients with MS.

Treatment options for both primary and secondary progressive MS are limited [31]. Dextromethorphan or quinidine is effective for treatment of pseudobulbar affect. Botulinum toxin injections are FDA-approved for urinary incontinence resulting from detrusor overactivity caused by multiple sclerosis. Non-pharmacologic interventions which may have efficacy in secondary MS (although rigorous controlled, large-scale trials are often lacking) include physiotherapy for balance; progressive resistance therapy for weakness; aerobic exercise for reduced cardiovascular fitness; energy conservation exercises for fatigue, bodyweight-supported treadmill training, transcutaneous electrical nerve stimulation, and exercise or massage for pain; cognitive retraining and exercise for cognitive dysfunction; and cognitive behavioral therapy for depression [31].

Stroke

Stroke is the fifth leading cause of death in the USA and is the leading cause of long-term disability [32]. Risk factors include age, previous history of stroke or transient ischemic attack (TIA), family history of stroke, African-American or Hispanic ethnicity, hypertension, dyslipidemia, diabetes mellitus (HgbA1c < 7%), cigarette smoking, excessive alcohol consumption, physical activity, diet, obesity, and illicit drug use (most notably intravenous drugs and cocaine) [33]. Stroke is identified as new-onset focal neurologic deficit(s) due to a disruption in the blood supply in the brain. When these focal neurologic deficits last longer than 24 h, this is defined as a stroke. If these deficits resolve within 24 h, then this is known as a transient ischemic attack (TIA). Stroke can be classified into two major types: ischemic and hemorrhagic. The diagnostic workup is fairly similar for both types. A clinical examination should be done, and neuroimaging (preferably an MRI but head CT when an urgent answer is needed or when MRI is unavailable or contraindicated) should be obtained.

Approximately 87% of strokes are classified as ischemic. Ischemic stroke occurs when a blood clot develops inside a cerebral blood vessel or when a blood clot embolizes from another part of the body (usually the heart). This cutting off of the blood supply creates two zones: the core ischemic zone and the ischemic penumbra. If the blood supply is not restored within a few hours of the stroke, the ischemic penumbra also dies. Treatments for ischemic stroke fall into two categories: (1) thrombolytic therapy to reperfuse the penumbra and possibly the core ischemic zone and (2) stroke prevention management. The stroke prevention depends on the subtype. The TOAST classification system designates the subtypes of ischemic stroke: small artery occlusion, large artery occlusion, cardioembolic, and others [34].

Tissue plasminogen activator (tPA) still remains the mainstay for clot thrombolysis in acute ischemic stroke; the window of use has increased from 3 to 4.5 h, but the sooner the tPA is administered, the better the likelihood of successful reperfusion. Mechanical thrombectomy can also be used to remove a blood clot but needs to be used after tPA administration and within 6 h of a stroke [35]. Secondary stroke prevention is the other key aspect to stroke treatment. All patients who have a stroke or TIA should have tight control of blood pressure, diabetes, and hyperlipidemia (with solid evidence for statin-lowering therapy) as per American Heart Association and American Diabetes Association guidelines [36]. Additional ischemic stroke prevention depends on subtype. Extracranial carotid disease should be treated with medical therapy (antiplatelet therapy, statin therapy, and risk factor modification); in certain cases, surgical interventions such as carotid endarterectomy and carotid angioplasty may also be appropriate. Intracranial atherosclerosis should be treated with appropriate medical therapy; surgical interventions are still under investigation. Cardioembolic stroke due to non-valvular atrial fibrillation (both paroxysmal and permanent types) should be treated with a vitamin K antagonist (target INR 2.5), apixaban, and dabigatran; rivaroxaban can be used to treat recurrent non-valvular atrial fibrillation (AF). Patients with non-cardioembolic ischemic stroke or TIA (e.g., lacunar stroke) should be treated with antiplatelet agents (initial options include aspirin monotherapy, the combination of aspirin, and extended-release dipyridamole and clopidogrel) [36]. Non-pharmacologic interventions for prevention of all types of stroke and TIA include smoking cessation, regular physical exercise (one to three times of intense exercise a week), and dietary modifications such as the Mediterranean diet or DASH diet.

Hemorrhagic stroke is divided into two categories: intracerebral hemorrhage (ICH), bleeding in the brain tissue, and subarachnoid hemorrhage (SAH), bleeding in the subarachnoid space, namely, the space between the brain and the surrounding tissue. Hemorrhagic stroke accounts for 13% of strokes and has a mortality of 33% in the first month [37]. Risk factors include age, hypertension, oral anticoagulants, and weakened blood vessels due to aneurysms and arteriovenous malformations. Hemorrhagic strokes occurs when a blood vessel inside the brain breaks, releasing blood and compressing the brain tissue. Treatments include endovascular coiling or surgical treatment (such as clipping the aneurysm). Patients with ICH should also undergo management of risk factors for bleeding (severe coagulation factor deficiency, severe thrombocytopenia, oral anticoagulants), intensive care unit monitoring, glucose monitoring, and treatment with antiepileptic drugs (AEDs) when appropriate [38].

Traumatic Brain Injury (TBI)

Traumatic brain injury (TBI) is a common disorder in older adults. In the USA from 2002 to 2006, the highest rate of TBI was among patients aged 75 years and older (339.3 per 100,000) [39]. The main reason for the higher prevalence of TBI in older adults is falls [39]. Classification criteria for possible, mild, and moderate-severe TBI are listed in Figure. 32-1 [40]. While neuroimaging can be helpful for diagnosing moderate-severe TBI, it can be normal in mild TBI although on neuropathological examination axonal shearing can be seen [41]. Complications from TBI include chronic subdural hematoma, epidural hematoma, and neuropsychiatric sequelae (such as cognitive decline, personality changes, apathy, impulsivity, mood and anxiety disorders, and, more rarely, psychosis and mania) [42]. Moderate and severe TBI are well-established risk factors for dementia. The long-term effects of mild TBI are under investigation [41].

No drugs are FDA-approved to treat the neuropsychiatric sequelae of TBI [43]. The evidence for acetylcholinesterase inhibitors and memantine for dementia secondary to TBI has not been well-demonstrated. Stimulants and dopaminergic agonists such as modafinil and bupropion can be used off-labeled for apathy and fatigue. Cognitive rehabilitation (problem-solving therapy and mne-

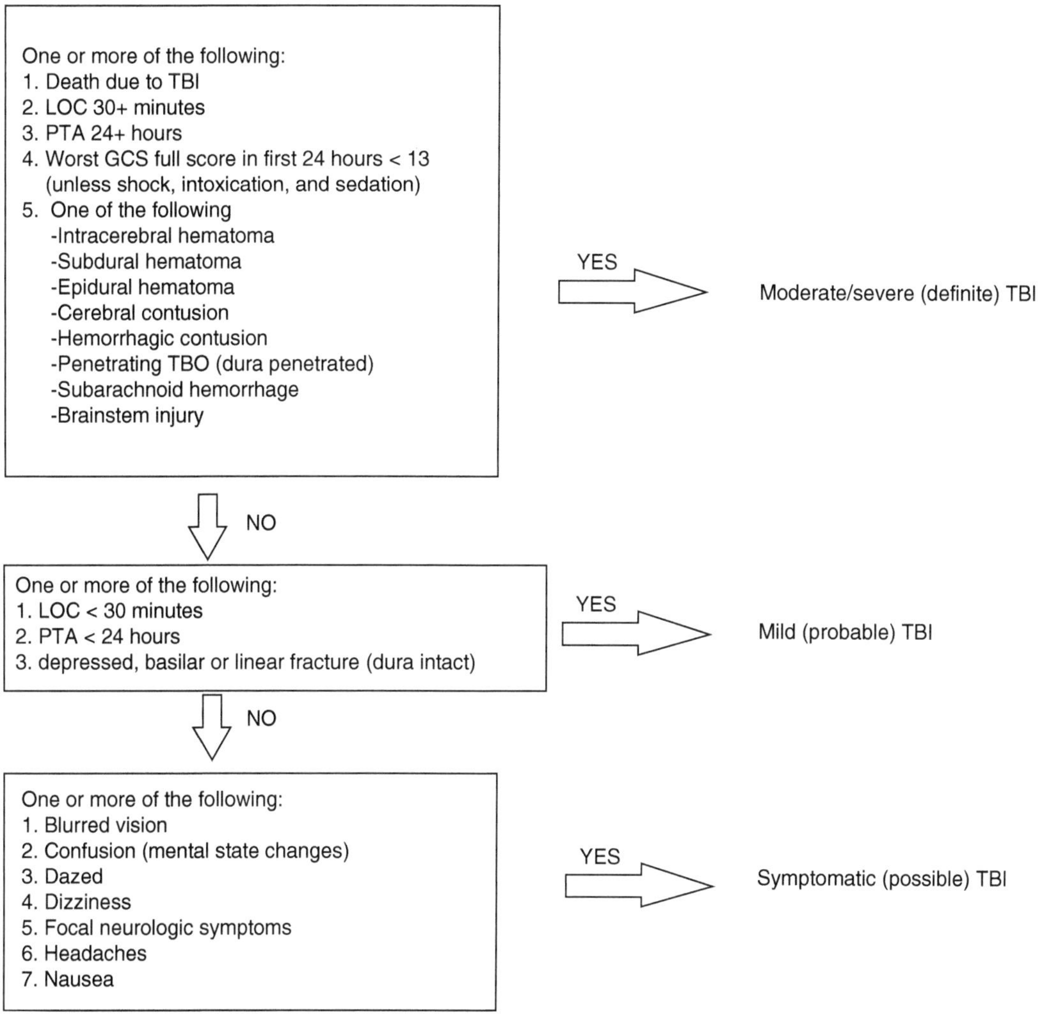

FIGURE. 32-1. Mayo classification of traumatic brain injury. Adapted from Malec JF, Brown AW, Leibson CL et al. The mayo classification system for traumatic brain injury severity. *J Neurotrauma* 2007;24(9):1417–24. *TBI* traumatic brain injury, *GCS* Glasgow coma scale, *LOC* loss of consciousness, *PTA* post-traumatic amnesia

monic devices such as handheld organizers) is crucial for addressing cognitive deficits from TBI. SSRIs can be helpful for treating depression [43]. In terms of non-pharmacologic interventions, environmental modifications to simplify the surroundings can also be helpful especially in cognitively impaired patients. In older adults, fall prevention measures can reduce future risk of TBI. All fall risk prevention measures include simplifying polypharmacy or discontinuing medications on the Beers criteria list and consulting occupational therapy for home and environmental modifications [44].

Seizures

The prevalence of seizures decreases with age, although dementia is a risk factor for epilepsy. Comorbid neuropsychiatric disorders such as mood symptoms and cognitive impairment are more common in older adults with epilepsy [45]. Non-epileptic behavioral disorders which include the paradoxically named "psychogenic seizure" are more common in older adults. The gold standard for diagnosis of seizures is video-EEG monitoring. Ambulatory EEG, however, can also be done and is more convenient. Antiepileptic drugs

(AEDs) fall into two categories: narrow-spectrum and broad-spectrum drugs. Narrow-spectrum drugs are more effective at treating specific seizure syndromes or certain types of seizures (partial or generalized), whereas broad-spectrum drugs can cover both partial and generalized seizures [46]. The broad-spectrum AEDs include phenytoin, levetiracetam, lamotrigine, phenytoin, topiramate, felbamate, zonisamide, valproic acid, and phenobarbital. Combinations of AEDs may be necessary for full seizure control, but at the same time, it increases the likelihood of side effects. Older adults are at higher risk for side effects from AEDs because of decreased hepatic and renal clearance; decreased serum albumin level can also result in increased levels of certain AEDs which are highly protein bound including valproic acid, phenytoin, and carbamazepine [46]. Certain AEDs such as valproic acid, lamotrigine, and carbamazepine are used in the management of bipolar disorder. Drug-drug interactions are common among these three drugs and can affect titration schedules and maximum recommended doses.

Headaches

Although the prevalence of headaches decreases with age [47], about 15% of headaches in older adults have a potentially serious medical or neurologic cause [48]. Therefore, clinicians need to obtain a detailed history and complete a physical examination to determine if older patients present with any of the ominous signs for underlying illness (red flags) (Table 32-1). Even when headaches are not a life-threatening emergency, they are still a significant cause of disability and a common reason for emergency room visits [47].

If a headache due to an emergent cause is suspected on history and/or physical examination, neuroimaging (usually a non-contrast head CT to detect bleeding) and lumbar puncture should be obtained immediately [49]. Additional tests and consultations should also be performed to confirm the suspected etiology. Temporal artery biopsy, erythrocyte sedimentation rate (which if elevated can be supportive of the diagnosis), and emergent rheumatologic and neurosurgical consultations should be obtained in suspected cases of giant cell arteritis (GCA). Tonometry and emergent ophthalmologic consultation should be obtained in suspected cases of acute angle-closure glaucoma (AACG). TIA needs to be ruled out before a patient is diagnosed with migraine with aura; since the incidence of migraine with aura is generally earlier in life, most patients will be able to identify whether the current attack is migraine or not. Once emergent, secondary causes have been ruled out; clinicians often rely on clinical history and physical examination to diagnose the cause of primary headaches.

TABLE 32-1. Red flags for headache emergencies

- Severe, persistent headache that reaches in maximal pain within seconds to minutes
- No similar headaches in the past
- ≥50 years in age
- Abnormal vital signs (e.g., fever, hypertension)
- Altered mental status (including syncope)
- New-onset neurologic signs (focal or non-focal)
- Seizure
- Rapid onset of headache with exertion (exercise or sexual activity)
- Immunosuppression (e.g., HIV and cancer)
- Visual disturbances or abnormal ophthalmologic findings
- Recent head trauma
- Pain spreading to the lower neck and between the shoulders
- Currently taking anticoagulants or sympathomimetics (both as prescribed medications and illicit drugs such as cocaine and methamphetamine)
- Signs of potentially increased intracranial pressure (e.g., nausea, vomiting, papilledema)

Adapted from Cutrer FM. Evaluation of the adult with headache in the emergency department. www.uptodate.com/

Secondary Headaches

Subarachnoid hemorrhage (SAH), intracranial hemorrhage (ICH), TBI, seizures, intracranial neoplasms, and central nervous system (CNS) infections can cause secondary headaches and are discussed in other sections. Giant cell arteritis (GSA or temporal arteritis) is characterized by inflammation of blood vessels in the scalp region. GCA is distinguished by headache, often in the temporal region and visual changes [50]. GCA is more likely in people of Northern European descent and is associated with HLA-DR4 and the alleles of locus HLA-DRB1 [51]. The mechanism is most likely due to autoimmune mechanisms, since people with GCA are at higher risk for another autoimmune disorder including polymyalgia rheumatic [51]. If GCA is suspected, clinicians should immediately initiate high doses of corticosteroids while they await confirmatory biopsy results. If left untreated, GCA can result in permanent blindness. Generally headache symptoms and elevated erythrocyte sedimentation rate (ESR) resolve with treatment.

Acute angle-closure glaucoma (AACG) is characterized by acute loss of vision due to sudden blockage of drainage of the aqueous humor in the eye. Tonometry can be used to detect the sudden increase in intraocular pressure, and physical exam can reveal eye pain and a hardened globe. AACG is an ophthalmologic emergency. Risk factors for AACG include family history of AACG, Asian ethnicity, female, age over 60, and farsightedness [52]. Treatment requires the removal of part of the iris with laser or conventional surgery.

Medication overuse headache (MOH) is often comorbid with tension-type headache (TTH) and migraines. International Classification of Headache Disorders (ICHD-3) criteria requires ≥15 days of headache per month in a patient with a pre-existing headache disorder and more than 3 months of medication overuse for headache management [53]. Risk factors include chronic use of substances (caffeine as part of daily intake or combination analgesics, ergots, triptans, opioids, butalbital, simple analgesics, and acetaminophen) which are often used inappropriately or excessively to manage chronic TTH or migraines. Treatment requires multicomponent interventions. First, patients must be weaned 100% of the offending medications. Second, patients need to be put on appropriate prophylactic medications and learn about non-pharmacologic interventions (see below). Third, clinicians should strictly limit the use of acute medications. Fourth, patients and families should be educated about reasonable expectations about headache medications [54].

Primary Headaches

TTH is the most common type of headache in older adults with an estimated prevalence of more than 30% [55]. TTH is generally a mild to moderate headache which often presents as a bilateral "band-like pressure" that can last from minutes to days and is usually not associated with nausea, photophobia, or phonophobia [53]. TTH is classified by frequency of the headache (infrequent, frequent, and chronic). Although TTH is quite common, the neurobiology of TTH is not well-understood. It is common for patients with TTH to have more than one headache disorder such as migraine and MOH. The first-line treatments for acute symptoms are NSAIDs, salicylates, and aspirin. Caffeine used in combination with analgesics may have some benefits. Butalbital and opioids should be avoided if at all possible to minimize the likelihood of developing headache secondary to substance use or withdrawal. In patients with frequent or chronic TTH, amitriptyline can be used, but it has anticholinergic effects. Second-line prophylactic medications include venlafaxine and mirtazapine [56].

Migraine is another common type of headache in older adults. The two most common types of migraine are without and with aura. Migraine without aura is characterized by at least five headaches that last 4–72 h; headaches usually are unilateral, pulsating, which are moderate to severe in intensity and are associated with nausea and/or photophobia and phonophobia [53]. Migraine with aura is characterized by at least two attacks which consist of an aura followed by a headache within 60 min or less. The aura is characterized by reversible neurologic symptoms (visual, sensory, speech/language, motor, brainstem, or retinal). Each aura symptom can last 5–60 min and at least one must be unilateral [53]. Risk factors include being female, having a family history, having changes in estrogen level (increased prevalence in middle age), and environmental factors such as exercise, skipping meals, and sleep disturbances. Cortical spreading depression is a phenomenon in which a wave of depolarization spreads slowly across the brain which is followed by a suppression of brain activity. This is thought to be a key mechanism for the development of migraine auras [57].

Table 32-2 describes abortive therapies for migraines all have potentially adverse effects in older adults [58]. Prophylactic treatments include first-line agents (strong evidence for efficacy) such as certain anticonvulsants (divalproex sodium and topiramate), certain

TABLE 32-2. Drug classes of abortive therapies for migraines and contraindications

Category of abortive therapies	Contraindications
• Triptans – Preferable in patients with nausea and – Vomiting	– Hemiplegic migraine – Basilar migraine – Ischemic stroke – Ischemic heart disease – Prinzmetal's angina – Uncontrolled hypertension – Pregnancy
• Dopaminergic blockers – Preferable in patients with nausea and – Vomiting – Can be co-administered with – Diphenhydramine to prevent extrapyramidal – Symptoms	– Extrapyramidal symptoms – Diphenhydramine—anticholinergic effects
• Dihydroergotamine with metoclopramide	– Ischemic vascular disease (cardiovascular, cerebrovascular, and peripheral)
• Ketorolac	– Renal dysfunction

Adapted from Bajwa ZH and Smith JH. Acute treatment of migraine in adults. www.uptodate.com/

beta-blockers (metoprolol, propranolol, and timolol), and second-line agents (moderate evidence for efficacy) such as certain antidepressants (amitriptyline and venlafaxine) and certain beta-blockers (atenolol and nadolol). Divalproex sodium, sodium valproate, beta-blockers (when not medically contraindicated), and venlafaxine are preferable in older adults because topiramate frequently causes cognitive slowing and amitriptyline has anticholinergic side effects. Fenoprofen, ibuprofen, ketoprofen, naproxen, and naproxen sodium are first-line prophylactic agents for episodic migraines [59].

Non-pharmacologic management for headaches includes headache diaries to identify and minimize triggers; regular exercise; healthy diet with complex carbohydrates and minimal use of caffeine and, in patients with migraines, tyramine-rich foods; weight loss when clinically indicated; regular sleep; biofeedback; and cognitive behavioral therapy. Alternative medications for migraine prevention include the first-line agent butterbur (which has toxic side effects which limit its use) and second-line agents such as riboflavin, magnesium, and feverfew [60].

References

1. de Lau LM, Breteler MM. Epidemiology of Parkinson's disease. Lancet Neurol. 2006;5(6):525–35.
2. Pringsheim T, Jette N, Frolkis A, Steeves TD. The prevalence of Parkinson's disease: a systematic review and meta-analysis. Mov Disord. 2014;29(13):1583–90.
3. Walker Z, Possin KL, Boeve BF, Aarsland D. Lewy body dementias. Lancet. 2015;386(10004):1683–97.
4. Aarsland D, Marsh L, Schrag A. Neuropsychiatric symptoms in Parkinson's disease. Mov Disord. 2009;24(15):2175–86.
5. Aminian KS, Strafella AP. Affective disorders in Parkinson's disease. Curr Opin Neurol. 2013;26(4):339–44.
6. Parkinson Disease. U.S. National Library of Medicine. http://ghr.nlm.nih.gov/condition/parkinson-disease. Published 1 Feb 2016, Updated May 2012, Accessed 8 Feb 2016.
7. Vasconcellos LF, Pereira JS. Parkinson's disease dementia: diagnostic criteria and risk factor review. J Clin Exp Neuropsychol. 2015;37(9):988–93.
8. Hughes AJ, Daniel SE, Kilford L, Lees AJ. Accuracy of clinical diagnosis of idiopathic Parkinson's disease. A clinico-pathological study of 100 cases. JNNP. 1992;55(3):181–4.
9. Coelho M, Ferreira JJ. Late-stage Parkinson's disease. Nat Rev Neurol. 2012;8(8):435–42.
10. Aarsland D, Pahlhagen S, Ballard OG, Ehrt U, Svenningsson P. Depression in Parkinson disease--epidemiology, mechanisms and management. Nat Rev Neurol. 2012;8(1):35–47.
11. Helmich RC, Toni I, Deuschl G, Bloem BR. The pathophysiology of essential tremor and Parkinson's tremor. Curr Neurol Neurosci Rep. 2013;13(9):378.
12. Edwards MJ, Deuschl G. Tremor syndromes. Continuum (Minneap Minn). 2013;19(5):1213–24.
13. Poston KL. Overview of rare movement disorders. Continuum (Minneap Minn). 2010;16(1):49–76.
14. Pringsheim T, Wiltshire K, Day L, Dykeman J, Steeves T, Jette N. The incidence and prevalence of Huntington's disease: a systematic review and meta-analysis. Mov Disord. 2012;27(9):1083–91.
15. Ross CA, Aylward EH, Wild EJ, et al. Huntington disease: natural history, biomarkers and prospects for therapeutics. Nat Rev Neurol. 2014;10(4):204–16.
16. Huntington disease. U.S. National Library of Medicine. http://ghr.nlm.nih.gov/handbook/inheritance/anticipation. Published 1 Feb 2016, Accessed 8 Feb 2016.
17. Papoutsi M, Labuschagne I, Tabrizi SJ, Stout JC. The cognitive burden in Huntington's disease: pathology, phenotype, and mechanisms of compensation. Mov Disord. 2014;29(5):673–83.

18. Paulsen JS, Hoth KF, Nehl C, Stierman L. Critical periods of suicide risk in Huntington's disease. Am J Psychiatry. 2005;162(4):725–31.
19. Epping EA, Kim JI, Craufurd D, et al. Longitudinal psychiatric symptoms in prodromal Huntington's disease: a decade of data. Am J Psychiatry. 2016; 173(2):184–92.
20. Mehta P, Anteo V, Kaye W, et al. Prevalence of amyotrophic lateral sclerosis- United States, 2010–2011. MMWR. 2014;63(Suppl 7):1–12.A.
21. Amyotrophic Lateral Sclerosis (ALS) Fact Sheet. NINDS. http://www.ninds.nih.gov/disorders/amyotrophiclateralsclerosis/detail_ALS.htm. Published June 2013, Updated 1 Feb 2016, Accessed 9 Feb 2016.
22. Tiryaki E, Horak HA. ALS and other motor neuron diseases. Continuum (Minneap Minn). 2014;20:1185–207.
23. Brooks BR, Miller RG, Swash M, Munsat TL, World Federation of Neurology Research Group on Motor Neuron Diseases. El Escorial revisited: revised criteria for the diagnosis of amyotrophic lateral sclerosis. Amyotroph Lateral Scler Other Motor Neuron Disord. 2000;1(5):293–9.
24. Rohrer JD, Isaacs AM, Mizielinska S, et al. C9orf72 expansions in frontotemporal dementia and amyotrophic lateral sclerosis. Lancet Neurol. 2015;14(3):291–301.
25. Borroni B, Bonvicini C, Alberici A, et al. Mutation within TARDBP leads to frontotemporal dementia without motor neuron disease. Hum Mutat. 2009;30(11):E974–83.
26. Koch-Henriksen N, Soelberg Sørensen P. The changing demographic pattern of multiple sclerosis epidemiology. Lancet Neurol. 2010;9(5): 520–32.
27. Awad A, Stűve O. Multiple sclerosis in the elderly patient. Drugs Aging. 2010;27(4):283–94.
28. Katz Sand IB, Lublin FD. Diagnosis and differential diagnosis of multiple sclerosis. Continuum (Minneap Minn). 2013;19(4):922–43.
29. Freedman MS. Present and emerging therapies for multiple sclerosis. Continuum (Minneap Minn). 2013;19(4):968–91.
30. Saidha S, Eckstein C, Calabresi PA. New and emerging disease modifying therapies for multiple sclerosis. Ann N Y Acad Sci. 2012;1247:117–37.
31. Feinstein A, Freeman J, Lo AC. Treatment of progressive multiple sclerosis: what works, what does not, and what is needed. Lancet Neurol. 2015;14(2): 194–207.
32. Stroke. Centers for Disease Control and Prevention. http://www.cdc.gov/stroke/. Published 3 Nov 2015. Accessed 9 Feb 2016.
33. Prabhakaran S, Chong JY. Risk factor management for stroke prevention. Continuum (Minneap Minn). 2014;20(2):296–308.
34. Adams HP, Bendixen BH, Kappelle LJ, et al. Classification of subtype of acute ischemic stroke: definitions for use in a Multicenter clinical trial. Stroke. 1993;24(1):35–41.
35. Khatri P. Evaluation and management of acute ischemic stroke. Continuum (Minneap Minn). 2014;20(2):283–95.
36. Kernan WN, Ovbiagele B, Black HR, et al. Guidelines for the prevention of stroke in patients with stroke or transient ischemic attack: a guideline for healthcare professionals from the American Heart Association/American Stroke Association. Stroke. 2014;45(7):2160–236.
37. González-Pérez A, Gaist D, Wallander MA, McFeat G, García-Rodríguez LA. Mortality after hemorrhagic stroke: data from general practice (The Health Improvement Network). Neurology. 2013;81(6):559–65.
38. Hemphill JC 3rd, Greenberg SM, Anderson CS, et al. Guidelines for the management of spontaneous intracerebral hemorrhage: a guideline for healthcare professionals from the American Heart Association/American Stroke Association. Stroke. 2015;46(7):2032–60.
39. Faul M, Xu L, Wald MM, Coronado VG. Traumatic brain injury in the United States: emergency department visits, hospitalizations and deaths 2002–2006. Atlanta, GA: Centers for Disease Control and Prevention, National Center for Injury Prevention and Control; 2010.
40. Malec JF, Brown AW, Leibson CL, et al. The mayo classification system for traumatic brain injury severity. J Neurotrauma. 2007;24(9):1417–24.
41. Levin HS, Diaz-Arrastia RR. Diagnosis, prognosis, and clinical management of mild traumatic brain injury. Lancet Neurol. 2015;14(5): 506–17.
42. McAllister TW. Neurobehavioral sequelae of traumatic brain injury: evaluation and management. World Psychiatry. 2008;7(1):3–10.
43. Rao V, Koliatsos V, Ahmed F, Lyketsos C, Kortte K. Neuropsychiatric disturbances associated with traumatic brain injury: a practical approach to evaluation and management. Semin Neurol. 2015; 35(1):64–82.
44. Stippler M, Holguin E, Nemoto E. Traumatic brain injury in elders. Ann Longterm Care. 2012; 20(5):41–6.
45. Haut SR, Katz M, Masur J, Lipton RB. Seizures in the elderly: impact on mental status, mood and sleep. Epilepsy Behav. 2009;14(3):540–4.

46. French JA, Gazzola DM. Antiepileptic drug treatment: new drugs and new strategies. Continuum (Minneap Minn). 2013;19(3):643–55.
47. Jensen R, Stovner LJ. Epidemiology and comorbidity of headache. Lancet Neurol. 2008;7(4):354–61.
48. Pascual J, Berciano J. Experience in the diagnosis of headaches that start in elderly people. J Neurol Neurosurg Psychiatry. 1994;57(10):1255–7.
49. Walker RA, Wadman MC. Headache in the elderly. Clin Geriatr Med. 2007;23(2):291–305.
50. Giant Cell Arteritis. American College of Rheumatology. http://www.rheumatology.org/I-Am-A/Patient-Caregiver/Diseases-Conditions/Giant-Cell-Arteritis. Updated 2013, Accessed 9 Feb 2016.
51. Carmona FD, González-Gay MA, Martín J. Genetic component of giant cell arteritis. Rheumatology. 2014;53(1):6–18.
52. Amerasinghe N, Aung T. Angle-closure: risk factors, diagnosis and treatment. Prog Brain Res. 2008;173:31–45.
53. Headache Classification Committee of the International Headache Society (IHS). The International Classification of Headache Disorders, 3rd edition (beta version). Cephalalgia. 2013;33(9):629–808.
54. Tepper SJ. Medication-overuse headache. Continuum (Minneap Minn). 2012;18(4):807–22.
55. Goldberg SW, Silberstein S, Grosberg BM. Considerations in the treatment of tension-type headache in the elderly. Drugs Aging. 2014;31:797–804.
56. Bendtsena L, Eversb S, Lindec M, Mitsikostasd DD, Sandrinie G, Schoenenf J. EFNS guideline on the treatment of tension-type headache – report of an EFNS task force. Eur J Neurol. 2010;17(11):1318–25.
57. Charles AC, Baca SM. Cortical spreading depression and migraine. Nat Rev Neurol. 2013;9(11):637–44.
58. Bajwa ZH, Smith JH. Acute treatment of migraines in adults. http://www.uptodate.com/contents/acute-treatment-of-migraine-in-adults. Reviewed 19 Jan 2016. Accessed 8 Feb 2016.
59. American Association of Neurology. Pharmacologic treatment for episodic migraine prevention in adults. Continuum (Minneap Minn) 2012;18(4): Appendix A.
60. American Association of Neurology. NSAIDs and complementary meds for episodic migraine. Continuum (Minneap Minn) 2012;18(4): Appendix C.

33
Psychiatric Disorders Due to a General Medical Condition

Michael C. Hann, Aaron Meyer, Evan N. Caporaso, and Thomas Wolfgang Klotz

Introduction

The geriatric proportion of the total population of the USA has increased as advances in medicine prolong the human life span. The population of adults older than 65 years is expected to reach 20% of the total population of the USA within the next 15 years [1]. The burden of chronic disease has likewise increased. Nearly a quarter of individuals aged 65 and over suffers from coronary disease, hypertension, or stroke [2]. Geriatric populations suffer from increased rates of conditions associated with cumulative lifetime exposures, such as emphysema and COPD. Nearly 20% of individuals in this age group also have some form of cancer. Overall the rates of chronic illness are higher among older adults when compared to the general population, with two thirds of these individuals suffering from multiple chronic conditions including cardiovascular disease, diabetes, renal disease, and other conditions that significantly affect the quality of life such as arthritis. In addition, the psychological toll posed by these disorders, the limitations imposed by their physiologic sequelae, and the secondary effects of their treatments can have a detrimental effect on the psychiatric well-being of older adults. Geriatric mental health has come under increased scrutiny as a growing domain of healthcare that requires increased clinical attention and research input. Recent estimates suggest that approximately 20% of individuals aged 55 and older have a mental health problem requiring clinical attention [2]. In this subchapter, causes of acute mentation changes will be discussed as it relates specifically to the elderly. Additionally, subacute and chronic causes of secondary psychiatric findings will be highlighted. At the conclusion of this subchapter, the reader will have a more solid grasp of neuropsychiatric manifestations of general medical conditions.

Aging and Physiology

The physiology of aging is associated with decreased physiologic reserve and diminished functional capacity in drug metabolism at both the cellular and the organ level. The volume of distribution for lipophilic drugs increases as lean body mass is supplanted with adipose tissue, slowing elimination rates for certain psychoactive medications such as benzodiazepines and morphine [3]. Progressive structural changes in the kidneys reflect a loss of glomeruli and decreased GFR over time, with accordant impairments in acid-base homeostasis and salt balance. First pass metabolism may be less efficient due to decreased hepatic size and blood flow, potentially amplifying the bioavailability (and physiologic effect) of certain medications [4, 5]. The neurons of the peripheral and central nervous system also degrade with age, a process mediated by the accumulation of abnormal proteins, oxidative injury, and mutations to genetic material. Certain phenotypes may dispose individuals to "selective neuron vulnerability" in old age or even adulthood, a phenomenon of CNS injury to discrete

R. R. Tampi et al. (eds.), *Psychiatric Disorders Late in Life*, https://doi.org/10.1007/978-3-319-73078-3_33

neuron populations as seen with Alzheimer's disease and the hippocampus, Parkinson's and the basal ganglia, and other neurodegenerative syndromes [6]. Multiple studies have shown that aging is associated with decrements in specific aspects of cognition such as working memory, which may in part reflect age-related changes to the prefrontal cortex [7]. Changes associated with significant pharmacodynamic impact include increased GABA-aminergic sensitivity, changes to dopamine metabolism exacerbating risk of drug-induced Parkinsonism, decreased cholinergi function potentially amplifying drug-related anticholinergic effects, and decreased serotonin reuptake and receptor frequency [8]. In totality, these changes in physiology, which may be exacerbated in the setting of chronic illness, render aged individuals especially vulnerable to adverse drug effects and harmful medication interactions.

Aging and Polypharmacy

The industry of medicine has met the rising tide of chronic diseases in the burgeoning geriatric population with a plethora of medications. This can lead to burdensome and complex medication regimens, especially for individuals who suffer from multiple illnesses, as is common among the sickest elderly individuals. Studies have suggested that polypharmacy is associated with increased rates of adverse drug reactions, medication nonadherence, and elevated risk for geriatric syndromes such as cognitive impairment, urinary incontinence, and impaired balance resulting in falls [9]. Although there is no strict numerical quantity of medications that represents a threshold for polypharmacy, a prospective study identified that, among a geriatric cohort, individuals prescribed eight or more medications were at significantly increased risk for re-hospitalization within 1 year [10]. Antipsychotic polypharmacy is a specific problem within the field of geriatric psychiatry and appears to be correlated with both living environment (skilled nursing facilities and other forms of long term care) and severity of mental illness [11]. This problem is potentiated by the utility of antipsychotics as an expeditious measure of behavioral control among the delirious elderly. Adding to the problem of polypharmacy, many drugs that are used routinely in medical management are associated with psychiatric side effects ranging from mood impairment to psychosis, which makes it difficult to differentiate them from non-iatrogenic endogenous illness. In one study, for example, corticosteroids were associated with psychiatric side effects in 6% of all patients treated [12]. Polypharmacy increases the likelihood of a psychiatric side effect as multiple medications inhibit hepatic metabolism, including statins, omeprazole, and certain antihypertensives, among others, creating a biologic environment where medication concentrations may insidiously rise to toxic levels [13]. Polypharmacy continues to present as a challenge in geriatric medicine. A research effort targeting polypharmacy found that specialized geriatric care in collaboration with dedicated clinical pharmacists reduced the rates of serious adverse drug reactions in older patients on multiple medications, suggesting the importance of a holistic team-based approach to the geriatric patient [14].

Cardiovascular Disease

Geriatric patients are increasingly vulnerable to issues pertaining to cardiovascular disease, with heart disease as a general category being the leading cause of death among adults older than 65 years in the USA. While the link between cardiac pathology and psychiatric comorbidity is perhaps most dramatically evident in Takotsubo cardiomyopathy, where psychiatric disorders are an independent predictor of the disease [15], the management of more common cardiac pathology carry substantial risk for the presentation of de novo psychiatric symptomatology. Management of conditions such as coronary artery disease, congestive heart failure, hypertension, valve disease, and cardiac arrhythmias are complicated by a substantial degree of comorbidity, with as many as 70% of patients having four additional chronic conditions requiring treatment [16]. Alone, these conditions produce functional impairment that often curtails ability to perform ADLs and IADLs, resulting in barriers to care, caregiver fatigue, inhibited physical activity, and decreased sense of self-worth. Medical management of these conditions can provide functional relief but can confer a risk of central nervous system side effects of their own accord, with agents such as beta-blockers having occasional side effects of increasing incidence of fatigue and confusion. Other mainstays of treatment of cardiac disease such as mineralocorticoid receptor antagonists, angiotensin-converting enzyme (ACE) inhibitors, and angiotensin receptor blockers have the potential to create substantial electrolyte imbalances which may present as altered mental status. Effective management of conditions such as hypertension carries the inherent risk of compensatory hypotension, dizziness, and syncope, which can limit functional ability and risk provoking anxiety, particularly the fear of falling. This is an important consideration when prescribing other medications that have the potential to predispose to syncope, including acetylcholinesterase inhibitors, peripheral alpha blockers such as prazosin, or tricyclic antidepressants [17]. In addition to the physiologic and metabolic strain produced by treatment of cardiovascular disease, the cost associated with complex procedures necessary to complete and sustain cardiovascular interventions can be detrimental to the socioeconomic standing of geriatric patients with subsequent stressors impacting their psychiatric well-being.

Orthopedic Injuries

Among the geriatric population, the most common cause of physical trauma is falls. Whether the cause is instability resulting from polypharmacy as discussed earlier or alterations in gait from a primary neurodegenerative disease, one third of adults over 65 years can be expected to suffer a fall each year, making falls the leading cause of physical trauma in the geriatric community [18]. Many subpopulations of the geriatric community are at increased risk for osteoporosis, vitamin D deficiency, and osteomalacia increasing the risk of fractures resulting from a mechanical fall. The resulting orthopedic injuries associated with falls carry with them substantial risk for complex medical management, which may be detrimental to the psychiatric well-being of geriatric patients. Among older adults, suffering long bone or pelvic fractures with need of orthopedic repair are increases the risk for fat embolization, which can occasionally present as isolated neuropsychiatric dysfunction. Among older individuals who are status post falls and deemed to be at risk of developing neurologic dysfunction would often be woken for neurologic exam every 1–2 h during the initial postoperative phase, substantially increasing the risk for the development of iatrogenic delirium. Management of postoperative pain in these settings often incorporates the use of narcotics, which increases the risk for a myriad of potential psychiatric manifestations. In the short to medium term following a fall and subsequent recovery, the immobility associated with orthopedic injury can be an independent stressor [19]. This can lead to physical and social isolation, further physical deconditioning, weight loss, and fatigue, which, taken as a whole, constitute a confluence of symptoms that are frequently associated with the onset of depression and increased mortality [20].

Delirium

Delirium is an acute impairment in cognitive functioning associated with medical or surgical insults. Delirium may closely mimic psychiatric pathology and is a widespread problem and is strongly associated with adverse outcomes among hospitalized geriatric patients. Delirium is defined by its time course (acuity of onset) paired specifically with attention deficits, although it may also be associated with disorganized thinking and an altered level of consciousness [12]. Delirium affects approximately 30% of hospitalized geriatric patients. The 2010 National Institute of Health and Care Excellence (NICE) delirium guidelines listed age > 65 as one of the primary risk factors in the development of delirium [21]. This diagnosis is marked by several key findings, the most common of which is "waxing and waning" attention. The American Psychiatric Association's *Diagnostic and Statistical Manual of Mental Disorders*, 5th edition (DSM-5), lists five key features, including (1) aforementioned attention deficits, (2) fluctuating course of awareness, (3) cognitive disturbances such as orientation changes and changes in perception (i.e., visual hallucinations), (4) absence of alternative diagnoses which would better explain mentation changes, and (5) supporting evidence (physical examination findings, pertinent laboratory values, etc.) [22]. These characteristics have been described in great detail in a variety of texts, but a more recently studied topic is the nature of delirium. Several theories have been raised with no unifying consensus. The multifactorial explanation of the etiology of delirium consists of abnormalities in the neurobiological components of attention, neuronal aging, physiologic stress, subcortical neural pathways (patients with Parkinson's are more susceptible to delirium), and contributions from various neurotransmitters such as inflammatory cytokines (implicated in sepsis) [23]. Factors implicated in the development of delirium are myriad (see Table 33-1).

Once delirium is recognized, prompt treatment is absolutely imperative. Unfortunately, ED physicians tend to miss 57–83% of delirium cases, and if admitted, physicians miss up to 90% of these cases. Thus, any abrupt change in mentation in a hospitalized elderly patient should require a thorough infectious evaluation, including urinalysis, complete blood count (CBC)/complete metabolic panel (CMP), and chest radiograph (at a minimum) [24]. Special attention needs to be paid to individual circumstances for each patient. As mentioned above, polypharmacy is a common contributing factor in acute mental status changes. Nearly 11% of ED visits among people older than 65 are due to adverse drug events when compared to 4% of general population [25]. Therefore, thorough medication reconciliation should be performed by multiple members of the healthcare team on admission and during outpatient encounters. Discussions with family members regarding how patients take medications (i.e., pill box, individual bottles), who is involved in medication dispensing, and prior history of medication administration errors are important considerations. After medication reconciliation, determining the potential risk of medication interactions and side effects are other necessary considerations, as even problems as non-specific as abdominal pain (common problem in medications like acetylcholinesterase inhibitors) can influence mentation changes. Moreover, metabolic changes such as hyperammonemia are common with certain psychotropic medications (valproic acid probably the most commonly considered) [25].

Following initial laboratory work-up for common laboratory abnormalities, consideration of patient's medical history can be revealing. For instance, a delirious patient with prior history of depression should have an updated thyroid panel to evaluate for metabolic derangements (to be discussed in upcoming section). Cirrhotic patients should have ammonia and platelet levels checked [24]. Patients presenting with acute chronic obstructive pulmonary disease (COPD) exacerbation should have an arterial blood gas (ABG), as hypercarbia can present with acute mentation changes. Of note, ABG is more sensitive than venous blood gas (VBG) to detect acute changes in carbon dioxide retention. Additionally, despite increased attention paid to opioid and benzodiazepine epidemics, there is a preponderance of complications associated with concurrent controlled substances prescriptions [26]. Of note, the 1980s and 1990s saw a dramatic, almost logarithmic increase in prescribing practices. Unfortunately, these medications are often continued unquestioningly until problems develop. Consider the patient who was initially prescribed benzodiazepines in their 50s and continue to receive these medications, without attention paid to adherence practicalities [27]. A thorough medical examination needs to incorporate regular checks of prescription drug monitoring programs (excluding states like Missouri which has not yet legalized such an important registry). Checking for concurrent opiate and benzodiazepine

TABLE 33-1. Factors implicated in the development of delirium

Drugs	Opioids, benzodiazepines, antihistamines, medication side effects
Infections	Urinary tract infection, upper respiratory infection, pneumonia
Metabolic	Thyroid derangements, electrolyte abnormalities, hypercarbia
Brain disorders	CNS infections, head injury
Organ failure	Renal failure, liver disease, pulmonary (hypoxemia)

prescriptions and discussing the possibility of mentation deficits from these medications are absolutely essential [28]. Practitioners have an obligation to raise difficult topics of conversation when patients present with delirium, which could be primarily attributed to controlled substances.

Of note, delirium can also be explained by substance intoxication or withdrawal [29]. As noted above, routine checking of prescription drug monitoring programs is essential. Geriatric patients with prior history of substance abuse require an in-depth evaluation of current use practices. For instance, methadone prescriptions due to opioid use disorder are not flagged in these prescription-monitoring programs. Special attention needs to be paid with methadone history, especially calling patient's clinic [30]. Routine urine toxicology studies can be particularly revealing [24]. Additionally, recent documentation of infectious disease screening can help rule out common infectious causes of delirium in this population. Specifically, screening for hepatitis C, human immunodeficiency virus (HIV), and syphilis can help in the secondary evaluation for delirium in patients without known source of common infections. This is increasingly pertinent given the increased rate of sexually transmitted infection risk in the geriatric population living at group facilities [31].

If these evaluations are negative, tertiary considerations involve anatomic and neurological causes of delirium. Computed tomography (CT) can help elucidate the possibility of ischemic etiology, with the caveat of no apparent acute focal neurologic findings. Electroencephalography (EEG) is helpful in the consideration of nonconvulsive status epilepticus. Lumbar puncture may be necessary as well if there is corresponding concern for meningitis or if hydrocephaly is suggested due to gait changes, incontinence, and/or enlarged ventricles on computerized tomography (CT) scan. As one can see, the differential diagnosis and accompanying evaluation possibilities are broad and require potentially wide-ranging approach.

Once delirium is suspected, physicians and nurses typically use the Confusion Assessment Method (CAM) to diagnose delirium (see Table 33-2). Diagnosis requires presence of features 1 and 2, along with either 3 or 4 [24].

TABLE 33-2. Confusion Assessment Method (CAM)

Feature	*Assessment*
1. Acute onset and fluctuating course	"Evidence of acute change in mental status from patient's baseline" "did the abnormal behavior fluctuate?"
2. Inattention	"Did patient have difficulty focusing attention, for example, being easily distracted?"
3. Disorganized thinking	"Is patient's thinking disorganized or incoherent, such as rambling or irrelevant conversation, unclear or illogical flow of ideas, unpredictable switching from subject to subject?"
4. Altered level of consciousness	Anything other than alert (i.e., vigilant, lethargic, stupor, or coma)

The annual cost of delirium in the USA is about $150 billion, which adds emphasis to the necessity for prompt management of delirium once diagnosed. Given the increased mortality associated with the delayed diagnosis and treatment of delirium, hospitals have begun paying increased attention to earlier recognition and the management of delirium. Apart from prompt diagnosis, there are essential environmental approaches that help mitigate psychiatric manifestations of delirium [26]. For instance, transferring patients to rooms with windows is especially helpful in promoting normal sleep-wake cycles. Additionally, administration of melatonin agents can aid in optimizing neurotransmitter-associated wakefulness pathways. Utilization of classical music can help calm patients. If possible, family members and hospital staff can aid in frequent reorientation of patient to the correct date and time. These factors help avoid deleterious effects of restraint use which increases agitation. Limiting the use of bladder catheters and nasogastric tubes are other important considerations in the management of delirium, as these devices are not only niduses for infection but often represent justification for physical restraints. Chemical restraints such as benzodiazepines and neuroleptics should also be avoided as much as possible given their association with the prolongation of delirium. If managed correctly, delirium is often correctable and patients may return to their cognitive baseline. However, for many patients recovery may be incomplete. Among 126 patients with documented in-hospital delirium who underwent intubation in the ICU, 79% and 71% of survivors had cognitive impairment at 3- and 12-month follow-up, respectively [32].

Thyroid Disorders

A smoldering, subacute cause of psychiatric abnormalities due to a medical condition is thyroid derangements. While a common consideration in patients with depression is hypothyroidism (and often presents similarly in geriatric patients), thyrotoxicosis in elderly patients has several unique attributes. Surprisingly, apathy may be presenting feature in elderly patients with hyperthyroidism. Although emotional lability and psychosis can be witnessed, apathy is one of the most defining features of hyperthyroidism in the elderly [33]. Additionally, memory changes and confusion are associated with thyroid abnormalities. The most worrisome though is the possible development of thyroid storm, which can progress to delirium, somnolence, and coma [34]. Etiology of cognitive disturbances due to thyroid abnormalities is multifactorial with theories varying from adrenergic pathways to neuronal injury [35]. Physical examination does not often include presence of goiter in this subset of patients [36]. Diagnostic considerations include the basic thyroid function tests (thyroid-stimulating hormone (TSH), T3, and T4). Electroencephalography (EEG) findings often demonstrate generalized slowing. Treatment involves correction of thyroid abnormalities. Unfortunately, mentation changes often lag behind normalization of thyroid hormones.

Neoplastic Processes

Psychiatric disorders are an under-recognized comorbidity among cancer patients. Psychiatric diagnoses among older adults with cancers are complicated by the natural process of bereavement associated with cancer diagnoses and confounded by overlap between depressive symptomatology and somatic symptoms rooted in the cancer or its treatment. Chemotherapeutic treatments for cancer are themselves associated with significant side effects including mental health problems. A study tracking symptoms among 472 patients newly initiated on chemotherapy identified that, among various symptom clusters, older patients (≥60 years of age) reported increased pain, nausea, and psychological distress at a statistically significant level [37]. Predominant concerns among all chemotherapy patients in the study included insomnia and distress over decision-making, nutritional concerns such as appetite loss and fatigue [37]. Radiotherapy, chemotherapy, and androgen deprivation therapy utilized in a study of breast and prostate cancer patients were found to significantly aggravate insomnia, a common psychiatric complaint [38]. Chemotherapy agents are a heterogeneous group and a description of each individual drug is beyond the scope of this text. Previous review articles have outlined the side effect profiles and depressogenic effects of specific chemotherapy agents [39].

There are several paraneoplastic processes associated with psychiatric findings, including leptomeningeal metastases, diffuse glioma, and central nervous system (CNS) lymphomas. While the majority of cases of CNS lymphoma occur in males between ages 45 and 65 years, this process can also occur among older adults. The immune system is thought to have a central role in pathogenesis of this disease, given the predominance in immunosuppressed individuals. Patients with CNS lymphoma often present with findings such as psychotic agitation, depression, apathy, as well as personality changes. MRI and lumbar puncture are often helpful in clarifying this diagnosis [40]. Leptomeningeal metastases are present in about 5% of metastatic diagnoses. Cancers most commonly associated with this type of metastasis are breast cancer, lung cancer, and melanoma. Patients usually present with headache but altered mentation is not uncommon [41]. Additionally, high-grade gliomas such as glioblastoma multiform and anaplastic gliomas present with subtle personality changes. Approximately 50% of patients with glioblastoma are older than 65 years of age. Older adults have a poorer prognosis than those with younger age with age and functional capacity being the two most important prognostic factors. However, the overall life expectancy after diagnosis does not vary by much, the best-case scenario has about an 8-month survival rate while worst-case scenario has about a 3-month survival. Radiation has demonstrated a life expectancy increase about 12 weeks [42].

Pain

Older adults often have verbal and cognitive impairments that make communication around pain difficult. This communication deficit can lead to behavioral manifestations of pain such as agitation and aggression. When there is a change in patient's behavior without a known cause, medical staff should perform a thorough pain assessment. Conducting a pain assessment or gathering input from caregivers can reduce psychiatric complaints. There are several tools which can be employed to address pain among individuals who have difficulty communicating, including The Critical Care Observation Tool and The Pain Assessment Checklist for Seniors with Severe Dementia [43]. In some instances, trial of pain relievers can be useful in assessing possibility of pain as a cause of psychiatric symptoms. Not surprisingly, symptoms of depression and anxiety are often found among patients suffering from pain. Treatment of pain also carries the aforementioned risk for mentation changes, especially those prescribed opiates [44].

Neuroophthalmic Disorders

Among patients who present with isolated visual hallucinations, often this finding is due to an underlying medical condition. The absence of auditory hallucinations helps distinguish these conditions from primary psychiatric disorders. The diagnoses can be divided based on the type of hallucination—simple versus complex [45]. In terms of simple hallucinations, retinal etiologies are most common. Visual hallucinations typically present for seconds with characteristic findings such as lights or whirling pinwheels. Prompt evaluation by ophthalmologist is essential [46]. Charles Bonnet syndrome is described by simple or complex hallucinations due to macular degeneration, glaucoma, diabetic retinopathy, or cerebral infarction [47]. Migraines typically involve simple hallucinations (aura). Narcolepsy often produces vivid visual hallucinations prior to sleep, occasionally leading to the sufferer dreading going to sleep. These visual findings are due to rapid eye movements (REM) blending with wakefulness. These patients should be managed by a sleep specialist [48].

Delusional Parasitosis

While primary delusional parasitosis is a psychiatric diagnosis, secondary delusional parasitosis is often a symptom of an underlying medical condition. This is a relatively rare disorder that is marked by the false belief that one is infested by insects [49]. The mean age for this diagnosis is 57 years and predominately affects females. Individuals at risk for this disorder are often socially isolated, a common concern for geriatric patients [50]. Patients usually present with pruritic symptoms with history marked by prior negative medical evaluations [51]. After psychiatric conditions are ruled out, full medical evaluation is indicated. Nutritional deficiencies such as vitamin B12 and folate deficiencies have been associated with secondary delusional parasitosis [52]. CNS disorders such as multiple sclerosis and prior neurosurgical procedures have been associated with this diagnosis. The use of certain prescription medications such as corticosteroids and ketoconazole is associated with this disorder. Substance abuse should also be a consideration in the evaluation when older adults present with delusional parasitosis [53].

Toxic-Metabolic Encephalopathy

There are several categories of encephalopathies, the most common of which is septic. The other notable causes are related to organ failure. All encephalopathies affect systems involved in arousal and awareness related due to disturbance of the blood-brain barrier, which can then lead to entry of inflammatory cytokines. In some cases of encephalopathy, specifically hepatic, neurologic manifestations are also related to the development of cerebral edema [54]. Neurohormonal differences are also noted with the different types of encephalopathy, specifically, uremic encephalopathy which has been associated with increase in parathyroid hormone [55]. Vitamin deficiencies are implicated in Wernicke's encephalopathy, most commonly associated with alcoholic nutritional states and patients receiving artificial nutrition. In management of these encephalopathies, care should be taken to minimize restraint use, as this has been associated with prolongation of mental status changes, increased aspiration risk, and loss of mobility [56].

HIV-Associated Neurocognitive Disorders (HAND)

Although the incidence of HIV-related dementias has dramatically declined since the introduction of antiretroviral therapy, research continues on the classification, mechanisms, and treatment of this disorder. Indirect mechanisms are implicated in the neurologic decline, as HIV is not known to directly affect neuronal pathways. The more severe forms of cognitive decline is associated with acquired immune deficiency syndrome (AIDS) (CD4 < 200 or presence of AIDS-defining illness) [57]. Interestingly, HIV dementia is distinguished from other forms of dementia due to the exclusion of cortical impairments (i.e., apraxia, aphasia, etc.). While depression is common in this subset, mania and psychosis have been documented as well. Regarding depressive findings, patients with HAND often describe an absence of sadness or crying spells, differentiating this condition from major depressive disorder. Neuropsychological testing is often required to make the diagnosis. Given the immunocompromised state of patients with HIV, other infectious etiologies (toxoplasmosis, cryptococcal infection, progressive multifocal leukoencephalopathy) must be excluded prior to the HAND diagnosis (along with other common causes of cognitive impairment) [58].

Depression Due to Chronic Medical Conditions

This subchapter would not be complete without a discussion of the association between chronic medical illness and depression. While the annual prevalence of major depressive disorder is approximately 7%, the prevalence leaps to 25% in those with chronic medical illness [59]. Mortality and hospitalization frequency increases in dialysis patients with depression when compared to those without mental illness. As an example, one study analyzing international cancer data generated using the World Mental Health Survey identified a mood disorder prevalence of 9.3% and an anxiety disorder prevalence of 14.9% in patients with active cancer [60]. These rates were elevated relative to cancer survivors who in turn had rates higher than that identified for individuals with no past cancer diagnosis. Past studies have investigated post-traumatic symptomatology in population of cancer survivors and identified symptomatology warranting diagnosis of post-traumatic stress syndrome with prominence of vigilance, insomnia, and cognitive deficits as primary complaints. This suggests the need for providers to be alert to this vein of pathology among geriatric cancer patients, including those who have undergone treatment [61]. Recent data has demonstrated the importance of targeted depression screenings for those individuals with chronic medical conditions along with provision of collaborative care interventions [62]. Depression screenings in this population yields less false-positive results due to the higher likelihood of depression. As cognitive impairment is implicated in depression as well as encephalopathy, care should be taken to diagnostically distinguish between the two conditions [63].

Conclusions

Older adults often present with multiple medical conditions that may result in or worsen preexisting psychiatric disorders. The presence of comorbid medical and psychiatric disorders often worsens the outcomes for the two conditions. Additionally, diagnoses may be missed or conditions misdiagnosed among the elderly due to lack of specificity of diagnostic symptoms, the poor awareness of these conditions among clinicians, and the unavailability of proper screening tools that are specific to older adults. However, the prompt diagnosis and treatment of the comorbid medical and psychiatric disorders may improve clinical outcomes and the quality of life among the older adults.

References

1. Centers ford Disease Control (CDC). The state of aging and health in America 2013. Atlanta, GA: US Department of Health and Human Services; 2013.
2. Centers ford Disease Control (CDC) & Directors NACD. The state of mental health and aging in America issue brief 1: what do the data tell us? Atlanta, GA: US Department of Health and Human Services; 2013.
3. Mangoni AA, Jackson SH. Age-related changes in pharmacokinetics and pharmacodynamics: basic principles and practical applications. Br J Clin Pharmacol. 2004;57(1):6–14.
4. Abou-Saleh MT, Katona C, Kumar A. Principles and practice of geriatric psychiatry. 3rd ed. Chichester, West Sussex: John Wiley & Sons; 2011.
5. Klotz U. Pharmacokinetics and drug metabolism in the elderly. Drug Metab Rev. 2009;41(2):67–76. https://doi.org/10.1080/03602530902722679.
6. Mattson MP, Magnus T. Ageing and neuronal vulnerability. Nat Rev Neurosci. 2006;7(4):278–94. https://doi.org/10.1038/nrn1886.
7. Mattay VS, Fera F, Tessitore A, Hariri AR, Berman KF, Das S, et al. Neurophysiological correlates of age-related changes in working memory capacity. Neurosci Lett. 2006;392(1–2):32–7. https://doi.org/10.1016/j.neulet.2005.09.025.
8. Varma S, Sareen H, Trivedi JK. The geriatric population and psychiatric medication. Mens Sana Monogr. 2010;8(1):30–51. https://doi.org/10.4103/0973-1229.58818.
9. Hajjar ER, Cafiero AC, Hanlon JT. Polypharmacy in elderly patients. Am J Geriatr Pharmacother. 2007;5(4):345–51. https://doi.org/10.1016/j.amjopharm.2007.12.002.
10. Sganga F, Landi F, Ruggiero C, Corsonello A, Vetrano DL, Lattanzio F, Cherubini A, Bernabei R, Onder G. Polypharmacy and health outcomes among older adults discharged from hospital: results from the CRIME study. Geriatr Gerontol Int. 2015;15(2):141–6. https://doi.org/10.1111/ggi.12241.
11. Dolder CR, Mckinsey J. Antipsychotic polypharmacy among patients admitted to a geriatric psychiatry unit. J Psychiatr Pract. 2011;17(5):368–74. https://doi.org/10.1097/01.pra.0000405368.20538.cd.
12. Casagrande Tango R. Psychiatric side effects of medications prescribed in internal medicine. Dialogues Clin Neurosci. 2003;5(2):155–65.
13. Inouye SK, van Dyck CH, Alessi CA, Balkin S, Siegal AP, Horwitz RI. Clarifying confusion: the confusion assessment method. A new method for detection of delirium. Ann Intern Med. 1990;113(12):941–8.
14. Schmader KE, Hanlon JT, Pieper CF, Sloane R, Ruby CM, Twersky J, et al. Effects of geriatric evaluation and management on adverse drug reactions and suboptimal prescribing in the frail elderly. Am J Med. 2004;116(6):394–401. https://doi.org/10.1016/j.amjmed.2003.10.031.
15. Templin C, Ghadri JR, Diekmann J, Napp LC, Bataiosu DR, Jaguszewski M, et al. Clinical features and outcomes of Takotsubo (stress) cardiomyopathy. N Engl J Med. 2015;373(10):929–38. https://doi.org/10.1056/NEJMoa1406761.
16. Bell SP, Orr NM, Dodson JA, Rich MW, Wenger NK, Blum K, et al. What to expect from the evolving field of geriatric cardiology. J Am Coll Cardiol. 2015;66(11):1286–99. https://doi.org/10.1016/j.jacc.2015.07.048.
17. By the American Geriatrics Society 2015 Beers Criteria Update Expert Panel. American Geriatrics Society 2015 updated beers criteria for potentially inappropriate medication use in older adults. J Am Geriatr Soc. 2015;63(11):2227–46. https://doi.org/10.1111/jgs.13702.
18. Bergen G, Stevens MR, Burns ER. Falls and fall injuries among adults aged ≥65 years – United States, 2014. MMWR Morb Mortal Wkly Rep. 2016;65(37):993–8. https://doi.org/10.15585/mmwr.mm6537a2.
19. Bower ES, Wetherell JL, Petkus AJ, Rawson KS, Lenze EJ. Fear of falling after hip fracture: prevalence, course, and relationship with one-year functional recovery. Am J Geriatr Psychiatry. 2016;24(12):1228–36. https://doi.org/10.1016/j.jagp.2016.08.006.
20. Brown PJ, Rutherford BR, Yaffe K, Tandler JM, Ray JL, Pott E, Chung S, Roose SP. The depressed frail phenotype: the clinical manifestation of increased biological aging. Am J Geriatr Psychiatry. 2016;24(11):1084–94. https://doi.org/10.1016/j.jagp.2016.06.005.
21. Scholz AF, Oldroyd C, McCarthy K, Quinn TJ, Hewitt J. Systematic review and meta-analysis of risk factors for postoperative delirium among older patients undergoing gastrointestinal surgery. Br J Surg. 2016;103(2):e21–8. https://doi.org/10.1002/bjs.10062.
22. American Psychiatric Association (APA). Diagnostic and statistical manual of mental

disorders: DSM-5. 5th ed. Washington, DC: American Psychiatric Association; 2013.
23. Sher Y, Miller Cramer AC, Ament A, Lolak S, Maldonado JR. Valproic acid for treatment of hyperactive or mixed delirium: rationale and literature review. Psychosomatics. 2015;56(6):615–25. https://doi.org/10.1016/j.psym.2015.09.008.
24. Odiari EA, Sekhon N, Han JY, David EH. Stabilizing and managing patients with altered mental status and delirium. Emerg Med Clin North Am. 2015;33(4):753–64. https://doi.org/10.1016/j.emc.2015.07.004.
25. Sikka V, Kalra S, Galwankar S, Sagar G. Psychiatric emergencies in the elderly. Emerg Med Clin North Am. 2015;33(4):825–39. https://doi.org/10.1016/j.emc.2015.07.009.
26. American Geriatrics Society Expert Panel on Postoperative Delirium in Older Adults. Postoperative delirium in older adults: best practice statement from the American Geriatrics Society. J Am Coll Surg. 2015;220(2):136–148.e131. https://doi.org/10.1016/j.jamcollsurg.2014.10.019.
27. Tannenbaum C, Martin P, Tamblyn R, Benedetti A, Ahmed S. Reduction of inappropriate benzodiazepine prescriptions among older adults through direct patient education: the EMPOWER cluster randomized trial. JAMA Intern Med. 2014;174(6):890–8. https://doi.org/10.1001/jamainternmed.2014.949.
28. Garrido MM, Prigerson HG, Penrod JD, Jones SC, Boockvar KS. Benzodiazepine and sedative-hypnotic use among older seriously ill veterans: choosing wisely? Clin Ther. 2014;36(11):1547–54. https://doi.org/10.1016/j.clinthera.2014.10.007.
29. Reinhardt MM, Cohen CI. Late-life psychosis: diagnosis and treatment. Curr Psychiatry Rep. 2015;17(2):1. https://doi.org/10.1007/s11920-014-0542-0.
30. Darker CD, Sweeney BP, Barry JM, Farrell MF, Donnelly-Swift E. Psychosocial interventions for benzodiazepine harmful use, abuse or dependence. Cochrane Database Syst Rev. 2015;5:CD009652. https://doi.org/10.1002/14651858.CD009652.pub2.
31. Bodley-Tickell AT, Olowokure B, Bhaduri S, White DJ, Ward D, Ross JD, Smith G, Duggal HV, Goold P. Trends in sexually transmitted infections (other than HIV) in older people: analysis of data from an enhanced surveillance system. Sex Transm Infect. 2008;84(4):312–7. https://doi.org/10.1136/sti.2007.027847.
32. Girard TD, Jackson JC, Pandharipande PP, Pun BT, Thompson JL, Shintani AK, et al. Delirium as a predictor of long-term cognitive impairment in survivors of critical illness. Crit Care Med. 2010;38(7):1513–20. https://doi.org/10.1097/CCM.0b013e3181e47be1.
33. Stern RA, Robinson B, Thorner AR, Arruda JE, Prohaska ML, Prange AJ. A survey study of neuropsychiatric complaints in patients with Graves' disease. J Neuropsychiatry Clin Neurosci. 1996;8(2):181–5. https://doi.org/10.1176/jnp.8.2.181.
34. Trasciatti S, Prete C, Palummeri E, Foppiani L. Thyroid storm as precipitating factor in onset of coma in an elderly woman: case report and literature review. Aging Clin Exp Res. 2004;16(6):490–4.
35. Fukui T, Hasegawa Y, Takenaka H. Hyperthyroid dementia: clinicoradiological findings and response to treatment. J Neurol Sci. 2001;184(1):81–8.
36. Boelaert K, Torlinska B, Holder RL, Franklyn JA. Older subjects with hyperthyroidism present with a paucity of symptoms and signs: a large cross-sectional study. J Clin Endocrinol Metab. 2010;95(6):2715–26. https://doi.org/10.1210/jc.2009-2495.
37. Yamagishi A, Morita T, Miyashita M, Kimura F. Symptom prevalence and longitudinal follow-up in cancer outpatients receiving chemotherapy. J Pain Symptom Manag. 2009;37(5):823–30. https://doi.org/10.1016/j.jpainsymman.2008.04.015.
38. Savard J, Ivers H, Savard MH, Morin CM. Cancer treatments and their side effects are associated with aggravation of insomnia: results of a longitudinal study. Cancer. 2015;121(10):1703–11. https://doi.org/10.1002/cncr.29244.
39. Celano CM, Freudenreich O, Fernandez-Robles C, Stern TA, Caro MA, Huffman JC. Depressogenic effects of medications: a review. Dialogues Clin Neurosci. 2011;13(1):109–25.
40. Bataille B, Delwail V, Menet E, Vandermarcq P, Ingrand P, Wager M, Guy G, Lapierre F. Primary intracerebral malignant lymphoma: report of 248 cases. J Neurosurg. 2000;92(2):261–6. https://doi.org/10.3171/jns.2000.92.2.0261.
41. Kesari S, Batchelor TT. Leptomeningeal metastases. Neurol Clin. 2003;21(1):25–66.
42. Scott JG, Bauchet L, Fraum TJ, Nayak L, Cooper AR, Chao ST, et al. Recursive partitioning analysis of prognostic factors for glioblastoma patients aged 70 years or older. Cancer. 2012;118(22):5595–600. https://doi.org/10.1002/cncr.27570.
43. Fuchs-Lacelle S, Hadjistavropoulos T. Development and preliminary validation of the pain assessment checklist for seniors with limited ability to communicate (PACSLAC). Pain Manag Nurs. 2004;5(1):37–49.

44. Herr K, Coyne PJ, Key T, Manworren R, McCaffery M, Merkel S, Pelosi-Kelly J, Wild L, American Society for Pain Management Nursing. Pain assessment in the nonverbal patient: position statement with clinical practice recommendations. Pain Manag Nurs. 2006;7(2):44–52. https://doi.org/10.1016/j.pmn.2006.02.003.
45. Wilkinson F. Auras and other hallucinations: windows on the visual brain. Prog Brain Res. 2004;144:305–20. https://doi.org/10.1016/S0079-6123(03)14421-4.
46. Hikichi T, Yoshida A. Time course of development of posterior vitreous detachment in the fellow eye after development in the first eye. Ophthalmology. 2004;111(9):1705–7. https://doi.org/10.1016/j.ophtha.2004.02.015.
47. Menon GJ, Rahman I, Menon SJ, Dutton GN. Complex visual hallucinations in the visually impaired: the Charles bonnet syndrome. Surv Ophthalmol. 2003;48(1):58–72.
48. Bódizs R, Sverteczki M, Lázár AS, Halász P. Human parahippocampal activity: non-REM and REM elements in wake-sleep transition. Brain Res Bull. 2005;65(2):169–76. https://doi.org/10.1016/j.brainresbull.2005.01.002.
49. Freinhar JP. Delusions of parasitosis. Psychosomatics. 1984;25(1):47–49, 53. https://doi.org/10.1016/S0033-3182(84)73096-9.
50. Foster AA, Hylwa SA, Bury JE, Davis MD, Pittelkow MR, Bostwick JM. Delusional infestation: clinical presentation in 147 patients seen at Mayo Clinic. J Am Acad Dermatol. 2012;67(4):673.e1–673.e10. https://doi.org/10.1016/j.jaad.2011.12.012.
51. Bhatia MS, Jagawat T, Choudhary S. Delusional parasitosis: a clinical profile. Int J Psychiatry Med. 2000;30(1):83–91. https://doi.org/10.2190/BBDT-CGB9-BB3L-8HM3.
52. Lyell A. The Michelson lecture. Delusions of parasitosis. Br J Dermatol. 1983;108(4):485–99.
53. Slaughter JR, Zanol K, Rezvani H, Flax J. Psychogenic parasitosis. A case series and literature review. Psychosomatics. 1998;39(6):491–500. https://doi.org/10.1016/S0033-3182(98)71281-2.
54. Ely EW, Stephens RK, Jackson JC, Thomason JW, Truman B, Gordon S, Dittus RS, Bernard GR. Current opinions regarding the importance, diagnosis, and management of delirium in the intensive care unit: a survey of 912 healthcare professionals. Crit Care Med. 2004;32(1):106–12. https://doi.org/10.1097/01.CCM.0000098033.94737.84.
55. Bolton C, Young G. Uremic encephalopathy. In: Neurological complications of renal disease. Stoneham: Buttersworth; 1990. p. 44.
56. Bommersbach TJ, Lapid MI, Rummans TA, Morse RM. Geriatric alcohol use disorder: a review for primary care physicians. Mayo Clin Proc. 2015;90(5):659–66. https://doi.org/10.1016/j.mayocp.2015.03.012.
57. Moroni M, Antinori S. HIV and direct damage of organs: disease spectrum before and during the highly active antiretroviral therapy era. AIDS. 2003;17(Suppl 1):S51–64.
58. Singer EJ, Thames AD. Neurobehavioral manifestations of human immunodeficiency Virus/AIDS: diagnosis and treatment. Neurol Clin. 2016;34(1):33–53. https://doi.org/10.1016/j.ncl.2015.08.003.
59. Meader N, Mitchell AJ, Chew-Graham C, Goldberg D, Rizzo M, Bird V, et al. Case identification of depression in patients with chronic physical health problems: a diagnostic accuracy meta-analysis of 113 studies. Br J Gen Pract. 2011;61(593):e808–20. https://doi.org/10.3399/bjgp11X613151.
60. Nakash O, Levav I, Aguilar-Gaxiola S, Alonso J, Andrade LH, Angermeyer MC, et al. Comorbidity of common mental disorders with cancer and their treatment gap: findings from the world mental health surveys. Psychooncology. 2014;23(1):40–51. https://doi.org/10.1002/pon.3372.
61. Cordova MJ, Andrykowski MA, Kenady DE, McGrath PC, Sloan DA, Redd WH. Frequency and correlates of posttraumatic-stress-disorder-like symptoms after treatment for breast cancer. J Consult Clin Psychol. 1995;63(6):981–6.
62. Unützer J, Katon W, Callahan CM, Williams JW, Hunkeler E, Harpole L, et al. Collaborative care management of late-life depression in the primary care setting: a randomized controlled trial. JAMA. 2002;288(22):2836–45.
63. Conde MV, Williams JW, Mulrow CD. Targeting depression interviewing: an exercise in diagnostic reasoning. J Gen Intern Med. 1998;13(4):262–5.

34 Psychological Factors Affecting Medical Conditions

Kalya Vardi

Introduction

It is now widely accepted that psychiatric disorders are associated with biological and behavioral changes which can negatively impact a person's physical health. None of us, however, are immune to psychological stress, and even in the absence of a psychiatric disorder, people often exhibit physiologic changes and maladaptive behaviors in response to stress. "Psychological factors affecting other medical conditions" is a diagnosis recognized by the DSM 5 and, despite its name, encompasses both psychological *and* behavioral factors which influence the course of a medical condition [1]. According to the DSM 5, the essential feature of this diagnosis is "the presence of one or more clinically significant psychological or behavioral factors that adversely affect a medical condition by increasing the risk for suffering, death or disability." The diagnosis can be applied to medical conditions with clear pathophysiology, as well as to functional disorders and idiopathic medical symptoms. The psychological or behavioral factors can be related to a psychiatric disorder, but the medical symptoms should not be a direct result of the psychiatric disorder (e.g., shortness of breath during a panic attack).

This section considers older age as a stage in the development of an individual and focuses on the most common or unique psychosocial features of this stage and their impact on health outcomes. Overall, the research in this area suffers from heterogeneous definitions of psychosocial experiences and physical health. Although higher quality research exists on the effects of specific psychiatric disorders on specific medical conditions (such as major depression and cardiovascular disease), this section will not cover these results in any depth in order to spotlight the broader psychosocial challenges of older adulthood, which affect many more people, including those with psychiatric disorders, and receive less attention elsewhere in this book and the medical literature overall.

Common Life Changes and Stressors in Older Adulthood

Retirement

Researchers have conceptualized retirement as a process which incorporates multiple phases, including decision-making, decreasing work activities, and adjusting to retirement. At each stage, multiple factors can influence a person's experience of retirement, so although retirement itself is a common life event, everyone's experience of retirement is unique. For some people, this experience is positive and contributes to increased psychosocial and physical well-being. However, longitudinal studies from the United States and Germany indicate that retirement has little to no effect on the psychological well-being of 70–75% of retirees and that 10–25% of people experience a decline in psychological well-being

R. R. Tampi et al. (eds.), *Psychiatric Disorders Late in Life*, https://doi.org/10.1007/978-3-319-73078-3_34

after retiring [2]. Focusing on the decision-making phase highlights the importance of people's motivations for retirement on their subsequent experience. For example, decisions motivated by health issues or family care needs suggest underlying stressors which may counteract or outweigh the benefits of retirement, such as decreased job stress and increased opportunity to pursue leisure activities.

Not surprisingly, retirees with better pre-retirement psychological well-being tend to have better post-retirement psychological well-being. Predictors of positive psychological well-being in retirement include being married (compared with being single or widowed), having a happier marriage, and having a spouse who is also retired (compared with one who is still working); retiring voluntarily or receiving financial incentives to retire; having planned for retirement; and pursuing leisure activities, bridge employment, or volunteer work in retirement [2]. Entering retirement with lower psychological well-being due to high levels of work stress or being unemployed right before retirement predicts lower psychological well-being in retirement [2].

Similarly, retirees' pre-retirement health status best predicts their physical health in retirement [2]. The relationship between the psychological effects of retirement and health outcomes has not been well studied; however, there is some evidence that psychosocial factors influence health outcomes in retirement. In particular, retiring from a physically demanding job has been associated with worse cardiovascular health in retirement, likely due to decreased physical activity [2]. Financial insecurity and more restrictive or expensive health insurance have also been associated with lower physical well-being in retirement [2].

Bereavement

Although bereavement can occur at any time throughout the life span, it is more common in older age. The death of a relative or close friend can lead to intense emotional suffering. Depressive symptoms may include decreased motivation to engage in self-care and health-promoting behaviors, decreased interest in social and physical activities, poor sleep, and increased or decreased appetite. In addition, bereavement can result in decreased social regulation of health behaviors by disrupting longstanding routines. For example, the death of a spouse is strongly associated with increased risk for unintentional weight loss and nutritional problems due to dietary behavioral changes, such as eating alone, skipping meals, eating fewer home cooked meals, and eating less fruits and vegetables [3]. A 2014 review by Stahl on the negative health effects of bereavement found large effects in studies that measured nutrition and sleep, medium effects in studies that measured weight status and tobacco use, and small effects in studies that measured physical activity and alcohol consumption [3].

Social Isolation and Loneliness

Social isolation is more common in older adulthood than at other points in development due to retirement and bereavement, as well as functional limitations. Social isolation is a risk factor for worse health, mortality, and cognitive decline [4]. In particular, research has shown that socially isolated adults are more likely to develop coronary artery disease and heart failure, and among adults with heart failure, socially isolated adults are more likely to be hospitalized [4].

Although loneliness and social isolation overlap, not all socially isolated people are lonely and vice versa. The data are mixed as to whether loneliness or social isolation is more important to well-being; nonetheless, several studies have identified loneliness as a risk factor for increased mortality independent of social isolation [4]. In addition, loneliness has been associated with decreased cellular immunity, as evidenced by lower natural killer cell activity and smaller increases in natural killer cell numbers in response to acute stress [5]. Loneliness and social isolation are both independent risk factors for depression, which in turn, has been associated with physiologic and behavioral changes that forebode poor health.

Awareness of Mortality

In general, the older we get, the more cognizant we are of our own mortality. Research has shown that older age is inversely correlated with estimates of future time (i.e., time until death) but also that these estimates vary considerably among adults in the same age group [6]. This increased awareness of our mortality is neither inherently good nor bad for our health. For some people, this awareness motivates them to engage in health promoting behaviors; for others, it discourages them. More often than not though, shorter future time expectancy is associated with lower subjective well-being and increased depressive symptoms [6]. Socioemotional selectivity theory (SST) suggests that limited future time perception motivates us to prioritize socioemotional goals [6]. The strength and vulnerability integration model reconciles SST with the data that subjective well-being tends to decrease with limited future time perspective by recognizing that cognitive and physical deficits can interfere with a person's ability to engage in effective strategies to enhance their well-being [6]. Research supports the idea that cognitive and physical functioning mediate the relationship between future time perspective and depression. Specifically, older adults who perceive their future time as limited are less likely to report depressive symptoms if their cognitive and physical functioning are good than if they are poor [6]. In summary, whether or not we choose to engage in positive health behaviors as we get older likely depends, at least in part, on whether or not we think we can achieve our socioemotional goals in the time we have left.

Ageism

Ageism refers to stereotyping of and discrimination against people or groups on the basis of their age. While ageism can apply to people of any age, the term is predominantly used to describe the stigmatization of older people. Ageism against older people is very common. In fact, research suggests that implicit (i.e., unconscious) ageism is more common than implicit sexism or racism [7]. For the most part, ageism is viewed as socially acceptable, which is unfortunate, because mounting evidence demonstrates that ageism negatively impacts the lives of older adults. When older adults are exposed to ageist stereotypes, they tend to internalize ageist beliefs and take on these qualities, as evidenced by worse performance on measures of memory, handwriting, and self-confidence [7]. Exposure to negative stereotypes about aging has also been associated with increased heart rate, blood pressure, and skin conductance, all of which are markers of cardiovascular stress [7]. Over the long term, older adults with negative perceptions about aging tend to have poorer functional health, recover from illness more slowly, and die younger [7].

Psychological Factors in Older Adulthood

Personality Traits

Personality traits are mostly stable from age 20 onward [8]. Multiple studies from around the world have examined the personality traits of centenarians to determine whether certain personality traits are associated with survival to older age. Although the methods and results vary across studies, the majority of studies suggest that centenarians have high levels of conscientiousness, extraversion, and optimism and low levels of neuroticism [9]. In separate studies of the relationship between personality traits and health outcomes, lower conscientiousness and higher neuroticism have been associated with higher body mass index, greater risk of metabolic syndrome, and greater risk of Alzheimer's disease [9]. Higher optimism has been associated with better cardiovascular health, including lower mortality from cardiovascular disease, lower incidence of coronary artery disease and stroke, and lower rates of re-hospitalization after coronary artery bypass surgery [10]. These findings are partially explained by the effects of personality on health behaviors. For example, higher conscientiousness is associated with lower rates of drug and alcohol use, risky driving, and unhealthy eating, as well as higher physical activity [9]. Nonetheless, multiple studies have shown that controlling for health behaviors does not eliminate the association between personality traits and mortality [9]. The health benefits of dispositional optimism persist even after controlling for living circumstances (such as institutionalization) and psychiatric illness (such as depressive or anxiety disorders) [9].

Purpose in Life

Purpose in life can be defined as "a self-organizing life aim that stimulates goals, manages behavior and provides a sense of meaning" [11]. Many people have theorized that having a strong sense of purpose in life increases psychological well-being and resilience to stress. Research has since demonstrated that higher purpose in life is associated not only with better psychological well-being but also with better health outcomes. For example, a 2016 meta-analysis of ten prospective studies found that having a high sense of purpose in life strongly predicts lower all-cause mortality even after adjusting for possible confounders, including age, sex, and cardiovascular risk factors [11].

As with other variables discussed in this chapter, purpose in life most likely exerts its effects on physical health via both behavioral and biological pathways. A 2014 study by Kim et al. found that, after adjusting for sociodemographic factors, each unit increase in sense of purpose on a six-point scale was associated with a significantly higher likelihood that people would obtain recommended health screenings, including cholesterol testing, colonoscopy, mammogram, Pap smear, and prostate examination [12]. At a biological level, greater purpose in life has been associated with better immune function and lower salivary cortisol levels [11]. Also of note, higher purpose in life reduces the risk of developing mild cognitive impairment and Alzheimer's disease [13] and modifies the association between Alzheimer's disease pathology and cognitive decline, such that people with higher purpose in life have better cognitive function than expected relative to their disease burden [14].

Fear of Falling

Falling is a common problem for older adults and can have serious consequences. Roughly one third of older people experience functional decline after a fall [15]. This decline is only partially explained by the direct physical consequences of a fall. Fear of falling is associated with decreased physical activity, which in turn, negatively impacts balance and gait, and increases the risk of future falls [15]. Fear of falling is also associated with decreased socialization, decreased quality of life, and increased incidence of depression [15]. The reported prevalence of fear of falling among older adults ranges from 20 to 85% [14]. Older adults who had a prior fall during activity are at the highest risk; however, people who have never fallen make up more than half of all older adults with fear of falling [15]. Other risk factors for developing fear of falling include older age, female sex, and subjective dizziness [15].

Differential Diagnosis

Cognitive Decline

The prevalence of cognitive problems increases with age. Cognitive deficits can interfere with treatment adherence by affecting understanding, motivation, and/or memory. Cognitive deficits can also manifest as poor self-care, including problems with nutrition and hygiene.

Financial Problems

Older adults are at risk for financial problems, especially if they have multiple medical conditions for which treatment can be costly. Financial problems can interfere with a patient's ability to pay for medications and care or obtain transportation to appointments. Healthy food can be prohibitively expensive, and in the absence of secure housing, health care becomes a lesser priority.

Elder Abuse

Elder abuse affects one in ten older adults [16]. Abuse can be physical, verbal-psychological, or sexual, or take the form of financial exploitation or neglect. Treatment nonadherence, weight loss, or frequent emergency visits may be the only signs of abuse [16]. Elder abuse predicts higher rates of hospitalization and nursing home placement, as well as increased mortality, even after controlling for chronic medical conditions [16].

Treatment

The diagnosis *psychological factors affecting other medical conditions* captures a wide variety of psychological and behavioral problems. This heterogeneity hinders development of specific treatment interventions, and not surprisingly, little research has been published on this topic. That said, the most important step in treatment is making the diagnosis and ruling out other causes. Cognitive decline, financial abuse, and elder abuse, if identified, should be addressed. If the patient has another psychiatric disorder, such as major depression, it should be treated as usual. Even if the patient does not meet criteria for another psychiatric disorder, they may benefit from psychotherapy to process stressors and improve coping skills. In cases of treatment nonadherence, motivational interviewing can facilitate change by helping patients resolve ambivalence and align their behavior with their goals and values.

We can also extrapolate from the available data on risk factors and protective factors to make general recommendations for how to improve psychological well-being in older adults. Encouraging older adults to engage in social activities may combat feelings of isolation and provide social regulation in favor of healthier behaviors. Engaging in volunteer or part-time work can provide a sense of purpose, in addition to increasing social interaction. As medical professionals, we can also help older adults by disseminating accurate information about aging in order to combat the many false, negative stereotypes which are pervasive in our society.

Conclusion

Psychological stress can negatively impact physical health via biological and behavioral mechanisms. In older adults, common stressors include the transition to retirement, bereavement, social isolation, and ageism. In addition, certain personality traits predispose to increased health problems and a shorter life span, while others are protective. Helping patients improve their coping skills, maintain social connections, and identify purpose in their lives may improve their health outcomes.

References

1. American Psychiatric Association. Somatic symptom and related disorders. In: Diagnostic and statistical manual of mental disorders. 5th ed. 2013. doi:https://doi.org/10.1176/appi.books.9780890425596.dsm09.
2. Wang M, Shi J. Psychological research on retirement. Annu Rev Psychol. 2014;65:209–33.
3. Stahl ST, Schulz R. Changes in routine health behaviors following late-life bereavement: a systematic review. J Behav Med. 2014;37(4):736–55.
4. Courtin E, Knapp M. Social isolation, loneliness and health in old age: a scoping review. Health Soc Care Community. 2017;25(3):799–812.
5. Mushtaq R, Shoib S, Shah T, Mushtaq S. Relationship between loneliness, psychiatric disorders and physical health: a review on the psychological aspects of loneliness. J Clin Diagn Res. 2014;8(9):WE01–4.
6. Hoppmann CA, Infurna FJ, Ram N, Gerstorf D. Associations among individuals' perceptions of future time, individual resources, and subjective well-being in old age. J Gerontol B Psychol Sci Soc Sci. 2017;72(3):388–99.
7. Allen JO. Ageism as a risk factor for chronic disease. Gerontologist. 2016;56(4):610–4.
8. Law J, Richmond RL, Kay-lambkin F. The contribution of personality to longevity: findings from the Australian centenarian study. Arch Gerontol Geriatr. 2014;59(3):528–35.
9. Andersen SL, Sun JX, Sebastiani P, et al. Personality factors in the long life family study. J Gerontol B Psychol Sci Soc Sci. 2013;68(5):739–49.
10. Avvenuti G, Baiardini I, Giardini A. Optimism's explicative role for chronic diseases. Front Psychol. 2016;7:295.
11. Cohen R, Bavishi C, Rozanski A. Purpose in life and its relationship to all-cause mortality and cardiovascular events: a meta-analysis. Psychosom Med. 2016;78(2):122–33.
12. Kim ES, Strecher VJ, Ryff CD. Purpose in life and use of preventive health care services. Proc Natl Acad Sci U S A. 2014;111(46):16331–6.
13. Boyle PA, Buchman AS, Barnes LL, Bennett DA. Effect of a purpose in life on risk of incident Alzheimer disease and mild cognitive impairment in community-dwelling older persons. Arch Gen Psychiatry. 2010;67(3):304–10.
14. Boyle PA, Buchman AS, Wilson RS, Yu L, Schneider JA, Bennett DA. Effect of purpose in life on the relation between Alzheimer disease pathologic changes on cognitive function in advanced age. Arch Gen Psychiatry. 2012;69(5):499–505.
15. Scheffer AC, Schuurmans MJ, Van Dijk N, Van der Hooft T, De Rooij SE. Fear of falling: measurement strategy, prevalence, risk factors and consequences among older persons. Age Ageing. 2008;37(1):19–24.
16. Lachs MS, Pillemer KA. Elder Abuse. N Engl J Med. 2015;373(20):1947–56.

Index

R. R. Tampi et al. (eds.), *Psychiatric Disorders Late in Life*, https://doi.org/10.1007/978-3-319-73078-3

MIX
Papier aus verantwortungsvollen Quellen
Paper from responsible sources
FSC® C105338

If you have any concerns about our products,
you can contact us on
ProductSafety@springernature.com

In case Publisher is established outside the EU,
the EU authorized representative is:
Springer Nature Customer Service Center GmbH
Europaplatz 3, 69115 Heidelberg, Germany

Printed by Libri Plureos GmbH
in Hamburg, Germany